Minimally Invasive Bariatric and Metabolic Surgery

Marcello Lucchese • Nicola Scopinaro
Editors

Minimally Invasive Bariatric and Metabolic Surgery

Principles and Technical Aspects

Springer

Editors
Marcello Lucchese
General and Emergency Surgery
Bariatric Surgery
Careggi University Hospital
Florence
Italy

Nicola Scopinaro
Department of Surgery
University of Genoa Medical School
Genoa
Italy

ISBN 978-3-319-15355-1 ISBN 978-3-319-15356-8 (eBook)
DOI 10.1007/978-3-319-15356-8

Library of Congress Control Number: 2015939892

Springer Cham Heidelberg New York Dordrecht London

Printed on acid-free paper

Springer International Publishing AG Switzerland is part of Springer Science+Business Media (www.springer.com)

Preface

Obesity affects millions of people worldwide with a negative impact on quality and duration of their lives.

This condition represents a major issue in terms of public health due to the cost of the many comorbidities often associated. Moreover, obesity has a multifactorial background, thus its treatment needs a multifactorial environment with several specialists involved in the course of evaluation, treatment, and follow-up of the patients.

Nevertheless, the role of the bariatric surgeon is still central in identifying a therapeutic strategy upon the suggestions provided by the multidisciplinary team. In fact, when asked to treat a condition of severe obesity, a surgeon cannot act directly on the primary cause of the obesity itself. This means that different techniques are still available to the surgeon's choice and that the best treatment for obese patients is to "tailor" a specific procedure according to the patient's expectations, the degree of overweight, the presence and type of comorbidities, and the expected postoperative compliance.

Therefore, the bariatric surgeon needs to know all the possible medical problems linked to obesity together with their implications and solutions.

A sudden innovation took place in the last years since it was observed that bariatric surgery could improve some metabolic conditions such as type 2 diabetes and metabolic syndrome, hypertension, impaired fertility, and sleep apnea, sometimes before achieving a significant weight loss.

Consequently, the aim of bariatric surgery was upgraded from just a weight loss surgery to a metabolic surgery suitable to manipulate all the possible hormonal and metabolic changes that can be responsible for the improvement of the abovementioned comorbidities. Therefore, bariatric surgeons started to be called more and more often to address a solution for some chronic diseases, sometimes not directly linked to the excess of weight.

On the one hand, this book frames out the evolution of bariatric surgery beyond the principles of surgical treatment, providing an overall picture of the evolution and treatment of medical, endocrine, and psychological aspects that must be considered in the multidisciplinary approach to the obese patients. On the other hand, the book provides some important technical principles addressed to both bariatric and general surgeons. In fact, even surgeons not directly involved in bariatrics will be called more and more often to treat patients who previously had a bariatric procedure.

The knowledge of bariatric techniques and their consequences would dramatically help in their work.

The present book is also addressed to all the health professionals and students who want to know more about the surgical treatment of obesity, and we hope that this will help to understand the real impact of this severe illness on patients' lives.

Finally, a special thanks to all the colleagues who contributed to realize the present book, investing a precious part of their time in building up this project.

Florence, Italy — Marcello Lucchese
Genoa, Italy — Nicola Scopinaro

Contents

Part I

Obesity

1 Historical Background: From the Past to Present

John B. Dixon and T. Rice

Obesity and conditions associated with it have been detailed for centuries, to the extent that little appears to be new, yet we are still struggling to answer the most basic questions. This chapter will deal with some of the key questions and challenges that present today from a historical perspective to examine just how far we have come, and will conclude with an historical overview of bariatric-metabolic surgery.

> The big questions
> Is obesity a disease?
> How much is known about the extent of obesity complications?
> What is the cause? And who is to blame?
> How are obese people perceived?
> How should obesity be managed?

Evidence of human obesity can be traced back 35,000 years to the time of the first human population in Europe. Statues in ivory, limestone, and terracotta of obese humans dating back 23–25 thousand years have been found through many areas of Europe. Perhaps the most famous of these is an Austrian figurine the "Venus of Willendorf". During the hunter-gatherer era humans were typically lean, and the overweight and obese state, with greater energy storage, may have represented a survival benefit during times of scarcity. However, since humans adopted agricultural practices and moved to settled societies, history has consistently portrayed obesity as a threat to health and moral substance, while at times also representing wealth and status.

1.1 Is Obesity a Disease?

On June 18, 2013, the American Medical Association (AMA) adopted a policy that recognises obesity as a disease that requires a range of medical interventions to advance treatment and prevention. The debate continues as many health care providers, professional organisations, and payors, take a philosophical approach that it is not a disease, and yet it would be difficult to find or design any definition of "disease" that could exclude obesity. Ancient Egyptians were thought to have perceived obesity as a disease, as stone reliefs showed sporadic obese individuals, often on walls portraying illness. The Aztecs believed obesity was supernatural, a misfortune of the Gods. Hippocrates (460–377 BCE), who correctly acknowledged the energy balance equation,

J.B. Dixon (✉) • T. Rice, MD
Clinical Obesity Research Laboratory,
Baker IDI Heart and Diabetes Institute,
St Kilda Road Central, PO Box 6492,
Melbourne, VIC 8008, Australia
e-mail: john.dixon@bakeridi.edu.au;
toni.rice@bakeridi.edu.au

M. Lucchese, N. Scopinaro (eds.), *Minimally Invasive Bariatric and Metabolic Surgery: Principles and Technical Aspects*, DOI 10.1007/978-3-319-15356-8_1,

recognised obesity as associated with death and infertility. "*Corpulence is not only a disease itself, but a harbinger of others*" – *Hippocrates*. Galen of Pergamon (AD 129–217), the Greek physician, surgeon, and philosopher, argued that excessive corpulence harmed the actions or functions of the body and thus was a disease. He considered obesity as a disease of size or quantity and declared that ridding the patient of excessive fat would provide the "cure". By the sixteenth and seventeenth century, accounts of obesity and its comorbidity were detailed and widely available for practitioners. Girolamo Mercuriale, writing in 1587, believed that when obesity only impacted upon the body's appearance, it was simply a symptom, but when it impacted upon the proper function of the body, it became a disease.

Disease

"A pathological condition with signs and symptoms"

"An abnormal or harmful condition"

"Impairment of function"

"A pathological condition resulting from various causes, such as infection, genetic defect, or environmental stress"

1.2 Obesity-Related Complications: Comorbidity

Perhaps in deference to a rigid denial of obesity as a disease, we have been driven to address the complications of obesity as comorbidities rather than accept the reality of a common origin of these issues. Generally, we regard disorders of regulation as causing complications, sometimes even without proof of specific causality, for example, the disorders associated with diabetes, hypertension, dyslipidaemia, renal dysfunction, neurological degeneration, and alcoholism. Yet historically, obesity was clearly described in terms of its associated complications.

The earliest recognition of type 2 diabetes was credited to Hindu physicians Sushrut and Charak (500–400 BCE). They observed that people with a sugary taste of urine were often indolent, *overweight* individuals who consumed excessive sweet and fatty foods, and recommended physical work as a cure.

Obesity has been repeatedly associated with both male and female infertility, for example, in Persian physician-philosopher Avicenna's (980–1037) renowned *Canon medicinae*. Descriptions of women with reduced or absent menstruation, together with masculine features and poor fertility, may be found in biblical records, works of Hippocrates, and throughout history in all global regions and ethnicities. Interestingly, the durability of the phenotype may suggest that the robust masculine features and reduced fertility provided survival advantage under stressful circumstances, so polycystic ovary syndrome may actually not have been considered a "disease" state in times gone by.

The common theory regarding the underlying pathophysiology of obesity during the sixteenth and seventeenth centuries was that excess fat caused tightness or constriction within the body, impeding the flow of blood, humours, and vital heat. The observations that obesity was associated with asthma, cardiac events, and obstructive sleep apnoea were actually quite consistent with this prevailing theory. Avicenna's *Canon* beautifully describes asthma, sudden death, and cardiovascular disease as complications of obesity. "Severe obesity restricts movement and causes breathlessness … breathing passages are obstructed and flow of air hindered leading to nasty temperament …. On the whole these people are at risk of sudden death … because their veins are small and compressed. They are vulnerable to stroke, hemiplegia …."

French physician Jean Fernel (1497–1555) also provided a graphic account of the dangers of overconsumption. "The vessels were overburdened with excrements which could not be sufficiently evacuated. Everything inside the body became compressed and tight. The pathways in the body were narrowed or obstructed and the body was no longer permeable and sufficiently ventilated. When the compression in the body reached a maximum, the innate heat could be extinguished or vessels could rupture, leading to sudden death".

Giovanni Argenterio (1566), in a commentary on Galen, warned "that people with 'too much fat' had shorter lives. Since most of their blood was transformed into fat, the body was robbed of its necessary nutrition and the fat also pressed on the vessels and suffocated the vital heat".

Sleep disturbances were also well recognised before the first medical description of sleep apnoea was made by Sidney Burwell and colleagues (1956), and the Dickens Pickwickian club papers (1837). Gosky (1658) described the obese as "'slow, lazy, and idle', they tired quickly or even developed an irresistibly strong propensity to fall asleep".

1.3 How Is Obesity Viewed by Society? What Is the Cause? Who Is to Blame?

Excess has historically dominated causal aspects of obesity. Hippocrates proposed that health consisted of balancing the body's four humours, and obesity is caused by a surplus of the humours.

Galen's writings *On the Power of Foods* (AD 180) suggested that digested food was converted to blood, and the more food consumed, the more blood is produced and the more obese a person becomes. This view had not changed in the seventeenth century, when obesity was being described as being due to abundant oily blood, derived from excessive food. By the early eighteenth century, Hossauer distinguished "obesitas haereditaria", a form with a familial susceptibility, from obesity acquired through an over-indulgent lifestyle.

Weakness of character, sloth, and gluttony have often dominated the Christian views of obesity. Obese people were commonly labelled as lazy, due to their reduced ability to move and function freely, without suffering shortness of breath. Mercuriale, writing in 1587, described that obesity impaired intellectual function, especially when obesity was not innate but acquired through gluttony. He felt the Lacedaemonians had been justified in condemning those who were fat as having little intelligence and courage. By the eighteenth century, it appears that physicians' dire warnings about the consequences of obesity were being promulgated, at least in part, in order to provide scientific justification for the accepted social values of diligence and temperance.

Yet the pejorative views of obesity as being representative of a lack of self-control and "impure spirit" were not universal, nor were they applied uniformly across the spectrum of overweight and obesity. Art indicates that at times throughout history, moderate degrees of corpulence were considered desirable, particularly among women, and so they chose to over-consume to obtain a more succulent beautiful body. It seemed that only severe, highly visible obesity, often associated with signs of illness such as shortness of breath and impaired mobility, were viewed as problematic. Indeed, even to the current day, there are tribes and nations in Africa that deliberately overfeed young women prior to marriage, in preparation for childbearing, and to enhance beauty and the appearance of wealth.

More widely however, obesity was associated with illness, impurity, decay, and putrefaction. As a result of the consumption of excessive food, the humours were thought to be over-burdened and the innate heat weakened, much like a fire being smothered, and the fat itself accumulated and stagnated in the vessels and cavities of the body. Until the eighteenth century, fat was not understood to be a biological fuel source that could be "burnt off", but was rather seen as a functional excrement, which could only be excreted with great difficulty. Those with excessive fat in their body were well advised to seek help from physicians to get rid of superfluous fat before there was any manifest harm.

Linked with the character judgements made about the obese, there was a clear perspective that fat people failed to address their issue, ignored their sickness until too late, and were difficult to treat, with therapies having reduced effect.

This context appears to be the basis for many physicians' attitudes and beliefs today. The concept that obesity may be more than simply an individual responsibility and should instead be considered a broader societal and public health issue appears to be limited to the last century and especially recent decades, and is still a contentious view in the present day.

1.4 Therapy for Obesity

Historical therapies for obesity have been designed to address the specific cause, and in many ways closely parallel today's dominant treatment options, involving changes to diet, sweating, hard work, and exercise. Soranus of Ephesus wrote about the treatment of obesity in the second century AD, with his work translated and expanded by Caelius Aurelianus in the fifth century. These prominent physicians described the need to both limit food intake and reduce the stored fat, by means of perspiration. Physical activity (including "passive exercise" such as riding in a chariot, or reading poetry aloud) and heat treatments (hot baths, massages) were recommended to induce sweating. Soranus and Caelius also advocated keeping the obese patient awake, in order to exhaust their bodies and generate more heat. While these measures were dubious in light of today's understanding, their dietary plan actually resonates quite closely with today's very low energy diet protocols, incorporating intermittent periods of significant food restriction, with a return to a more stable diet in between, and complete avoidance of fatty foods.

By the fifteenth and sixteenth centuries, dietary manipulations were taking more questionable turns, with physicians prescribing dietary components known to stimulate the innate heat, such as spicy and sour foods. Foods with diuretic properties were also heavily prescribed. Perhaps, one of the first comprehensive weight management programs followed the successful self-treatment of the Scottish physician, George Cheyne (1671–1743), who used major changes to his diet, hot foods, hot baths (springs), and physical activity to alter his excessive weight.

William Banting's "Letter on Corpulence Addressed to the Public", with four editions published in the 1860s, described the first widely-circulated low-carbohydrate diet for the treatment of obesity. Banting had overcome obesity with the help of physician William Harvey through, among other measures, eliminating bread, butter, milk, sugar, beer, and potatoes from his diet.

The health (hot) spa, healthy lifestyle, heavy sweating, healthy diet, and vegetarian approaches have continued to be mainstays of therapy up to the present day. Many still feel that this methodology forms the only morally appropriate therapy today.

1.5 Complementary, Traditional, and Drug Therapies

It seems logical to target obesity, a chronic disease resulting from dysfunctional energy regulation, with drug therapy. However, the road to delivering effective drug therapy has been littered with disappointment, failure, and drug withdrawals. This has been attributed to unacceptable side effects and difficulty targeting key central energy balance pathways. Central energy balance pathways contain redundant protective elements common to other essential processes of living including control of blood pressure, oxygen saturation, temperature, blood glucose, and electrolytes, so their manipulation has been challenging.

As already mentioned, treatments were historically aimed at enhancing the excretion of excess fat through the urine, faeces, and sweat, so were predominantly laxatives, diuretics, and stimulants that increased body temperature and promoted sweating. Soranus of Ephesus again seems to be the forefather of the use of laxatives and purgatives. Many of the traditional medicine streams including Chinese Traditional Medicine and Ayurvedic Medicine also include such agents. One example is Brindleberry (Garcinia cambogia, hydroxycitric acid), which has featured in the culinary and medicine traditions of Asian countries for centuries, as an agent to sour food, control appetite, and prevent the accumulation of excess fat. Despite Garcinia and its active components showing no efficacy for weight management in modern clinical trials, it is still widely available today and publicised as a natural therapy for weight loss, touted as a stimulant of fat-burning.

Interestingly, one of the only pharmacotherapies available to treat obesity today, orlistat (Xenical), could actually be considered as falling into this category of "fat excretion enhancers". Its action as a lipase inhibitor prevents the absorption of ingested fat, resulting in the excretion of dietary fat in the faeces. Of course, we now understand that it is not the excretion of internal fat stores that brings about weight loss, as was thought in the seventeenth century, but rather the prevention of fat absorption from the diet. While its effects are modest (average 5 % weight loss) and side effects are unfavourable, in today's environment of rigorous drug approval it is one of the few options considered to be sufficiently safe and effective.

The seventeenth-century Tibetan medical treatise *The Blue Beryl*, written by Sangye Gyamtso, included such measures as massaging the body vigorously with pea flour, and consuming gullet, hair, and flesh of a wolf. Odd as this remedy sounds, it is actually not so far removed from the use of porcine thyroid extracts, which began in the 1890s, in response to much more scientifically sound observation and reasoning. Given that hypothyroid patients who received the extract began to lose weight as their other symptoms improved, it seemed a logical extension to try the same therapy in obese patients. While later recognised to be dangerous in euthyroid individuals, this line of hormonal manipulation to effect weight loss has continued, with growth hormone and more recently human chorionic gonadotropin also being tried as effective obesity therapies, but found wanting. The discoveries of leptin and ghrelin also initially brought great hopes of finding "the cause of obesity" and effective therapies, yet these failed to lead to any useful treatments.

Many of the more recent therapies have targeted the reduction of hunger, increased early satiation and satiety, and increased energy expenditure. In the 1930s, dinitrophenol, an uncoupler of oxidative phosphorylation, was introduced as an obesity treatment. Its toxic side effects (including sometimes fatal hyperthermia, neuropathy, and cataracts) saw it banned by the FDA in 1938 however. Amphetamines then became the drugs of choice for a multitude of "diet pills" which reached the height of their popularity in the 1960s and 1970s, but were still being used and abused in various forms until the 1990s (Obetrol, which was later rebranded as Adderall, is one notable example). The amphetamines and several more contemporary sympathomimetics acted primarily through appetite suppression, effectively targeting the noradrenaline and serotonin systems. Unfortunately, most of these agents have now been withdrawn due to neurological and cardiovascular side effects, including fenfluramine (developed in 1973), dexfenfluramine (mid-1990s), the fen-phen combination of fenfluramine and phentermine, Ephedra (ma huang, a Traditional Chinese Medicine), and most recently sibutramine (approved 1997), which was available until 2010. Phentermine is still available for short-term use as a single therapy, and has most recently been approved in the USA in combination with topiramate (Qsymia) for the treatment of chronic severe obesity.

The few modern drug therapies available are moderately effective, generally allowing 2–10 % of body weight loss, but have never had major uptake or been able to be used continuously, as would be needed to treat a chronic condition, due to the side effects. Further complicating the matter, as a result of past disappointments such as those described above, it is extraordinarily difficult to get new preparations approved. The literature throughout the twentieth century was continually optimistic and promoted the long list of potential targets that would change the game in the future. This approach continues today, yet history would suggest the current optimism is misplaced, but for a set of critical observations regarding bariatric-metabolic surgery.

1.6 Bariatric-Metabolic Surgery

By last century, with sound scientific reasoning, obesity was well understood and the solutions seemed obvious, but treatments continually failed. However, one therapeutic modality, bariatric-metabolic surgery, bucked the trend and is now helping to advance our understanding of the whole disease of obesity. Bariatric surgery started in the early 1950s, with various intestinal bypass procedures, and has been gradually evolving since. Surgery has evolved largely through an extraordinary group of committed surgeons whose innovation and determination has generated so much more than the range of safe and effective procedures that we have today. This surgical innovation preceded knowledge of the key hormones and mechanistic pathways known to be critical in the regulation of human energy balance, yet still effectively acted upon them. Surgery, perhaps naively, targeted "restriction" of intake with gastric procedures and "reduced absorption" with diversionary procedures.

Edward Mason, known as the father of obesity surgery, provided enormous impetus to modern bariatric surgery in 1967 with the loop gastric bypass, and later developed and championed the vertical banded gastroplasty. These were important nutritional and metabolic departures from intestinal bypass procedures which had proved problematic. Nicola Scopinaro, using insights into intestinal physiology, developed the biliopancreatic diversion which provided selective and limited intestinal malabsorption that when combined with partial gastric resection was extraordinarily successful for weight loss, dyslipidaemia, and type 2 diabetes. Numerous versions of the gastric bypass and gastroplasties dominated bariatric surgery until the early 1990s. Fixed gastric bands had never been popular, but then two surgeons recognised the importance of stomal adjustability – Dag Hallberg, in trying to optimise the restriction of vertical banded gastroplasty, and Ivor Kuzmak, in modifying fixed banding. The adjustable gastric band was developed during the early general laparoscopic surgery era and heralded the revolution of laparoscopic bariatric surgery. Within a short period Wittgrove and Clarke were performing laparoscopic Roux-en-Y gastric bypass and it was clear that laparoscopic surgery was the way forward in bariatric surgery. The major advances in bariatric surgery over the last decade have been related to standardisation and quality control, major reductions in operative morbidity and mortality, the publication of credible high quality research and monitoring through national and international registries (Fig. 1.1).

The extraordinary observation that bariatric surgical interventions not only worked but the effect was durable was perhaps the greatest moment in the "history of obesity", certainly for the management of obesity. But it was an observation that was largely missed; it was well ahead of its time, and it challenged the most fundamental societal attitudes and beliefs about obesity. Gastro-intestinal procedures, some with very simple changes, could transform the severely obese ill person into a leaner healthier functional individual who never looked back. Was it curing the sloth and gluttony, strengthening the intellect and the character, and providing courage? Or was it effectively treating a disease of disordered regulation of energy balance? Bariatric surgery demonstrated for the first time that there was an effective therapy in humans, but it would take almost 50 years before the critical questions of just how it worked would adequately be scientifically addressed. The process of investigation was actually the reverse of the familiar steps used in developing most novel therapies – "This surgery clearly works in humans, but we need definitive proof so let's see if it works in rodents". The procedures do work, and this model is now providing mechanistic insights. We are now starting to understand the mechanisms involved in bariatric surgery, and by extension some of the processes involved in the development and treatment of obesity-related metabolic disease.

It's not a disease
Comorbidity not complications
Weakness of character
Personal responsibility–Poor choices
Personal rather than a public health issue
The correct therapy is obvious

Today, the challenge of obesity and the diseases that it causes such as type 2 diabetes has never been greater. Despite important insights provided through bariatric-metabolic surgery, population perceptions regarding the cause, who is to blame, and solutions for management have changed little in thousands of years. To tackle this epidemic we need to change these perceptions and embrace the

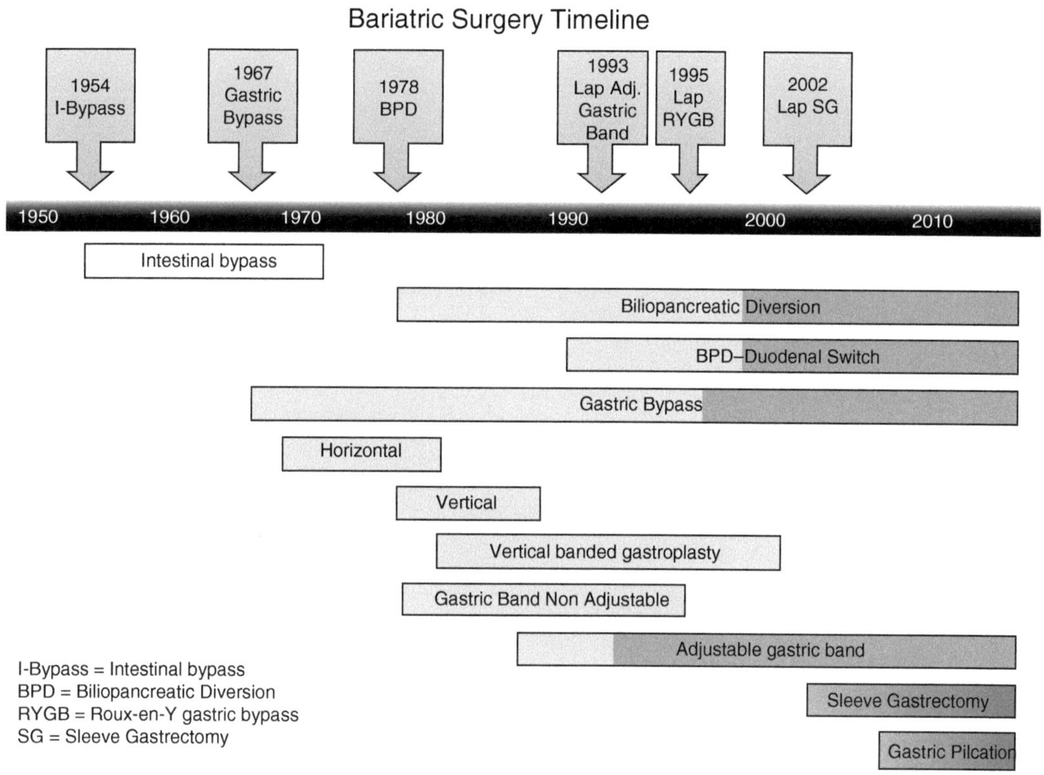

Fig. 1.1 Bariatric surgery timeline

epidemic as a whole-of-society/environmental issue, with victims that have an incurable chronic disease that reduces the length and quality of life. The problem is obvious; the solutions are not. There have been no serendipitous moments or paradigm shifts that have changed our societal focus and perceptions about obesity – which is in fact a serious disease. Findings regarding the genetic and epigenetic aspects of obesity and metabolic programming, our current understanding central control of energy balance and defence of body weight (fat), and the evidence that bariatric surgery provides a durable weight change should have changed these societal perceptions and driven a fundamental change in our search for solutions. The future will depend on understanding and exploring the facts, rather than beliefs, and designing solutions that work rather than holding on to solutions that should work, but never will.

Suggested Reading

1. Azziz R, Dumesic DA, Goodarzi MO. Polycystic ovary syndrome: an ancient disorder? Fertil Steril. 2011;95:1544–8.
2. Bray G. Chapter 1. History of obesity. In: Williams G, Frühbeck G, editors. Obesity: science to practice. Chichester: Wiley; 2009.
3. Dossey L. Gluttony and obesity. Explore (NY). 2010; 6:1–6.
4. Haslam D. Obesity: a medical history. Obes Rev. 2007;8 Suppl 1:31–6.
5. Papavramidou N, Christopoulou-Aletra H. Management of obesity in the writings of Soranus of Ephesus and Caelius Aurelianus. Obes Surg. 2008;18:763–5.
6. Park RJ. Historical reflections on diet, exercise, and obesity: the recurring need to "put words into action". Can Bull Med Hist. 2011;28:383–401.
7. Stolberg M. 'Abhorreas pinguedinem': fat and obesity in early modern medicine (c. 1500-1750). Stud Hist Philos Biol Biomed Sci. 2012;43:370–8.

2 Incidence and Prevalence of Obesity

Luca Busetto and Stefania Maggi

2.1 Introduction

In the recent years, obesity has received considerable attention as a major health problem worldwide. Obesity is now the most prevalent form of malnutrition in the industrialized countries and it is rapidly becoming highly prevalent also in the developing world. The relevance of obesity as a *risk factor* for several medical conditions and diseases is well known. Obesity is linked to various disabling and/or life-threatening conditions, such as heart disease, diabetes, hypertension, stroke, certain cancers, osteoarthritis, respiratory abnormalities, gastro-esophageal reflux disease (GERD), and liver disease (nonalcoholic fatty liver disease, cirrhosis, and hepatocellular carcinoma). Therefore, *obesity epidemic* was numbered as one of the major contributors to the global burden of disease and disability [1]. According to some predicting models, the rapidly increasing prevalence of obesity and related comorbidities can reverse in some countries the current prevailing trend of increasing life expectancy [2].

L. Busetto (✉)
Department of Medicine, University of Padova, Via Giustiniani, 2, Padova 35128, Italy
e-mail: luca.busetto@unipd.it

S. Maggi
CNR, Neuroscience Institute, Aging Branch, Padova, Via Giustiniani, 2, Padova 35128, Italy
e-mail: stefania.maggi@in.cnr.it

2.2 Definition of Overweight and Obesity

According to the World Health Organization, overweight and obesity are defined as an abnormal or excessive fat accumulation that presents a risk to health. A crude population measure of overweight and obesity is the *body mass index* (BMI), a person's weight (in kilograms) divided by the square of his height (in metres). BMI (kg/m^2) is used in epidemiology and in clinical practice to define underweight, normal weight, overweight (pre-obesity), and obesity [3]. However, the use of BMI as a proxy for adiposity, the true determinant of the obese state, has been criticized, given that body weight is the sum of individual organs and tissues and therefore it includes adipose tissue, skeletal muscle mass, and organs mass. Moreover, BMI does not convey any information on fat distribution (e.g., visceral fat accumulation and fatty infiltrations in individual organs) that is now considered an important determinant of metabolic and cardio-vascular risk [4]. On the other hand, current reference methods for the direct measurement of fat mass (underwater-weighing; total body densitometry) or total and regional adipose tissue volumes (CT or MRI) are costly and not applicable in large epidemiologic investigations or in routine clinical practice.

On a population level, a strong positive correlation between BMI and overall *body fat* content has been extensively reported [5]. However, this

M. Lucchese, N. Scopinaro (eds.), *Minimally Invasive Bariatric and Metabolic Surgery: Principles and Technical Aspects*, DOI 10.1007/978-3-319-15356-8_2,

Table 2.1 Classification of weight category by BMI

Classification	BMI (kg/m^2) general cut-off points	BMI (kg/m^2) cut-off points for Asian populations
Underweight	<18.5	<18.5
Normal range	18.5–24.9	18.5–22.9
Pre-obese	25.0–29.9	23.0–27.4
Obese class I	30.0–34.9	27.5–32.4
Obese class II	35.0–39.9	32.5–37.4
Obese class III	≥40.0	≥37.5

Source: Adapted from WHO [3, 8]

can mask significant variations in the relationship between BMI and adiposity on an individual level. For instance, the body fat content of a healthy subject with a normal BMI value has been demonstrated to vary from 8 to 38 % in men and from 30 to 44 % in women [6]. This large variability implies that an individual subject may have a BMI corresponding to an obese state both having a low fat-free mass and a substantial fat accumulation or having a large skeletal muscle mass and normal fat mass. This latter condition typically occurs in athletes, in which high BMI may simply reflect increased muscle mass, which does not have anything to do with obesity and associated diseases. Even at an epidemiological level, the poor performance of BMI as a marker adiposity is emphasized by the large differences in percentage body fat observed between men and women having the same BMI level, with women having a higher percentage of body fat than men [7]. Ethnical factors also play a role. A BMI of 20–25 kg/m^2, which is considered normal and healthy in a Caucasian subject, correspond to an elevated body fat content and is associated to an increased disease risk in people belonging to other ethnic groups, and particularly in Asian subjects. This observation prompted the WHO to adopt different cut-off points for overweight and obesity in people of Asian origin (Table 2.1) [8].

2.3 Prevalence of Obesity Worldwide

The *prevalence of obesity* around the world is monitored by the WHO through the Global Database on BMI, which gathered data from surveys or population studies, where weight and height are measured or self-reported [9]. According to WHO database, 34.5 % of the world adults (age ≥ 20 years) were overweight and 11 % were obese in 2008 [9]. This means that in the world there were more than 1.4 billion overweight adults in 2008. Of these over 200 million men and nearly 300 million women were obese [9]. The prevalence of overweight and obesity was higher in women than in men (overweight: 35.1 vs. 33.8 %; obesity 14.0 vs. 10.0 %) [9]. Prevalence of obesity varies greatly across the WHO regions. Obesity is much more prevalent in the Americas (29.7 % in women and 23.5 % in men), in the WHO region of Europe (23.1 % in women and 20.4 % in men), and in the Eastern Mediterranean region (24.5 % in women and 13.0 % in men). Prevalence of obesity are lower in the WHO regions of Africa (11.1 % in women and 5.3 % in men), Western Pacific (6.8 % in women and 5.1 % in men), and South East Asia (3.7 % in women and 1.7 % in men). In all WHO regions women were more likely to be obese than men, and in the WHO regions for Africa, Eastern Mediterranean, and South East Asia, women had roughly double the obesity prevalence of men [9]. At a national level, the nations with the higher prevalence of overweight/obesity are represented by Pacific Islands (Nauru, Cook Islands, Tonga, Samoa, Palau, Kiribati), where the prevalence stands over 80 %. High-income Arabic Kingdoms in the Persian Gulf region (Kuwait, Qatar, United Arab Emirates, Saudi Arabia, and Bahrain) had overweight prevalence between 70 and 80 % and represents the second group of nations with the highest prevalence in the world. The only world three nations with a prevalence of overweight in 2008 lower than 10 % were represented by very poor low-income states (Bangladesh, Ethiopia, and Nepal) [9]. Besides ethnic factors, the economic levels play a crucial role in determining overweight/obesity prevalence worldwide. Indeed, the prevalence rates increase with *income level* of countries up to upper middle-income levels. The prevalence of overweight in high and upper middle-income countries was more than double that of low- and lower middle-income countries. For obesity, the difference is more than triple

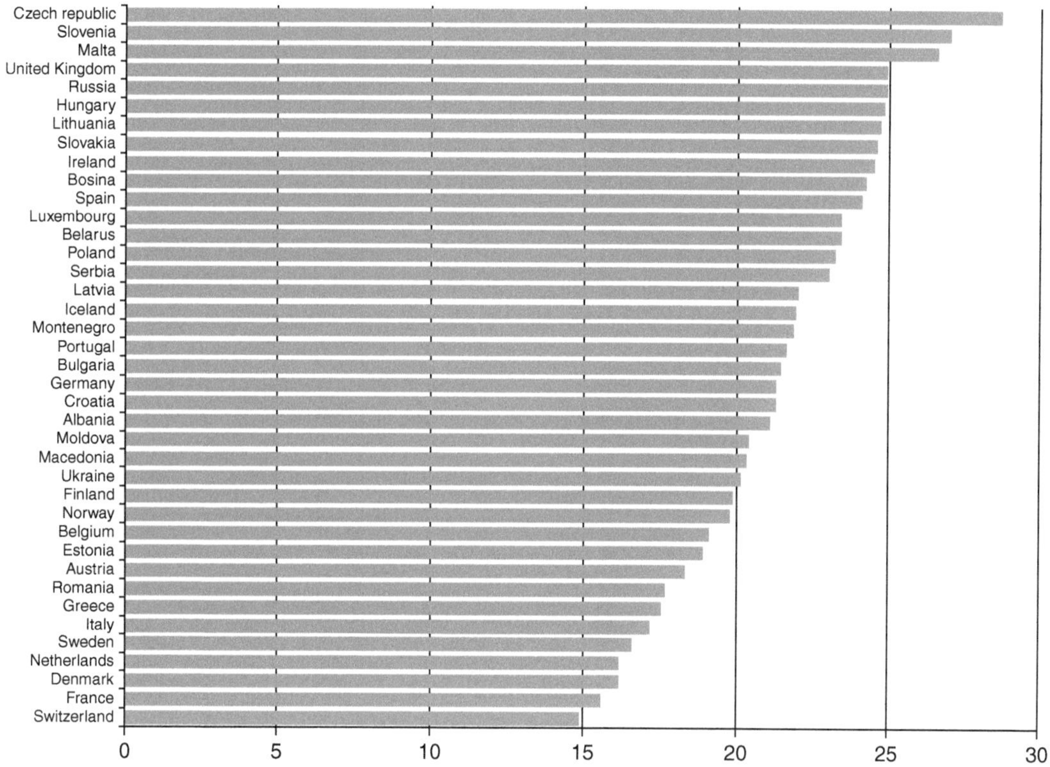

Fig. 2.1 The prevalence (%) of obesity in adults in European nations, according to WHO database 2008 [9]

from lower middle-income countries to upper middle-income countries [9].

The USA has a high prevalence of overweight and obesity. The more recent US data are from the National Health and Nutrition Examination Survey, 2011–2012 [10]. According to this survey, more than one-third (34.9 %) of adults were obese. Prevalence of obesity was higher among middle-aged adults (39.5 %) than among younger (30.3 %) or older (35.4 %) adults. The overall prevalence of obesity did not differ between men and women. However, large racial differences were observed. The prevalence of obesity was higher among non-Hispanic black (47.8 %), Hispanic (42.5 %), and non-Hispanic white (32.6 %) adults than among non-Hispanic Asian adults (10.8 %). Among non-Hispanic black adults, 56.6 % of women were obese compared with 37.1 % of men [10].

In 2008, the general prevalence of obesity in the WHO region for Europe was lower (21.9 %) than the prevalence observed in the US (31.8 %) [9]. However, the prevalence of overweight and obesity varies greatly across the European countries, with countries having obesity figures closer to the US values and countries having much lower figures. The prevalence of obesity in European nations ranked according to the WHO levels in 2008 [9] is represented in Fig. 2.1.

In Italy, prevalence of overweight according to WHO database was 49.2 % in 2008, and prevalence of obesity was 17.2 % [9]. These estimates are largely based on data collected by the Cardiovascular Epidemiologic Observatory of the Italian Health Institute (Istituto Superiore di Sanità – Progetto Cuore). A more detailed analysis of this database demonstrated an overweight prevalence of 50 % in men and 34 % in women. In the same sample, the prevalence of obesity was 17 % in men and 21 % in women [11]. Overweight and obesity prevalence was higher in the southern regions of Italy, where 19 % of men and 30 % of women were obese, and 52 % of men and 35 % of women are overweight [11].

Alarming prevalence of obesity has been observed also in *children and adolescents* in several countries worldwide. A study comparing data from large nationwide surveys, has shown that the combined prevalence of obesity and overweight in children was high in the USA (25 %), moderate in Russia (16 %), and low in China (7 %) [12]. In 2011–2012, the prevalence of obesity in the USA was 16.9 % in subjects 2- to 19-year-olds [13]. In Italy, 22.2 % of children in primary school were overweight and 10.6 % had obesity in 2012 [14]. Alarming data have been observed in the southern regions of Italy where more than 40 % of 6–10-year-old children were overweight or obese [14]. A high percentage of obese children and adolescents nowadays present complications that, until a decade ago, characterized only adulthood: insulin resistance, type 2 diabetes, dyslipidemia, nonalcoholic fatty liver disease, metabolic syndrome, and hypertension [15]. These complications are associated in children and adolescents to cardiovascular events, cancer, and premature death as in adult [15]. Obese children are also at higher risk of precocious puberty, polycystic ovary syndrome, sleep apnea, orthopedic complications, and psychological and social disturbances [16]. Finally, obese children have a higher probability of becoming obese adults, thus fueling current epidemic of obesity and related diseases [16].

2.4 Incidence and Time Trends

The prevalence of obesity has increased steadily in the past 30 years, configuring an unprecedented "epidemic" for a non-communicable disease. The worldwide prevalence of obesity had nearly doubled since 1980 (10 % of men and 14 % of women were obese in 2008, compared with 5 % for men and 8 % for women in 1980) [9]. In the early 1960s, the prevalence of obesity in the USA was 11 % among men and 16 % among women, and it changed relatively little until 1980. Data from NHANES II (between 1976 and 1980) and NHANES III (between 1988 and 1994) demonstrate that the prevalence rates of obesity increased considerably, to about 21 % in men and 26 % in women. By 2003–2004 the prevalence had increased further to almost 32 % in men and 34 % in women [10]. An even greater increase in prevalence has been observed for the most severe forms of obesity: whereas the general prevalence of obesity (BMI >30 kg/m^2) doubled in the last 15 years of the twentieth century in the USA, the prevalence of morbid obesity (BMI >40 kg/m^2) had a fourfold increase and the prevalence of super-obesity (BMI >50 kg/m^2) had a sixfold increase [17]. However, these *secular trends* on the prevalence of obesity must be considered with caution: a continuous variable, such as body weight, is used to classify dichotomous variables such as obesity and overweight. This could imply that an average modest weight gain might lead to a relevant increase in the incidence of overweight and obesity. However, in the USA it has been reported that the average increase of BMI has been very relevant, changing from 25.6 kg/m^2 in 1976–1980 to 27.9 kg/m^2 in 1999–2004 in men, and from 25.3 to 28.7 kg/m^2 in women [18]. The increase in the prevalence of obesity has been observed worldwide and most countries had rising trends of obesity. Only 2 of the 28 countries in the Global database on BMI showed a falling trend in the prevalence of obesity in men (Denmark and Saudi Arabia), and 5 of the 28 countries showed a falling trend in the prevalence of obesity in women (Denmark, Ireland, Saudi Arabia, Finland, and Spain) [9].

This discouraging global picture of the "obesity epidemic" may be partially ameliorated by the fact that recent data seem to suggest a stabilization of prevalence after years and years of progressive increment in some industrialized countries with high prevalence of overweight and obesity. In the USA, there was no significant change in obesity prevalence in the total adult population between 2003–2004 and 2011–2012 (+2.8 percentage points) [13]. A significant increase in prevalence was observed only among adults aged 60 years and older (+4.4 percentage points) [13].

Obesity trends in *children and adolescents* seem to parallel trends of overweight and obesity in adults. Previous studies indicate that in many developed countries children obesity has reached levels similar to those in the USA and that obesity prevalence is rapidly increasing in developing countries (e.g., in Brasil, has tripled from 1970 (4 %) to 1990 (14 %)). On the other hand, more recent trend seems to stabilize in the US children and this might be due to the aggressive campaign against obesity and unhealthy dietary patterns. Among American children and adolescents aged 2–19 years, there was no significant change in obesity prevalence between 2003–2004 and 2011–2012 overall (−0.2 percentage points) [13], but there was a significant decrease in obesity prevalence among 2–5-year-old American children (−5.5 percentage points) [13]. Data from other countries also have shown a decline or stabilization of obesity levels in children. In Germany, a significant decline in overweight or obesity in children aged 4–7 years and a stabilization in children from 8 to 16 years of age have been observed between 2004 and 2008 [13]. Results of an Italian survey on prevalence of overweight and obesity in primary school children demonstrated a trend to stabilization in prevalence in the very recent years [14].

Conclusion

The prevalence of obesity has increased dramatically in the last decades in both adults and children, with evidence of possible recent stabilization in some industrialized countries. Nevertheless, the prevalence rates continue to be greater than one third of the population and the obesity epidemic is still escalating in the developing world. The reduction of the prevalence rate of obesity is a public health priority. Obesity is the result of a complex interaction between the environment, genetic predisposition, and human behavior. It is associated with an increased risk of numerous chronic diseases, disability, and death. In addition, the obesity epidemic represents a heavy burden on the economy with its massive health care costs. The problem of overweight and obesity has therefore emerged as one of the most pressing global issues that we will continue to face during the next several decades.

References

1. Peeters A, Backholer K. Is the health burden associated with obesity changing? Am J Epidemiol. 2012; 176:840–5.
2. Olshansky SJ, Passaro DJ, Hershow RC, et al. A potential decline in life expectancy in the United States in the 21st century. N Engl J Med. 2005;352:1138–45.
3. WHO. Obesity: preventing and managing the global epidemic. Report of a WHO consultation. World Health Organ Tech Rep Ser. 2000;894:1–253.
4. Müller MJ, Lagerpusch M, Enderle J, et al. Beyond the body mass index: tracking body composition in the pathogenesis of obesity and the metabolic syndrome. Obes Rev. 2012;13:6–13.
5. Okorodudu DO, Jumean MF, Montori VM, et al. Diagnostic performance of body mass index to identify obesity as defined by body adiposity: a systematic review and meta-analysis. Int J Obes (Lond). 2010; 34:791–9.
6. Thomas EL, Frost G, Taylor-Robinson SD, Bell JD. Excess body fat in obese and normal-weight subjects. Nutr Res Rev. 2012;25:150–61.
7. Karastergiou K, Smith SR, Greenberg A. Sex differences in human adipose tissues – the biology of pear shape. Biol Sex Differ. 2012;3:13.
8. WHO. Appropriate body-mass index for Asian populations and its implications for policy and intervention strategies. Lancet. 2004;363:157–63.
9. World Health Organization. Obesity. 2008. [Accessed 7 Apr 2014]. Available at: http://www.who.int/topics/obesity/en/.
10. Ogden CL, Carroll BK, Flegal KM. Prevalence of obesity among adults: United States, 2011-2012. NCHS Data Brief. 2013;131:1–8.
11. Progetto Cuore. Istituto Superiore di Sanità. 2014. [Accessed 7 Apr 2014]. Available at: http://www.cuore.iss.it/eng/.
12. Wang Y. Cross-national comparison of childhood obesity: the epidemic and the relationship between obesity and socioeconomic status. Int J Epidemiol. 2001;30:1129–36.
13. Ogden CL, Carroll MD, Kit BK, Flegal KM. Prevalence of childhood and adult obesity in the United States, 2011-2012. JAMA. 2014;311:806–14.
14. Okkio alla Salute. Ministero dell'Istruzione, dell'Università e della Ricerca. 2014. [Accessed 7 Apr 2014]. Available at: http://www.okkioallasalute.iss.it/.
15. Weiss R, Dziura J, Burgert TS, et al. Obesity and the metabolic syndrome in children and adolescents. N Engl J Med. 2004;350:2362–74.
16. Han JC, Lawlor DA, Kimm SYS. Childhood obesity. Lancet. 2010;375:1737–48.
17. Sturm R. Increases in clinically severe obesity in the United States, 1986-2000. Arch Intern Med. 2003;163: 2146–8.
18. Finucane MM, Stevens GA, Cowan MJ, et al. National, regional, and global trends in body-mass index since 1980: systematic analysis of health examination surveys and epidemiological studies with 960 country-years and 9.1 million participants. Lancet. 2011;377:557–67.

3 The Pathophysiology of Obesity

Geltrude Mingrone and Marco Castagneto

The *New York Times* announced in June 2013 that millions of Americans contracted a disease [1]. This was not caused by any peculiar pathogen, but occurred because the American Medical Association had declared obesity a "multimetabolic and hormonal disease state". In spite of this, the debate on whether and/or when this statement applies will likely continue also because many more millions of people worldwide are facing the same problem. Perhaps, when we will have achieved a better understanding of the etiology and pathophysiology of obesity, it will be possible to answer this question.

3.1 Etiology

The simplest explanation of the mechanisms which lead to weight gain and to obesity is that of a caloric intake in excess of energy expenditure used for thermogenesis, body functions, and physical activity (Fig. 3.1). The calories in excess of requirements are then stored as triglycerides in the fat cells of the adipose tissue or, more appropriately, of the adipose organ [2]: the fat cells enlarge and can also proliferate by differentiation of precursors. However, there is a very remarkable variability among individuals of the metabolic response to the increased energy intake in relation to environmental, life style, genetic, and neuro-hormonal factors which should be taken into consideration and will be discussed in this chapter.

G. Mingrone, MD, PhD (✉)
Department of Internal Medicine, Catholic University, Largo A. Gemelli 8, Rome 00168, Italy
e-mail: gmingrone@rm.unicatt.it

M. Castagneto, MD
Department of Surgery, Catholic University, Largo A. Gemelli 8, Rome 00168, Italy
e-mail: mcastagneto@rm.unicatt.it

3.2 Physiology of Caloric Intake and Energy Expenditure

The basic physiological mechanisms that regulate the energy balance in the central nervous system (CNS) derive from the afferent signals from the periphery regarding satiety and adiposity, which trigger efferent neuro-hormonal activation aimed at reducing appetite and maintaining energy balance [3, 4].

Afferent signals derive from the gastrointestinal tract, including pancreas and liver, in the form of autonomic stimulation by physical and chemical food ingestion [5]. Even more importantly, a series of hormones are released by the gut which assist in nutrient digestion and absorption and regulate through the vagus satiety feeling. Among them there are cholecystokinine (CCK) which stimulates exocrine pancreas function, peptide YY (PYY) which increases energy expenditure and slows gastric emptying as well

M. Lucchese, N. Scopinaro (eds.), *Minimally Invasive Bariatric and Metabolic Surgery: Principles and Technical Aspects*, DOI 10.1007/978-3-319-15356-8_3,

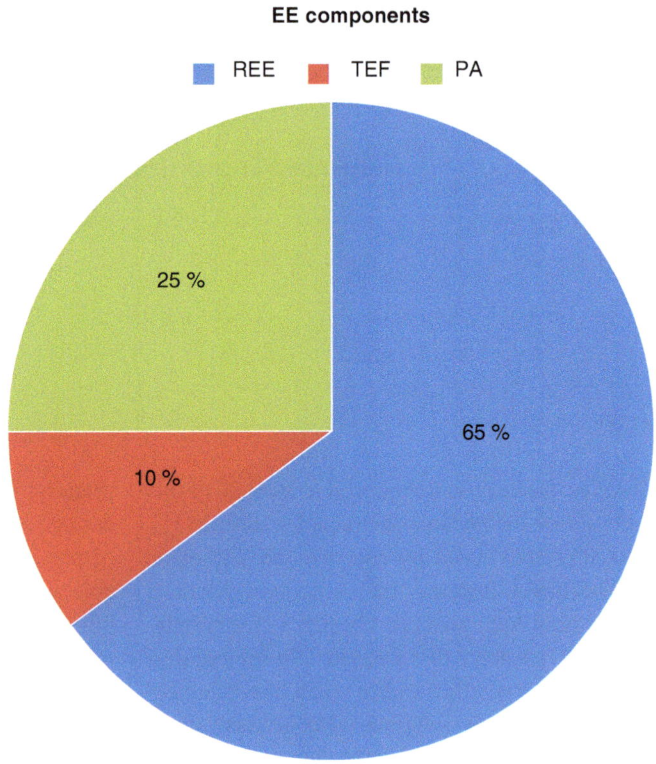

Fig. 3.1 Partitioning of daily energy expenditure (*EE*). Resting energy expenditure (*REE*) represents 65 % of daily EE, thermic effect of food (*TEF*) or food thermogenesis 10 %, and physical activity (*PA*) the remaining 25 %

as it is done by glucagon-like peptide 1 (GLP1) which, in addition, has a potent effect on endocrine pancreatic function [6, 7]. Finally, insulin, glucagon and amylin, beside their effects on carbohydrates metabolism, act on the hypothalamus stimulating satiety. On the contrary, ghrelin, a potent orexigenic peptide, secreted by the fundus of the stomach when empty, is suppressed by food ingestion. The other type of afferent signals regulating food intake, comes from the adipose tissue which is not only a fat storage compartment but, as it has been progressively recognized, plays an active role in maintaining energy balance. In fact, the adipose organ produces a number of mediators with important physiological functions and impacts in the development of diseases linked to obesity [8–10].

More than 50 adipose tissue hormones and cytokines have been described including acute phase proteins, complement-like factors and adhesion molecules. These so-called adipokines are involved in the regulation of satiety, energy balance, lipid and glucose metabolism, and inflammation [11]. There are two types of adipose tissues, the "white" and the "brown" [12]. The former is prevalent in mammals and is made of round adipocytes containing a large fat droplet which displaces the small nucleus to the periphery. The brown adipocyte is smaller with many small fat accumulations and is rich of mitochondria which are responsible for the darker appearance. Thermogenesis is the primary function of this type of adipose tissue and, in fact, contrary to the white one, it contains uncoupling proteins which prevent storage of energy in the ATP molecules. It is also highly vascularized and innervated by sympathetic fibers. On the other hand, the white adipose tissue, which is widely prevailing in the adult, beside adipocyte, contains macrophages, fibroblasts, leukocytes, and endothelial cells which are responsible for the secretion of additional mediators to those peculiar of adipose tissue. The most well known adipokines are leptin, adiponectin, tumor necrosis factor α (TNFα), interleukin 6 (IL6), and resistin.

Leptin is a peptide with a central function in the regulation of body weight through limitation of food intake and enhancement of energy expenditure. Being produced by adipocytes, its blood level is directly proportional to the fat mass. In turn, leptin binds to the leptin receptor in the hypothalamus with the activation of anorexigenic response. Leptin and its receptor are regulated by separate genes whose mutation leads to endocrine abnormalities including obesity similar to the one observed in the *ob/ob* mice, deficient in leptin, and in the *db/db* mice that have a deficit of leptin receptors [13]. The relative interplay between leptin production and leptin receptor expression may partly explain the so-called leptin resistance phenomenon which is commonly observed in patients who are obese in the face of high circulating levels of leptin [14]. Another very interesting action of leptin, beside the regulation of appetite and of energy expenditure, is a direct stimulation of T lymphocytes with increased inflammatory cytokines production such as TNFα and IL6.

Adiponectin is a cytokine-like molecule that interacts with its specific receptor on the cell membrane of the central nervous system, of the muscles and of the liver. The action of the adiponectin is antithetic to leptin being reduced in obesity, increasing glucose and fatty acids uptake and reducing production of TNFα and IL6 and of other inflammatory mediators [15].

Resistin is a protein which is secreted mainly by adipocytes and macrophages, and owes its name to its enhancing effect on insulin resistance. This might be due, at least partially, to the increased hepatic glucose production and to the impaired glucose uptake and glycogen synthesis effect. In addition, it displays an inflammatory action especially on smooth muscle cells through stimulation of the immune system [16].

3.3 Central Regulation of Energy Homeostasis and Efferent Signaling

The central nervous system is the site where converge afferent nervous and hormonal signals so far described, providing information on satiety and adiposity and where effector neuro-chemical signals are activated in order to maintain the energy balance.

The appetite brain network includes the insula, the amygdala/hippocampus, the orbitofrontal cortex with the ventromedial prefrontal cortex and the nucleus striatum (Fig. 3.2). Relevant information, in particular sight and smell, reaches the brain as external cues acting on the amygdala and insula; interoceptive information from the gut is sensed by the insula, while circulating peptides and nutrients are sensed by the hypothalamus and brainstem, as well as by the ventral tegmental area and the substantia nigra. The amygdala encodes the current incentive value of food cues, while the insula conveys sensory features of foods and its activity is modulated by hunger. The cognitive control over appetite regions, either to enhance or to suppress appetite, is mediated mainly via the frontal lobes. Fasting increases activation of the hypothalamus, insula, and striatum, while meal consumption increases activation of the prefrontal cortex. A recent review [17] has highlighted how obesity is consistently associated with heightened or abnormal responses to visual food cues in a distributed network of brain regions involved in reward/motivation and emotion/memory and how a prolonged long-term exposure to highly palatable, high-calorie foods may cause decreased reward area activation following food intake. By using a positron emission tomography (PET) approach, Del Parigi et al. [18] found that obese individuals showed a greater activation in the midbrain and middle-dorsal insula that are areas involved in the cerebral reward response, and a lesser activation in the posterior cingulate cortex, which is associated with awareness state. PET studies demonstrated that obese adults show a lower postprandial activation of the cognitive control areas than lean individuals. EEG studies described the temporal evolution of the brain responses to face and food pictures, highlighted differences in resting state cortical networks among underweight, normal-weight, and overweight/obese subjects and changes in responses of the obese subjects with respect to the normal-weight individuals.

In the arcuate nucleus, there are two types of neurons [19]: the first with anorexigenic and the second with orexigenic effects. The first type produces pro-opiomelanocortin peptide which interacting with the ventromedial as well as the other hypothalamic nuclei reduces food intake and increases energy expenditure. On the contrary,

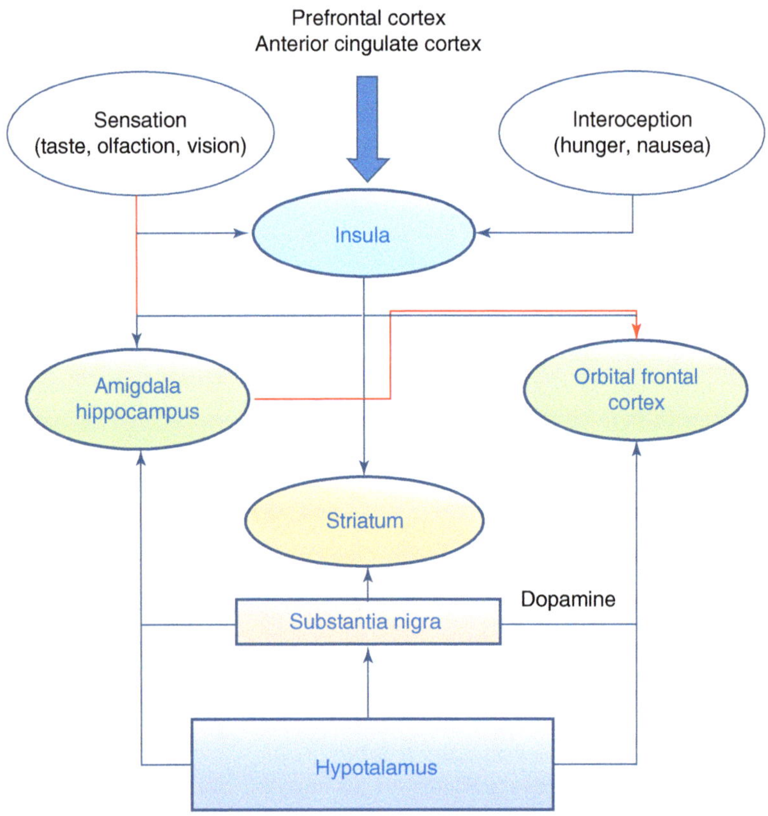

Fig. 3.2 Appetite Brain Network. Information from the prefrontal cortex and the anterior cingulated cortex arrive to the insula, which receives also afferences relative to food sensations like taste, olfaction and vision, and interoceptive sensation, such as hunger. Efferences from the insula reach the amigdala and hippocampus and the orbital frontal cortex and the striatum. The latter has also afferences from the substantia nigra that reach also the orbital frontal cortex and the striatum. Finally, the hypothalamus sends information to the substantia nigra, the orbital frontal cortex, and the striatum. In red are highlightened the inhibitory actions

the orexigenic neurons synthesize PYY and aguti-related peptide which increase food intake and reduce energy consumption (Fig. 3.3). The hypothalamus receives sensory satiety signals from the peripheral organs through the vagal complex in the hindbrain and also directly from the blood carrying nutrients and peptides from the digestive system as well as from the adipose tissue. Finally, additional signal are acquired from limbic and cortical areas regarding cognitive and reward response to food intake [4].

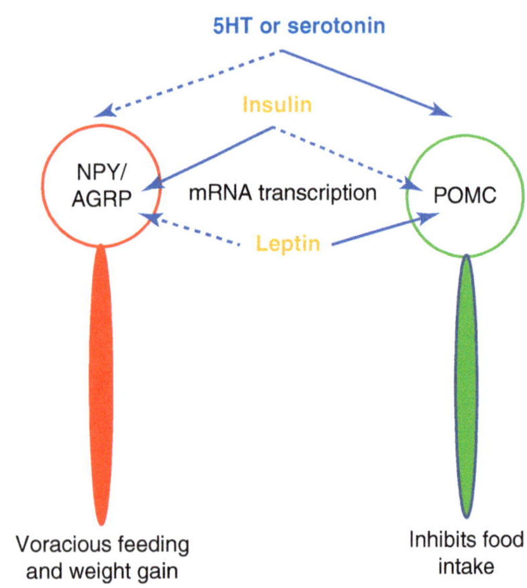

Fig. 3.3 Stimulatory effects are indicated by solid lines and inhibitory effects by dashed lines. 5-hydroxytryptamine or serotonine as well as leptin stimulates pro-opiomelanocortin (*POMC*) neurons and inhibits the neuropetide Y(NPY)/agouti related protein neurons. Insulin does the contrary. Therefore, insulin stimulates appetite while serotonin and leptin do the opposite

3.4 Pathophysiology of Obesity

3.4.1 Environmental and Genetic Factors

Regardless of whether obesity is a condition or a disease, it arises from multiple etiologic determinants, either inherited or acquired. In particular, the strict interplay of environmental and genetic factors is strongly correlated to obesity development. Environment contributes providing and advertising easy access to calorie-dense and palatable food, facilitating sedentary lifestyle, while increasing prevalence of mental distress or illness either by itself or because of related medications [20]. It represents an important determinant of the obesity epidemics especially in the western countries. Environmental factors act on individual genetic background which animal as well as human family studies have shown to be a major determinant of obesity. Indeed, weight is a highly inheritable trait although greatly polymorphic and polygenic. More than 40 genes have been so far linked to obesity which, interacting with the environment, may result in its relevant phenotypic expression [21]. At the present time, however, carrying obesity genes have little recognizable effect and, therefore, should be considered as more of a risk factor than a determinant [22]. Thus, an epigenetic component in the pathophysiology of obesity should be taken into consideration. In fact, recent works have shown how genome mutations, that do not involve changes in DNA sequence, could explain how environmental conditions, like maternal food intake during pregnancy and overfeeding during infancy have an impact on obesity susceptibility [23, 24]. However, there are some monogenic obesity syndromes with well characterized single locus mutations especially in the pediatric population. Among them it should be mentioned the Prader-Willis syndrome (in which seven genes of paternal origin are deleted), the Bordet-Biedl syndrome, the leptin deficiency syndrome, and other rare diseases all associated with complex neurological abnormalities.

3.4.2 Obesity as Derangement of Central Regulation of Energy Balance

When the fine neuro-hormonal control of food intake and energy expenditure, which takes place predominantly at the CNS level, fails then alterations in neuro-chemical signaling ensues that affect the adiposity and satiety feedback mechanism. Animal and human studies on obese and lean subjects lend support to this standpoint [25]. As a consequence, the energy in excess is stored as fat in the adipose organ which, beside subcutaneous tissue, includes the visceral and pelvic fat and also the peri-muscular, peri-vascular, and peri-osteal areas. As mentioned before, the adipocyte responds to fat accumulation with enlargement and also with proliferation thus representing the core pathology of obesity [25]. The pathophysiology, on the other hand, encompasses the inappropriate secretion of hormones and mediators associated with the central feedback satiety signaling as well as the numerous cytokines produced by fat cells. As illustrated before, the adipose tissue, especially when it is expanded, represents a major component of the endocrine and reticuloendothelial system.

In fact, in addition to the adipokines specifically produced by the expanded fat cells, macrophages and T and B lymphocytes also increase and secrete inflammatory cytokines such as TNFα, IL1, IL6, and acute phase proteins [26]. The inflammatory action of adipose tissue spreads to other organs, like the liver, the pancreas or like the vascular system, contributing to the well-known clinical manifestations of obesity. Among them hypertension, atherogenesis, atherosclerosis, fatty liver dysfunction (non-alcoholic fatty liver disease, NAFLD, and non-alcoholic steatohepatitis, NASH), insulin resistance, and type 2 diabetes mellitus are the commonest [27].

From the metabolic point of view, it should be underlined that the excessive burden of fat, which is stored in the adipocytes as triglycerides, implicates increased circulating free fatty acid levels which in turn are responsible for the lipotoxicity effect at organ level like the liver and the pancreas [28]. The latter occurs especially on the β-cells which progressively go into exhaustion.

3.4.3 Clinical Correlates of Obesity

3.4.3.1 Impaired Glucose Tolerance and Type 2 Diabetes Mellitus

This is one of the most common co-morbidities of obesity which affects over 80 % of diabetic patients. The basic pathophysiological mechanism of this disease is strictly related to the increased insulin resistance requiring enhanced insulin secretion with eventual β-cell exhaustion [29]. There are many causative factors of insulin resistance even though not all of them are fully understood. However, the chronic low grade inflammation state of obesity, which is caused by the enhanced production of cytokines and other mediators, are a major determinant of insulin resistance. For instance, TNFα activates intracellular kinases which inhibit insulin receptors making them less responsive to insulin signaling [30]. Another mechanism of insulin resistance is the previously reported excessive level of circulating free fatty acids which, in addition to the mentioned lipotoxicity effect, by accumulating in the muscle cells and hepatocytes impair insulin sensitivity probably through the impairment of the insulin signaling cascade [31, 32]. Finally, the gastrointestinal microbiota, which is different in lean or obese subjects, may play a role also in decreasing insulin sensitivity by modifying intestinal immunologic and permeability milieu with the resulting additional energy absorption and translocation of inflammatory bacterial products [33].

3.4.4 Cardiovascular Disease

Type 2 diabetes and insulin resistance, together with hypertension and dyslipidemia, represent the features of the so-called metabolic syndrome which is mediated by excessive inflammatory adipokine production coupled with the lipotoxicity effect. In the end, the generalized endothelial damage results in atherogenesis, atherosclerosis, and multiple organ dysfunctions. Coronary artery disease has a primary place in the morbidity of obesity since each of the conditions of the metabolic syndrome are independent risk factors [27]. To this should be added the renal functional impairment, the fatty liver dysfunction, the obstructive sleep apnea, and finally the chronic abdominal compartment syndrome with the elevated central venous pressure producing dysfunction of the abdominal organs as well as impairment of CNS circulation [34].

3.4.5 Obesity and Cancer

Epidemiological studies [35] have shown that obesity is associated with increased rates of cancers affecting breast, endometrium, esophagus, colon, and kidney. It is estimated that in the obese population, the risk is 1.5–3.5 folds higher respect to the lean subjects. Multiple factors can explain the association between obesity and cancer depending on the type of tumor, the age, and the sex of the subject. Possible mechanisms of carcinogenesis include hyperinsulinemia and high level of insulin-like growth factor as well as sex hormones. Also the chronic adipokine-mediated inflammation state with the ensuing oxidative stress plays a role [36].

Conclusions

The homeostatic neuro-hormonal mechanisms which maintain a correct balance between energy intake and energy expenditure may become disrupted for genetic and environmental factors in the obese population. The excessive accumulation of fat in the enlarged adipocytes triggers the production of inflammatory factors which progressively lead to serious comorbidities and eventually a reduced life expectancy.

References

1. Hoyt l, Burnett L. Should obesity be a disease? N.Y. Times. 2014, Feb. 23, SR 12.
2. Cinti S. The adipose organ at a glance. Dis Model Mech. 2012;5(5):588–94.
3. Morton GJ, Cummings DE, Baskin DG, Barsh GS, Schwartz MW. Central nervous system control of food intake and body weight. Nature. 2006;443(7109):289–95.
4. Lenard NR, Berthoud HR. Central and peripheral regulation of food intake and physical activity: pathways and genes. Obesity (Silver Spring). 2008;16 Suppl 3:S11–22.
5. Owyang C, Heldsinger A. Vagal control of satiety and hormonal regulation of appetite. J Neurogastroenterol Motil. 2011;17(4):338–48.
6. Stengel A, Taché Y. Interaction between gastric and upper small intestinal hormones in the regulation of hunger and satiety: ghrelin and cholecystokinin take the central stage. Curr Protein Pept Sci. 2011;12(4):293–304.

7. Rehfeld JF. Incretin physiology beyond glucagon-like peptide 1 and glucose-dependent insulinotropic polypeptide: cholecystokinin and gastrin peptides. Acta Physiol (Oxf). 2011;201(4):405–11.
8. Burger KS, Berner LA. A functional neuroimaging review of obesity, appetitive hormones and ingestive behavior. Physiol Behav. 2014;136:121–7.
9. Mason BL, Wang Q, Zigman JM. The central nervous system sites mediating the orexigenic actions of ghrelin. Annu Rev Physiol. 2014;76:519–33.
10. Mietlicki-Baase EG, Hayes MR. Amylin activates distributed CNS nuclei to control energy balance. Physiol Behav. 2014;136:39–46.
11. Cao H. Adipocytokines in obesity and metabolic disease. J Endocrinol. 2014;220(2):T47–59.
12. Trayhurn P, Wood IS. Adipokines: inflammation and the pleiotropic role of white adipose tissue. Br J Nutr. 2004;92(3):347–55.
13. Jéquier E. Leptin signaling, adiposity, and energy balance. Ann N Y Acad Sci. 2002;967:379–88.
14. Mark AL. Selective leptin resistance revisited. Am J Physiol Regul Integr Comp Physiol. 2013;305(6):R566–81.
15. Turer AT, Scherer PE. Adiponectin: mechanistic insights and clinical implications. Diabetologia. 2012;55(9):2319–26.
16. Lazar MA. Resistin- and obesity-associated metabolic diseases. Horm Metab Res. 2007;39(10):710–6.
17. Carnell S, Gibson C, Benson L, Ochner CN, Geliebter A. Neuroimaging and obesity: current knowledge and future directions. Obes Rev. 2012;13(1):43–56.
18. Del Parigi A, Gautier JF, Chen K, Salbe AD, Ravussin E, Reiman E, Tataranni PA. Neuroimaging and obesity: mapping the brain responses to hunger and satiation in humans using positron emission tomography. Ann N Y Acad Sci. 2002;967:389–97.
19. Miras AD, le Roux CW. Mechanisms underlying weight loss after bariatric surgery. Nat Rev Gastroenterol Hepatol. 2013;10(10):575–84.
20. d'Autume C, Musher-Eizenman D, Marinier E, Viarme F, Frelut ML, Isnard P. Eating behaviors and emotional symptoms in childhood obesity: a cross-sectional exploratory study using self-report questionnaires in 63 children and dolescents. Arch Pediatr. 2012;19(8):803–10.
21. O'Rahilly S, Farooqi IS. Human obesity as a heritable disorder of the central control of energy balance. Int J Obes (Lond). 2008;32 Suppl 7:S55–61.
22. Rhee KE, Phelan S, McCaffery J. Early determinants of obesity: genetic, epigenetic, and in utero influences. Int J Pediatr. 2012;2012:463850.
23. Drummond EM, Gibney ER. Epigenetic regulation in obesity. Curr Opin Clin Nutr Metab Care. 2013;16(4):392–7.
24. Mingrone G, Manco M, Mora ME, Guidone C, Iaconelli A, Gniuli D, Leccesi L, Chiellini C, Ghirlanda G. Influence of maternal obesity on insulin sensitivity and secretion in offspring. Diabetes Care. 2008;31(9):1872–6.
25. Bray GA. Obesity is a chronic, relapsing neurochemical disease. Int J Obes Relat Metab Disord. 2004;28(1):34–8.
26. Schäffler A, Müller-Ladner U, Schölmerich J, Büchler C. Role of adipose tissue as an inflammatory organ in human diseases. Endocr Rev. 2006;27(5):449–67.
27. Redinger RN. The pathophysiology of obesity and its clinical manifestations. Gastroenterol Hepatol (N Y). 2007;3(11):856–63.
28. Griffin ME, Marcucci MJ, Cline GW, Bell K, Barucci N, Lee D, Goodyear LJ, Kraegen EW, White MF, Shulman GI. Free fatty acid-induced insulin resistance is associated with activation of protein kinase C theta and alterations in the insulin signaling cascade. Diabetes. 1999;48(6):1270–4.
29. DeFronzo RA, Tripathy D. Skeletal muscle insulin resistance is the primary defect in type 2 diabetes. Diabetes Care. 2009;32 Suppl 2:S157–63.
30. Johnson AM, Olefsky JM. The origins and drivers of insulin resistance. Cell. 2013;152(4):673–84.
31. Mingrone G, Henriksen FL, Greco AV, Krogh LN, Capristo E, Gastaldelli A, Castagneto M, Ferrannini E, Gasbarrini G, Beck-Nielsen H. Triglyceride-induced diabetes associated with familial lipoprotein lipase deficiency. Diabetes. 1999;48(6):1258–63.
32. Mingrone G, Castagneto M. Role of lipids in insulin resistance and type 2 diabetes mellitus development. Nutrition. 1999;15(1):64–6.
33. Kootte RS, Vrieze A, Holleman F, Dallinga-Thie GM, Zoetendal EG, de Vos WM, Groen AK, Hoekstra JB, Stroes ES, Nieuwdorp M. The therapeutic potential of manipulating gut microbiota in obesity and type 2 diabetes mellitus. Diabetes Obes Metab. 2012;14(2):112–20.
34. Frezza EE, Shebani KO, Robertson J, Wachtel MS. Morbid obesity causes chronic increase of intraabdominal pressure. Dig Dis Sci. 2007;52(4):1038–41.
35. Calle EE, Rodriguez C, Walker-Thurmond K, Thun MJ. Overweight, obesity, and mortality from cancer in a prospectively studied cohort of U.S. adults. N Engl J Med. 2003;348(17):1625–38.
36. Pischon T, Nöthlings U, Boeing H. Obesity and cancer. Proc Nutr Soc. 2008;67(2):128–45.

Obesity-Related Comorbidities

4

Paola Fierabracci, Anna Tamberi, and Ferruccio Santini

4.1 Introduction

Obesity contributes to the development of many diseases that increase the risk of mortality and worsen the quality of life. Recent studies indicate that, relative to the normal weight category, the main contribution to excess mortality in obesity comes from higher levels of BMI, while overweight (defined as a BMI of 25–<30 kg/m^2) appears associated with significantly lower all-cause mortality [1]. However, BMI does not take into account body composition and body distribution and it has been clearly established that the preferential accumulation of fat in the upper body and visceral districts is more harmful because it is associated with an increased risk of developing diabetes, dyslipidemia, hypertension, and cardiovascular disease. The main obesity-related comorbidities are depicted in Fig. 4.1.

4.2 The Metabolic Syndrome (MetS)

The metabolic syndrome is defined by a cluster of interconnected biochemical and clinical parameters associated with visceral obesity, which increase the risk of mortality for all causes. The main factors that contribute to the syndrome are insulin resistance, dyslipidemia, endothelial dysfunction, elevated blood pressure, a hypercoagulable and inflammatory state. Several definitions of MetS have been proposed (Table 4.1) [1–6], many of them being focused on insulin resistance. The ATPIII and IDF definitions employ measures that are readily available to physicians, thus facilitating their clinical application, although discrepancies may arise when the definition is applied to different ethnic groups [7]. In particular, the risk of type 2 diabetes mellitus (T2DM) increases at much lower levels of obesity in Asians compared to Europeans. Therefore, a new set of criteria with ethnic/racial specific cutoffs has been recently proposed [8].

4.2.1 Visceral Obesity

The white adipose tissue (WAT) includes white adipocytes and stromal vascular cells (preadipocytes, endothelial cells, pericytes, and various immune cells) [9]. In lean subjects, most WAT is localized at subcutaneous sites while only minor

P. Fierabracci • A. Tamberi • F. Santini (✉)
Obesity Center at the Endocrinology Unit, University Hospital of Pisa, Via Paradisa 2, Pisa 56100, Italy
e-mail: pfierab2001@yahoo.it; annatamberi84@gmail.com; ferruccio.santini@med.unipi.it

M. Lucchese, N. Scopinaro (eds.), *Minimally Invasive Bariatric and Metabolic Surgery: Principles and Technical Aspects*, DOI 10.1007/978-3-319-15356-8_4,

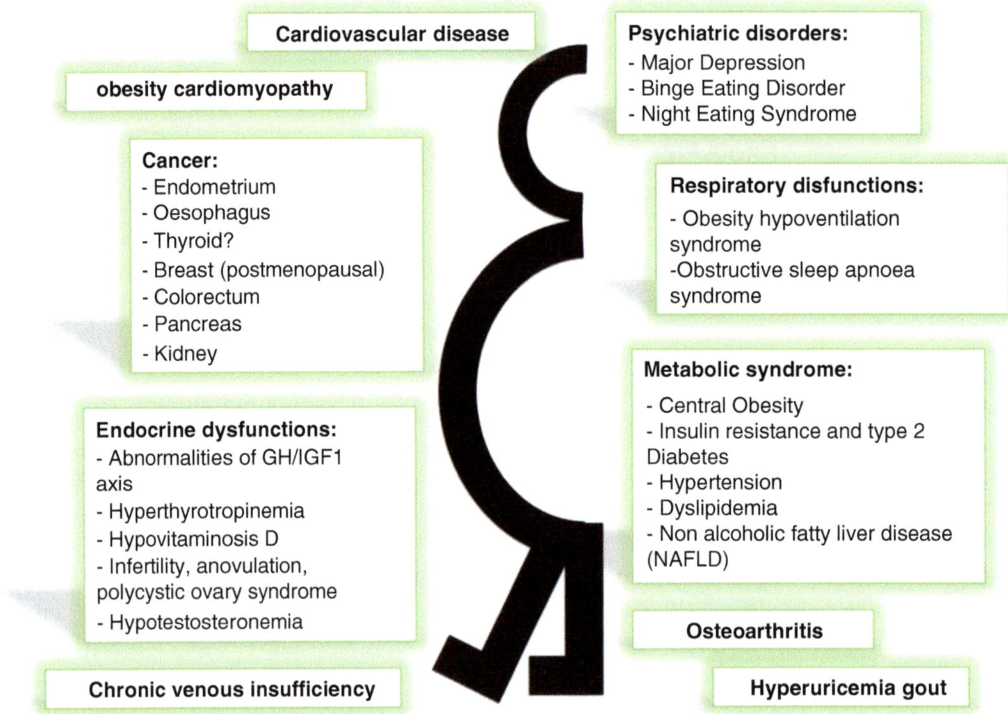

Fig. 4.1 Main obesity-related comorbidities

adipose tissue depots are associated with internal organs including the omental, mesenteric, epiploic, retroperitoneal, and intrathoracic fat. A gender-related difference in fat deposition has been described, prior to and during the development of obesity. Women have generally higher adiposity than men. Furthermore, women accumulate more in subcutaneous sites whereas men accumulate more fat within the central area. In response to a positive energy balance, when physiological fat depots cannot further expand, fat accumulation may occur at undesired sites such as the liver, the heart, the skeletal muscle, and the pancreas. Ectopic fat deposition is predictive of insulin resistance and related metabolic abnormalities referred to as the metabolic syndrome. The adipose tissue is an endocrine organ producing adipokines, like adiponectin and leptin, and inflammatory cytokines such as interleukin (IL-6) and tumor necrosis factor (TNF)-α. Ectopic/visceral obesity is associated with hypoxic, inflamed, and dysfunctional adipose tissue that modifies its secretion thus contributing to the insulin resistant, proinflammatory, prothrombotic, and pro-hypertensive state of the metabolic syndrome.

4.2.2 Insulin Resistance and Type 2 Diabetes

Insulin resistance is a pathophysiological condition in which peripheral tissues such as the adipose tissue, the muscle, and the liver are less sensitive to insulin action. Therefore, pancreatic beta cells have to secrete more insulin to overcome the hyperglycemia of insulin-resistant individuals. The resulting hyperinsulinemia may compensate for insulin resistance to some biological actions of the hormone (e.g., maintenance of normoglycemia) but it may cause an overexpression of insulin activity in normally sensitive tissues. The clinical manifestations of MetS are the result of some insulin actions associated with a resistance to other actions [10]. In the long term, the inability by pancreatic beta cells to

Table 4.1 Criteria for the diagnosis of metabolic syndrome

	WHO (1998) [2]		EGIR (1999) [3]		ATPIII (2001) [4]		AACE (2003) [5]		IDF (2005) [6]	
Insulin resistance	IGT, IFG, T2DM, or lowered insulin sensitivity[a] plus any two of the following		Plasma insulin >75th percentile plus any two of the following		None, but any three of the following five features		IGT or IFG plus any of the following based on the clinical judgment		None	
Hyperglycemia	**Male and female**		**Male and female**		**Male and female**		**Male and female**		**Male and female**	
	IGT, IFG, or T2DM		IGT or IFG (but not diabetes)		>110 mg/dl (includes diabetes)		IGT or IFG (but not diabetes)		≥100 mg/dl (includes diabetes)	
Obesity	**Male**	**Female**	**Male**	**Female**	**Male**	**Female**	**Male and Female**		**Male and Female**	
	Waist-to-hip ratio >90 and/or: BMI > 30 kg/m^2	Waist-to-hip ratio >0.85	Waist circumf. ≥ 94 cm	Waist circumf. ≥ 80 cm	Waist circumf. ≥ 102 cm	Waist circumf. ≥ 88 cm	BMI ≥ 25 kg/m^2		Increased waist circumference (population specific) plus any two of the following	
Dyslipidemia	**Male and female**		**Male and female**		**Male and female**		**Male and female**		**Male and female**	
	Triglycerides ≥ 150 mg/dl		Triglycerides ≥ 150 mg/dl		Triglycerides ≥ 150 mg/dl		Triglycerides ≥ 150 mg/dl		Triglycerides ≥ 150 mg/dl or receiving treatment	
			and/or:		and HDL cholesterol:		and HDL cholesterol:		and HDL cholesterol:	
	Male	**Female**	HDL cholesterol <39 mg/dl		**Male**	**Female**	**Male**	**Female**	**Male**	**Female**
	<35 mg/dl	<39 mg/dl			<40 mg/dl	<50 mg/dl	<40 mg/dl	<50 mg/dl	<40 mg/dl	<50 mg/l
Hypertension	**Male and female**		**Male and female**		**Male and female**		**Male and female**		**Male and female**	
	≥140/90 mmHg		≥140/90 mmHg or on hypertension treatment		≥130/85 mmHg		≥130/85 mmHg		Systolic ≥130 mm Hg or Diastolic ≥85 mm Hg or on hypertension treatment	
Others	**Male and female**									
	Microalbuminuria: Urinary excretion rate of >20 mg/min or: Albumin:creatinine ratio of >30 mg/g.									

[a]Insulin sensitivity measured under hyperinsulinemic euglycemic conditions, glucose uptake below lowest quartile for background population under investigation
BMI body mass index, *IFG* impaired fasting glucose, *IGT* impaired glucose tolerance, *T2DM* type 2 diabetes mellitus

produce sufficient hormone to correct insulin resistance may lead to hyperglycemia and type 2 diabetes [11].

The action of insulin is expressed through binding to specific receptors that determine the activation of a cascade involved in the control of cell metabolism, including the synthesis of glycogen, triglycerides (TG), and proteins, as well as other biological responses specific of each cell-type. Insulin resistance may occur at multiple levels, including desensitization of the insulin receptors, inhibition of the signaling cascade and effects on gene transcription. Insulin resistance is not necessarily associated with obesity, but appears with abnormal fat distribution (i.e., visceral fat accumulation) [12].

4.2.3 Dyslipidemia

The "atherogenic dyslipidemia" is characterized by an increase of lipoproteins containing apolipoprotein B (apoB), elevated fasting and postprandial triglycerides, with the preponderance of small dense lipoprotein and low levels of high density lipoprotein cholesterol (HDL-C). This pattern appears to be heritable, but several nongenetic factors, such as abdominal adiposity, influence the expression of this phenotype. Insulin resistance may lead to atherogenic dyslipidemia by several mechanisms, including increased lipolysis with excessive delivery of free fatty acids to the liver that uses them as substrate for the synthesis of TG [13, 14].

4.2.4 Hypertension

Essential hypertension is a common feature of the metabolic syndrome [15]. Current evidence suggests that visceral obesity is characterized by an activation of the renin-angiotensin system (RAS), resulting in increased expression of angiotensinogen, angiotensin II (AT II), and AT1 receptor, which, in concert, contribute to the development of hypertension [16]. In addition, insulin resistance and hyperinsulinemia lead to activation of the sympathetic nervous system, leading to increased sodium reabsorption at kidney level [17]. Furthermore, adipose tissue produces aldosterone in response to AT II [18] and adipocytes can be considered a renin-angiotensin-aldosterone miniature.

4.3 The Obesity Cardiomyopathy

The obese status is associated with a spectrum of cardiovascular disorders ranging from a hyperdynamic circulation with subclinical myocardial structural changes to overt heart failure. Occurrence of obesity cardiomyopathy as a distinct entity has been proposed. Obesity cardiomyopathy may result from a complex interaction between functional, metabolic, and toxic factors, including an expansion of the blood volume, insulin resistance, activation of the sympathetic nervous system, and cardiac lipotoxicity.

Study performed by ultrasonic tissue characterization in a series of severely obese healthy subjects showed early myocardial structural and functional alterations that were almost completely normalized after weight loss achieved by bariatric surgery [19, 20].

4.4 The Nonalcoholic Fatty Liver Disease (NAFLD)

Increasing evidence suggests that NAFLD represents the hepatic component of the metabolic syndrome and the most common cause of abnormal liver tests in the adult population of Western countries. NAFLD is a consequence of visceral fat accumulation and is defined by a lipid accumulation >5 % in hepatic tissue in the absence of chronic alcohol consumption [21]. NAFLD is characterized by a wide spectrum of liver damage ranging from simple steatosis to advanced fibrosis and to cryptogenic cirrhosis through steatohepatitis (NASH), and, ultimately, to hepatocellular carcinoma [22, 23]. The prevalence and severity of NAFLD increases with increments of body mass index. NAFLD is usually asymptomatic, and hepatomegaly can be the only objective sign. No combination of clinical or biochemical abnormalities can accurately differentiate the spectrum of NAFLD, and only liver biopsy can establish the diagnosis. Whole hepatic enlargement is proportional to the severity of the metabolic syndrome, and various imaging methodologies can be used for the estimation of liver volume. Recently, an ultrasound technique has been introduced, which measures the hepatic left lobe volume (HLLV) [24, 25]. HLLV was tightly correlated to intra-abdominal fat and an excellent indicator of visceral adiposity, clustering with the parameters defining the metabolic syndrome. Furthermore, after weight loss achieved by gastric banding, reduction of the HLLV was the best single predictor of improvement of various cardiometabolic risk factors.

4.5 Respiratory Dysfunctions

Obesity hypoventilation syndrome (OHS) and obstructive sleep apnea syndrome (OSAS) are the main pulmonary dysfunctions associated with obesity [26]. Fat accumulation in the upper site of the body leads to reduction in chest wall compliance and respiratory muscle performance, with consequent hypoxemia and progressively worsening disability. OHS is defined as the combined presence of obesity and awake arterial hypercapnia ($PaCO_2$ >45 mmHg) in the absence of other causes of hypoventilation.

OSAS is characterized by repetitive upper airway occlusion episodes leading to apnea with arousal being required to reestablish airway patency. OSAS affects up to 7 % of the adult male population, and its prevalence increases with age. The apnea/hypopnea index (AHI) that indicates the frequency of the apnea/hypopnea episodes per hour of sleep, is commonly used to quantify the severity of OSAS. The pathophysiology of OSAS is mainly based on the imbalance between the collapsing forces of the upper airway during inspiration and the counteracting forces of the upper airway dilating muscles [27]. Obesity and male gender are the most important risk factors for sleep apnea [28]. The OSAS prevalence is 12- to 30-fold higher among morbidly obese patients than in the general population [29] with visceral obesity being more strictly associated to OSAS; the accumulation of adipose tissue in the neck and in the pharyngeal structures is one of the main mechanisms involved in this association. Noteworthy, OSAS itself may predispose individuals to worsening obesity because of sleep deprivation, daytime somnolence, and disrupted metabolism [30]. Sleep fragmentation and chronic intermittent hypoxia are likely to play a prevalent role in causing the increased morbidity and mortality in comparison with simple obesity [31], and OSAS is indeed associated [32] with an increased prevalence of metabolic syndrome, hypertension, insulin resistance and T2DM, and cardiovascular illness, such as transient ischemic attacks, stroke, cardiac arhythmias, myocardial infarction, and pulmonary hypertension [33, 34].

4.6 Psychiatric Disorders

Major depression, binge eating disorder (BED), and night eating syndrome (NES) are commonly associated with obesity. Current evidence suggests that there is a temporal association between obesity and depression, which would make obesity a risk factor for the development of the disease. However, a temporal depression to obesity relationship has also been observed, which may be due to eating and sleeping disturbances as well as the use of antidepressant medications [35].

Early-onset obesity is associated with the development of eating disorders, body-dysmorphic disorders, and low self-esteem. In a recent study including 280 obese subjects, patients with early onset obesity displayed a higher burden of depressive spectrum symptomatology than patients who developed obesity only during adulthood [36].

BED, defined as the ingestion of large amount of food in a short period of time (>2H) accompanied by a sense of loss of control over eating, is another psychiatric disorder independently associated with obesity and depression. Its prevalence increases with severity of the obese state. NES is characterized by evening hyperphagia, meaning that at least 25 % of the daily caloric intake is consumed after the last evening meal or that two or more nocturnal eating episodes occur per week. NES is more common among obese persons although it is not exclusive to them [37]. About one in five obese subjects assessed for eligibility for bariatric surgery present with mood and/or personality disorders [38, 39]. A careful psychological and/or psychiatric assessment and treatment should always be provided to establish the eligibility for bariatric surgery, to improve the postoperative outcome and to reduce the risk of complications.

4.7 Osteoarthritis

Osteoarthritis (OA) is the most important musculoskeletal disease associated with obesity [40]. It is a disabling degenerative joint disorder characterized by pain, limitation of mobility, and an overall negative impact on quality of life. The incidence and progression of OA in obese subjects is increased both in weight-bearing and non-weight-bearing joints. Weight loss contribute to improve symptoms and to delay the progression of joint disease. The pathogenesis of obesity-related OA is multifactorial: Both mechanical factors as well as metabolic factors appear to be involved, including the low-grade inflammatory state associated with obesity and the abnormal expression of adypokines. Weight loss may improve both pain and joint function, and osteoarthritis should be considered when assessing the indications of obese candidates to bariatric surgery.

4.8 Cancer

The International Agency for Research into Cancer and the World Cancer Research Fund (WCRF) [41] have reported a strong association of obesity with the endometrial, esophageal adenocarcinoma, colorectal, postmenopausal breast, prostate, and renal cancers, whereas other types of malignancies such as leukemia, non-Hodgkin's lymphoma, multiple myeloma, malignant melanoma, and thyroid tumors are less frequent [42]. The main pathogenic mechanisms include BMI, excess weight, particularly visceral fat accumulation, diet, and lifestyle factors. Furthemore, biological mechanisms appear to be involved, such as hyperinsulinemia and insulin resistance, the activities of IGFs and IGF binding proteins, sex hormones and SHBG, low-grade inflammation, changes in adipose tissue production of adipokines and vascular growth factors, oxidative stress, endocrine disruptors, and alterations in immune function.

The Swedish Obese Subjects (SOS) study, reporting the long-term effects of bariatric surgery on morbidity and mortality in a follow-up period longer than 10 years, showed a significant reduction in cancer incidence in association with substantial weight loss [43].

4.9 Endocrine Dysfunctions

4.9.1 The Thyroid

The relationships between serum thyroid hormones, body weight, and feeding have been extensively investigated. A reciprocal interaction between the hypothalamus-pituitary-thyroid axis and the adipose tissue is required for the proper homeostasis of energy balance. In both lean and obese subjects, thyroid hormone and TSH levels are strongly influenced by the individual nutritional status [44]. Fasting is characterized by a reduction of T3 in the bloodstream, while the production rate of the hormone is significantly increased during overfeeding, thus explaining increased serum levels of T3 observed in some obese cohorts compared to controls. A slight elevation of serum TSH has been described in obese subjects. However, these changes are usually within the normal range and current evidence suggests that they may represent an adaptive response of the hypothalamus-pituitary-thyroid axis to weight gain. The increased rate of thyroid hormone disposal occurring in obese individuals would be the primary event promoting an activation of the hypothalamus-pituitary-thyroid axis, aimed at maintaining serum thyroid hormones within the euthyroid range. While thyroid hormone replacement therapy is required if obesity is associated with subclinical or overt hypothyroidism, no specific intervention is required for minor TSH changes, not related to a specific thyroid disease. In a large series of severely obese subjects evaluated before bariatric surgery [45], thyroid disease was by far the most frequent among endocrine diseases, including primary hypothyroidism, non-autoimmune nodular disease, and thyroid cancer. Although these prevalence rates did not substantially differ from those observed in a comparable population of normal weight subjects, we suggest that routine screening for thyroid dysfunction should be always performed during the preoperative evaluation of bariatric patients.

4.9.2 Vitamin D

An inverse relationship between obesity and serum 25-OH vitamin D has been consistently reported, and vitamin D deficiency leading to secondary hyperparathyroidism is a common finding in obese candidates to bariatric surgery. Putative pathogenic mechanisms of vitamin deficiency in obese individuals include: poor sunlight exposure, reduced 25-OH vitamin D synthesis at hepatic level, diminished vitamin D bioavalaibility due to increased uptake by the adipose tissue, and inadequate dietary intake. In some studies, hypovitaminosis D has been linked with obesity-related comorbidities such as hypertension and type 2 diabetes mellitus [46].

4.9.3 The GH/IGF I Axis

Obesity is associated with abnormalities of the growth hormone/insulin-like growth factor-1 (GH/IGF-1) axis. Both GH secretion rate and burst frequency are reduced in obese as compared to lean subjects [47]. Furthermore, morbidly obese patients show reduced GH secretion after pharmacological stimulation, with serum peak GH levels frequently comparable to those found in adult patients with organic GH deficiency [48, 49]. Serum concentrations of IGF-1 reflect the combined effects of integrated GH secretion and tissue responsiveness to GH. Low serum IGF-1 concentrations have been consistently reported in severe obesity [50–53]. Improvement of GH/IGF-1 activity after weight loss [54] suggests a reversible defect of this axis, strictly related to body weight.

A recent study [55] performed in obese women demonstrated that the extent of IGF-1 deficiency is proportional to increased BMI; after laparoscopic adjustable gastric banding a spontaneous raise of serum IGF-1 occurred, proportional to the extent of weight reduction. Overall, these observations indicate that, beside age, body weight is a major determinant of serum IGF-1 levels in obesity.

4.9.4 The Adrenal Gland

The abdominal fenotype of obesity with associated metabolic and cardiovascular alterations may resemble hypercortisolism, thus providing the basis for a role of glucocorticoids on the development of human obesity [56, 57]. In obese individuals, daily variations of serum adrenocorticotropin hormone (ACTH) and cortisol are usually maintained. At variance, dynamic studies suggest the presence of a hyperresponsiveness of the hypothalamic–pituitary–adrenocortical (HPA) axis to various stimuli [58]. Density of the glucocorticoid receptor in the visceral adipose tissue appears to be higher than in peripheral subcutaneous fat [59], suggesting a pathogenic role of cortisol in the development of abdominal obesity.

Stress adaptation requires a series of responses that include an activation of the HPA axis [60, 61]. Abdominal obesity and its metabolic comorbidities are significantly associated with stress-related conditions such as adverse life events, psychological disturbances, and psychosocial distress [62–68]. Chronic hyperactivation of the HPA axis due to the inability to cope with long-term environmental adverse events has been advocated among the mechanisms leading to abdominal obesity in susceptible individuals [69, 70].

Cushing's syndrome has been detected in 0.8 % obese subjects candidates to bariatric surgery, a prevalence greater than that reported in the general population. Considering the possible lack of distinguishable features of hypercortisolism in obese patients, we believe that screening of Cushing's disease by a simple overnight 1 mg dexamethasone test may be performed to avoid improper bariatric surgery [44].

4.9.5 The Gonads

Fertility can be negatively affected by obesity in both genders. In women, early onset of obesity favors the development of menses irregularities, chronic oligo-anovulation and infertility in the adult age. In addition, increased risk of miscarriage and impairment of the outcome of assisted reproductive technologies and pregnancy have been reported. The main factors implicated in these associations may be insulin resistance and compensatory hyperinsulinemia. The adverse effects of obesity are specifically evident in polycystic ovary syndrome. In men, obesity is associated with low testosterone levels. In severely obese individuals, reduced spermatogenesis associated with severe hypotestosteronemia may favor infertility. Moreover, the frequency of erectile dysfunction increases with increasing BMI. The impact of obesity on fertility appears to be particularly important before assisted reproductive technologies are used [71].

References

1. Flegal KM, Kit BK, Orpana H, Graubard BI. Association of all-cause mortality with overweight and obesity using standard body mass index categories: a systematic review and meta-analysis. JAMA. 2013;2(309):71–82.
2. Alberti KG, Zimmet PZ. Definition, diagnosis and classification of diabetes mellitus and its complications. Part 1: diagnosis and classification of diabetes mellitus provisional report of a WHO consultation. Diabet Med. 1998;15:539–53.
3. Balkau B, Charles MA. Comment on the provisional report from the WHO consultation. European Group for the Study of Insulin Resistance (EGIR). Diabet Med. 1999;16:442–3.
4. Expert Panel on Detection, Evaluation, and Treatment of High Blood Cholesterol in Adults. Executive Summary of The Third Report of The National Cholesterol Education Program (NCEP) Expert Panel on Detection, Evaluation, And Treatment of High Blood Cholesterol In Adults (Adult Treatment Panel III). JAMA. 2001;285:2486–97.
5. Einhorn D, Reaven GM, Cobin RH, Ford E, Ganda OP, Handelsman Y, Hellman R, Jellinger PS, Kendall D, Krauss RM, Neufeld ND, Petak SM, Rodbard HW, Seibel JA, Smith DA, Wilson PW. American College of Endocrinology position statement on the insulin resistance syndrome. Endocr Pract. 2003;9:237–52.
6. International Diabetes Federation: The IDF consensus worldwide definition of the metabolic syndrome. http://www.idf.org/metabolic-syndrome.
7. Ritchie SA, Connell JM. The link between abdominal obesity, metabolic syndrome and cardiovascular disease. Nutrition, metabolism and cardiovascular disease. Nutr Metab Cardiovasc Dis. 2007;17:319–26.
8. Alberti KG, Eckel RH, Grundy SM, Zimmet PZ, Cleeman JI, Donato KA, Fruchart JC, James WP, Loria CM, Smith Jr SC, International Diabetes Federation Task Force on Epidemiology and Prevention, Hational Heart, Lung, and Blood Institute, American Heart Association, World Heart Federation; International Atherosclerosis Society, International Association for the Study of Obesity. Harmonizing the metabolic syndrome: a joint interim statement of the international diabetes federation task force on epidemiology and prevention; National heart, lung, and blood institute; American heart association; World heart federation; International atherosclerosis society; And international association for the study of obesity. Circulation. 2009;20(120):1640–5.
9. Proença AR, Sertié RA, Oliveira AC, Campaña AB, Caminhotto RO, Chimin P, Lima FB. New concepts in white adipose tissue physiology. Braz J Med Biol Res. 2014;47:192–205.
10. Gill H, Mugo M, Whaley-Connell A, Stump C, Sowers JR. The key role of insulin resistance in the cardiometabolic syndrome. Am J Med Sci. 2005;330:290–4.
11. Petersen K, Shulman GI. Etiology of insulin resistance. Am J Med. 2006;420:125–6.
12. Jensen MD, Haymond MW, Rizza RA, Cryer PE, Miles JM. Influence of body fat distribution on free fatty acid metabolism in obesity. J Clin Invest. 1989;83:1168–73.
13. Lewis GF, Steiner G. Acute effects of insulin in the control of VLDL production in humans: implications for the insulin-resistant state. Diabetes Care. 1996;19:390–3.
14. Ginsberg HN, Zhang YL, Hernandez-Ono A. Regulation of plasma triglycerides in insulin resistance and diabetes. Arch Med Res. 2005;36:232–40.
15. Ferrannini E, Natali A. Essential hypertension, metabolic disorders, and insulin resistance. Am Heart J. 1991;121:1274–82.
16. Malhotra A, Kang BP, Cheung S, Opawumi D, Meggs LG. Angiotensin II promotes glucose-induced

activation of cardiac protein kinase C isozymes and phosphorylation of troponin I. Diabetes. 2001;50: 1918–26.
17. Morse SA, Zhang R, Thakur V, Reisin E. Hypertension and the metabolic syndrome. Am J Med Sci. 2005; 330:303–10.
18. Briones AM, Nguyen Dinh Cat A, Callera GE, Yogi A, Burger D, He Y, Corrêa JW, Gagnon AM, Gomez-Sanchez CE, Gomez-Sanchez EP, Sorisky A, Ooi TC, Ruzicka M, Burns KD, Touyz RM. Adipocytes produce aldosterone through calcineurin-dependent signaling pathways: implications in diabetes mellitus-associated obesity and vascular dysfunction. Hypertension. 2012;59:1069–78.
19. Di Bello V, Santini F, Di Cori A, Pucci A, Palagi C, Delle Donne MG, Fierabracci P, Marsili A, Talini E, Giannetti M, Biadi O, Balbarini A, Mariani M, Pinchera A. Obesity cardiomyopathy: is it a reality? An ultrasonic tissue characterization study. J Am Soc Echocardiogr. 2006;19:1063–71.
20. Di Bello V, Santini F, Di Cori A, Pucci A, Talini E, Palagi C, Delle Donne MG, Marsili A, Fierabracci P, Valeriano R, Scartabelli G, Giannetti M, Anselmino M, Pinchera A, Mariani M. Effects of bariatric surgery on early myocardial alterations in adult severely obese subjects. Cardiology. 2008;109:241–8.
21. Brunt EM, Tiniakos DG. Histopathology of nonalcoholic fatty liver disease. World J Gastroenterol. 2010; 14(16):5286–96.
22. Caldwell S, Argo C. The natural history of non-alcoholic fatty liver disease. Dig Dis. 2010;28:162–8.
23. Musso G, Gambino R, Cassader M, Pagano G. Meta-analysis: natural history of non-alcoholic fatty liver disease (NAFLD) and diagnostic accuracy of non-invasive tests for liver disease severity. Ann Med. 2011;43:617–49.
24. Santini F, Giannetti M, Mazzeo S, Fierabracci P, Scartabelli G, Marsili A, Valeriano R, Pucci A, Anselmino M, Zampa V, Vitti P, Pinchera A. Ultrasonographic evaluation of liver volume and the metabolic syndrome in obese women. J Endocrinol Invest. 2007;30:104–10.
25. Giannetti M, Piaggi P, Ceccarini G, Mazzeo S, Querci G, Fierabracci P, Salvetti G, Galli G, Ricco I, Martinelli S, Di Salvo C, Anselmino M, Landi A, Vitti P, Pinchera A, Santini F. Hepatic left lobe volume is a sensitive index of metabolic improvement in obese women after gastric banding. Int J Obes (Lond). 2012;36:336–41.
26. Al Dabal L, Bahammam AS. Obesity hypoventilation syndrome. Ann Thorac Med. 2009;4:41–9.
27. Malhotra A, White DP. Obstructive sleep apnoea. Lancet. 2002;360:237–45.
28. Palla A, Digiorgio M, Carpenè N, Rossi G, D'Amico I, Santini F, Pinchera A. Sleep apnea in morbidly obese patients: prevalence and clinical predictivity. Respiration. 2009;78:134–40.
29. Young T, Peppard PE, Taheri S. Excess weight and sleep-disordered breathing. J Appl Physiol (1985). 2005;99:1592–9.
30. Zamarron C, García Paz V, Riveiro A. Obstructive sleep apnea syndrome is a systemic disease. Current evidence. Eur J Intern Med. 2008;19:390–8.
31. Lanfranco F, Motta G, Minetto MA, Baldi M, Balbo M, Ghigo E, Arvat E, Maccario M. Neuroendocrine alterations in obese patients with sleep apnea syndrome. Int J Endocrinol. 2010;2010:474518.
32. Vgontzas AN, Bixler EO, Chrousos GP. Metabolic disturbance in obesity versus sleep apnea: the importance of visceral obesity and insulin resistance. J Intern Med. 2003;254:32–44.
33. Alam I, Lewis K, Stephens JW, Baxter JN. Obesity, metabolic syndrome and sleep apnea: all pro-inflammatory states. Obes Rev. 2007;8:119–27.
34. Knutson KL, Zhao X, Mattingly M, Galli G, Cizza G. Predictors of sleep disordered breathing in obese adults who are chronic short sleepers. Sleep Med. 2012;13:484–9.
35. Heo M, Pietrobelli A, Fontaine KR, Sirey JA, Faith MS. Depressive mood and obesity in US adults: comparison and moderation by sex, age, and race. Int J Obes (Lond). 2006;30:513–9.
36. Mauri M, Calderone A, Fagiolini A, Santini F, Borri C, Oppo A, Romano A, Rinaldi S, Polini M, Lippi C, Pinchera A, Cassano GB. Psychiatric disorders and lifetime mood spectrum symptoms in early and late onset obesity. Obes Metab. 2008;4:99–105.
37. Cassidy K, Kotynia-English R, Acres J, Flicker L, Lautenshlager N, Almeida OP. Association between lifestyle factors and mental health measures among community-dwelling older women. Aust N Z J Psychiatry. 2004;38:940–7.
38. Mauri M, Rucci P, Calderone A, Santini F, Oppo A, Romano A, Rinaldi S, Armani A, Polini M, Pinchera A, Cassano GB. Axis I and II disorders and quality of life in bariatric surgery candidates. J Clin Psychiatry. 2008;69:295–301.
39. Vincent HK, Heywood K, Connelly J, Hurley RW. Obesity and weight loss in the treatment and prevention of osteoarthritis. PM R. 2012;4:S59–67.
40. Glade MJ. Food, nutrition, and the prevention of cancer: a global perspective. American Institute for Cancer Research/World Cancer Research Fund, American Institute for Cancer Research, 1997. Nutrition. 1999;15:523–6.
41. De Pergola G, Silvestris F. Obesity as a major risk factor for cancer. J Obes. 2013;2013:291546.
42. Sjöström L, Gummesson A, Sjöström CD, Narbro K, Peltonen M, Wedel H, Bengtsson C, Bouchard C, Carlsson B, Dahlgren S, Jacobson P, Karason K, Karlsson J, Larsson B, Lindroos AK, Lönroth H, Näslund I, Olbers T, Stenlöf K, Torgerson J, Carlsson LM. Swedish Obese Subjects Study. Effects of bariatric surgery on cancer incidence in obese patients in Sweden (Swedish Obese Subjects Study): a prospective, controlled intervention trial. Lancet Oncol. 2009;10:653–62.
43. Bray GA, Fisher DA, Chopra IJ. Relation of thyroid hormones to body-weight. Lancet. 1976;1:1206–8.
44. Fierabracci P, Pinchera A, Martinelli S, Scartabelli G, Salvetti G, Giannetti M, Pucci A, Galli G, Ricco I, Querci G, Rago T, Di Salvo C, Anselmino M, Vitti P, Santini F. Prevalence of endocrine diseases in

morbidly obese patients scheduled for bariatric surgery: beyond diabetes. Obes Surg. 2011;21:54–60.
45. Ybarra J, Sánchez-Hernández J, Pérez A. Hypovitaminosis D and morbid obesity. Nurs Clin North Am. 2007;42:19–27.
46. Veldhuis JD, Iranmanesh A, Ho KK, Waters MJ, Johnson ML, Lizarralde G. Dual defects in pulsatile growth hormone secretion and clearance subserve the hyposomatotropism of obesity in man. J Clin Endocrinol Metab. 1991;72:51–9.
47. Maccario M, Valetto MR, Savio P, Aimaretti G, Baffoni C, Procopio M, Grottoli S, Oleandri SE, Arvat E, Ghigo E. Maximal secretory capacity of somatotrope cells in obesity: comparison with GH deficiency. Int J Obes Relat Metab Disord. 1997;21:27–32.
48. Makimura H, Stanley T, Mun D, You SM, Grinspoon S. The effects of central adiposity on growth hormone (GH) response to GH-releasing hormone-arginine stimulation testing in men. J Clin Endocrinol Metab. 2008;93:4254–60.
49. Juul A. Serum levels of insulin-like growth factor I and its binding proteins in health and disease. Growth Horm IGF Res. 2003;13:113–70.
50. Brick DJ, Gerweck AV, Meenaghan E, Lawson EA, Misra M, Fazeli P, Johnson W, Klibanski A, Miller KK. Determinants of IGF1 and GH across the weight spectrum: from anorexia nervosa to obesity. Eur J Endocrinol. 2010;163:185–91.
51. Kreitschmann-Andermahr I, Suarez P, Jennings R, Evers N, Brabant G. GH/IGF-I regulation in obesity–mechanisms and practical consequences in children and adults. Horm Res Paediatr. 2010;73:153–60.
52. Rasmussen MH. Obesity, growth hormone and weight loss. Mol Cell Endocrinol. 2010;316:147–53.
53. Rasmussen MH, Hvidberg A, Juul A, Main KM, Gotfredsen A, Skakkebaek NE, Hilsted J, Skakkebae NE. Massive weight loss restores 24-hour growth hormone release profiles and serum insulin-like growth factor-I levels in obese subjects. J Clin Endocrinol Metab. 1995;80:1407–15.
54. Belobrajdic DP, Frystyk J, Jeyaratnaganthan N, Espelund U, Flyvbjerg A, Clifton PM, Noakes M. Moderate energy restriction-induced weight loss affects circulating IGF levels independent of dietary composition. Eur J Endocrinol. 2010;162:1075–82.
55. Galli G, Pinchera A, Piaggi P, Fierabracci P, Giannetti M, Querci G, Scartabelli G, Manetti L, Ceccarini G, Martinelli S, Di Salvo C, Anselmino M, Bogazzi F, Landi A, Vitti P, Maffei M, Santini F. Serum insulin-like growth factor-1 concentrations are reduced in severely obese women and raise after weight loss induced by laparoscopic adjustable gastric banding. Obes Surg. 2012;22:1276–80.
56. Bjorntorp P. Centralization of body fat. Chichester: Wiley; 2001.
57. Pasquali R, Cantobelli S, Casimirri F, Capelli M, Bortoluzzi L, Flamia R, Labate AM, Barbara L. The hypothalamic-pituitary-adrenal axis in obese women with different patterns of body fat distribution. J Clin Endocrinol Metab. 1993;77:341–6.
58. Schiffman SS, Graham BG, Sattely-Miller EA, Peterson-Dancy M. Elevated and sustained desire for sweet taste in african-americans: a potential factor in the development of obesity. Nutrition. 2000;16:886–93.
59. Björntorp P, Rosmond R. Neuroendocrine abnormalities in visceral obesity. Int J Obes Relat Metab Disord. 2000;24 Suppl 2:S80–5.
60. Pasquali R, Gagliardi L, Vicennati V, Gambineri A, Colitta D, Ceroni L, Casimirri F. ACTH and cortisol response to combined corticotropin releasing hormone-arginine vasopressin stimulation in obese males and its relationship to body weight, fat distribution and parameters of the metabolic syndrome. Int J Obes Relat Metab Disord. 1999;23:419–24.
61. Pasquali R, Ambrosi B, Armanini D, Cavagnini F, Uberti ED, Del Rio G, de Pergola G, Maccario M, Mantero F, Marugo M, Rotella CM, Vettor R, Study Group on Obesity of the Italian Society of Endocrinology. Cortisol and ACTH response to oral dexamethasone in obesity and effects of sex, body fat distribution, and dexamethasone concentrations: a dose-response study. J Clin Endocrinol Metab. 2002;87:166–75.
62. Bale TL. Stress sensitivity and the development of affective disorders. Horm Behav. 2006;50:529–33.
63. Ghitza UE, Gray SM, Epstein DH, Rice KC, Shaham Y. The anxiogenic drug yohimbine reinstates palatable food seeking in a rat relapse model: a role of CRF1 receptors. Neuropsychopharmacology. 2006;31:2188–96.
64. Adam TC, Epel ES. Stress, eating and the reward system. Physiol Behav. 2007;91:449–58.
65. Viau V. Functional cross-talk between the hypothalamic-pituitary-gonadal and -adrenal axes. J Neuroendocrinol. 2002;14:506–13.
66. Das UN. Obesity: genes, brain, gut, and environment. Nutrition. 2010;26:459–73.
67. Gibson EL, Checkley S, Papadopoulos A, Poon L, Daley S, Wardle J. Increased salivary cortisol reliably induced by a protein-rich midday meal. Psychosom Med. 1999;61:214–24.
68. Slag MF, Ahmad M, Gannon MC, Nuttall FQ. Meal stimulation of cortisol secretion: a protein induced effect. Metabolism. 1981;30:1104–8.
69. Vicennati V, Ceroni L, Gagliardi L, Gambineri A, Pasquali R. Comment: response of the hypothalamic-pituitary-adrenocortical axis to high-protein/fat and high-carbohydrate meals in women with different obesity phenotypes. J Clin Endocrinol Metab. 2002;87:3984–8.
70. Vicennati V, Pasquali R. Abnormalities of the hypothalamic-pituitary-adrenal axis in nondepressed women with abdominal obesity and relations with insulin resistance: evidence for a central and a peripheral alteration. J Clin Endocrinol Metab. 2000;85:4093–8.
71. Pasquali R, Patton L, Gambineri A. Obesity and infertility. Curr Opin Endocrinol Diabetes Obes. 2007;14:482–7.

5 Hypogonadism and Obesity

Mario Maggi, Annamaria Morelli, Micaela Luconi, Francesco Lotti, Marcello Lucchese, Enrico Facchiano, and Giovanni Corona

5.1 Introduction

Obesity is a complex condition virtually affecting all ages and socioeconomic groups [1, 2]. Excess body weight is a crucial risk factor for mortality and morbidity not only for cardiovascular diseases but also for type 2 diabetes mellitus (T2DM), cancer, and musculoskeletal disorders which cause nearly three million deaths every year worldwide [1, 2]. Despite this evidence, however, obesity is still one of today's most blatantly visible – yet most neglected – public health problems. A great amount of evidence has documented that obesity represents an important risk factor also for male hypogonadism [2–6]. The specific pathogenetic mechanisms involved in this phenomenon are complex and not completely understood. Evidence indicates that T deficiency induces increased adiposity and, at the same time, increased adiposity induces hypogonadism [2–6]. In line with these data, few randomized clinical studies (RCTs) have documented a possible improvement of fat mass and metabolic control in men with obese T2DM and metabolic syndrome (MetS) [7, 8]. On the other hand, weight loss is able to increase testosterone (T) levels in men [6]. All the aforementioned issues will be better analyzed in the following sections.

5.2 Definition of Male Hypogonadism

Male hypogonadism is defined as the failure of the testes to produce sperm, sex steroids (T being the most abundant), or both, because of a central (pituitary/hypothalamus) or peripheral (testicular) deficiency [3–5]. The latter condition is termed primary (hypergonadotropic) hypogonadism, while the former is known as

M. Maggi • F. Lotti
Sexual Medicine and Andrology Unit, Department of Experimental, Clinical and Biomedical Sciences "Mario Serio", University of Florence, Florence, Italy

A. Morelli
Anatomy and Histology Unit, Department of Experimental and Clinical Medicine "Mario Serio", University of Florence, Florence, Italy

M. Luconi
Endocrinology Unit, Department of Experimental, Clinical and Biomedical Sciences "Mario Serio", University of Florence, Florence, Italy

M. Lucchese • E. Facchiano
Bariatric and Metabolic Surgery Unit, University of Florence, Florence, Italy

G. Corona (✉)
Endocrinology Unit, Medical Department, Azienda Usl, Maggiore-Bellaria Hospital, Bologna, Italy
e-mail: jocorona@libero.it

M. Lucchese, N. Scopinaro (eds.), *Minimally Invasive Bariatric and Metabolic Surgery: Principles and Technical Aspects*, DOI 10.1007/978-3-319-15356-8_5,

secondary (hypogonadotropic, HH) hypogonadism. This classical dichotomic nosography in hypo- and hypergonadotropic hypogonadism retains a practical utility for treatment purpose. In fact, while hypogonadal patients with hypothalamic or pituitary diseases can be successfully treated with either gonadotropin/gonadotropin releasing hormone (GnRH) or T, for those affected by primary testicular failure, only T substitution can be considered. However, the aforementioned classification of hypogonadism does not take into consideration T-deficiency related symptoms. It is well known that both primary and secondary hypogonadism, if not treated, are characterized by symptoms and signs of dramatically different severity, depending on the age of onset. We have provided our classification based on time of symptom onset, as reported in Fig. 5.1 [9]. In the case of very early onset hypogonadism (VEOH), i.e., during early fetal life, symptoms can be very severe, ranging from an almost complete feminine body shape to various defects in virilization [3–5]. In the case of a peri-pubertal appearance of hypogonadism (early onset hypogonadism, EOH), because of central (e.g., pituitary tumors, as germinoma) or peripheral defects (e.g., Klinefelter's syndrome), there might be a slowing or delaying in puberty progression, with a eunuchoidal phenotype, including scant body hair, high-pitched voice, microorchidism, and prostate hypoplasia. Late onset hypogonadism (LOH) is the most frequent form of T deficiency and indicates a form of syndromic male hypogonadism with a clinical exordium in young adulthood or later on [3–5]. In the latter condition, hypogonadal symptoms will be relatively mild, insidious, and difficult to recognize, but often bothersome and frustrating, such as weakness and fatigue, reduced libido and erectile dysfunction, mood symptoms, low bone mineral density, mild anemia, all of which

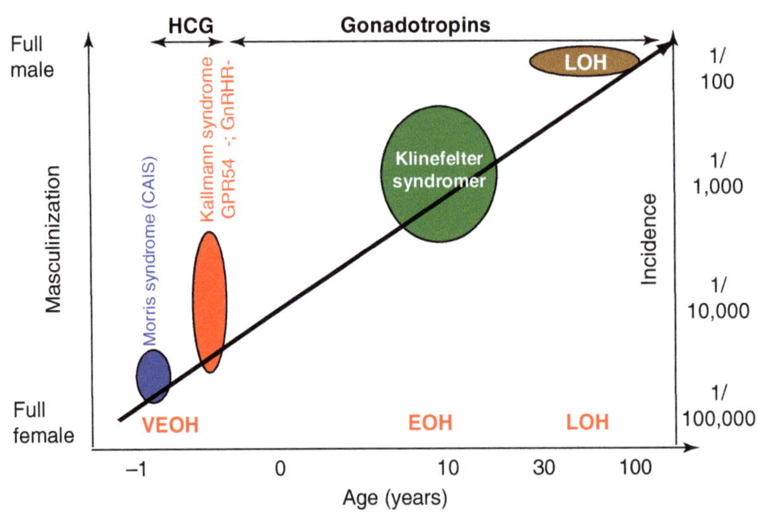

Fig. 5.1 Classification of male hypogonadism as a function of age of onset and patient's phenotype. Schematic prevalence in male population is also shown. Size of ellipsis reflects on abscissa (log scale): age of onset and on ordinates (log scale): incidence (right axis) or female to male phenotype (left axis, arbitrary unit). *VEOH*: very early onset hypogonadism, i.e., starting during fetal life for absence of testosterone formation or activity (e.g., complete androgen insensitivity or Morris' Syndrome, *blue ellipsis*) or impaired secretion or activity of GnRH (e.g., Kallmann's syndrome or mutation in GPR54 and GnRH receptor, *red ellipsis*). *EOH* early onset hypogonadism (i.e., peri-pubertal onset, such as in Klinefelter's syndrome, *green ellipsis*). *LOH* late onset hypogonadism, i.e., in adulthood or aging (*brown ellipsis*) (Adapted from Ref. [9])

Table 5.1 More and less specific clinical symptoms and signs associated with hypogonadism

	Symptoms	Clinical signs
More specific	Sexual Reduced sexual desire (libido) Erectile dysfunction Decreased spontaneous erections Physical Decreased vigorous activity Difficulty walking >1 km Inability to bend Psychological Sadness Loss of energy Fatigue	Increased body fat, body mass index Very small (especially <5 ml) or shrinking testes Decreased prostate size
Less specific	Sexual Decreased frequency of intercourse Decreased autoeroticism Delayed ejaculation Physical Hot flushes, sweats Decreased energy, motivation, initiative, and self-confidence Reduced muscle bulk and strength Diminished physical or work performance Psychological Poor concentration and memory Sleep disturbance, increased sleepiness	Loss of body (axillary and pubic) hair, reduced shaving Gynecomastia

can contribute to decreasing the overall quality of life ([3–5, 10], see also Table 5.1).

5.3 Definition of Late Onset Hypogonadism

Different T thresholds have been proposed for the biochemical definition of low T [3–5]. According to major international guidelines, T substitution has to be offered to symptomatic individuals when circulating total T is below 8 nmol/L (231 ng/dL). In addition, there is also general agreement that a total T level above 12 nmol/L (346 ng/dL) does not require substitution. When total T is repetitively >8 and <12 nmol/L, in the presence of typical hypogonadal symptoms (as listed before), a T treatment trial might be considered [3–5]. In addition, it should be recognized that a pathological valuate of T must be confirmed in a second sample before prescribing T replacement therapy (TRT) [3–5].

5.4 LOH and Obesity, Clinical Evidence

The association between LOH, obesity, MetS, insulin resistance, and T2DM is well known [5–7, 11–14]. Accordingly, in two independent meta-analyses of the available evidence, we reported that subjects with MetS and T2DM have significantly reduced T levels (about 3 nmol/l lower) [15, 16]. Zumoff et al. [17] and ourselves [18] previously showed that SHBG-bound and unbound testosterone levels decreased in obese males in proportion to the degree of their obesity, even after adjustment for obesity-related conditions (see also Fig. 5.2). In addition, data from morbidly obese men indicate that LH levels and pulse amplitude were attenuated when compared to normal weight controls [19, 20]. These observations support the concept of a true obesity-associated HH. The specific pathogenetic mechanisms linking LOH with insulin resistance, MetS, and T2DM appear to be complex and often multi-directional (see Fig. 5.3).

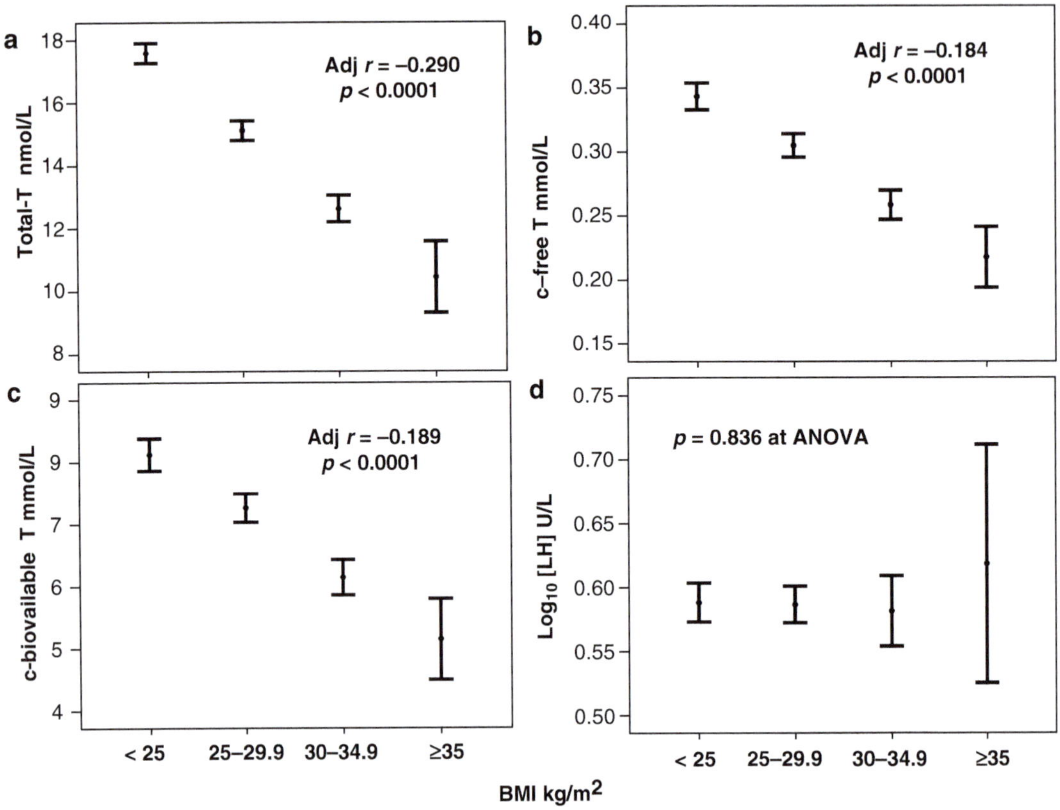

Fig. 5.2 Testosterone (T; panels **a–c**) and luteinizing hormone (LH, panel **d**) levels as a function of obesity classification. *T* testosterone, c-free-T and c-bioavailable-T = calculated free and bioavailable testosterone according to Vermeulen formula. *BMI* body mass index. Data are expressed as mean [95 % confidence interval]. Data are derived from a consecutive non-selected series of men (mean age = 51.3 ± 13.3 years) attending our Sexual Medicine & Andrology Clinic for sexual dysfunction between 2000 and 2013 (unpublished). The inset indicates the age adjusted data. BMI was considered as a continuous value

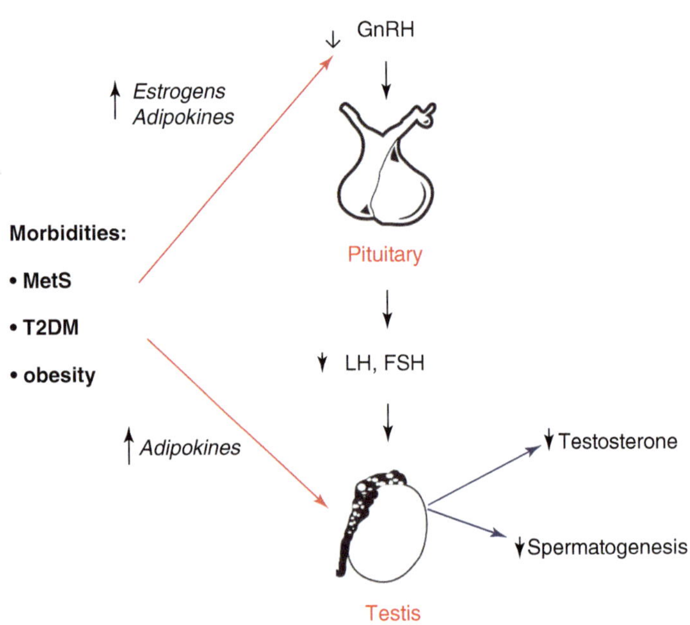

Fig. 5.3 Proposed interactions between increased visceral fat and hypogonadism. *MetS* metabolic syndrome, *T2DM* type 2 diabetes mellitus, *LH* luteinizing hormone, *FSH* follicle stimulating hormone, *GnRH* gonadotropin-releasing hormone, *T* testosterone

Obesity is characterized by a relative abundance of estrogens since P450 aromatase is highly expressed by fat tissue. The increased amount of estrogen levels, might, in turn, have a negative effect on both the hypothalamus and the pituitary, leading to decreased LH secretion [6, 7]. Accordingly, it has been reported that the use of the aromatase inhibitor letrozole can restore T levels and increase LH levels in severely obese hypogonadal men [21]. In line with this view, we now show that body weight loss, obtained either through lifestyle or bariatric intervention, is associated to a fall in estrogen levels and with a rise in gonadotropins and T [6]. However, other fat-associated factors, besides estrogens, have been proposed as a link between obesity and reproductive axis disorders: a series of adipokines and among them, the most extensively studied are leptin, ghrelin, and adiponectin ([22] see also Fig. 5.3).

5.5 LOH and Obesity: Experimental Studies

The contribution of the different metabolic derangements on the related condition of HH has been recently investigated in an animal model of high fat diet (HFD)-induced MetS [23]. The model, established in adult male rabbits fed a HFD for 3 months, has been largely characterized by our group [24–30] and recapitulates the human phenotype, including visceral obesity, hypertension, dyslipidemia, and glucose intolerance. Moreover, as in humans, HFD rabbits exhibit an overt HH, with low plasma levels of testosterone, luteinizing hormone (LH), and follicle-stimulating hormone (FSH), and reduced androgen-dependent organ weight. In this experimental model, sex hormone imbalance was associated with MetS severity, since T decreased and estrogen increased as a function of the number of MetS components [23]. Also, gonadotropin plasma levels were negatively associated with MetS and, among MetS factors, hyperglycemia and hypercholesterolemia resulted as being the major determinants for the negative association with LH levels, while the dyslipidemic component (high cholesterol and triglycerides) appeared to be associated with FSH reduction [23]. Moreover, hormonal alterations also correlated with glucose intolerance severity. Since the pituitary gonadotropins are positively controlled by GnRH and a reduced content of GnRH neurons was demonstrated in the hypothalamus from HFD rabbits [24], the role of HFD-related alterations in the hypothalamic area in determining the documented dysfunctions of the gonadotropic axis have been extensively investigated. A close association of MetS – and in particular the related altered glucose and lipid metabolism – has been identified with peculiar hypothalamic alterations, including increased expression of the glucose transporter 4 (GLUT4) and inflammation. Indeed, HFD determined a low-grade inflammation in the hypothalamus, significantly inducing microglial activation and interleukin-6 (IL-6) expression. Interestingly, all these hypothalamic derangements were, in turn, associated with LH and FSH reduction, and occurred in the preoptic area of the hypothalamus, lining the third ventricle, where GnRH neurons reside. Accordingly, the same hypothalamic area was characterized by a reduced immunopositivity not only for GnRH [24], but also for Kisspeptin-1 receptor (KISS1R; 23), which along with its natural ligand kisspeptin represents the most characterized system mediating, at central level, the effects of a range of metabolic inputs known to regulate GnRH secretion [31, 32]. However, a not fully clarified issue is whether metabolic alterations act directly on GnRH neurons or are mediated by other integrating factors. Indeed, recent findings demonstrated that a subpopulation of GnRH neurons projects dendrites in regions outside the blood–brain barrier, where they may directly sense molecules circulating in the bloodstream [33]. Hence, the range of factors that are integrated by GnRH neurons for the control of the GnRH/gonadotropin secretion could be extended. Using a well characterized cellular model, we identified a direct inhibitory action of increasing glucose concentrations on human fetal GnRH-secreting neurons, the FNC-B4 cells [34–37], thus opening new mechanistic insights into the direct metabolic control of GnRH release [38]. FNC-B4 cells express glucose transporters (GLUT1, GLUT3, and GLUT4) and may respond to changes in glucose concentrations. Exposing FNC-B4 cells to high glucose significantly reduced the expression not only of GnRH but also of genes relevant for GnRH neuron function, such as KISS1R and leptin receptor. Even if obtained in vitro, these findings support the idea of a direct, deleterious contribution of hyperglycemia on human GnRH neurons, thus improving our understanding about the pathogenic mechanisms linking HH to metabolic disorders. Overall, in vitro and in vivo experimental studies indicate that metabolic derangements may activate proinflammatory pathways within the hypothalamus, thus compromising a key brain area involved in the control of reproduction. In agreement with this possibility, in vivo treatment with obeticholic acid, a drug that ameliorates glucose metabolism in the rabbit MetS model [24, 29], not only reverted all the HFD-induced hypothalamic alterations – including GLUT4 induction and inflammatory response – but also increased GnRH mRNA expression [23].

5.6 Testosterone Therapy and Obesity

In obese individuals, several studies have demonstrated that intense lifestyle intervention, along with nutritional counseling and physical activity, is able to reduce weight loss and to conjointly raise T levels. A recent meta-analysis, in fact, showed that weight loss is associated with an increase of bound and unbound T levels, along with gonadotropin levels, and that the final effect is directly related to the amount of body mass index (BMI) reduction [6]. Accordingly, the analysis of longitudinal data of the European Male Aging Study demonstrated that weight loss was associated with a proportional increase – and weight gain with a proportional decrease – in total T and sex hormone binding globulin [39]. Based on this evidence, lifestyle modifications should be strongly encouraged in hypogonadal subjects with obesity, T2DM, and MetS.

Unfortunately, diet and behavioral therapies often ultimately fail. Several uncontrolled studies have shown that T replacement therapy (TRT) could improve body composition and reduced fat mass (see Ref. [4, 5, 7, 8] for review). The International, multicenter, Post-Authorization Surveillance Study (IPASS) on long-acting-intramuscular T undecanoate conducted on 1,493 hypogonadal men showed that after 9–12 months waist circumference decreased from 100 to 96 cm and blood pressure and lipid parameters were altered in a favorable and significant manner [40]. Another more recent open-label, single-center, cumulative, prospective registry study of 255 hypogonadal men (aged 33–69 years) showed that normalizing serum T to normal physiological levels produced consistent loss of body weight, waist circumference, and BMI over the full 5 years of the study [41]. Despite this evidence, unfortunately, only few RCTs have evaluated the impact of TRT in patients with MetS and T2DM. By meta-analyzing available evidence, we found that TRT was associated with a significant reduction of fasting glycemia, HOMA index, triglyceride levels, and waist circumference in patients with MetS [8]. Accordingly, an improvement of fasting glycemia, HbA1c, and triglyceride levels was observed in subjects with T2DM [8]. Hence, TRT and lifestyle modifications can also be combined, and this is strongly recommended in LOH obese individuals. However, this strategy has been tested only in two placebo-RCTs (92 and 93). By meta-analyzing the results of these studies, we report here that the combination of TRT and lifestyle modifications is able to improve waist line, HOMA index, and lipid profile (reducing triglycerides and increasing HDL cholesterol levels) when compared to both placebo and lifestyle modifications alone [42].

Conclusions

Several clinical and experimental data have documented a strong inverse relationship between obesity and testosterone levels. The underlying pathogenetic mechanisms appear to be complex and often multi-directional. According to the current guidelines [5], intense lifestyle intervention, along with nutritional counseling and physical activity should be the first approach to obese individuals with hypogonadism. However, since diet and behavioral therapies often fail, TRT and lifestyle modifications can also be combined. In fact, several uncontrolled studies have shown that TRT could improve body composition and reduced fat mass. Conversely, only limited RCTs are available. Longer and larger studies are advisable to better clarify the role of TRT in obese men.

References

1. Finucane MM, Stevens GA, Cowan MJ, Danaei G, Lin JK, Paciorek CJ, Singh GM, Gutierrez HR, Lu Y, Bahalim AN, Farzadfar F, Riley LM, Ezzati M, Global Burden of Metabolic Risk Factors of Chronic Diseases Collaborating Group (Body Mass index). National, regional, and global trends in body-mass index since 1980: systematic analysis of health examination surveys and epidemiological studies with 960 country-years and 9.1 million participants. Lancet. 2011;377:557–67.
2. Corona G, Rastrelli G, Filippi S, Vignozzi L, Mannucci E, Maggi M. Erectile dysfunction and central obesity: an Italian perspective. Asian J Androl. 2014. doi:10.4103/1008-682X.126386 [Epub ahead of print].
3. Corona G, Rastrelli G, Forti G, Maggi M. Update in testosterone therapy for men. J Sex Med. 2011;8:639–54.
4. Corona G, Rastrelli G, Vignozzi L, Maggi M. Emerging medication for the treatment of male hypogonadism. Expert Opin Emerg Drugs. 2012;17:239–59.
5. Buvat J, Maggi M, Guay A, Torres LO. Testosterone deficiency in men: systematic review and standard operating procedures for diagnosis and treatment. J Sex Med. 2013;10:245–84.
6. Corona G, Rastrelli G, Monami M, Saad F, Luconi M, Lucchese M, Facchiano E, Sforza A, Forti G, Mannucci E, Maggi M. Body weight loss reverts obesity-associated hypogonadotropic hypogonadism: a systematic review and meta-analysis. Eur J Endocrinol. 2013;168(6):829–43.
7. Saad F, Aversa A, Isidori AM, Gooren LJ. Testosterone as potential effective therapy in treatment of obesity in men with testosterone deficiency: a review. Curr Diabetes Rev. 2012;8:131–43.
8. Corona G, Rastrelli G, Maggi M. Diagnosis and treatment of late-onset hypogonadism: systematic review and meta-analysis of TRT outcomes. Best Pract Res Clin Endocrinol Metab. 2013;27:557–79.
9. Morelli A, Corona G, Filippi S, Ambrosini S, Forti G, Vignozzi L, Maggi M. Which patients with sexual dysfunction are suitable for testosterone replacement therapy? J Endocrinol Invest. 2007;30:880–8.
10. Corona G, Rastrelli G, Vignozzi L, Mannucci E, Maggi M. How to recognize late-onset hypogonadism in men with sexual dysfunction. Asian J Androl. 2012;14:251–9.
11. Wu FC, Tajar A, Pye SR, Silman AJ, Finn JD, O'Neill TW, Bartfai G, Casanueva F, Forti G, Giwercman A, Huhtaniemi IT, Kula K, Punab M, Boonen S, Vanderschueren D, European Male Aging Study Group. Hypothalamic-pituitary-testicular axis disruptions in older men are differentially linked to age and modifiable risk factors: the European Male Aging Study. J Clin Endocrinol Metab. 2008;93:2737–45.
12. Corona G, Mannucci E, Lotti F, Fisher AD, Bandini E, Balercia G, Forti G, Maggi M. Pulse pressure, an index of arterial stiffness, is associated with androgen deficiency and impaired penile blood flow in men with ED. J Sex Med. 2009;6(1):285–93.
13. Corona G, Rastrelli G, Silverii A, Monami M, Sforza A, Forti G, Mannucci E, Maggi M. The identification of prediabetes condition with ARIC algorithm predicts long-term CV events in patients with erectile dysfunction. J Sex Med. 2013;10(4):1114–23.
14. Corona G, Rastrelli G, Balercia G, Lotti F, Sforza A, Monami M, Forti G, Mannucci E, Maggi M. Hormonal association and sexual dysfunction in patients with impaired fasting glucose: a cross-sectional and longitudinal study. J Sex Med. 2012;9(6):1669–80.
15. Corona G, Monami M, Rastrelli G, Aversa A, Sforza A, Lenzi A, Forti G, Mannucci E, Maggi M. Type 2 diabetes mellitus and testosterone: a meta-analysis study. Int J Androl. 2011;34(6 Pt 1):528–40.
16. Corona G, Monami M, Rastrelli G, Aversa A, Tishova Y, Saad F, Lenzi A, Forti G, Mannucci E, Maggi M. Testosterone and metabolic syndrome: a meta-analysis study. J Sex Med. 2011;8(1):272–83.
17. Zumoff B, Strain GW, Miller LK, et al. Plasma free and non-sex-hormone-binding-globulin-bound testosterone are decreased in obese men in proportion to their degree of obesity. J Clin Endocrinol Metab. 1990;71:929–31.
18. Corona G, Mannucci E, Fisher AD, Lotti F, Petrone L, Balercia G, Bandini E, Forti G, Maggi M. Low levels of androgens in men with erectile dysfunction and obesity. J Sex Med. 2008;5:2454–63.
19. Giagulli VA, Kaufman JM, Vermeulen A. Pathogenesis of the decreased androgen levels in obese men. J Clin Endocrinol Metab. 1994;79:997–1000.
20. Vermeulen A, Kaufman JM, Deslypere JP, Thomas G. Attenuated luteinizing hormone (LH) pulse amplitude but normal LH pulse frequency, and its relation to plasma androgens in hypogonadism of obese men. J Clin Endocrinol Metab. 1993;76:1140–6.
21. Loves S, de Jong J, van Sorge A, Telting D, Tack CJ, Hermus A, Westerterp K, de Boer H. Somatic and psychological effects of low-dose aromatase inhibition in men with obesity-related hypogonadotropic hypotestosteronemia. Eur J Endocrinol. 2013;169:705–14.
22. Michalakis K, Mintziori G, Kaprara A, Tarlatzis BC, Goulis DG. The complex interaction between obesity, metabolic syndrome and reproductive axis: a narrative review. Metabolism. 2013;62:457–78.
23. Morelli A, Sarchielli E, Comeglio P, et al. Metabolic syndrome induces inflammation and impairs gonadotropin-releasing hormone neurons in the

preoptic area of the hypothalamus in rabbits. Mol Cell Endocrinol. 2014;382:107–19.

24. Filippi S, Vignozzi L, Morelli A, et al. Testosterone partially ameliorates metabolic profile and erectile responsiveness to PDE5 inhibitors in an animal model of male metabolic syndrome. J Sex Med. 2009;6:3274–88.
25. Vignozzi L, Morelli A, Filippi S, et al. Farnesoid X receptor activation improves erectile function in animal models of metabolic syndrome and diabetes. J Sex Med. 2011;8:57–77.
26. Vignozzi L, Morelli A, Sarchielli E, et al. Testosterone protects from metabolic syndrome-associated prostate inflammation: an experimental study in rabbit. J Endocrinol. 2012;212:71–84.
27. Vignozzi L, Filippi S, Comeglio P. Nonalcoholic steatohepatitis as a novel player in metabolic syndrome-induced erectile dysfunction: an experimental study in the rabbit. Mol Cell Endocrinol. 2014;25:143–54.
28. Vignozzi L, Filippi S, Comeglio P, et al. Tadalafil effect on metabolic syndrome-associated bladder alterations: an experimental study in a rabbit model. J Sex Med. 2014. doi:10.1111/jsm.12478.
29. Morelli A, Comeglio P, Filippi S, et al. Testosterone and farnesoid X receptor agonist INT-747 counteract high fat diet-induced bladder alterations in a rabbit model of metabolic syndrome. J Steroid Biochem Mol Biol. 2012;132:80–92.
30. Morelli A, Comeglio P, Filippi S, et al. Mechanism of action of phosphodiesterase type 5 inhibition in metabolic syndrome-associated prostate alterations: an experimental study in the rabbit. Prostate. 2013;73:428–41.
31. Pinilla L, Aguilar E, Dieguez C, et al. Kisspeptins and reproduction: physiological roles and regulatory mechanisms. Physiol Rev. 2012;92:1235–316.
32. George JT, Millar RP, Anderson RA. Hypothesis: kisspeptin mediates male hypogonadism in obesity and type 2 diabetes. Neuroendocrinology. 2010;91:302–7.
33. Herde MK, Geist K, Campbell RA, Herbison AE. Gonadotropin-releasing hormone neurons extend complex highly branched dendritic trees outside the blood-brain barrier. Endocrinology. 2011;152:3832–41.
34. Vannelli GB, Ensoli F, Zonefrati R, et al. Neuroblast long-term cell cultures from human fetal olfactory epithelium respond to odors. J Neurosci. 1995;15:4382–94.
35. Maggi M, Barni T, Fantoni G, et al. Expression and biological effects of endothelin-1 in human gonadotropin-releasing hormone-secreting neurons. J Clin Endocrinol Metab. 2000;85:1658–65.
36. Morelli A, Fibbi B, Marini M, et al. Dihydrotestosterone and leptin regulate gonadotropin-releasing hormone (GnRH) expression and secretion in human GnRH-secreting neuroblasts. J Sex Med. 2009;6:397–407.
37. Morelli A, Marini M, Mancina R, et al. Sex steroids and leptin regulate the "first Kiss" (KiSS 1/G-protein-coupled receptor 54 system) in human gonadotropin-releasing-hormone-secreting neuroblasts. J Sex Med. 2008;5:1097–113.
38. Morelli A, Comeglio P, Sarchielli E, et al. Negative effects of high glucose exposure in human gonadotropin-releasing hormone neurons. Int J Endocrinol. 2013. doi:10.1155/2013/684659.
39. Camacho EM, Huhtaniemi IT, O'Neill TW, et al. Age-associated changes in hypothalamic-pituitary-testicular function in middle-aged and older men are modified by weight change and lifestyle factors: longitudinal results from the European Male Ageing Study. Eur J Endocrinol. 2013;168:445–55.
40. Zitzmann M, Mattern A, Hanisch J, Gooren L, Jones H, Maggi M. IPASS: a study on the tolerability and effectiveness of injectable testosterone undecanoate for the treatment of male hypogonadism in a worldwide sample of 1,438 men. J Sex Med. 2013;10:579–88.
41. Saad F, Haider A, Doros G, Traish A. Long-term treatment of hypogonadal men with testosterone produces substantial and sustained weight loss. Obesity (Silver Spring). 2013. doi:10.1002/oby.20407 [Epub ahead of print].
42. Corona G, Vignozzi L, Sforza A, Maggi M. Risks and benefits of late onset hypogonadism treatment: an expert opinion. World J Mens Health. 2013;31(2):103–25. doi:10.5534/wjmh.2013.31.2.103. Epub 2013 Aug 31.

6 Microbiota Organ and Bariatric Surgery

Nicola Basso, Giovanni Casella, Emanuele Soricelli, Geltrude Mingrone, and Adriano Redler

The gastrointestinal tract is known to be a complex and finely balanced ecosystem. It is one of the largest interfaces between the outside world and the human internal environment.

The human gut hosts 100 trillion (100^{14}) microorganisms, encompassing hundreds of phylotypes composed of approximately 1,100 prevalent species, with approximately 160 such species per individual. Density of bacterial cells in the colon is estimated to be 10^{12} per ml, making it one of the most densely populated microbial habitats on Earth. In its entirety, the microflora is estimated to contain 150-fold more genes than our own host genomes and this bacterial genome (microbiome) contributes a broad range of biochemical and metabolic functions that the host could not otherwise perform. Microbiota, in total, weighs up to 2 kg. One-third of our gut microbiota is common to most people, two-thirds are specific for each individual being a sort of identity card. This separate ecosystem contributes substantial beneficial functions to the host: digestion of otherwise indigestible plant polysaccharides, development of the mucosal and systemic immune system, and control of the regeneration of the intestinal epithelium. The definition "microbiota organ" (Fig. 6.1) seems to be appropriate [1, 2].

Different species and quantities of bacteria are found at different points along the digestive tract. The stomach pH is deadly for most microbes, the acid-resistant *Lactobacillus* and *Streptococcus* are predominant and account for 10^{2-3}/ml. In the duodenum and jejunum up to 10^{4-5} bacteria/ml (*Lactobacillus*, *Escherichia coli*, *Enterococcus faecalis*) can be found despite the toxicity of bile and pancreatic secretions. The number of bacteria rises in the ileum (10^7 bacteria/ml) and in the colon (10^{12} bacteria/ml). The large intestine contains the largest number of bacteria, and is characterized by a complex and dense microbial community mainly made up of anaerobic species [3].

Three bacterial divisions, the Firmicutes (Gram-positive), Bacteroidetes (Gram-negative), and Actinobacteria (Gram-positive) dominate the adult human gut microbiota. The Firmicutes is the largest bacterial phylum (60 %) and contains more than 200 genera, including *Lactobacillus*, *Mycoplasma*, *Bacillus*, and *Clostridium*; the

N. Basso (✉)
Department of Surgical Sciences, "Sapienza" University of Rome, Via Napoli, 51, Rome 00184, Italy
e-mail: nicola.basso@uniroma1.it

G. Casella • E. Soricelli • A. Redler
Department of Surgical Sciences, "Sapienza" University of Rome, Vle Regina Elena, 324, Rome 00161, Italy
e-mail: Giovanni.casella@uniroma1.it; lelesori@hotmail.com; adriano.redler@uniroma1.it

G. Mingrone
Department of Internal Medicine, Catholic University, Largo A. Gemelli 8, Rome 00168, Italy
e-mail: gmingrone@rm.unicatt.it

M. Lucchese, N. Scopinaro (eds.), *Minimally Invasive Bariatric and Metabolic Surgery: Principles and Technical Aspects*, DOI 10.1007/978-3-319-15356-8_6,

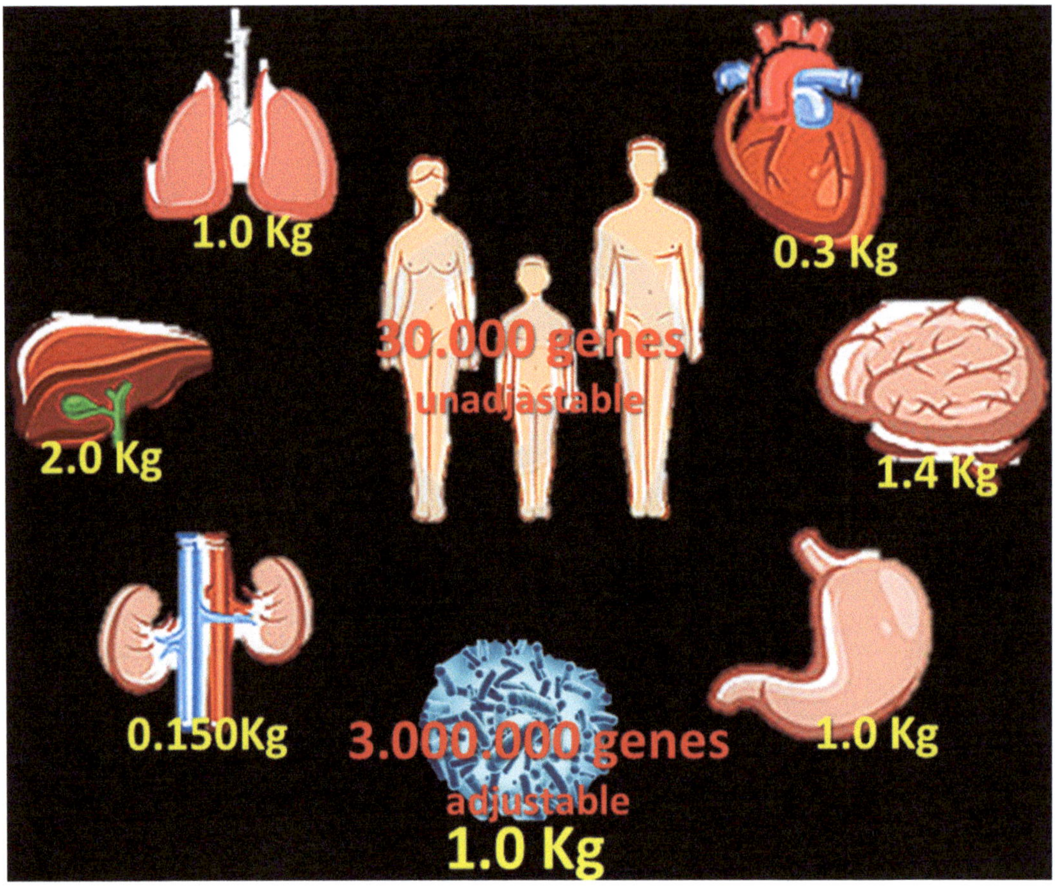

Fig. 6.1 The microbiota organ

Bacteroidetes (20 %) include about 20 genera; the Actinobacteria (Gram-positive) are frequently missed by RNA gene sequencing and can be detected only by fluorescent in situ hybridization (FISH). It is worth noting that human species and murine species have similar microbiota composition [4].

Newborn babies are germ free. The development of the gut microbiota starts at birth and its composition changes substantially at three stages in life: from birth to weaning; from weaning to attaining a "normal" diet; during old age. Sterile inside the uterus, the newborn's digestive tract is quickly colonized by microorganisms from the mother (vagina, feces, skin, breast, etc.) and from the environment in which the delivery takes place. Nutrition is a driving factor in shaping gut microbiota composition and its functional maturation, from birth to adulthood. From the third day, the composition of the intestinal flora is directly dependent on how the infant is fed: in breastfed babies, compared to infant formulas nourished babies, gut microbiota is dominated by Bifidus bacteria. Breast milk is rich in oligosaccharides, fermented in the distal gut and promoting the growth of beneficial microbes as bifidobacteria. At the age of 4 years, the gut microbiota in host individuals has fully matured.

Transformation to the adult-type microbiota is triggered by multiple host and external factors. Carnivore microbiomes are enriched in protein degradation genes, while herbivore microbiomes are enriched in genes necessary to break down starch, thus, a Prevotella-type community is associated with fiber intake and a Bacteroides-type community with high protein intake.

After transformation to the adult type and until the seventh decade, the gut microbiota remains remarkably constant. However, the inter phyla *numerical proportions* may have important fluctuations around an individual core of stable colonizers. Microbes in the human gut undergo selective pressure from the host as well as from microbial competitors. This typically leads to a homeostasis of the ecosystem in which some species occur in high and others in low abundance (the "long-tail" effect), with some low abundance species, like methanogens, performing specialized functions beneficial to the host [5, 6].

6.1 Functions of Microbiota

The gut microbiota has multiple functions related not only to the gastro-intestinal system but also to the central and autonomic nervous system, the immune system. Alterations of the microbiota may lead to anxiety and depressive status: a significant correlation between gut inflammatory status and anxiety traits has been documented [7, 8].

Although the most abundant molecular functions generally trace back to the most dominant species, some of them may be contributed to primarily by low-abundance genera. Because of this factor and of additional ones such as the elevated number of species, the numerical variations induced by host and external factors, the multiple functions, investigations on microbiota are difficult and necessitate specific and sophisticated methods to answer specific questions: nucleic acid studies (which are they?), metatranscriptomics, metaproteomics, metabolomics (what are they doing?), and metagenomics. The study of "clusters" of functionally related groups is of help in elucidating microbiota's role [5, 9].

6.2 Microbiota and Obesity

The gut microbiota is highly vulnerable to changes in the gut microenvironment. Under normal conditions, commensal microbes and their hosts enjoy a symbiotic relationship. A qualitative and/or quantitative imbalance in the intestinal flora, in their metabolic activities or changes in their local distribution leads to a condition known as *dysbiosis* where microbial imbalance exerts adverse effects on the host. A pivotal role of gut microbiota has been evidenced in the development of gastrointestinal diseases, such as *Clostridium difficile* infection (CDI), other inflammatory bowel diseases, and colorectal cancer [10, 11].

Recent studies have highlighted a role for gut microbiota dysbiosis in the genesis of obesity and of the metabolic syndrome. There are a number of linking arguments: dysbiosis occurs in diabetic and obese versus lean individuals; some components of the gut microbiota (e.g., lipopolysaccharides, LPS) play a harmful role in obesity and diabetes; the diet takes part in the modulation of the gut microbiome and microbiota composition/function in obesity and metabolic syndrome [12–20].

In obese subjects (human and murine), the gut microbiota has a higher proportion of the phylum Firmicutes and a lower proportion of the phylum Bacteroidetes, the reverse occurs in lean subjects [15, 16]. A direct relationship between Bacteroidetes abundance and body weight has been demonstrated.

Gnotobiology, which is the selective colonization of germ-free animals, has given insight into the role covered by the commensal microbiota in a series of patho-physiological mechanisms, such as obesity, insulin resistance, and diabetes.

The host-bacterial association possesses a beneficial mutuality enhancing the host digestive and metabolic efficiency and ensuring a stable metabolic supply for the microorganisms.

In fact, germ-free mice show a less body fat content than conventional raised mice. High-fat Western-type diet in conventional mice induces obesity and insulin resistance. When given the same diet, germ-free mice are resistant to obesity and to insulin resistance. The effect is FIAF (fasting-induced adipose factor) dependent (Fig. 6.2) [12, 17].

Colonization of germ-free mice with conventional microbiota leads to a 60 % increase in the body fat that likely depends on the greater capacity to extract energy from food which, otherwise,

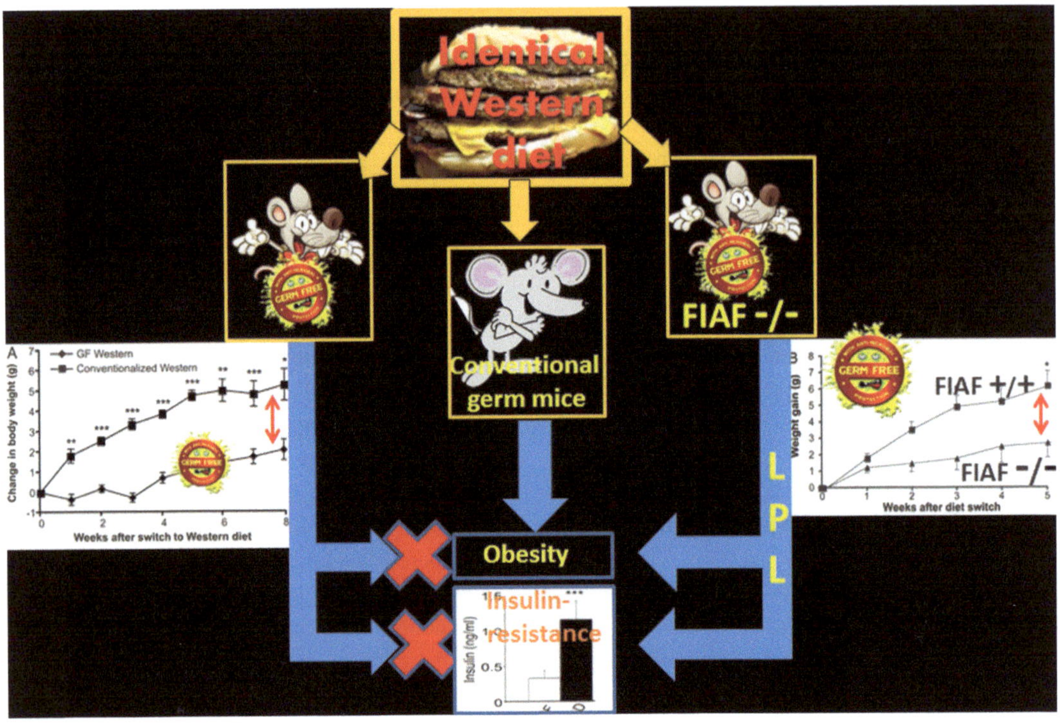

Fig. 6.2 Germ-free mice are resistant to obesity and to insulin resistance. The effect is fasting-induced adipose factor (*FIAF*) dependent [12, 15, 46]

would be only partially utilized, together with an increased insulin resistance [12, 13].

In fact, the microbiota metabolizes complex carbohydrates present in the fibers, which could not be otherwise digested, to oligo- and mono-saccharides, which in turn are fermented to short-chain fatty acids, including butyrate, propionate, and acetate. Short-chain fatty acids are absorbed in the colon, where butyrate provides energy for colonic epithelial cells. Through the portal circulation acetate and propionate reach the liver and peripheral organs, where they become substrates for gluconeogenesis and de novo lipogenesis, thus determining the accumulation of triglycerides in the liver [12, 18, 21] (Fig. 6.3).

Besides representing an energy source, short-chain fatty acids modulate intestinal gene expression by inhibiting the enzyme histone deacetylase and regulate energy metabolism through G-protein-coupled receptors (GPCRs), such as GPR41 or GPR43 [17, 18].

The effect of increasing body weight is enhanced if germ-free mice are colonized with flora derived from obese rather than from lean donors (Fig. 6.4) [14].

Furthermore, germ-free mice "humanized" by microbiota from human donors become sensible to western-type high-fat diet (Fig. 6.5) [22].

In addition, obese mice have an inversion of the proportional intestinal content of Bacteroidetes and Firmicutes with a net reduction of the former and an increase of the latter [15, 16]. Interestingly, germ-free animals show a decreased lipogenic-related gene expression which can contribute to their leaner shape [13].

6.3 Microbiota and Metabolic Syndrome

High-fat diet induces significant changes in the composition of the gut microbiota by decreasing the population of bifidobacteria. Decreased bifidobacteria determine loosening of the tight junctions between cells thus being responsible for increased gut permeability to a major component

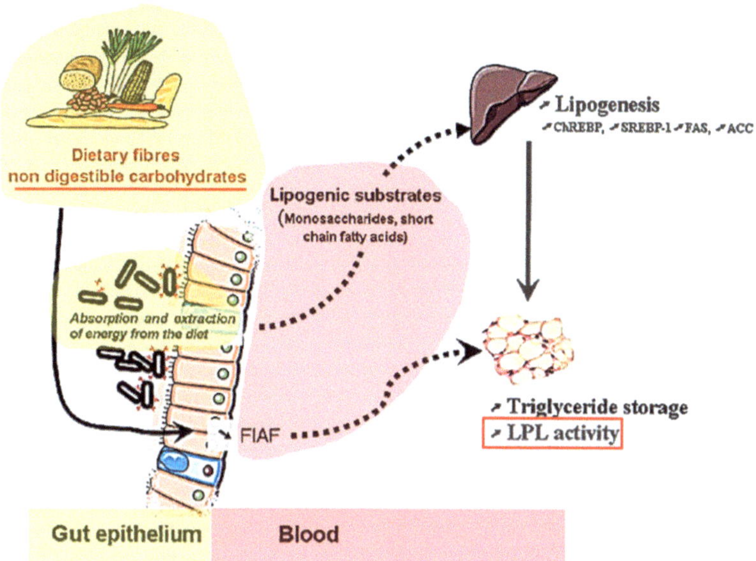

Fig. 6.3 In obese individuals, the microbiota is capable of extracting extra energy from the food by fermenting, otherwise indigestible, carbohydrates to mono saccharides and to short-chain fatty acids (SCFA) thus increasing fat storage [12, 21]. *FIAF*: fasting-induced adipose factor; *LPL*: Lipoprotein Lipase (from Cani and Delzenne [21] modified)

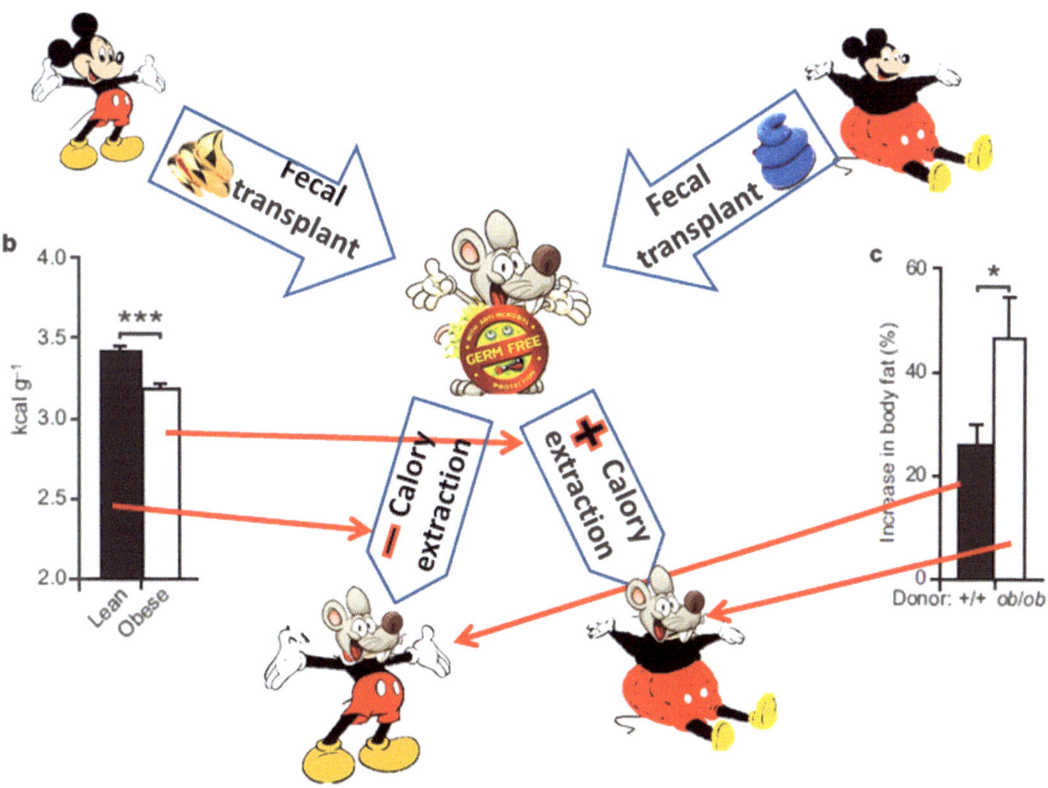

Fig. 6.4 Germ-free mice colonized with microbiota derived from obese donors gain more weight than germ-free mice colonized from lean donors [14]

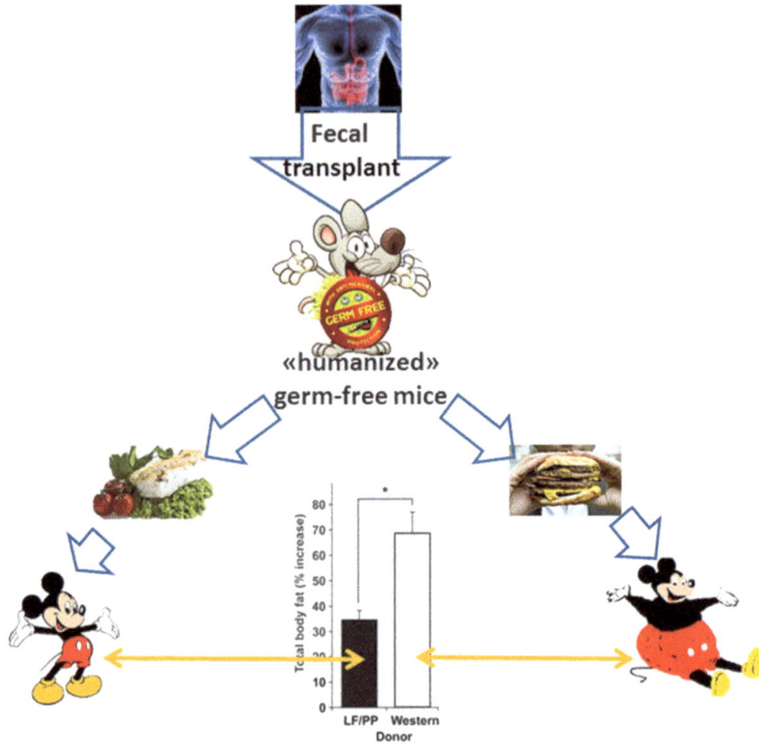

Fig. 6.5 Germ-free mice "humanized" by microbiota from human donors become sensible to western-type high-fat diet [22]

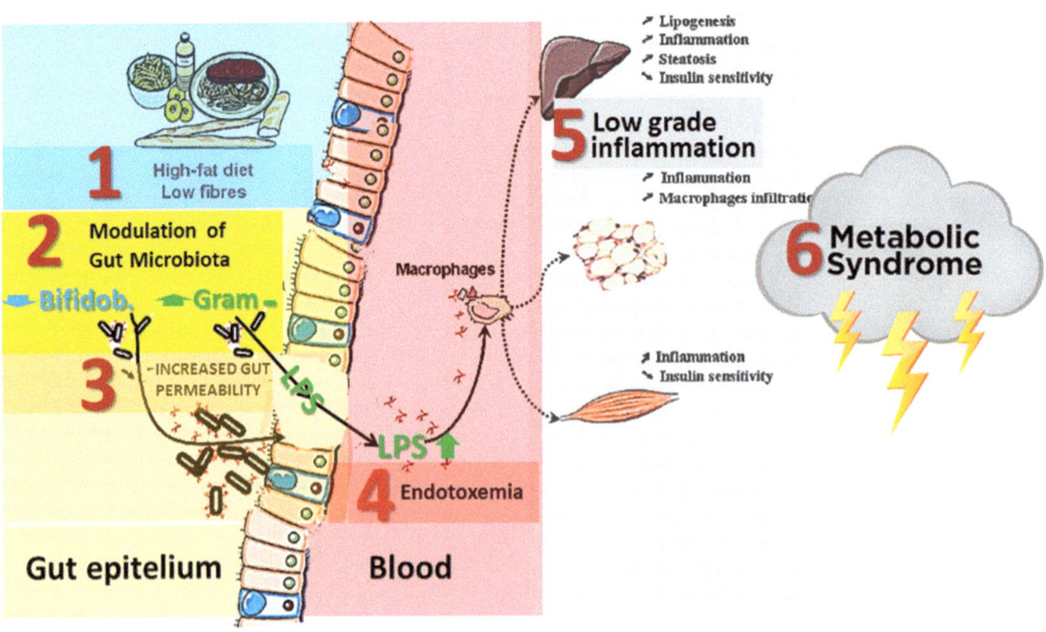

Fig. 6.6 Microbiota modulation is responsible for increased gut permeability to lipopolysaccharides (LPS), thus inducing endotoxiemia, low-grade inflammation and metabolic syndrome (From Cani and Delzenne [21] modified)

of the outer membrane of Gram-negative bacteria, the LPS (Fig. 6.6), an endotoxin that possesses pro-inflammatory actions and blunts insulin signaling [18], ensuing low-grade inflammation (metabolic endotoxemia), diminished insulin sensitivity and, finally, metabolic syndrome.

Table 6.1 From high-fat diet to the metabolic syndrome [14]

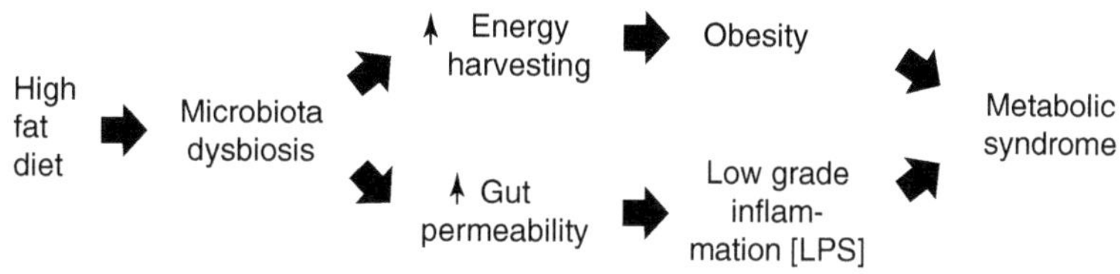

Correlation between LPS endotoxemia and fasting insulinemia, glycemia, and triglycerides has been demonstrated in type 2 diabetic patients [23].

The two driving factors of the metabolic syndrome, energy harvest and gut permeability, are dependent on gut microbiota dysbiosis [14] (Table 6.1).

6.4 Microbiota and Surgery

Bariatric surgery results in weight loss, reduced adiposity, and improved glucose metabolism, not simply attributable to decreased caloric intake or absorption. Gut microbiota share some of these effects.

Surgery induces changes in environmental and systemic factors, as well as in the anatomy of the digestive tract, all of which might have an effect on the composition of the gut microbiota [24].

- *Acid production*: the diminished acid secretion, because of gastric resection (sleeve gastrectomy [SG], bilio-pancreatic diversion [BPD]) or gastric bypass [GBP]), determines marked changes in the intestinal pH that affect genus and species relative proportions of the intestinal flora rather than the overall cell number. Achlorhydria is associated with an increased number of Gram-positive bacteria and with modifications of microbiota ecology in the lower gastrointestinal tract: microbial community composition and short-chain fatty acid production [25].
- *Food transit time*: in SG and in GBP the food reaches rapidly in the small intestine stimulating the secretion of entero-hormones (PYY, GLP-1). In malabsorption operations, portions of the small bowel are bypassed and undigested food reaches the colon.
- *Entero-hepatic cycle*: in operations with Roux limb (GBP, BPD) the bile acids follow a different route from that of food. GBP seems to be associated with increased primary bile acids in the blind loop and secondary bile acids further down in the gastrointestinal tract, both of which have antimicrobial properties.
- Antimicrobial prophylaxis for patients undergoing bariatric surgical procedures determines an acute although transient effect on microbiota composition.
- Time spent masticating: in all procedures with a restrictive component, increased chewing time produces larger quantities of saliva and promotes gastric secretion and motility.
- Food choices and preferences: after bariatric surgery diet changes in terms of quantity and quality. From soft diet in the first weeks, the patients switch gradually to a regular diet but with foods different from those consumed before surgery.

The mechanisms linking rearrangement of the gastrointestinal tract to the metabolic outcomes are largely unknown, a role for microbiota has been advocated.

Very few studies report the effect of bariatric surgery on the microbiota composition. To date only four studies in humans and five studies in animals have been reported (Table 6.2).

In 2009, Zhang et al. were the first to report on the effect of GBP on gut microbiota in man [26]. They examined microbial 16S rRNA genes from PCR amplicons by using the pyrosequencing technology to compare the microbial community structures of nine individuals, three normal weight, three morbidly obese, and three post-GBP. In normal-weight and in obese individual Firmicutes were dominant, in GBP patients Firmicutes were significantly decreased with a proportional increase of Gammaproteobacteria. Most importantly, in obese subjects, the population number of Archaea hydrogen utilizing H^+ extracted from indigestible polysaccharides and thus increasing energy uptake, was higher than in normal weight subjects and in subjects with GBP (Fig. 6.7).

These results suggest that microbiota play a significant role in the genesis of the GBP-induced EWL. However, the work has an important bias: the three studied groups were composed of separate subjects without longitudinal preoperative and postoperative assessments.

In 2010, Furet confronted the microbiota profiles in the feces of morbidly obese patients before, 3, and 6 months after GBP and associated these data to body composition, metabolic data, and inflammatory markers [27]. He confirmed the augmented Firmicutes/Bacteroidetes ratio in obese patients; at 3 and 6 months post-GBP this ratio diminished in direct relationship to patient's weight loss (body weight, BMI, body fat mass, and serum leptin concentrations). A significant negative relationship between the amount of *Faecalibacterium prausnitzii* and metabolic and inflammatory parameters was found. Furthermore, the weight loss was positively correlated to the amount of *Bifidobacterium* population.

Table 6.2 Literature overview on bariatric surgery and microbiota

Author	Year	Subjects	*N*	Type of surgery
Zhang et al. [26]	2009	Humans	9	GBP
Furet et al. [27]	2010	Humans	43	GBP
Graessler et al. [28]	2013	Humans	6	GBP
Kong et al. [31]	2013	Humans	15	GBP
Li et al. [29]	2011	Rats		GBP
Li et al. [31]	2011	Rats		GBP
Liuo et al. [32]	2013	Mice		GBP
Osto et al. [44]	2013	Rats		GBP
Ryan et al. [33]	2014	Mice		SG

More recently, these data have been confirmed by Graessler in six obese patients submitted to GBP [28].

Li et al. showed a substantial higher concentration of gut Proteobacteria, especially *Enterobacter hormaechei*, and a proportionate lower concentration of Firmicutes and Bacteroidetes in rats after GBP in comparison with sham-operated rats [29, 30]. In a similar study in man, Kong et al. investigated the gut microbiota from fecal samples and adipose tissue samples in severely obese individuals, before and after GBP 31]. Early after surgery a remarkable 37 % increase in gut bacteria belonging to the phylum Proteobacteria occurred. The researchers also found a significant association between gut microbiota composition and adipose tissue gene expression (including metabolic and inflammatory genes) as well as clinical phenotype – as substantial proportion of which were independent from changes in caloric intake.

In a recent intriguing study, Liou et al. demonstrated that the implantation by gastric gavage of gut microbiota from GBP-operated mice into germ-free mice, triggered decreased host weight and adiposity [32]. GBP was associated with increased populations of Proteobacteria (*Escherichia*) and Verrucomicrobia (*Akkermansia*), and a reduction in Firmicutes compared to sham surgery or to food restriction. Mice that underwent GBP extracted significantly less energy from the diet than mice that underwent sham surgery or calorie-restricted

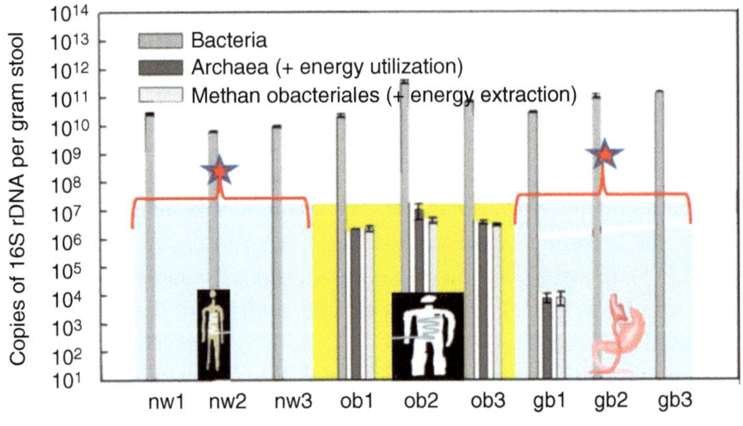

Fig. 6.7 Obese subjects (*ob*) had a higher number of hydrogen utilizing Archaea than normal weight subjects (*nw*) and subjects with Roux-en-Y gastric bypass (*gb*) (From Zhang et al. [26] modified)

mice. This effect may have been mediated by gut restructuring and by changes in the intestinal microbiota (Fig. 6.8).

Most important, germ-free mice on HFD, when colonized with microbiota from GBP mice, had a significant weight loss and exhibited a trend toward lower fasting insulin levels. In mice colonized with microbiota from sham surgery animals no effect was apparent. These data indicate that the decreased host adiposity is transmissible through the GBP altered microbiota and that it plays an active role in weight loss and metabolic status [32].

The possibility of transplantation of the beneficial effects of GBP on weight and metabolism through the gut microbiota as reported by Liou opens new exciting perspectives in the treatment of obesity and related diseases.

The relationship between bariatric surgery and gut microbiota has been investigated taking into account one type of procedure, GBP. Only recently a study concerns the effects of SG on bile acids circulation and associated changes to gut microbiota [33]. After SG, in HFD mice the increase of circulating bile acids was associated to a substantial reduction of the relative abundance of Bacteroides and to an increase in the relative abundance of *Lactobacillus* and *Lactococcus* and of Enterobacteriaceae (genus *Escherichia coli*). Concomitantly decrease in adiposity and improvement in glucose tolerance occurred. These effects were dependent on

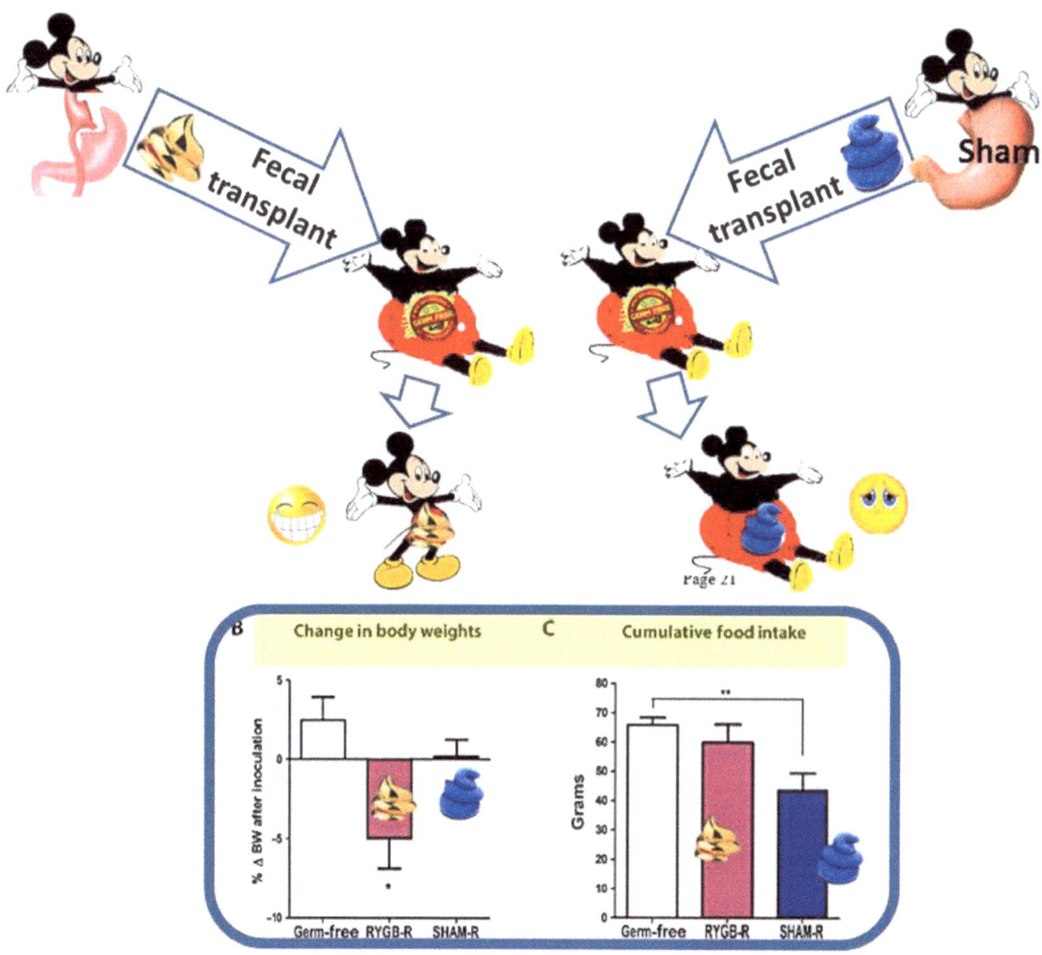

Fig. 6.8 Microbiota altered by Roux-en-Y gastric bypass, when transferred to intact germ-free animals, induced in the host phenotypic and metabolic changes mimicking the effects of surgery in the operated subject [32]

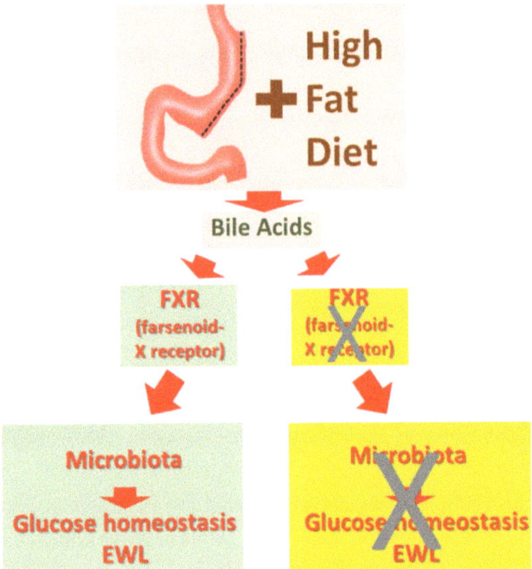

Fig. 6.9 The effects of sleeve gastrectomy on metabolism and microbiota are mediated by Farsenoid-X receptors (*FXR*)

Farsenoid-X receptor (FXR) signaling molecule. While microbiota is modified and modifies bile acids, FXR represents a link both to microbiota changes and to surgery benefits [33] (Fig. 6.9).

6.5 Probiotics and Prebiotics

Manipulation of the gut microbiota to prevent obesity and/or to control the glycemic metabolism has been investigated in animals and humans using prebiotics and probiotics.

According to the 2001 FAO/WHO definition, probiotics are "live micro-organisms which, when administered in adequate amounts, confer a health benefit on the host" [34]. The rationale for the use of probiotics for the treatment of gut microbiota-related diseases is the restoration of intestinal homeostasis by beneficial microbes. Probiotics are *Lactobacilli* and *Bifidobacteria*, but also yeasts such as *Saccharomyces boulardii*, *Streptococci*, and nonpathogenic strains of *Escherichia coli* [35].

Prebiotics (mostly oligosaccharides) are nondigestible but fermentable food ingredients that selectively stimulate the growth or activity of one or more gut microbes beneficial to the human host. At present, only inulin and trans-galacto-oligosaccharides are used as prebiotics having as main target two bacterial genera, *Lactobacilli* and *Bifidobacteria*. Cani demonstrated that *Bifidobacteria* are capable of lowering LPS levels by reducing intestinal permeability and thus preventing the low-grade inflammation. Inulin treatment in high-fat-fed diabetic mice restored *Bifidobacteria* levels, diminished body weight, normalized low-grade inflammation, improved glucose-tolerance, and glucose-induced insulin secretion. These effects were mediated via a GLP-1- and PYY-dependent pathway (Fig. 6.10). Use of prebiotics to modify gut microbiota to favor the beneficial bifidobacteria was hypothesized [36–39] (Fig. 6.10).

In a RCT by Woodard, daily use of probiotics (*Lactobacillus*) in patients submitted to GBP, at 6 months post-op, determined significant reduction in bacterial overgrowth (measured with H_2 breath levels), greater although not significant percent of excess weight loss (EWL), and significantly higher postoperative vitamin B12 levels when compared to the control group [40].

6.6 Fecal Transplant in Clinics

In the fourth century in China, the use of human fecal suspension by mouth for patients with severe diarrhea has been described. Recent literature reports the implantation of microbiota from human feces by naso-gastric tube, colonoscopy, or enema in the therapy of recurrent *Clostridium difficile* infection (CDI), after failed antibiotic therapy. A total of 317 patients were treated with a 93 % resolution rate. In 2013, in a RCT reported by Van Noon in the *NEMJ*, fecal transplant (FT) was confronted to vancomycin therapy in CDI patients [41]. Cured patients were 94 % in the FT group and 31 % in the vancomycin group. In another study, CDI resolution was stable at 17 months follow-up in 91 % of patients and the host gut microbiota was similar to the donor microbiota at 24 months follow-up [42]. In 2013, the FDA accepted FT as an investigational therapy.

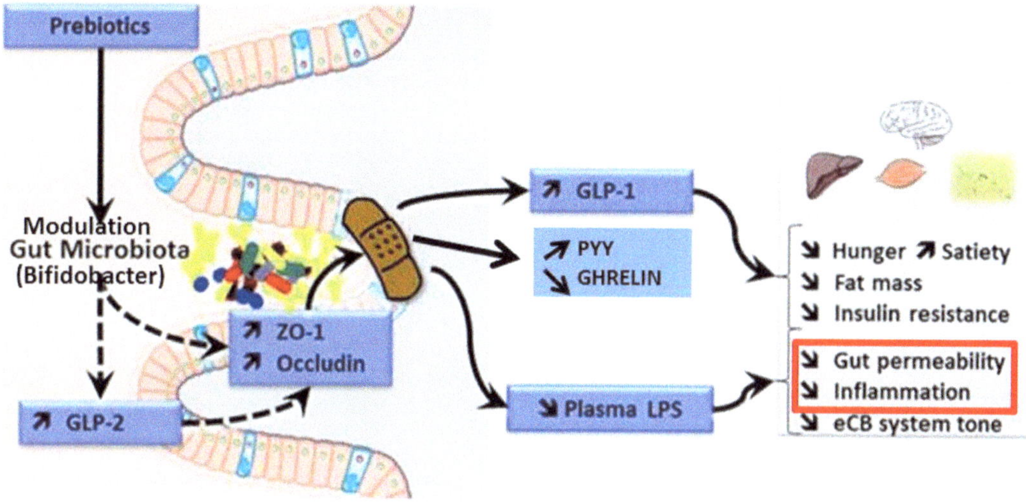

Fig. 6.10 Prebiotics act by increasing *Bifidobacterium* population, decreasing gut permeability and modulating gut peptides endogenous production (From Delzenne et al. [45]). *eCB* endocannabinoid, *GLP-1* glucagon-like peptide 1, *GLP-2* glucagon-like peptide 2, *LPS* lipopolysaccharides, *ZO-1* zonula occludens 1, *PYY* Peptide YY

More interesting for the purpose of this chapter is the 2010 work by Vrieze. A double-blind RCT was conducted on 18 obese patients with the metabolic syndrome [43]. Nine patients received FT from lean donors and nine patients received their own feces (control). After 6 weeks, in the FT from lean donors group fasting triglycerides levels were markedly reduced and peripheral and hepatic insulin sensitivity was markedly improved; no effect was apparent in the control group. Although the beneficial effects remitted after 12 weeks, it is not known whether repeated FT would be beneficial.

6.7 Summary

Gut microbiota composition and its metabolites are different in obese and lean individuals.

Gut microbiota plays a central role in energy harvesting and storage and in the pathogenesis of low-grade inflammation and hence in the genesis of obesity and of the metabolic syndrome.

Bariatric surgery (GBP and SG) determines significant changes in the composition of gut microbiota. The exact significance of these changes remains to be determined.

The beneficial effects of gut microbiota can be transferred from lean to obese subjects.

Gut microbiota can be modulated by pro- and prebiotics and by FT.

The therapeutic value of FT deserves investigation.

More conclusive studies in the experimental animal and especially in man are needed.

Conclusions

While there are only few firm data on the relationship between microbiota and the obesity and metabolic syndrome problem, it is undoubtable that the "microbiota organ," rich of more than three million genes deserves a greater attention.

A tremendous lack of data limits our current knowledge of the complexity of gut microbiota-host interactions and the exact mechanisms linking dietary habits, gut microbiota, and metabolic disorders.

Investigations centered on the relationship between bariatric surgery and gut microbiota are very scarce, do not encompass the different bariatric procedures, and need systematic controlled human studies to confirm the clinical relevance of the observed laboratory data.

However, experimental and clinical studies, although in a very preliminary manner, indicate that bariatric surgery affects gut microbiota both in the experimental and in the clinical setup determining microbiota changes that induce less energy harvesting and less chronic inflammation. As a consequence, the metabolic syndrome is positively influenced. In addition, the demonstrated possibility of transferring the "beneficial" effects of microbiota from lean or surgically treated subjects to patients with the metabolic syndrome not only may be advantageous in elucidating the mechanisms of "metabolic surgery," but also may indicate new promising therapeutic means for the third millennium "diabesity epidemic."

References

1. Savage DC. Microbial ecology of the gastrointestinal tract. Annu Rev Microbiol. 1977;31:107–33.
2. Frank DN, St Amand AL, Feldman RA, Boedeker EC, Harpaz N, Pace NR. Molecular-phylogenetic characterization of microbial community imbalances in human inflammatory bowel diseases. Proc Natl Acad Sci U S A. 2007;104:13780–5.
3. Flint HJ, Scott KP, Louis P, Duncan SH. The role of the gut microbiota in nutrition and health. Nat Rev Gastroenterol Hepatol. 2012;9(10):577–89.
4. Eckburg PB, Bik EM, Bernstein CN, et al. Diversity of the human intestinal microbial flora. Science. 2005;308:1635–8.
5. Arumugam M, et al. Enterotypes of the human gut microbiome. Nature. 2011;473:174–80.
6. Wu GD, Chen J, Hoffmann C, Bittinger K, et al. Linking long-term dietary patterns with gut microbial enterotypes. Science. 2011;334:105–8.
7. Foster JA, McVey Neufeld KA. Gut-brain axis: how the microbiome influences anxiety and depression. Trends Neurosci. 2013;36(5):305–12.
8. Maes M, Kubera M, Leunis JC. The gut-brain barrier in major depression: intestinal mucosal dysfunction with an increased translocation of LPS from gram negative enterobacteria (leaky gut) plays a role in the inflammatory pathophysiology of depression. Neuro Endocrinol Lett. 2008;29:117–24.
9. Hold GL, Pryde SE, Russell VJ, Furrie E, Flint HJ. Assessment of microbial diversity in human colonic samples by 16S rDNA sequence analysis. FEMS Microbiol Ecol. 2002;39(1):33–9.
10. Power SE, O'Toole PW, Stanton C, Ross RP, Fitzgerald GF. Intestinal microbiota, diet and health. Br J Nutr. 2014;111(3):387–402.
11. Tamboli CP, Neut C, Desreumaux P, Colombel JF. Dysbiosis in inflammatory bowel disease. Gut. 2004; 53(1):1–4.
12. Backhed F, Ding H, Wang T, et al. The gut microbiota as an environmental factor that regulates fat storage. Proc Natl Acad Sci U S A. 2004;101:15718–23.
13. Rabot S, Membrez M, Bruneau A, et al. Germ-free C57BL/6J mice are resistant to high-fat-diet-induced insulin resistance and have altered cholesterol metabolism. FASEB J. 2010;24:4948–59.
14. Turnbaugh PJ, Ley RE, Mahowald MA, et al. An obesity-associated gut microbiome with increased capacity for energy harvest. Nature. 2006;444:1027–31.
15. Ley RE, Backhed F, Turnbaugh P, et al. Obesity alters gut microbial ecology. Proc Natl Acad Sci U S A. 2005;102:11070–5.
16. Ley RE, Turnbaugh PJ, Klein S, et al. Microbial ecology: human gut microbes associated with obesity. Nature. 2006;444:1022–3.
17. Samuel BS, Shaito A, Motoike T, et al. Effects of the gut microbiota on host adiposity are modulated by the short-chain fatty-acid binding G protein-coupled receptor, Gpr41. Proc Natl Acad Sci U S A. 2008;105(43):16767–72.
18. Tremaroli V, Bäckhed F. Functional interactions between the gut microbiota and host metabolism. Nature. 2012;489(7415):242–9.
19. Cox LM, Blaser MJ. Pathways in microbe-induced obesity. Cell Metab. 2013;17(6):883–94.
20. Tilg H, Kaser A. Gut microbiome, obesity, and metabolic dysfunction. J Clin Invest. 2011;121(6):2126–32.
21. Cani PD, Delzenne NM. The role of the gut microbiota in energy metabolism and metabolic disease. Curr Pharm Des. 2009;15(13):1546–58.
22. Turnbaugh PJ, Ridaura VK, Faith JJ, Rey FE, Knight R, Gordon JI. The effect of diet on the human gut microbiome: a metagenomic analysis in humanized gnotobiotic mice. Sci Transl Med. 2009;1(6):6ra14.
23. Creely SJ, McTernan PG, Kusminski CM, et al. Lipopolysaccharide activates an innate immune system response in human adipose tissue in obesity and type 2 diabetes. Am J Physiol Endocrinol Metab. 2007;292(3):E740–7.
24. Aron-Wisnewsky J, Doré J, Clement K. The importance of the gut microbiota after bariatric surgery. Nat Rev Gastroenterol Hepatol. 2012;9(10):590–8.
25. Walker AW, et al. pH and peptide supply can radically alter bacterial populations and short-chain fatty acid ratios within microbial communities from the human colon. Appl Environ Microbiol. 2005;71:3692–700.
26. Zhang H, DiBaise JK, Zuccolo A, et al. Human gut microbiota in obesity and after gastric bypass. Proc Natl Acad Sci U S A. 2009;106(7):2365–70.
27. Furet JP, Kong LC, Tap J, et al. Differential adaptation of human gut microbiota to bariatric surgery-induced weight loss: links with metabolic and low-grade inflammation markers. Diabetes. 2010;59(12):3049–57.
28. Graessler J, Qin Y, Zhong H, et al. Metagenomic sequencing of the human gut microbiome before and after bariatric surgery in obese patients with type 2 diabetes: correlation with inflammatory and metabolic parameters. Pharmacogenomics J. 2013;13(6): 514–22.

29. Li JV, Ashrafian H, Bueter M, et al. Metabolic surgery profoundly influences gut microbial-host metabolic cross-talk. Gut. 2011;60(9):1214–23.
30. Li JV, Reshat R, Wu Q, et al. Experimental bariatric surgery in rats generates a cytotoxic chemical environment in the gut contents. Front Microbiol. 2011; 2:183.
31. Kong LC, Tap J, Aron-Wisnewsky J, et al. Gut microbiota after gastric bypass in human obesity: increased richness and associations of bacterial genera with adipose tissue genes. Am J Clin Nutr. 2013;98(1):16–24.
32. Liou AP, Paziuk M, Luevano Jr JM, Machineni S, Turnbaugh PJ, Kaplan LM. Conserved shifts in the gut microbiota due to gastric bypass reduce host weight and adiposity. Sci Transl Med. 2013;5(178):178ra41.
33. Ryan KK, Tremaroli V, Clemmensen C, et al. FXR is a molecular target for the effects of vertical sleeve gastrectomy. Nature. 2014;509(7499):183–8.
34. Schlundt J. Health and nutritional properties of probiotics in food including powder milk with live lactic acid bacteria. Report of a Joint FAO/WHO Expert Consultation on Evaluation of Health and Nutritional Properties of Probiotics in Food including Powder Milk with Live *Lactic Acid Bacteria, 1–4 October 2001. FAO Food and Nutrition Paper 85. FAO and WHO, 2006.*
35. Cammarota G, Ianiro G, Bibbò S, Gasbarrini A. Gut microbiota modulation: probiotics, antibiotics or fecal microbiota transplantation? Intern Emerg Med. 2014; 9(4):365–73.
36. Cani PD, Bibiloni R, Knauf C, et al. Changes in gut microbiota control metabolic endotoxemia-induced inflammation in high-fat diet-induced obesity and diabetes in mice. Diabetes. 2008;57:1470–81.
37. Cani PD, Neyrinck AM, Fava F, et al. Selective increases of bifidobacteria in gut microflora improves high-fat diet-induced diabetes through a mechanism associated with endotoxemia. Diabetologia. 2007;50:2374–83.
38. Aronsson L, Huang Y, Parini P, et al. Decreased fat storage by Lactobacillus paracasei is associated with increased levels of angiopoietin-like 4 protein (ANGPTL4). PLoS One. 2010;5:13087.
39. Lee HY, Park JH, Seok SH, et al. Human originated bacteria, Lactobacillus rhamnosus PL60, produce conjugated linoleic acid and show antiobesity effects in diet-induced obese mice. Biochim Biophys Acta. 2006;1761:736–44.
40. Woodard GA, Encarnacion B, Downey JR, et al. Probiotics improve outcomes after Roux-en-Y gastric bypass surgery: a prospective randomized trial. J Gastrointest Surg. 2009;13(7):1198–204.
41. van Nood E, Vrieze A, Nieuwdorp M, et al. Duodenal infusion of donor feces for recurrent Clostridium difficile. N Engl J Med. 2013;368(5):407–15.
42. Brandt LJ, Aroniadis OC, Mellow M, et al. Long-term follow-up of colonoscopic fecal microbiota transplant for recurrent Clostridium difficile infection. Am J Gastroenterol. 2012;107(7):1079–87.
43. Vrieze A, Van Nood E, Holleman F, et al. Transfer of intestinal microbiota from lean donors increases insulin sensitivity in individuals with metabolic syndrome. Gastroenterology. 2012;143(4):913–6.
44. Osto M, Abegg K, Bueter M, le Roux CW, Cani PD, Lutz TA. Roux-en-Y gastric bypass surgery in rats alters gut microbiota profile along the intestine. Physiol Behav. 2013;119:92–6.
45. Delzenne NM, Neyrinck AM, Cani PD. Modulation of the gut microbiota by nutrients with prebiotic properties: consequences for host health in the context of obesity and metabolic syndrome. Microb Cell Fact. 2011;10 Suppl 1:S10.
46. Bäckhed F, Manchester JK, Semenkovich CF, Gordon JI. Mechanisms underlying the resistance to diet-induced obesity in germ-free mice. Proc Natl Acad Sci U S A. 2007;104(3):979–84.

Part II

Surgery of Obesity

The "Bariatric Multidisciplinary Center"

7

John Melissas

Obesity (BMI ≥30 kg/m$^{2)}$ is a worldwide epidemic that currently affects 500 million adults and 40–50 million children, according to the World Health Organization (WHO), becoming one of the leading causes of death and disability in Europe and worldwide [1–3].

In the USA, the age-adjusted prevalence of obesity was 35.5 % among adult men and 35.8 % among adult women in 2009–2010, with the prevalence of obesity in children and adolescents being 16.9 % [4].

The prevalence of obesity has tripled since the 1980s in many European countries, with overweight and obesity affecting 50 % of the population [1–3].

More alarming is the rapidly growing prevalence of severe obesity (SO) (BMI ≥ 40 kg/m^2 or BMI ≥ 35 kg/m^2 with manifest of serious co-morbidities) which is increasing faster than obesity in adults and in children [5].

In Sweden, young adult men exhibited a five-fold increase in moderate obesity over the 30-year period ending in 2005, whereas SO increases ten-fold and is projected to affect 4 % of the adult Swedish population by the year 2020 [6]. Studies in the UK showed that adult SO doubled in the period 1995–2008 with higher level in women and models predict a tripling of SO prevalence for English women by the year 2030 [7].

J. Melissas
Bariatric Unit, Heraklion University Hospital, University of Crete, 164 Erythreas Street, Heraklion, Crete 71409, Greece
e-mail: melissas@med.uoc.gr

7.1 Obesity Burden and Cost

Obesity is a gateway to ill health and excess weight has proven to drastically elevate a person's risk of developing debilitating diseases, such as diabetes, hypertension, dyslipidemia, sleep apnea, vascular occlusion, nonalcoholic steatohepatitis, cancer, infertility, and pregnancy complications [4, 8, 9].

Overall, obesity reduces life-expectancy, quality of life and is a major cause of disability being extremely costly for the health system worldwide [4, 8–10]. Estimated direct costs for obesity and related co-morbidities treatment exceed 5 % of the total health care costs in both the USA and Europe [7, 8, 11]. Additionally, obesity-related indirect costs from work absence, reduction of productivity, etc. may exceed the direct medical costs [12]. Both direct and indirect expenditures correlate with the degree of obesity. As BMI increases, the number and severity of metabolic derangements increase in adults and children [9, 13]. The impact of obesity in women in reproductive age is of particular concern, because of the association between maternal pre-pregnancy obesity with serious pregnancy complications, greater fetal adiposity, and development of childhood obesity in the offspring [9].

M. Lucchese, N. Scopinaro (eds.), *Minimally Invasive Bariatric and Metabolic Surgery: Principles and Technical Aspects*, DOI 10.1007/978-3-319-15356-8_7,

In the USA, annual direct costs are three times higher for SO workers than for obese workers and more than ten times higher than for overweight employees. Absence from work is estimated to be 5.9 more days/year in SO workers compared to men with normal weight. Reduced productivity estimated in American SO workforce is equivalent to 1 month lost productivity per year [10, 14].

Obviously, weight management is going to play a major role in reducing both morbidity and mortality and health care costs in Europe and worldwide [4, 9, 11, 13].

7.2 Bariatric Surgery

Bariatric surgery is now recognized as the only effective treatment for severe obese (SO) patients with long-term sustained weight-loss and postoperative resolution or significant improvement in the obesity co-morbidities, being an interval part of the comprehensive management of SO patients [4, 9, 15]. Current evidence points to major benefits in terms of prevention of type 2 diabetes, important gains regarding cardiovascular risk and cancer reduction and suggests longevity [4, 9, 16].

Bariatric operations are preventive as well as therapeutic. Weight-loss achieved postoperatively may forestall or stop development of a significant number of obesity co-morbidities [4, 15, 16]. It is notable, particularly for its economic significance, that bariatric surgery can obviate the need for other major procedures, such as kidney, heart and liver transplantation, hip replacement, and cancer surgery [9]. Early intervention in any disease process provides greater likelihood of achieving partial or total remission and this is of great importance, when considering bariatric surgery at the younger age group and in those with BMI 30–35 kg/m^2 [9].

Heath care system benefits from bariatric surgery are enormous. A study from England suggested that if only 5 % of the eligible patients were to have bariatric surgery, the net saving for the NHS over 3 years would be nearly 400 million GB pounds. Additionally, the authors estimate that these savings would triple if 25 % of eligible SO patients were subjected to surgical intervention. That estimate does not include additional economic benefits associated with decrease in work absence and increase in workers' productivity [11].

7.3 Multidisciplinary Obesity Approach

Since obesity is a complex condition where biological, psychological, and social factors interfere to lead to excess body weight, its management cannot focus only on weight reduction. The improvement of body composition with fat-free mass maintenance, co-morbidities management, and quality of life improvement are also included in treatment terms. [8, 17, 18]

Therefore, comprehensive obesity management by either conservative or surgical method is "by definition" a multidisciplinary effort and should be undertaken by a team of different professionals able to tackle with the different aspects of obesity and its related disorders [4, 8, 17, 18].

Bariatric surgery has rapidly evolved into metabolic surgery. Type 2 diabetes, a primarily medical disease which evolved into a condition where surgeons may play a more active role in the diabetic patient management, is an excellent example. Bariatric-metabolic procedures can now be utilized to treat metabolic conditions even without direct relation to weight-loss [19]. This is further emphasizing the need of a holistic interdisciplinary approach for the management of the disorders that fall into the bariatric-metabolic surgery field [4, 19, 20].

The interdisciplinary guidelines and metabolic and bariatric surgery have been described in detail [4, 21–23]. It is remarkable to mention that for a given patient, the risk-benefit ratio requires an experienced multidisciplinary bariatric team to be carefully evaluated. The team providing such assessment should consist of the following specialists with experience in the management of the bariatric patient:

Physician
Surgeon
Anesthetist

Psychologist or psychiatrist
Nutritionist and/or dietician
Nurse practitioner/social worker

Additional consultation with endocrinologist, cardiologist, respiratory physician, ICU expert, interventional gastroenterologist, radiologist, and other specialists would be obtained as indicated [4, 23].

7.4 Safety and Efficacy of Surgical Intervention

Bariatric surgery needs to be safe and effective [24, 25]. This highly demanding challenging therapy necessitates the appropriate training and experience from the surgeon's part. It is vital that beyond the optimal therapeutic knowledge, the surgeon should also have the technical skills in the open and/or the laparoscopic surgery. Apart from performing meticulous pre- and post-operative care, the surgeon has to be committed to long-term patient follow-up [23, 24].

Additionally, institutional commitment to the excellent multidisciplinary care of the SO patient who has an exceptional surgical and anesthetic risk is essential to ensure safe and effective performance of bariatric surgery. The ancillary services including specialized nursing staff, dieticians, exercise advisors, and multidisciplinary medical team are extremely valuable and necessary [23, 24].

Medical and surgical facilities, such as operating room tables, surgical instruments, furniture, and radiology equipment capable of handling morbidly obese patients are "sine qua non" resources for any institution that seeks to treat bariatric patients [4, 23, 24].

Several parameters can be associated with extended hospital stay, higher complication rate and increased mortality after bariatric surgery. Advanced age, male gender, high BMI, inadequate training, and inexperienced surgeon may contribute to poor outcome of the surgical intervention. Although the first three parameters cannot be changed, the effort should focus on continuous improvement of the bariatric surgeon's training and experience [23, 24].

7.5 Surgeon's Training

The need for adequate training of the bariatric surgeon, particularly for those entering the field, has long before been recognized by the International Federation for the Surgery of Obesity and related Metabolic Disorders (IFSO) [25] and the American Society for Metabolic and Bariatric Surgery (ASMBS) [26].

Surgeons with comprehensive training are able to manage morbidly obese and super-obese patients with low morbidity and mortality and outcome results similar to those reported by experienced surgeons.

In a study by Kothori et al. [27], following completion of an advanced laparoscopic fellowship, a surgeon was evaluated for 125 consecutive patients. He performed gastric bypasses with mean operative time of 123 min, mean hospital stay of 2.2 days, anastomotic leak in 2.6 %, and intestinal obstruction in 0.6 % during the immediate post-operative period. The authors concluded that after a full training in bariatric laparoscopic surgery, results were similar and comparable to those published in the literature.

Re-operative bariatric surgery is an even more complex and demanding field. This type of surgery requires years of experience, more detailed preoperative patients' evaluation and should be practiced preferably by surgeons with extensive experience and in institutions with all the necessary facilities, equipment and multidisciplinary expertise [23].

7.6 Surgeon-Institution Volume

The relation between volume of patients managed per year and mortality for most procedures is well-known [28]. In a study of 474,108 patients subjected to eight cardiovascular operations or cancer resections, the surgeon's volume was inversely related to the operative mortality for all eight procedures [29].

In another study, 197 surgeons who performed 19,174 gastric bypass operations were evaluated in terms of relation between volume of surgeries with the incidence of complications and mortality.

The reported mortality rates were 1.3 % for surgeons performing 1–5 procedures over a 5-year period, 0.5 % for those performing 6–99 procedures, 0.3 % for those with 200–499 and 0.2 % for those performing ≥500 bariatric operations over 5 years. Similar results in favor of those surgeons with higher volume were found when complications rates were assessed [30].

Therefore, it is obvious that surgeons and institution should undertake the management of a minimum number of bariatric patients per year, to optimize the results of treatment offered.

7.7 Pre-operative Evaluation

The pre-operative evaluation of the bariatric patient covers a complete history, including previous weight-loss attempts and results. Obviously, the selection of patients for bariatric and metabolic surgery should follow the universally accepted indications, described by International Organizations, such as EASO, IFSO, IFSO-EC [4, 21, 22]. A complete physical examination should follow to assess surgical risk and guide in planning the appropriate pre-operative investigations and consultations.

Extra attention should be given to the presence of serious obesity co-morbidities, and at this stage the value of the multidisciplinary bariatric team is extremely important [4, 23, 24]. Conditions, such as type 2 diabetes, sleep apnea syndrome, hypertension, gastro-esophageal reflux disease, chronic anemia, previous deep venous thrombosis or pulmonary embolism and serious psychological disorders should be diagnosed and controlled. The addition to the standard multidisciplinary bariatric team of ICU specialist, endocrinologist, respiratory physician, hematologist, and gastroenterologist is both required and necessary, depending on the presence of certain co-morbidities in each patient [23, 24, 31].

It is extremely difficult to recommend standard pre-operative laboratory teams. The fact that potential bariatric patients may belong to different categories, such as low-risk obese patients, high-risk with underlying medical conditions, patients with serious psychological problems and patients for revisional bariatric surgery, creates further difficulties to advise a common barrage of tests [31].

However, all efforts should be made for the optimum control of all underlined medical conditions and for the reduction of surgical risk and complications [32, 33].

7.8 Post-operative Care and Follow-up

The post-operative follow-up consists of office visits at 1st, 3rd, 6th, 9th, 12th, 18th, and 24th month as common practice. Annual follow-up visits are recommended after the first 2 post-operative years. Additional visits depending on the patient's condition and the existence of co-morbidities should be considered necessary [24].

The patient is not only evaluated by the bariatric surgeon, but also by the entire multidisciplinary bariatric team. These office visits include history and clinical examination, laboratory tests as required, and consultations by experts depending on the procedure performed. Recording the outcome of existing co-morbidities, measuring weight, waist and hip parameters and offering dietary advices, behavioral modification techniques, encouraging participation in exercise programs and support groups are included in the long-term follow-up [4, 8, 9, 24, 25].

7.9 The Center of Excellence (COE) Concept

Experience in the USA and Europe has shown that the combination of a good surgeon operating in a good, well-equipped institution can ensure safe and effective management of the bariatric patient. Excellence in the surgical management of severely obese patients should be associated with permanent weight-loss, good quality of life, low short- and long-term complications, amelioration of obesity co-morbidities in the vast majority of patients and all those goals to be achieved with low morbidity and mortality [23, 34, 35].

When a bariatric center can prove that it has the necessary multilevel resources to undertake the management of severely obese patients with outstanding results, it can be accredited as a Center of Excellence (COE) in Bariatric and Metabolic Surgery [23, 24, 36].

The evaluation of centers is carried out by independent bodies and the COE designation is administered by a professional organization such as IFSO or the American College of Surgeons (ACS) or the ASMBS.

The philosophy of COE accreditation is simple: A well-trained and competent surgeon operating in a well-equipped and serviced institution with sufficient volume of patients, would be able to offer safe and efficient management of patients with metabolic disorders. Efficacious treatment of the bariatric/metabolic diseases would be beneficial to patients and health care systems.

Table 7.1 Surgeon's requirements

1. Appropriate certification to perform general surgery
2. Training and experience in gastrointestinal surgery
3. Successful completion of a training course in bariatric surgery
4. Testimonials by mentors (proctors) of satisfactory bariatric surgical ability
5. Careful maintenance of a database of all bariatric cases, including outcomes
6. Commitment to postoperative life-time follow-up of the patients
7. Have performed at least 25 bariatric cases per year (50 cases are required when adjustable gastric banding is most commonly utilized)
8. Be able to perform revisional surgery
9. Attend bariatric meetings regularly and subscribe to at least one bariatric journal
10. Perform at least 25 bariatric cases per year including a number of revisional cases among them (50 cases are required when adjustable gastric banding is most commonly utilized)
11. Be involved in the training and the accreditation of less-experienced bariatric surgeons
12. Follow-up for at least 75 % of the operated patients

7.10 The COE Program in Europe, Middle East, and Africa

In Europe, the establishment of a Center of Excellence program under the guidance of the European Chapter of IFSO (IFSO-EC) was appropriate and indicated [24, 35]. In May 2008, during the General Assembly of IFSO-EC in Capri, the concept of a COE program was unanimously endorsed by the representatives of all the European National Bariatric Societies. Thus, the European Accreditation Council for Bariatric Surgery (EAC-BS) was formed. Leading bariatric surgeons from the area of Europe, Middle East, and Africa are participating in the organization, either as members of the Scientific Board or the Review Committee [35]. In August 2009, during the General Council meeting in Paris, the COE program was endorsed by IFSO. Institutions and surgeons fulfilling the IFSO requirements (Tables 7.1 and 7.2) for safe and effective management of the morbidly obese patients could now apply (www.EAC-BS.com) for participation to the COE program [36].

7.11 The European Accreditation Council

EAC-BS examines the institutional facilities and the surgeon's qualifications and experience in order to ensure that they offer safe and efficient management to severely obese and patients with other metabolic disorders. EAC-BS utilizes the requirements set by IFSO [23] for surgeons [7] and institutions (Table 7.2) in order to accept them for participation in the COE program.

The management offered to the patients by the participating institutions and surgeons (Table 7.1) is carefully observing patients' outcome which is recorded in the International Bariatric Registry (IBAR™).

Indexes of excellence, such as intra- and postoperative complications, re-admissions, long-term complications, mortality, excess weight loss and co-morbidities outcome, are evaluated for each participating center.

Finally, a site visit by experienced auditor will follow to verify the reported patients' data and

Table 7.2 Institution's requirements

1. Ensure that surgeons performing bariatric surgery have the appropriate certification, training, and experience.
2. Provide ancillary services such as specialized nursing care, dietary instruction, counseling, and psychological assistance if and when needed
3. Have readily available consultants in cardiology, pulmonology, psychiatry, and rehabilitation with previous experience in treating bariatric surgery patients
4. Have trained anesthesiologists with experience in treating bariatric surgery patients
5. Ensure that a recovery room capable of providing critical care to morbidly obese patients and an intensive care unit with similar capacity are available
6. Ensure that radiology department facilities can perform emergency chest x-rays with portable machinery, abdominal ultrasonography, and upper GI series
7. Ensure that blood tests can be performed on a 24-h basis
8. Ensure that blood bank facilities are available and blood transfusion can be carried out at any time
9. Have comprehensive and full in-house consultative services required for the care of the bariatric surgical patients, including critical care services
10. Have the complete line of necessary equipment, instruments, items of furniture, wheel chairs, operating room tables, beds, radiology facilities such as CT scan, lifts, and other facilities specially designed and suitable for morbidly and super obese patients
11. Have a written informed consent process that informs each patient of the surgical procedure, the risk for complications and mortality rate, alternative treatments, the possibility of failure to lose weight and his/her right to refuse treatment
12. Maintain details of the treatment and outcome of each patient in a digital database.
13. Have experienced interventional radiologists available to take over the non-surgical management of possible anastomotic leaks and strictures
14. Performs at least 50 bariatric surgical cases per year including revisional cases. The peri-operative care and the surgical procedures have to be standardized for each surgeon.
15. Provides life-time follow-up for the majority and not less than 75 % of all bariatric surgical patients. Patients' data should be available on request by EAC-BS authorities.

examine the institutional equipment, facilities, resources and services. The auditor will construct a detailed report which is then forwarded to two Review Committee members for evaluation. Both reviewers will then submit their opinion to the Scientific Board, the final decision-making body. If everything is in order, EAC-BS will suggest to IFSO-EC that the center/surgeon is good enough to receive the COE designation (Table 7.3).

7.12 Results of IFSO-EC Center of Excellence Program

The program is evolving in a very satisfactory way. Seventy-two institutions and 118 surgeons from 22 countries from the region of Europe, Middle East, and Africa are participating.

Since January 2010, data from more than 22,881 bariatric patients have been entered in the IBAR. In 84.4 % of them, the applied treatment was a primary bariatric procedure, in 5.9 % a two-stage procedure and in 9.7 % a re-do for failure of the original operation.

From the primary procedures, 55.18 % were gastric bypass, 24.68 % sleeve gastrectomy, 11.52 % band, 0.50 % gastric plication, 1.15 % mini gastric bypass, 0.86 % biliopancreatic diversion (Scopinaro), 2.05 % biliopancreatic diversion (duodenal switch), 0.02 % gastroplasty, and 4.04 % "other" bariatric procedure.

Early (≤30 days) post-operative mortality was as low as 0.07 % for all procedures including the re-operations. Mortality for primary procedures was 0.04 %, for 2-stage 0.30 % and for re-do procedures 0.14 %.

Re-admissions for complications in the early (≤30 days) post-operative period was 1.69 % among all operated patients with primary procedures, and for the late (≥30 days) post-operative period 2.26 %. For the 2-stage and the re-do procedures the incidence of re-admissions for early complications was 1.28 and 4.24 % and for late complications 2.22 and 3.42 %, respectively.

Weight-loss as assessed by % EWL and % EBL for patients subjected to primary bariatric procedures at 12th post-operative month was 68.81 and 70.83 %, respectively. At 24th post-operative month, it was 70.83 and 78.71 %, respectively. Cure or significant improvement of obesity co-morbidities were observed in 79.4 %

Table 7.3 COE evaluation procedure

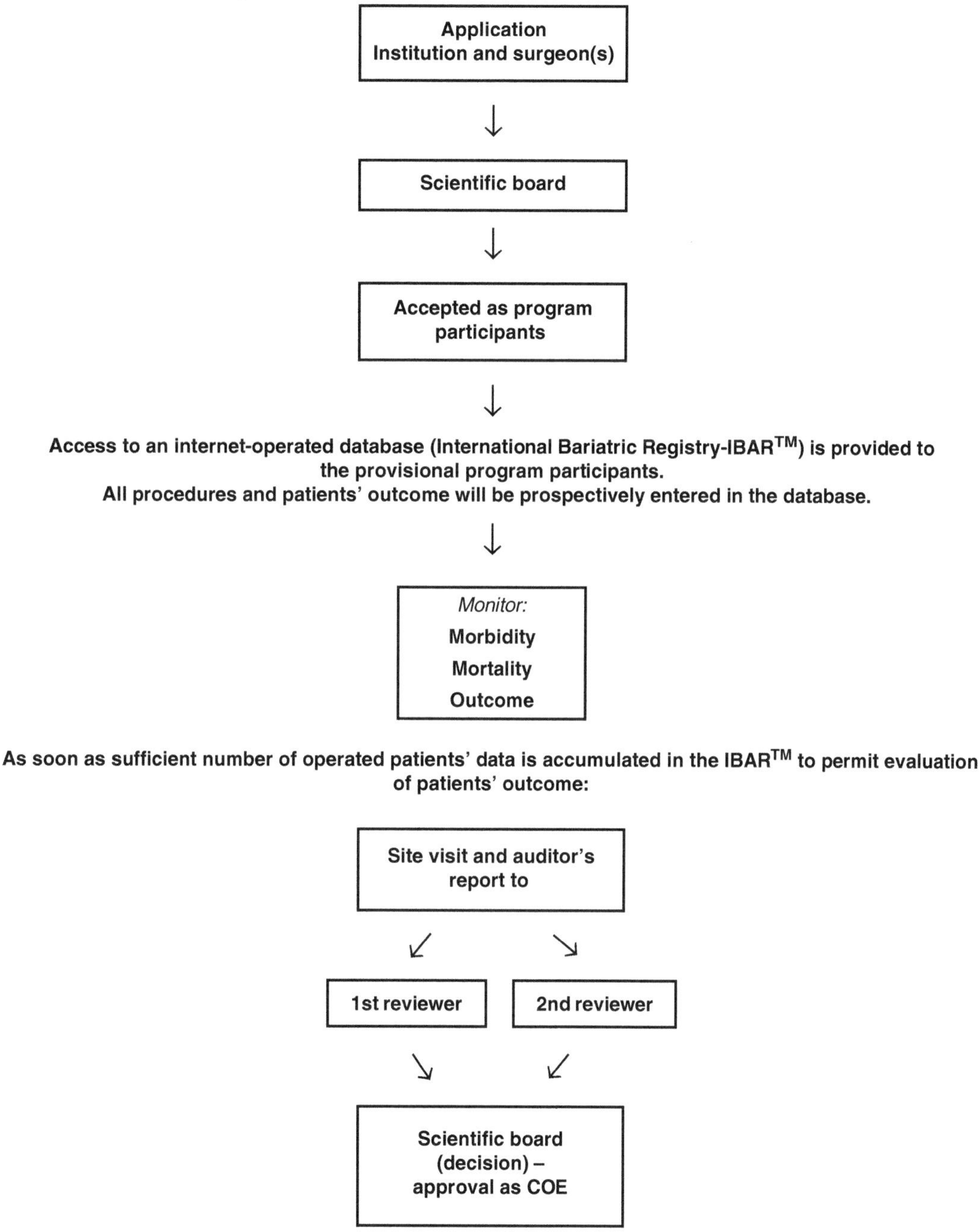

for diabetes, 77.2 % for hypertension, 84.6 % for osteo-articular diseases, 93.6 % for sleep apnea syndrome, and 80.8 % for dyslipidemia.

In conclusion, IFSO-EC COE program, administered in this geographic region by EAC-BS, offered significant incentives for safe and effective multidisciplinary management of morbidly obese patients in participating provisional and designated Center of Excellence institutions.

References

1. World Health Organization (WHO). Available at: http://www.euro.who.int/en/what-we-do/health-topics/noncommunicable-diseases/obesity. Accessed Apr 2013.
2. World Health Organization (WHO). Fact sheet No. 311 (updated March 2013) available at: http://www.who.int/mediacentre/factsheets/fs311/en/. Accessed Apr 2013.
3. Frühbeck G, Toplak H, Woodward E, et al. Obesity: the gateway to ill health - an EASO position statement on a rising public health, clinical and scientific challenge in Europe. Obes Facts. 2013;6:117–20.
4. Fried M, Yumuk V, Oppert JM, et al. Interdisciplinary European guidelines on metabolic and bariatric surgery. Obes Surg. 2014;24:42–55.
5. National Center for Health Statistics NCHS Health E-Stat: prevalence of overweight, obesity and extreme obesity among adults. United States, Trends 1976-80 through 2005-2006. Available at www.cdc.gov/nhs/fastats/overwt.htm. Last accesses 26 Jan 1012.
6. Neovius M, Teixeria-Pinto A, Rasmussen F. Shift in the composition of obesity in young adult men in Sweden over a third of a century. Int J Obes Surg. 2008;32:832–6.
7. The National Obesity Observatory (NOO). The epidemiology of morbid obesity. www.noo.org.uk/NOO_about_obesity/Morbid_obesity. Last accessed 6 Dec 2011.
8. Yumuk V, Frühbeck G, Oppert JM, et al. An EASO position statement on multidisciplinary obesity management in adults. Obes Facts. 2014;7:96–101.
9. Kral JG, Kava RA, Catalano PM, et al. Severe obesity: the neglected epidemic. Obes Facts. 2012;5:254–69.
10. Hensrud DD, Klein S. Extreme obesity: a new medical crisis in the United States. Mayo Clin Proc. 2006;81(10 suppl):S5–10.
11. Office of Health Economics (OHE): Shedding the pounds: Obesity Management, NICE Guidance and Bariatric Surgery in England. November 2010. Office of Health economics 12 Whitehall, London SW1A2DY. Available at www.ohe.org. Last accessed 12 Nov 2011.
12. Finkelstein EA, DiBonaventura M, Burgess SM, et al. The costs of obesity in the work place. J Occup Environ Med. 2010;52:971–6.
13. Picot J, Jones J, Colquitt JL, et al. The clinical effectiveness and cost-effectiveness of bariatric (weight loss) surgery for obesity: a systematic review and economic evaluation. Health Technol Assess (Winchester). 2009;13:1–190.
14. Durden ED, Huse D, Ben-Joseph R, et al. Economic costs of obesity to self-insured employers. J Occup Environ Med. 2010;52:991–7.
15. Sjöström L. Review of the key results from the Swedish Obese Subject trial-a prospective controlled intervention study of bariatric surgery. J Intern Med. 2013;273:219–34.
16. Buchwald H, Rudster KD, Williams SE, et al. Overall mortality, incremental life expectancy, and cause of death at 25 years in the program on the surgical control of the hyperlipidemia. Ann Surg. 2010;251:1034–40.
17. Tsigos C, Hainer V, Basdevant A, et al. Criteria for EASO-collaborating centres for obesity management. Obes Facts. 2011;4:329–33.
18. Tsigos C, Hainer V, Basdevant A, et al. Management of obesity in adults. European clinical practice guidelines. Obes Facts. 2008;1:106–16.
19. Fried M. Bariatric and metabolic surgery. Minerva Endocrinol. 2013;38:237–44.
20. Damaso AR, de Piano A, Campos RM, et al. Multidisciplinary approach to the treatment of obese adolescence: effects on cardiovascular risk factors, inflammatory profile, and neuroendocrine regulation of energy balance. Int J Endocrinol. 2013;2013:541032. doi:10.1155/2013/541032. Epub 2013 Oct 27.
21. Sauerland S, Angrisani L, Belachew M, et al. Obesity surgery: evidence-based guidelines of the European Association for Endoscopic surgery (EAES). Surg Endosc. 2005;19:200–21.
22. Guidelines Committee SAGES. SAGES guidelines for clinical application of laparoscopic bariatric surgery. Surg Endosc. 2008;22:2281–300.
23. Melissas J. IFSO guidelines for safety, quality and excellence in bariatric surgery. Obes Surg. 2008;18:497–500.
24. Melissas J. Safety, quality and excellence in bariatric surgery. Minerva Chir. 2009;64:239–52.
25. Cowan Jr GS. The Cancun IFSO statement on bariatric surgery qualifications. International Federation for the Surgery of Obesity. Obes Surg. 1998;8:86.
26. Inabnet 3rd WB, Bour E, Carlin AM, et al. Joint task force recommendations for credentialing of bariatric surgeons. Surg Obes Relat Dis. 2013;9:595–7.
27. Kothari SN, Boyd WC, Larson CA, et al. Training of a minimally invasive bariatric surgeon: are laparoscopic fellowships the answer? Obes Surg. 2005;15:323–9.
28. Nguyen NT, Paya M, Stevens CM, et al. The relationship between hospital volume and outcome in bariatric surgery at academic medical centers. Ann Surg. 2004;240:586–93.
29. Birkmayer JD, Stukel TA, Siewers AE, et al. Surgeon volume and operative mortality in the United States. N Engl J Med. 2003;349:2117–27.
30. Murr MM, Martin T, Haines K, et al. A state-wide review of contemporary outcomes of gastric bypass in Florida: does provider volume impact outcomes? Ann Surg. 2007;245:699–706.
31. Eldar S, Heneghan HM, Brethauer S, et al. A focus on surgical preoperative evaluation of the bariatric patient–the Cleveland Clinic protocol and review of the literature. Surgeon. 2011;9:273–7.

32. Ray EC, Nickels MW, Sayeed S, et al. Predicting success after gastric bypass: the role of psychosocial and behavioural factors. Surgery. 2003;134:555–64.
33. Ferrado DR. Preparing patients for bariatric surgery-the clinical considerations. Clin Rev. 2004;14:57–63.
34. Pratt GM, McLees B, Pories WJ. The ASMBS bariatric surgery Centers of Excellence program: a blueprint for quality improvement. Surg Obes Relat Dis. 2006;2:497–503.
35. Melissas J. IFSO European Chapter Centre of Excellence Program. In: Deitel M, Gagner M, Dixon J, Himpens J, Madan AK, editors. Handbook of obesity surgery. Toronto: FD-Communications Inc; 2010. p. 437–8.
36. European Accreditation Council for Bariatric Surgery. Homepage (Cited 26 May 2009). Available at www.EAC-BS.com.

Metabolic Surgery

8

Henry Buchwald

> Metabolic surgery [is] the operative manipulation of a normal organ or organ system to achieve a biological result for a potential health gain (Buchwald and Varco, 1978).

The above definition is from the foreword to our 1978 text titled *Metabolic Surgery* [1]. This concept of metabolic surgery is a broad interpretation of the role of the surgeon in medicine's battle against disease and the capability of surgery to contribute to proactive health care.

The discipline of surgery had its roots in incisional surgery, for example, the draining of boils in the days of the sixteenth-century guild of barber-surgeons. It rapidly became a craft, almost exclusively, of extirpative procedures. Radical and then ultraradical cancer resections exemplified this era. As surgical techniques matured and prosthetic materials and devices became available, reconstructive surgery was born and came to fruition in cardiac, orthopedic, and transplantation surgery. At present, we have firmly entered the realm of metabolic surgery, more by a realization of past and current accomplishments than by a dramatic evolution.

The 11 chapters written by prominent surgeons in our 1978 book talked of results and sequelae of operations for gastric ulcer disease (René Mengy), gastric bypass for obesity (Edward E. Mason), jejunoileal bypass in patients with morbid obesity (H. William Scott), partial ileal bypass for hyperlipidemia management (Henry Buchwald and Richard L. Varco), metabolic consequences of pancreatectomy (Ward O. Griffin, Jr), metabolic surgical significance of the spleen (Earl N. Metz, G. James Cerilli, Robert M. Zollinger), portal diversion for inborn errors of metabolism (Charles W. Putman, Thomas E. Starzl), ablation of normal endocrine glands as treatment of benign and malignant disease (Edward L. Kaplan), transplantation in metabolic disease (Arthur J. Matas, Richard L. Simmons, Robert J. Desnick), functional neurosurgery (Donlin N. Long), and pulsing electromagnetic fields (C. Andrew L. Bassett).

Today, 25 years later, we could more than double the number of chapters on metabolic surgery to include indirect and direct vagal nerve electronic stimulation for type 2 diabetes [2, 3], duodenal stimulation for type 2 diabetes [4], perirenal sympathetic nerve ablation for type 2 diabetes [5], pancreas transplantation and islet cell autotransplantation for type 2 diabetes [6, 7], carotid body procedures for hypertension [8], deep brain stimulation for refractory depression [9], unilateral cervical vagal stimulation for refractory depression [10], central nervous stimulation for epilepsy [11], intrathecal implantable pump infusions for pain and spasticity [12],

H. Buchwald, MD, PhD
Department of Surgery, University of Minnesota, 420 Delaware Street SE, MMC 290, Minneapolis, MN 55455, USA
e-mail: buchw001@umn.edu

M. Lucchese, N. Scopinaro (eds.), *Minimally Invasive Bariatric and Metabolic Surgery: Principles and Technical Aspects*, DOI 10.1007/978-3-319-15356-8_8,

implantable pump insulin infusion for type 2 diabetes [13], and the myriad of bariatric surgery procedures that have been introduced into the field since 1978 and are discussed in this volume (for example laparoscopic adjustable gastric banding, sleeve gastrectomy, biliopancreatic diversion, duodenal switch, gastric plication), as well as the experimental approaches to bariatrics and type 2 diabetes management (e.g., direct hypothalamic stimulation or ablation [14], truncal vagotomy [15], electronic gastric stimulation [16], duodeno-jejunal bypass [17, 18], ileal transposition [19–21], endoluminal sleeves [22]).

All of these procedures, and more, are examples of metabolic surgery and in their entirety encompass this field. Let it be emphasized, therefore, that bariatric surgery has not transitioned into being metabolic surgery but that bariatric surgery and its offshoots are all, and have always been, part of the discipline of metabolic surgery. Awareness of this concept by bariatric surgeons was greatly enhanced by the prescient work of Scopinaro and Pories, who about 20 years ago showed normalization of blood glucose values after biliopancreatic diversion [23] and gastric bypass [24]. A 2004 meta-analysis clearly emphasized that bariatric operations were also metabolic surgery by resolving or mitigating type 2 diabetes, hyperlipidemia, and hypertension, generally as a function of percentage excess weight loss (Table 8.1) [25].

This volume is primarily concerned with the metabolic surgery procedures of bariatric surgery, which, in turn, have given rise to metabolic operations specifically designed to mitigate certain of the comorbidities of obesity, with or without weight loss, in particular type 2 diabetes. This chapter will, therefore, discuss the old and newly proposed mechanisms of action for these procedures, the specific neurologic networks and hormones involved, the energy metabolism of obesity, the involvement of inflammation, and the present and future outcomes for this acquired knowledge.

8.1 Mechanisms of Action

Traditionally, the weight loss achieved by bariatric surgery has been attributed to either a restriction of food intake or malabsorption of unrestricted oral consumption. This simplistic approach, of course, ignores the minimal weight loss success achieved by electronic stimulation procedures [2, 3, 16] that employ no overt restriction of eating or of absorption. In the final analysis, at the level of caloric absorption from the intestinal tract, all the common bariatric surgery procedures are restrictive. This principle is illustrated in Fig. 8.1a of the steps in ostensibly restrictive bariatric surgery and in Fig. 8.1b of the steps in ostensibly malabsorptive bariatric surgery. Caloric intake can be restricted by the inhibition of eating caused by a gastric balloon, a gastric band, a sleeve gastrectomy, or a gastric bypass. Caloric intake can be equally restricted by the insufficient intestinal absorptive surface available in the so-called malabsorptive procedures. Since the bariatric surgery operations, even those with the ultrashort common channels of a biliopancreatic diversion or duodenal switch, extremely rarely cause excessive weight loss,

Table 8.1 Summary findings Ref. [25]

	Gastric banding (%)	Gastroplasty (%)	Gastric bypass (%)	Biliopancreatic division/duodenal switch (%)	Total (%)
% excess weight loss	−47.45	−68.17	−61.56	−70.12	−61.23
Resolution type 2 diabetes	47.9	71.6	83.7	98.9	76.8
Resolution hyperlipidemia	58.9	73.6	96.9	99.1	79.3
Resolution hypertension	43.2	69.0	67.5	83.4	61.7

Buchwald et al. [25]

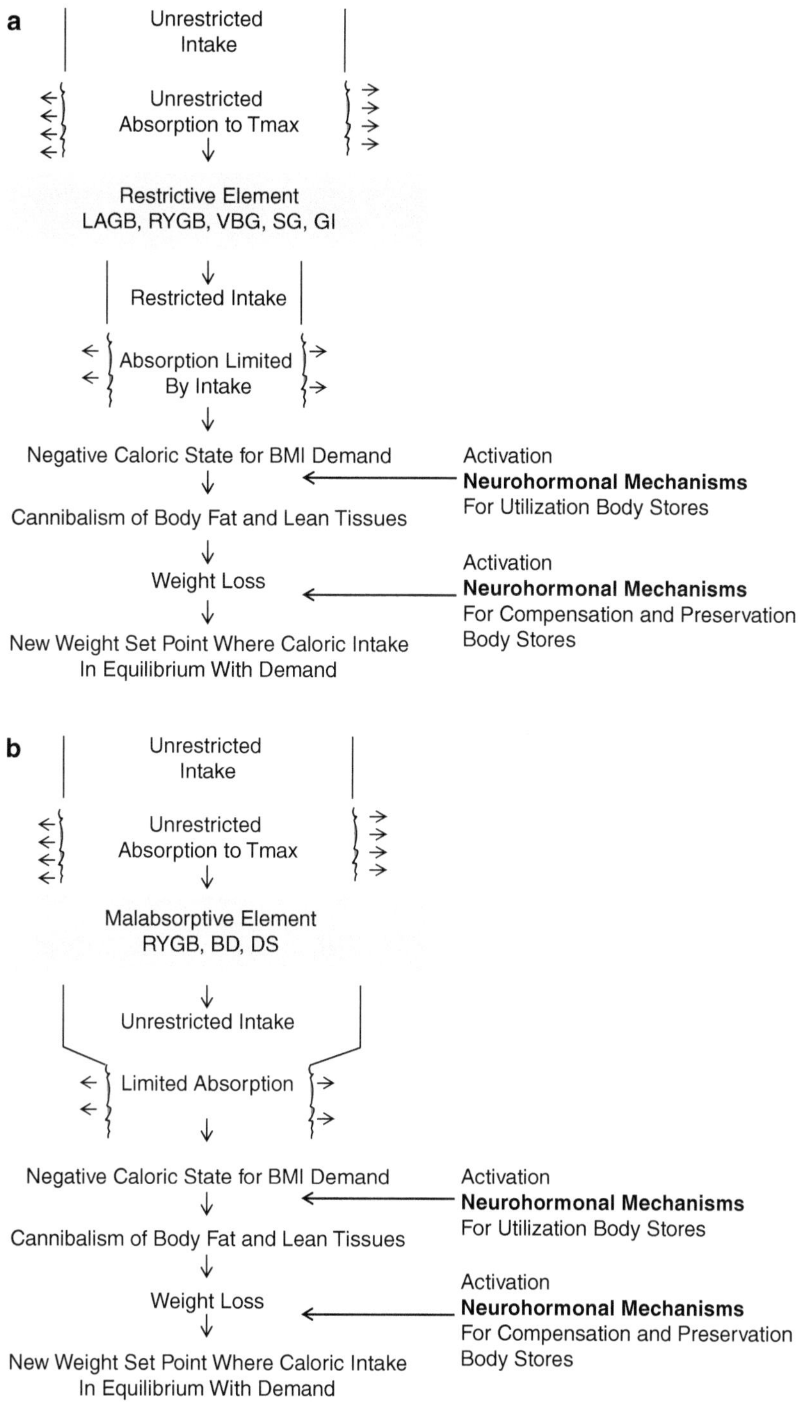

Fig. 8.1 Traditional explanatory mechanisms for bariatric operations: (**a**) Restrictive, (**b**) malabsorptive. Key: *LAGB* laparoscopic adjustable gastric band, *RYGB* Roux-en-Y gastric bypass, *VBG* vertical banded gastroplasty, *SG* sleeve gastrectomy, *GI* gastric imbrication, *BPD* biliopancreatic diversion, *DS* duodenal switch

there must be a brake effect in body metabolism not explainable by the old mechanisms of action concepts. Further, there are many nonobese, even lean, individuals who have undergone gastric or massive intestinal resections for various reasons and who subsequently maintained their body weight. It is time, therefore, in order to understand the changes we are eliciting by metabolic bariatric surgery, that we acknowledge that we do restrict the ability to eat and that we do restrict body caloric intake, but that we must look to more sophisticated explanations for the true mechanisms of action of these procedures. We need to investigate the complex neurohormonal networks that control weight, certain weight-related diseases, and the disease of obesity itself.

8.1.1 Neural Networks

There exists vigorous parasympathetic and sympathetic innervation to the intestinal tract. Old and extensive teaching of vagal nerve function concentrated on efferent stimulation of acid/pepsinogen secretion by the stomach, control of bile production and gallbladder function, and output of pancreatic exocrine enzymes [26, 27]. However, only 10–20 % of vagal fibers are efferent; 80 % or more are afferent. We know that these afferent connections go to the brain, primarily to the hypothalamus and medulla oblongata [28]. These fibers are intimately associated with hypothalamic functional centers related to hunger, appetite (post-hunger satisfaction eating behavior), and satiety [29]. Prosthetic gastric volume restrictors, gastric imbrication, adjustable gastric bands, Roux-en-Y gastric bypass, biliopancreatic diversion/duodenal switch, and simple sleeve gastrectomy, as well as the experimental procedures of gastric and vagal stimulation, duodeno-jejunal bypass, and endoluminal sleeves, all influence vagal, in particular afferent vagal, nerve function.

Sympathetic gut innervation is primarily mediated via the celiac plexus. Efferent sympathetic fibers are involved in glucose production and release, inhibition of gastrointestinal enzymes, and inhibition of peristalsis [30]; afferent sympathetic fibers are traceable to cerebral pain receptors. Roux-en-Y gastric bypass, biliopancreatic diversion/duodenal switch, and certain of the other metabolic/bariatric procedures, can be expected to induce a sympathetic neurologic response.

There is also an intrinsic nerve syncytium, primarily in the submucosal layer of the intestinal tract, extending from the esophagus to the anus [31] (Fig. 8.2). Surely, this network is altered by many of the metabolic/bariatric operations, for example, Roux-en-Y gastric bypass, biliopancreatic diversion/duodenal switch, and ileal transposition. The density of the submucosal neural fibers has been demonstrated to be an indicator of type 2 diabetes severity [32]. Finally, with respect to the participation of intestinal neurogenic pathways in the mechanisms of action of the metabolic/bariatric operations, there exists the high fundic gastric pacemaker [33], which is disconnected by a Roux-en-Y gastric bypass and biliopancreatic diversion, and totally extirpated by sleeve gastrectomy and duodenal switch.

8.1.2 Gut and Fat Derived Hormones

Complementing the neural network in influencing weight and obesity control mechanisms, as well as intimately involved in the obesity comorbidity of type 2 diabetes, are the gut and the fat derived hormones. Over the course of time, more and more individual intestinally and fat secreted hormones have and are being identified. Currently, there are about 100 of these unique peptides and they each have one or several functions [34]. Due to the concentrated efforts of dedicated investigators, the role and significance of specific gut hormones in the responsible mechanisms for the metabolic/bariatric procedures have been emphasized. Over time, the popularity of these individual hormones has risen and fallen, and possibly risen again. The true importance of each documented hormone in obesity and type 2 diabetes is as yet not pre-

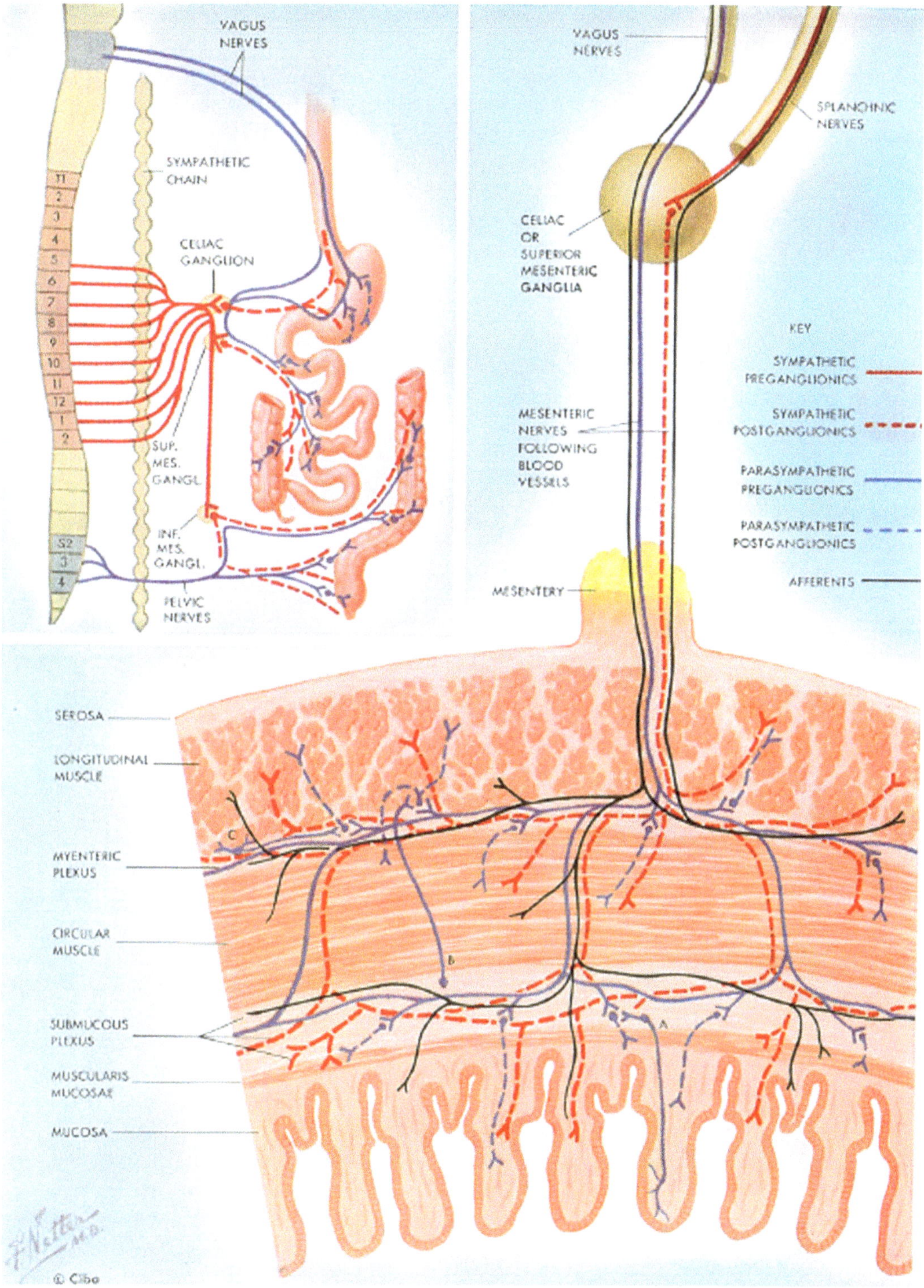

Fig. 8.2 Vagal and sympathetic innervation of the stomach and intestine; intestinal wall nerve syncytium (Reprinted from Netter [31], with permission from Elsevier)

cise. It is also likely that mechanisms of action are never dependent on a single hormone but rather on a mosaic of hormonal interactions. It is, therefore, pertinent to review the actions and properties of certain of the better understood hormones. Primary interest by metabolic/bariatric surgeons on hormonal mechanisms has focused on glucagon-like peptide-1 (GLP-1), peptide YY (PYY), leptin, ghrelin, and glucose-dependent insulinotropic peptide (formerly gastric inhibitory peptide) (GIP).

GLP-1 and PYY are both elaborated by the L-cells of the intestinal mucosa and seem to work in concert, eliciting the same metabolic responses or augmenting the actions of the other. Their gastrointestinal properties include the reduction of hunger and an increase in the sensation of satiety, resulting from stimulation of the arcuate nucleus of the hypothalamus [35–37]. They are also responsible for the "ileal brake" effect of delayed gastric emptying, delayed mouth-to-cecum transit time, and decreased jejunal wave pressure [38–40]. Regarding pancreatic endocrine function, GLP-1 and PYY contribute significantly to the incretin effect, defined as the concentration of insulin release by oral glucose stimulation that exceeds the insulin concentration elicited by the same amount of intravenous glucose [41]. The influence of GLP-1 on pancreatic endocrine function is direct and appears to be more powerful than that of PYY. GLP-1 stimulates glucose-dependent insulin secretion, preinsulin gene expression, β-cell proliferation and antiapoptotic pathways, and inhibits glucagon release [42, 43]. It has been shown that GLP-1 secretion is reduced in patients with type 2 diabetes [44, 45], which may be responsible for the hyperglycemia of this disease [46]. The PYY effect on insulin secretion is indirect by inhibiting the action of gastrin-stimulating peptide and gastrin-releasing peptide [47, 48].

It is interesting that PYY exhibits two active circulating forms: PYY (1-36) and PYY (3-36). PYY (1-36) increases appetite and promotes weight gain, and is not the PYY hormone that interests metabolic/bariatric surgeons. PYY (3-36) is the form cited in metabolic mechanisms literature and is responsible for centrally decreasing appetite and promoting weight loss [49–53]. PYY (3-36) also inhibits pentagastrine-stimulated gastric acid secretion [54] and the cephalic phase of pancreatic exocrine secretion [55, 56].

Both GLP-1 and PYY are secreted in increasing amounts as a function of the caloric content of ingested food [57]. Other influencing factors include the intestinal site of stimulation [58–60], bile acids [61], central neural and vagal mechanisms [62–64], and other hormones (vasoactive intestinal peptide [65], gastrin [66]). Leptin forms a triad with GLP-1 and PYY in weight regulating mechanisms, possibly providing for an autoregulatory feedback loop. Leptin stimulates GLP-1 secretion and GLP-1 suppresses leptin levels [67].

Leptin, a peptide hormone synthesized and released by adipocytes, has been implicated, by its action on mediobasal hypothalamic receptors, in maintaining a body weight set point [68–70]. When fat mass falls, plasma leptin levels fall as well, stimulating appetite and suppressing energy expenditure; when fat mass increases, plasma leptin levels increase, suppressing appetite and increasing energy expenditure [71–73]. Thus, apart from its reciprocal autoregulation mechanism with GLP-1, leptin's specific hypothalamic effect on suppressing eating is parallel to that of GLP-1. Leptin's relationship to obesity, however, is far from clear cut. Much of the leptin physiologic data were derived from rodent models and have not been equivalently substantiated in humans. Obese individuals generally have a high, not low, circulating concentration of leptin [73] and are stated to be leptin-resistant [71]. It is apparent, therefore, that the normal leptin feedback control in obese humans is flawed.

In addition to its action on the circulatory system, lung surfactant activity, bone, reproduction, and areas of the brain not involved in weight regulation, leptin is an inflammatory marker responding specifically to adipose-derived cytokines [74–77]. Increases in leptin levels in response to overeating may, therefore, play a role in inflammation-related diseases, including not only obesity but diabetes, hypertension, and cardiovascular disease.

Ghrelin is a peptide hormone produced by P/D1 cells in the fundus of the stomach and the episilon cells of the pancreas [78]. There are ghrelin receptors in the pituitary, stomach, intestine, pancreas, thymus, gonads, and heart [79]. Some of ghrelin's actions may be due to its potent stimulation of growth hormone secretion from the anterior pituitary [80]. Most interestingly, ghrelin selectively reduces mechanosensitivity of upper gastrointestinal vagal afferents [81]. Ghrelin's actions are in opposition to those of leptin: it increases hunger and eating [82, 83]. Circulating ghrelin levels are the highest before a meal and at their lowest thereafter [84]. Intravenously administered ghrelin increases food intake in a dose-dependent manner [85]. However, plasma ghrelin levels in the obese are lower than in lean individuals [86], suggesting that ghrelin does not contribute to obesity. An exception is Prader–Willi Syndrome where ghrelin levels are high [87, 88]. Ghrelin appears to be an anti-inflammatory hormone in opposition to the cytokine properties of leptin [89, 90].

GIP, secreted by the K-cells of the duodenum, along with GLP-1, is an incretin hormone [91]. In the past, it was believed that GIP neutralized and inhibited stomach acid, decreased gastric transit time, and retarded intestinal motility; however, recent information attributes these actions to secretin and not to physiologic levels of GIP. Thus, GIP is really not a gastric inhibitory hormone. It is now believed that the primary function of GIP is to induce insulin secretion via glucose hyperosmolarity in the duodenum [92]. Hence, a name change to glucose-dependent insulinotropic peptide, allowing for retention of the acronym "GIP." Type 2 diabetics are not responsive to GIP administration and have lower postprandial levels of GIP secretion compared to nondiabetics [93].

As our knowledge base evolves, other hormones will arouse interest and controversy with respect to their effects on normal body weight, obesity, type 2 diabetes, and other comorbidities of obesity. At present, attention is being paid to pancreatic polypeptide, cholecystokinin, oxyntomodulin, and adipose-derived adiponectin and resistin.

8.2 Energy Metabolism of Obesity

Having defined metabolic surgery, we should now more closely examine the energy metabolism of obesity, the primary working domain of metabolic/bariatric surgery. Past knowledge of obesity causation and mechanisms of action focused on genetics and energy balance [94, 95]. The genetics of obesity is not truly a subject to be covered under metabolic surgery or metabolics; however, energy balance is appropriately considered under metabolic mechanisms.

Total body metabolic processes in kinetic terms can be defined as total energy expenditure (TEE), which is equal to the basal metabolic rate (BMR), the energy of activity expenditure, the thermal effect of food (TEF), and adaptive thermogenesis (AT). The BMR is the lowest level of energy needed to maintain life (e.g., autonomic cardiorespiratory functions). The TEF is the body heat produced and the AT is the fluctuation in TEF produced by environmental temperature and humidity [95]. The homeostatic responses to increased food intake in normal individuals essentially is an attempt to resist weight gain; whereas, in obese individuals these mechanisms appear to be blunted resulting in a decrease in the TEF and a subsequent decrease in the TEE [96].

The nature of energy metabolism after metabolic/bariatric surgery has not been extensively studied and is not well understood. The preoperative TEE of patients undergoing gastric bypass can vary from normal to hypermetabolic. In the former, there appears to be no change postoperatively; in the latter, normalization of TEE seems to occur postoperatively [97]. Further, preservation of energy economy is reciprocal to the degree of weight loss [98]. After gastric bypass, both TEE and resting energy expenditure are decreased by about 25 % [99].

8.3 Inflammation

Currently, underlying causative mechanisms for obesity and type 2 diabetes are often focused on the state of inflammation. An increase in energy (caloric) intake over energy expenditure leads to an increase in the size of the adipocytes. Once the adipocyte volume exceeds 1 μl of lipid, the number of fat cells increases. The ensuing leptin response in non-obese individuals reduces hunger and downregulates caloric intake. In the obese, with a blunted leptin response [71], the unchecked caloric load overtaxes the adipocytes' ability to grow larger or increase in number resulting in a state of inflammation at the cellular level and ectopic fat storage in internal organs, including the liver and muscle [76]. In addition, the consumption of high volumes of fructose, absent in our ancestral diets, has been suggested to cause leptin resistance and elevated triglycerides, which result in weight gain [72, 100, 101] and a state of generalized inflammation.

The inflammation rationale carries over to obesity-induced type 2 diabetes. The increased fat cell mass results in an increase in free fatty acids, which, in turn, reduce glucose utilization by the liver and peripheral tissues, thereby reducing insulin clearance by the liver and increasing insulin delivery to the periphery, resulting in peripheral insulin resistance. Adipocyte-secreted cytokines contribute to the inflammatory state as well. The reactive oxygen species engendered by the inflammatory process are then responsible for endothelial damage, impaired beta cell function and, in general, play a cardinal role in the long-term complications of type 2 diabetes [102].

Conclusion

The epidemics of obesity and the obesity comorbidities, in particular type 2 diabetes, remain unchecked. Indeed, they have become global pandemics. The nonsurgical community has failed to treat effectively or to prevent these metabolic diseases. It is even more disturbing, that this body of individuals, who literally control the world's research resources, have not advanced scientifically cohesive, noncontradictory theories of causation that would allow for rational and successful therapeutic interventions. In contrast, metabolic/bariatric surgery has proven to be highly efficacious in treating obesity and its comorbidities. Metabolic/bariatric surgery today resolves upwards of 75 % of morbid obesity and super obesity, and does likewise for the obesity comorbidities. Our surgical tools, in contrast to unifocal pharmaceuticals, are more complex and multifaceted in what they engender in the neurohormonal mechanisms of the diseases of the metabolic syndrome. We are, however, learning to unravel the consequences of our operations, what metabolic parameters they influence, and what hormonal and inflammatory processes they alter. With this knowledge, we can eventually not only learn how our current procedures actually work but how to modify them and plan future procedures based on sound insights and experimental data. In addition, our gained understanding may allow us to help in the development of nonsurgical therapies. Over 200,000 new patients receive metabolic/bariatric operations annually. These individuals need to become our co-investigators in human basic science research. We must view metabolic surgery not as a compilation of operations but as a means to unravel the etiology of obesity and, in particular, its comorbidity type 2 diabetes. In the final analysis, metabolic surgery is cognitive surgery.

References

1. Buchwald H, Varco RL, editors. Metabolic surgery. New York: Grune & Stratton Inc; 1978.
2. Bohdjalian A, Prager G, Aviv R, et al. One-year experience with Tantalus: a new surgical approach to treat morbid obesity. Obes Surg. 2006;16:627–34.
3. Shikora S, Toouli J, Herrera MF, et al. Vagal blocking improves glycemic control and elevated blood pressure in obese subjects with type 2 diabetes mellitus. J Obes. 2013. doi:10.1155/2013/245683.
4. Khawaled R, Blumen G, Fabricant G, Ben-Arie J, Shikora S. Intestinal electrical stimulation decreases postprandial blood glucose levels in rats. Surg Obes Relat Dis. 2009;5:692–7.
5. Mahfoud F, Schlaich M, Kindermann I, et al. Effect of renal sympathetic denervation on glucose metabolism in patients with resistant hypertension: a pilot study. Circulation. 2011;123:1940–6.
6. Sener A, Cooper M, Bartlett ST. Is there a role for pancreas transplantation in type 2 diabetes mellitus? Transplantation. 2010;90:121–3.

7. Echeverri GJ. Type 2 diabetes mellitus: metabolic surgery and gastric submucosal islet transplantation, is there a connection? Transplantation. 2010;90:1036.
8. McBryde FD, Ap A, Hendy EB, et al. The carotid body as a putative therapeutic target for the treatment of neurogenic hypertension. Nat Commun. 2013;4:2395. doi:10.1038/ncomms3395.
9. Mayberg HS, Lozano AM, Voon V, McNeely HE, et al. Deep brain stimulation for treatment-resistant depression. Neuron. 2005;45:651–60.
10. Yuan W, Williams B. Long-term vagus nerve stimulation for severe refractory depression: a case study with a six-year follow-up. J Neuropsychiatry Clin Neurosci. 2012;24(4):E50–1.
11. Ge Y, Hu W, Zhang J, Meng F. Brain stimulation for treatment of refractory epilepsy. Chin Med J. 2013;126:3364–70.
12. Onofrio BM, Yaksh TL, Arnold PG. Continuous low-dose intrathecal morphine administration in the treatment of chronic pain of malignant origin. Mayo Clin Proc. 1981;56:516–20.
13. Rupp WM, Barbosa JJ, Blackshear PJ, et al. The use of an implantable insulin pump in the treatment of Type II diabetes. N Engl J Med. 1982;307:265–70.
14. Quaade F, Vaernet K, Larsson S. Stereotaxic stimulation and electrocoagulation of the lateral hypothalamus in obese humans. Acta Neurochir. 1974;30:111–7.
15. Kral JG. Vagotomy for treatment of severe obesity. Lancet. 1978;311:307–8.
16. Cigaina V, Pinato GP, Rigo V, et al. Gastric peristalsis control by *mono situ* electrical stimulation: a preliminary study. Obes Surg. 1996;6:247–9.
17. Klein S, Fabbrini E, Patterson BW, et al. Moderate effect of duodenal-jejunal bypass surgery on glucose homeostasis in patients with type 2 diabetes. Obesity. 2012;20:1266–72.
18. Cohen R, Caravatto PP, Correa JL, et al. Glycemic control after stomach-sparing duodenal-jejunal bypass surgery in diabetic patients with low body mass index. Surg Obes Relat Dis. 2012;8:375–80.
19. Mason EE. Ilial transposition and enteroglucagon/GLP-1 in obesity (and diabetic?) surgery. Obes Surg. 1999;9:223–8.
20. Gagner M. Surgical treatment of nonseverely obese patients with type 2 diabetes mellitus: sleeve gastrectomy with ileal transposition (SGIT) is the same as the neuroendocrine brake (NEB) procedure or ileal interposition associated with sleeve gastrectomy (II-SG), but ileal interposition with diverted sleeve gastrectomy (II-DSG) is the same as duodenal switch. Surg Endosc. 2001;25:655–6.
21. DePaula AL, Stival AR, DePaula CC, Halpern A, Vencio S. Surgical treatment of type 2 diabetes in patients with BMI below 35: mid-term outcomes of the laparoscopic ileal interposition associated with a sleeve gastrectomy in 202 consecutive cases. J Gastrointest Surg. 2012;16:967–76.
22. Rodriguez-Grunert L, Galvao Neto MP, Alamo M, Ramos AC, Baez PB, Tarnoff M. First human experience with endoscopically delivered and retrieved duodenal-jejunal bypass sleeve. Surg Obes Relat Dis. 2008;4:55–9.
23. Scopinaro N, Adami GF, Marinari GM, et al. Biliopancreatic diversion. World J Surg. 1998;22:936–46.
24. Pories WJ, Swanson MS, MacDonald KG, et al. Who would have thought it? An operation proves to be the most effective therapy for adult-onset diabetes mellitus. Ann Surg. 1995;222:339–52.
25. Buchwald H, Avidor Y, Braunwald E, et al. Bariatric Surgery: a systematic review and meta-analysis. JAMA. 2004;292:1724–37.
26. Gershon MD. Enteric nervous system: neural connections, neurotransmitters, and the function of 5-hydroxytryptamine. In: Kamm MA, Lennard-Jones JE, editors. Gastrointestinal transit, pathophysiology and pharmacology. Petersfield/Hampshire: Wrightson Biomedical Publishing Ltd; 1991. p. 21–32.
27. Brodal P. The cranial nerves, the vagus nerve. In: The central nervous system: structure and function. Oxford/New York: Oxford University Press; 2004. p. 355–6.
28. Brierley SM, Hughes P, Harrington A, Blackshaw LA. Innervation of the gastrointestinal tract by spinal and vagal afferent nerves. In: Johnson LR, Ghishan FK, Kaunitz JD, Merchant JL, Said HM, Wood JD, editors. Physiology of the gastrointestinal tract, vol. 1. 5th ed. San Diego: Elsevier Inc.; 2012. p. 703–31.
29. Johnson LR. Regulation of food intake. In: Johnson LR, editor. Gastrointestinal physiology. 7th ed. Philadelphia: Mosby/Elsevier; 2000. p. 137–42.
30. Brodal P. The peripheral autonomic nervous system, effects of sympathetic fibers in the gastrointestinal tract. In: The central nervous system: structure and function. Oxford/New York: Oxford University Press; 2004. p. 385–6.
31. Netter FH. The CIBA collection of medical illustrations. In: Nervous system, vol. 1. Summit: CIBA; 1962. p. 95.
32. Selim MM, Wendelschafer-Crabb MS, Redmon JB, et al. Gastric mucosal nerve density: a biomarker for diabetic autonomic neuropathy? Neurology. 2010;75:973–81.
33. Sanders KM, Koh SD, Ward SM. Organization and electrophysiology of interstitial cells of cajal and smooth muscle cells in the gastrointestinal tract. In: Johnson LR, Ghishan FK, Kaunitz JD, Merchant JL, Said HM, Wood JD, editors. Physiology of the gastrointestinal tract, vol. 1. 5th ed. San Diego: Elsevier Inc.; 2012. p. 511–56.
34. Berthoud HR, Shin AC, Zhen H. Obesity surgery and gut-brain communication. Physiol Behav. 2011;105:106–19.
35. Hernandez EJ, Whitcomb DC, Vigna SR, Taylor IL. Saturable binding of circulating peptide YY in the dorsal vagal complex of rats. Am J Physiol Gastrointest Liver Physiol. 1994;226:G511–6.
36. Druce MR, Small CJ, Bloom SR. Minireview: gut peptides regulating satiety. Endocrinology. 2004;145:2660–5.

37. Korner J, Leibel RL. To eat or not to eat – how the gut talks to the brain. N Engl J Med. 2003;349:926–8.
38. Savage AP, Adrian TE, Carolan G, Chatterjee VK, Bloom SR. Effects of peptide YY (PYY) on mouth to caecum intestinal transit time and on the rate of gastric emptying in healthy volunteers. Gut. 1987;28:166–70.
39. Spiller RC, Trotman IF, Adrian TE, et al. Further characterization of the 'ileal brake' reflex in man – effect of ileal infusion of partial digests of fat, protein, and starch on jejunal motility and release of neurotensin, enteroglucagon, and peptide YY. Gut. 1988;29:1042–51.
40. Spiller RC, Trotman IF, Higgins BE, et al. The ileal brake–inhibition of jejunal motility after ileal fat perfusion in man. Gut. 1984;25:365–74.
41. Tolhurst G, Reimann F, Gribble FM. Nutritional regulation of glucagon-like peptide-1 secretion. J Physiol. 2009;587:27–32.
42. Lim GE, Brubaker PL. Glucagon-like peptide 1 secretion by the L-cell. The view from within. Diabetes. 2006;55:S70–7.
43. Drucker DJ. The biology of incretin hormones. Cell Metab. 2006;3:153–65.
44. Toft-Nielsen MB, Damholt MB, Madsbad S, et al. Determinants of the impaired secretin of glucagon-like peptide-1 in type 2 diabetic patients. J Clin Endocrinol Metab. 2001;86:3717–23.
45. Mannucci E, Ognibene A, Cremasco F, et al. Glucagon-like peptide (GLP)-1 and leptin concentrations in obese patients with type 2 diabetes mellitus. Diabet Med. 2000;17:713–9.
46. Nauck M, Stockmann F, Ebert R, Creutzfeldt W. Reduced incretin effect in type 2 (non-insulin-dependent) diabetes. Diabetologia. 1986;29:46–52.
47. Lius F, Salva JA, Thompson JC. Peptide YY inhibits the insulinotropic action of gastric inhibitory polypeptide. Gastroenterology. 1989;96:690–4.
48. Guo YS, Singh P, DeBouno JF, Thompson JC. Effect of peptide YY on insulin release stimulated by 2-deoxyglucose and neuropeptides in dogs. Pancreas. 1988;3:128–34.
49. Ballantyne GH. Peptide YY(1-36) and peptide (YY(3-36): part I. Distribution, release and actions. Obes Surg. 2006;16:651–8.
50. Sileno AP, Brandt GC, Spann BM, Quay SC. Lower mean weight after 14 days intravenous administration peptide YY(3-36) (PYY(3-36)) in rabbits. Int J Obes. 2006;30:68–72.
51. Batterham RL, Cowley MA, Small CJ, et al. Gut hormone PYY(3-36) physiologically inhibits food intake. Nature. 2002;418:650–4.
52. Batterham RL, Cohen MA, Ellis SM, et al. Inhibition of food intake in obese subjects by peptide YY3-36. N Engl J Med. 2003;349:941–8.
53. Neary NM, Small CJ, Druce MR, et al. Peptide YY3-36 and glucagon-like peptide-17-36 inhibit food intake additively. Endocrinology. 2005;146:5120–7.
54. Adrian TE, Savage AP, Sagor GR, et al. Effect of peptide YY on gastric, pancreatic, and biliary function in humans. Gastroenterology. 1985;89:484–9.
55. Lluis F, Gomez G, Fujimura M, Greeley Jr GH, Thompson JC. Peptide YY inhibits nutrient-, hormonal-, and vagally-stimulated pancreatic exocrine secretion. Pancreas. 1987;2:454–62.
56. Hosotani R, Inoue K, Kogire M, et al. Effect of natural peptide YY on pancreatic secretion and cholecystokinin release in conscious dogs. Dig Dis Sci. 1989;34:468–73.
57. Adrian TE, Ferre G-L, Bacarese-Hamilton AJ, Fuessl HS, Polak JM, Bloom SR. Human distribution and release of a putative new gut hormone, peptide YY. Gastroenterology. 1985;89:1070–7.
58. Greeley Jr GH, Hashimoto T, Izukura M, et al. A comparison of intraduodenally and intracolonically administered nutrients on the release of peptide-YY in the dog. Endocrinology. 1989;125:1761–5.
59. Zhang T, Brubaker PL, Thompson JC, Greeley Jr GH. Characterization of peptide-YY release in response to intracolonic infusion of amino acids. Endocrinology. 1993;132:553–7.
60. Aponte GW, Fink AS, Meyer JH, Tatemoto K, Taylor IL. Regional distribution and release of peptide YY with fatty acids of different chain length. Am J Physiol. 1985;249:G745–50.
61. Adrian TE, Ballantyne GH, Longo WE, et al. Deoxycholate is an important releaser of peptide YY and enteroglucagon from the human colon. Gut. 1993;34:1219–24.
62. Onaga T, Zabielski R, Kato S. Multiple regulation of peptide YY secretion in the digestive tract. Peptides. 2002;23:279–90.
63. Zhang T, Uchida T, Gomez G, Lluis F, Thompson JC, Greeley Jr GH. Neural regulation of peptide YY secretion. Regul Pept. 1993;48:321–8.
64. Rudnicki M, Rigel DF, McFadden DW. Vagal cooling blocks circulating neuropeptide Y (NPY), peptide YY (PYY), and pancreatic polypeptide (PP) release. J Surg Res. 1991;51:40–5.
65. Ballantyne GH, Goldenring JR, Savoca PE, et al. Cyclic AMP-mediated release of peptide YY (PYY) from the isolated perfused rabbit distal colon. Regul Pept. 1993;47:117–26.
66. Greeley Jr GH, Jeng YJ, Gomez G, et al. Evidence for regulation of peptide-YY release by the proximal gut. Endocrinology. 1989;124:1438–43.
67. Anini Y, Brubaker PL. Role of leptin in the regulation of glucagon-like peptide-1 secretion. Diabetes. 2003;52:252–9.
68. Williams KW, Scott MM, Elmquist JK. From observation to experimentation: leptin action in the mediobasal hypothalamus. Am J Clin Nutr. 2009;89:9855–905.
69. Ahima RS, Flier JS. Leptin. Annu Rev Physiol. 2000;62:413–37.
70. Considine RV, Considine EL, Williams CJ, Hyde TM, Caro JF. The hypothalamic leptin receptor in humans: identification of incidental sequence polymorphisms and absence of the db/db mouse and fa/fa rat mutations. Diabetes. 1996;45:992–4.
71. Friedman JM. Leptin at 14 y of age: an ongoing story. Am J Clin Nutr. 2009;89:973S–9.

72. Ahima RS. Revisiting leptin's role in obesity and weight loss. J Clin Invest. 2008;118:2380–3.
73. Sinha MK, Opentanova I, Ohannesian JP, et al. Evidence of free and bound leptin in human circulation. Studies in lean and obese subjects and during short-term fasting. J Clin Invest. 1996;98:1277–82.
74. Fantuzzi G, Faggioni R. Leptin in the regulation of immunity, inflammation, and hematopoiesis. J Leukocyte Biol. 2000;68:437–46.
75. Perrier S, Caldefie-Chézet F, Vasson MP. IL-1 family in breast cancer: potential interplay with leptin and other adipocytokines. FEBS Lett. 2009;583:259–65.
76. Wabitsch M, Jensen PB, Blum WF, et al. Insulin and cortisol promote leptin production in cultured human fat cells. Diabetes. 1996;45:1435–8.
77. LaPensee CR, Hugo ER, Ben-Jonathan N. Insulin stimulates interleukin-6 expression and release in LS14 human adipocytes through multiple signaling pathways. Endocrinology. 2008;149:5415–22.
78. Inui A, Asakawa A, Bowers CY, et al. Ghrelin, appetite, and gastric motility: the emerging role of the stomach as an endocrine organ. FASEB J. 2004;18:439–56.
79. Howard AD, Feighner SD, Cully DF, et al. A receptor in pituitary and hypothalamus that functions in growth hormone release. Science. 1996;273:974–7.
80. Kojima M, Hosoda H, Date Y, Nakazato M, Matsuo H, Kangawa K. Ghrelin is a growth-hormone-releasing acylated peptide from stomach. Nature. 1999;402:656–60.
81. Page AJ, Slattery JA, Milte C, et al. Ghrelin selectively reduces mechanosensitivity of upper gastrointestinal vagal afferents. Am J Physiol Gastrointest Liver Physiol. 2007;292:G1376–84.
82. Lall S, Tung LY, Ohlsson C, Jansson JO, Dickson SL. Growth hormone (GH)-independent stimulation of adiposity by GH secretagogues. Biochem Biophys Res Commun. 2001;280:132–1138.
83. Tschöp M, Smiley DL, Heiman ML. Ghrelin induces adiposity in rodents. Nature. 2000;407:908–13.
84. Cummings DE, Frayo RS, Marmonier C, Aubert R, Chapelot D. Plasma ghrelin levels and hunger scores in humans initiating meals voluntarily without time- and food-related cues. Am J Physiol Endocrinol Metab. 2004;287:E297–304.
85. Wren AM, Small CJ, Ward HL, et al. The novel hypothalamic peptide ghrelin stimulates food intake and growth hormone secretion. Endocrinology. 2000;141:4325–8.
86. Cummings DE, Weigle DS, Frayo RS, et al. Plasma ghrelin levels after diet-induced weight loss or gastric bypass surgery. N Engl J Med. 2002;346:1623–30.
87. Goldstone AP, Thomas EL, Brynes AE, et al. Elevated fasting plasma ghrelin in prader-willi syndrome adults is not solely explained by their reduced visceral adiposity and insulin resistance. J Clin Endocrinol Metab. 2004;89:1718–26.
88. DelParigi A, Tschöp M, Heiman ML, et al. High circulating ghrelin: a potential cause for hyperphagia and obesity in prader-willi syndrome. J Clin Endocrinol Metab. 2002;87:5461–4.
89. Waseem T, Duxbury M, Ito H, et al. Ghrelin ameliorates TNF-a induced anti-proliferative and pro-apoptotic effects and promotes intestinal epithelial restitution. J Am Coll Surg. 2004;199(3 Suppl):16. doi:10.1016/j.jamcollsurg.2004.05.018.
90. Waseem T, Duxbury M, Ito H, Ashley SW, Robinson MK. Eogenous ghrelin modulates release of pro- and anti-inflammatory cytokines in LPS-stimulated macrophages through distinct signaling pathways. Surgery. 2008;143:334–42.
91. Meier JJ, Nauck MA. Glucagon-like peptide 1(GLP-1) in biology and pathology. Diabetes Metab Res Rev. 2005;21:91–117.
92. Thorens B. Glucagon-like peptide-1 and control of insulin secretion. Diabetes Metab. 1995;21:311–8.
93. Skrha J, Hilgertová J, Jarolímková M, Kunešová M, Hill M. Meal test for glucose-dependent insulinotropic peptide (GIP) in obese and type 2 diabetic patients. Physiol Res. 2010;59:749–55.
94. Lakka H-M, Bouchard C. Etiology of obesity. In: Buchwald H, Cowan GSM, Pories WJ, editors. Surgical management of obesity. Philadelphia: Elsevier; 2007. p. p18–28.
95. Ikramuddin S. Energy metabolism and biochemistry of obesity. In: Buchwald H, Cowan GSM, Pories WJ, editors. Surgical management of obesity. Philadelphia: Elsevier; 2007. p. 29–33.
96. Leibel RL, Rosenbaum M, Hirsch J. Changes in energy expenditure resulting from altered body weight. N Engl J Med. 1995;332:621–8.
97. Flancbaum L, Choban PS, Bradley LR, et al. Changes in measured resting energy expenditure after Roux-en-Y gastric bypass for clinicall severe obesity. Surgery. 1997;122:943–9.
98. Bobbioni-Harsch E, Morel P, Huber O, et al. Energy economy hampers body weight loss after gastric bypass. J Clin Endocrinol Metab. 2000;85:4695–700.
99. Das SK, Robert SB, McCrory MA, et al. Long-term changes in energy expenditure and body composition after massive weight loss induced by gastric bypass surgery. Am J Clin Nutr. 2003;78:22–30.
100. Shapiro A, Mu W, Roncal C, Cheng KY, Johnson RJ, Scarpace PJ. Fructose-induced leptin resistance exacerbates weight gain in response to subsequent high-fat feeding. Am J Physiol Regul Integr Comp Physiol. 2008;295:R1370–5.
101. Obici S, Rossetti L. Minireview: nutrient sensing and the regulation of insulin action and energy balance. Endocrinology. 2003;144:5172–8.
102. Boden G. Lipids and glucose in type 2 diabetes: what is the cause and effect? Diabetes Care. 2004;27:2253–9.

Diabetes Surgery

9

Francesco Rubino

9.1 Introduction

Bariatric surgery was originally designed to induce weight-reduction in morbidly obese patients. Benefits of bariatric surgery, however, extend well beyond weight loss and include dramatic improvement of type 2 diabetes, hypertension, dyslipidaemia and reduction of overall mortality. Studies in rodents and humans have shown that the anti-diabetes effects of certain bariatric procedures are not just secondary to weight loss and result from a variety of neuroendocrine and metabolic mechanisms, which are direct consequence of changes in gastrointestinal (GI) anatomy [1]. This knowledge provides a rationale for the use of gastrointestinal surgery as both, a treatment of type 2 diabetes and a tool to elucidate the elusive pathophysiology of this disease [2].

The exact molecular mechanism of action of surgery on diabetes remains unknown, but changes in intestinal glucose metabolism, gut hormones, bile acids (BAs), microbiota and nutrient sensing have been suggested to play a role [3–9]. These physiologic mechanisms provide a rational target for the design of new surgical techniques, gastrointestinal devices and for novel pharmaceuticals.

The broad implications for the care of diabetes and the fascinating mechanisms of action of bariatric surgery have attracted the interest of physicians, scientists and policy makers. This has transformed, over the past decade, an underappreciated surgical specialty, practised by only a few, dedicated and passionate surgeons into one of the fastest growing areas of twenty-first-century medicine.

As a result of an intense, multidisciplinary research effort over the past 10-years, a substantial body of level-1 evidence has now accumulated showing that surgical treatment of type 2 diabetes controls hyperglycaemia and improves quality of life more than lifestyle modifications and available drugs [10–13]. Several professional organizations already recommend consideration of surgery in the management of obese type 2 diabetes [14], and it is plausible that a surgical or interventional approach to this disease will become increasingly popular in the years to come.

The implementation of a surgical approach to type 2 diabetes, however, poses numerous challenges. Consistent with the goals of improving glycaemic and metabolic control, not merely weight loss, a surgical approach to type 2 diabetes requires the development of a new model of care

F. Rubino, MD
Bariatric and Metabolic Surgery,
The James Black Centre, King's College London,
Denmark Hill Campus, 125 Coldharbour Lane,
London SE5 9NU, UK

King's College Hospital, London, UK

Catholic University of Rome, Rome, Italy
e-mail: Francesco.rubino@kcl.ac.uk

M. Lucchese, N. Scopinaro (eds.), *Minimally Invasive Bariatric and Metabolic Surgery: Principles and Technical Aspects*, DOI 10.1007/978-3-319-15356-8_9,

distinct from traditional bariatric surgery. Surgical treatment of T2DM in fact cannot be based on the weight-centric model of bariatric surgery and requires disease-based criteria for surgical indication, diagnostics and outcome measures. The shift in the primary aim of treatment, from obesity to type 2 diabetes, also has ramifications for the definition of research priorities and for health care policies. For all the aforementioned reasons, "diabetes surgery" needs to be considered as a new surgical discipline, contiguous but distinct from traditional bariatric surgery [15].

Despite the challenges ahead, diabetes surgery has the potential to revolutionize diabetes care at large and change the way we look at this disease. This chapter presents an overview of this new discipline, from historical aspects to future directions.

9.2 History of Diabetes Surgery: From Heretical Suggestion to Accepted Treatment Option

In 1925, a case report in *The Lancet* documented rapid resolution of diabetes as a serendipitous observation in a patient with peptic ulcer days after gastrectomy and gastrojejunostomy [16]. The author asked: "what can we account for the apparent improvement (of diabetes)? The glycosuria was absent after the operation in spite of a diet containing a fair amount of carbohydrate". Several other clinical observations of dramatic improvement of diabetes after partial or total gastrectomies were reported throughout the first half of the twentieth century [17, 18]. With the advent of bariatric surgery for morbid obesity in the late 1950s, similar modifications of GI anatomy started to be performed in subjects with morbid obesity, a population with high prevalence of type 2 diabetes; as a result, reports of surgically induced control of type 2 diabetes became increasingly common [19, 20]. Dramatic improvements or even resolution of diabetes symptoms were observed with almost all types of bariatric operations, including vertical banded gastroplasty, jejuno-ileal bypass, gastric bypass and biliopancreatic diversion [19–24]. Elegant reports by Pories and colleagues in the early 1990s provided detailed descriptions of the clinical remission of hyperglycaemia after gastric bypass surgery [22, 23], emphasizing both the magnitude and the rapidity of this effect. Scopinaro and co-workers reported resolution of hyperglycaemia and discontinuation of diabetes medication in over 90 % of diabetic patients undergoing biliopancreatic diversion [24].

Although clinical observations of post-surgery remission of hyperglycaemia were consistently reported for more than half a century, such remarkable phenomenon remained substantially unknown to the rest of the scientific community. Even after the advent of electronic consultation of medical literature, diabetes experts were largely unaware that a surgical operation on the alimentary tract could exert such a profound effect on the disease.

Many factors have likely acted as a barrier for the dissemination of this knowledge and for the consideration of surgery as a diabetes treatment. First, segmentation of medical specialties and lack of interdisciplinary communication, an increasing phenomenon in twentieth-century medicine, may have played a role. Also, the observation of resolution of hyperglycaemia challenged the traditional teaching that diabetes is an invariably chronic and progressive disease and things that cannot be explained are often looked with skepticism in medicine. On the other hand, the prevailing view that obesity leads to diabetes and that weight loss improves hyperglycaemia provided a straightforward explanation for the effect of bariatric surgery in morbidly obese patients; in this context, the improvement of diabetes after gastrointestinal surgery could not be seen as an incongruous observation to inspire new hypothesis. Furthermore, as an implicitly organ-focused intervention, surgery could not be seen as a rational solution for a systemic disease such as diabetes. Perhaps most importantly, for most of the twentieth-century, the gastrointestinal tract was regarded as merely a tube for digestion and absorption of nutrients; this means that the surgical control of diabetes by gastrointestinal surgery could only be interpreted as an indirect result of restriction of energy intake.

My personal interest for the subject started in July 1999. I was spending an afternoon in the library of Mount Sinai Medical Center in New York researching on matters of surgical anatomy and technique to see if it was possible to simplify some procedures and facilitate a laparoscopic approach. Accidentally, I came across a table in a paper that summarized results of 1-month postoperative laboratory tests after biliopancreatic diversion. The vast majority of patients had normal plasma glucose levels despite many of them were reported to be diabetic prior to surgery. Although metabolic outcomes were not the scope of my research, I was puzzled by the idea that patients with diabetes could have normal glucose levels without using glucose-lowering drugs: how could such a radical and rapid effect be explained by weight loss alone? Given the role of the GI tract in the regulation of glucose insulin secretion through the so-called entero-pancreatic axis, I hypothesized that the anti-diabetic effect of bariatric surgery may result from neuroendocrine and/or metabolic mechanisms secondary to the anatomic rearrangement of GI anatomy. I thought that if this were true, there would be two important implications: first, gastrointestinal surgery could be used to intentionally treat diabetes ("diabetes surgery"), not only in the morbidly obese. Second, the gastrointestinal tract could represent a valuable target for other forms of intervention and possibly even harbour mechanisms of disease in diabetes [2].

With the visionary support of my mentor at the time, Dr. Michel Gagner, we submitted a protocol for a randomized clinical trial (RCT) comparing Roux-en-Y gastric bypass versus medical therapy for patients with BMI <35 kg/m^2. Perhaps ahead of its time, this protocol did not receive the approval of the Institutional IRB. Frustrated, but conscious that offering a surgical approach to diabetes for non-morbidly obese patients was, in fact, "unthinkable" for the knowledge of the time, and indeed also concerning for a number of reasonable objections, we decided to share the idea with other researchers and to pursue other forms of investigation. In a review/hypothesis paper published in the *Annals of Surgery* in 2002 [2], we presented data from the medical literature documenting efficacy of gastrointestinal surgery, particularly gastric bypass and biliopancreatic diversion, in both obese and non-obese diabetic subjects. Accordingly, we suggested that GI surgery could be a legitimate intervention to intentionally treat diabetes ("diabetes surgery") and that the GI tract could be an ideal target for interventions of curative intent [2].

Unable to test the hypothesis in humans, I turned to animal experiments to investigate whether a rearrangement of gastrointestinal anatomy could per se improve diabetes. Experiments using a modified version of human gastric bypass (duodenal-jejunal bypass – DJB) in Goto-Kakizaki rats, a non-obese model of type 2 diabetes provided the first experimental evidence that gastrointestinal surgery can directly improve type 2 diabetes by weight-independent mechanisms [1]. Clinical case-reports and case-series showing improvement of diabetes by a variety of gastrointestinal operations in non-obese individuals provided further support for the weight-independent effects of surgery [25, 26].

The idea of diabetes surgery gained acceptance particularly after a landmark 2007 international consensus conference in Rome (the "Diabetes Surgery Summit" [DSS]), where a group of leading international scholars discussed available evidence and recommended, for the first time, consideration of gastrointestinal surgery for type 2 diabetes including in selected patients with moderate obesity (BMI 30–35) [27]. After the Rome's DSS, the concept of "metabolic surgery" has rapidly emerged to more broadly indicate a surgical approach aimed at treating diabetes and obesity. The DSS also encouraged further clinical and mechanistic research in metabolic surgery and was instrumental in attracting physicians, as well as clinical and basic scientists to this emerging discipline. This has contributed to raising standards of research and practice and to a phenomenal growth in knowledge that has perhaps no parallel in any other field of surgery.

Over the past few years, research by several independent investigators has corroborated the finding that gastrointestinal surgery can directly improve diabetes [28–30] suggesting that a variety of GI mechanisms, including changes in gut hormones, bile acids, gut microbiota, duodenal-jejunal nutrient sensing and intestinal glucose uptake can play a role in the control of diabetes and obesity by gastrointestinal surgery [3–9]. Furthermore, there has also been a substantial improvement of the quality and level of clinical evidence in this field. At the time of this writing, there are at least eight reports in the literature from randomized clinical trials, all consistently showing that bariatric procedures can improve diabetes more than drugs and lifestyle interventions at least 1- to 3-years after surgery [10–13, 31–34]. A number of well-conducted case-control studies have also documented that surgery can reduce cardiovascular disease (CVD) and death associated with diabetes [35–37].

This growing body of evidence has led several professional organizations to recognize the role of surgery in diabetes. In 2009, the American Diabetes Association introduced surgery for the first time in its "Standards of Medical Care for Diabetes" [38]. In 2011, a landmark position statement by the interventional Diabetes Federation [14], an umbrella organization representing over 200 national diabetes societies, recommended that surgical treatment be considered in the management algorithm of diabetes care and emphasized the need to go beyond weight-centric criteria for surgical indication. Many surgical organizations (i.e. ASMBS, IFSO) and diabetes organizations (IDF) today recommend that surgery be considered for patients with type 2 diabetes that is difficult to control by medical therapies or when associated with conditions that increase risks of cardiovascular disease. In 2014, the question is no longer if surgery should be considered a diabetes treatment but when it should be offered and who are the patients for whom access to this form of treatment should be prioritized.

Clearly, in little more than a decade, diabetes surgery has progressed from a sort of heretical suggestion to an accepted treatment option in selected patients.

9.3 Mechanisms of Action of Gastrointestinal Operations on Glucose Metabolism: The Physiologic Rational for Diabetes Surgery

9.3.1 Effects of Surgery on Pathophysiologic Aspects of Type 2 Diabetes

Examining the mechanisms by which surgery can improve diabetes may help understand the physiology and pathophysiology of diabetes and inform the choice of surgical procedure for the treatment of T2DM as well as the design of new operations, devices and pharmaceutical therapies. The pathophysiology of T2DM is characterized by a combination of insulin resistance and inadequate insulin secretion; treatments of curative intent would need to address both defects. Gastrointestinal (GI) bypass procedures can improve both insulin sensitivity and insulin production [39–42] suggesting that interventions on the GI tract represent a rational and physiologic approach for diabetes treatment [43]. In particular, Roux-en-Y gastric bypass (RYGB) restores first-phase insulin response and results in hyper secretion of C-peptide and insulin following nutrient ingestion suggesting enhancement of beta-cell function [40–43]. Increased beta-cell mass has also been hypothesized following reports of nesidioblastosis complicating RYGB [44], observations of increased PDX1 levels [45] and prevention of beta-cell loss after experimental duodenal-jejunal bypass in rodents [46], and increased beta-cell mass after RYGB in pigs [47].

9.3.2 Role of Gut Hormones

9.3.2.1 Ghrelin

Ghrelin is a hormone chiefly synthesized by the gastric antrum and fundus and involved in regulation of both hunger and glucose homeostasis [48]. With sleeve gastrectomy (SG), RYGB and BPD-duodenal switch (which includes a SG), ghrelin-synthesizing cells of the gastric fundus are either resected or excluded from nutrient contact, whereas the fundus remains intact after traditional BPD (Scopinaro's procedure) and laparoscopic adjustable gastric banding (LAGB). Ghrelin levels decrease maximally after SG. After RYGB and BPD, ghrelin levels tend to decrease but the changes are not as consistent as after SG [49–52]. In contrast with the effects of other operations, ghrelin levels are most commonly increased after LAGB [53–56].

9.3.2.2 PYY

PYY is a 36-amino acid compound released from L-type endocrine cells in the lower intestine. It exists in two forms: PYY1–36 (total) and PYY3–36 (active), with the latter being the most common circulating form [22]. PYY acts on the arcuate nucleus inhibiting appetite and promoting weight loss [57]. Physiologically, PYY levels increase immediately after meals – a response that is blunted in obese patients. Following diversionary procedures (i.e. RYGB, BPD) and to some extent after sleeve gastrectomy, postprandial PYY response is increased, possibly contributing to early satiety and overall restriction of food intake [58–60].

9.3.2.3 Glucagon-Like Peptide 1 (GLP1)

GLP1 is an incretin hormone released together with GLP 2, oxyntomodulin and PYY from intestinal L-cells, which are more common in the ileum and colon. GLP-1 potentiates glucose-stimulated insulin secretion, inhibits glucagon release and suppresses gastric emptying ("ileal brake") [61]. Following gastrointestinal bypass procedures and sleeve gastrectomy, a postprandial rise in GLP1 is observed almost immediately after surgery and this effect is sustained over time [62, 63] whereas no changes in plasma GLP-1 are seen after LAGB [64]. Given the role of GLP-1 in the control of insulin secretion as well as gastric emptying and energy intake, the changes in GLP-1 response could plausibly play a role both in weight-reduction and improvement of hyperglycaemia after RYGB and SG.

The exact mechanism that causes such a change in GLP1 concentrations is unclear. Two hypotheses have been suggested. The hindgut hypothesis", holds that a faster presentation of nutrients to the distal bowel due the anatomic shortcut imposed by gastrointestinal bypass procedures may enhance secretion of GLP-1 by local L-cells [65]. The hindgut hypothesis is often presented as alternative to the "foregut" or "proximal" bowel hypothesis, which postulates that the exclusion of the duodenum and proximal jejunum may prevent secretion of a putative signal that promotes insulin resistance and type 2 diabetes [2, 3]. It is likely that the two mechanisms (enhancement of distal bowel physiology and reduction of proximal signals from the excluded bowel) are not mutually exclusive.

The "hindgut hypothesis", however, has been recently called into question by a number of observations. First, the hypothesis would not explain why similar changes in postprandial GLP-1 response occur after sleeve gastrectomy without shortcut for nutrients. Recent experiments in rodents show, in fact, that isolated duodenal bypass without gastric restriction/resection (DJB) does not cause the same postprandial increase of GLP-1 seen after RYGB or sleeve gastrectomy, suggesting that changes in GLP-1 observed after the latter operations may be related to disruption of the physiologic gastric phase of nutrient passage rather than to the bypass of the small bowel [66]. Furthermore, evidence from both human and animal studies show that blockage of GLP-1 action only modestly reduces the effect of surgery on glucose tolerance and diabetes control. In fact, the effect of RYGB on glucose metabolism is not substantially reduced in genetic mice models with attenuated GLP-1 secretion, in GLP-1-receptor deficient mice and after administration of GLP-1-receptor antagonist exendin-9,39 in human subjects [67, 68]. Altogether, these findings question the hindgut hypothesis as the primary mechanism for the improvement of diabetes after surgery.

9.3.2.4 Leptin

Leptin is primarily an adipocyte-derived hormone, but is also produced by the stomach. Circulating leptin levels contribute to the regulation of appetite and energy homeostasis. The role of gastric leptin, however, has remained unclear. A recent study in rodents suggests that endoluminal leptin could activate a neuroendocrine response through the jejunal leptin receptor – PI3K to lower glucose levels. In fact, enhanced activation of this jejunal leptin signaling was found to play a role in the rapid antidiabetic effect of DJB [69].

9.3.3 Role of Bile Acids (BAs)

The role of BAs in physiology is not limited to their contribution to digestion/absorption of nutrients. In fact, BAs have also hormonal activity; through the interaction with specific receptors, they contribute to the regulation of various metabolic pathways. BAs act through FXR receptors, which in turn regulate lipid and glucose metabolism [70]. Through these receptors in brown adipose tissue, BAs can also attenuate diet-induced obesity [71]. BAs can also activate the G protein-coupled receptor TGR5, through which they can influence insulin sensitivity. TGR5 receptors are also present in the L-cells of the distal bowel.

Procedures involving exclusion of the proximal bowel alter the physiologic mix of bile and nutrients, leading to presentation of undiluted bile acids to the distal intestine. This may result in an increase of circulating levels of BAs and also stimulate local L-cells via TGR5, possibly contributing to enhanced GLP-1 response. Serum bile acid (BA) levels increase following RYGB. An increase in bile acid levels, however, is also seen after sleeve gastrectomy and recent experiments implicate bile acid–FXR signaling in the improvement of glucose homeostasis after SG [72].

9.3.4 Role of Intestinal Flora (Microbiota)

The intestinal flora contributes to carbohydrate metabolism and energy production. Obese subjects have different gut flora compared to lean subjects. In particular, Firmicutes to Bacteroidetes ratio is elevated in the obese subjects. Following gastric bypass, the Firmicutes group decrease while Bacteroides increase at 3 and 6 months after surgery [73] In an interesting animal study by Kaplan and colleagues [5], RYGB led to a rapid and sustained increase in the relative abundance of certain microbes (*Escherichia* and *Akkermansia*) throughout the GI tract, independent of weight loss and calorie restriction. Transfer of these organisms into non-operated germ-free mice led to a decrease in weight and body fat mass. Altogether, these findings demonstrate that gastrointestinal surgery can dramatic alter the composition of intestinal microbiota, which may play a role in the improvement of metabolism.

9.3.5 Role of Changes in Intestinal Glucose Metabolism and Nutrient Sensing

Lipid and glucose sensing in the jejunum can activate a gut–brain–liver response that reduces hepatic glucose production, thus exerting a glucose-lowering effect. This mechanism does not require insulin and is enhanced after DJB [6]. Enhanced nutrient sensing appears to play a role in the rapid improvement of hyperglycaemia in insulin-deficient rodent models after DJB [6].

A recent study in rodents has also implicated re-programming of intestinal glucose metabolism in the glucose-lowering effects of RYGB. In particular, increased glucose metabolism is observed in the Roux-limb of rodents undergoing RYGB [7].

9.3.6 Surgical Anatomy and Anti-diabetes Effect

While all procedures result in variable degree of improvement of T2DM, meta-analysis of observational studies and results of randomized clinical trials suggest that procedures involving intestinal rerouting, like BPD and RYGB, have the greatest effect on diabetes [34, 74] and that longer intestinal bypass (such as in BPD) is associated with greater rates of remission of hyperglycaemia [11]. Studies in rodents [66] also show that while both gastric and intestinal mechanisms may contribute to improved glucose tolerance, intestinal mechanisms seem to play a major role in the improvement of glucose tolerance.

9.3.7 The Anti-incretin Theory

This theory [2, 43] provides a coherent theoretical model that could explain observations of physiologic response to nutrient ingestion as well as effects of gastrointestinal bypass surgery. According to the anti-incretin theory, nutrient passage through the GI-tract physiologically activates negative feedback mechanisms (anti-incretins) to balance the short- and long-term effects of incretins (GLP-1, GIP) thus preventing postprandial hyperinsulinaemic hypoglycaemia and proliferative disorders of the beta-cell. An excess of anti-incretin signals, possibly stimulated by specific macronutrient composition of modern diet or chemical additives, could cause insulin resistance, reduced insulin secretion and β-cell depletion, leading to T2DM. Conversely, reduction of nutrient stimuli on the gut through the exclusion of large portions of the upper small bowel from nutrient transit (i.e. RYGB, duodenal-jejunal bypass, biliopancreatic diversion) could reduce excess anti-incretin and restore appropriate incretins/anti-incretins balance, thus explaining improvement and remission of T2DM ("foregut hypothesis" or "proximal intestine hypothesis") [43].

The anti-incretin theory may explain the superior control of diabetes by diversionary procedures but also the efficacy of procedures that do not include duodenal exclusion such as, for instance, sleeve gastrectomy. In fact, any reduction of food stimulation on the proximal gastrointestinal tract, whether due to diet, mechanical gastric restriction (banding), anatomical exclusion (i.e. RYGB, BPD, DJB) or accelerated transit (i.e. sleeve gastrectomy) may reduce production of anti-incretin (diabetogenic) signals thereby improving glucose homeostasis.

The anti-incretin theory needs further experimental verification; however, a number of recent studies provide preliminary, supporting evidence. For instance, in a study by Salinari and co-workers, protein extracts from the duodenum and/or jejunum of diabetic rodents and humans induced insulin resistance in cell-based assays and in normal rats [75]. This observation supports the hypothesis that the proximal small bowel of subjects with type 2 diabetes may produce diabetogenic factor(s), consistent with one of the predictions made by the anti-incretin theory.

9.4 Current Clinical Evidence: The Clinical Rational for Diabetes Surgery

9.4.1 Durability of Glycaemic Control After GI Surgery

Long-term control of glycaemia and normal levels of glycosylated haemoglobin have been observed in obese diabetic patients for up to 15 years follow-up. According to a meta-analysis involving 22,094 patients with T2DM, procedure-specific rates of disease remission (defined as persistent normoglycaemia without diabetes medications) were 48 % for LAGB, 68 % for VBG, 84 % for RYGB and 98 % for BPD [76]. However, most of the studies involved in this meta-analysis were retrospective in nature and with relatively short-follow-up (1- to 3-year). A large multicenter, prospective observational study – the Swedish Obese Subjects (SOS) study – [77] compared bariatric surgery (LAGB $n=156$, VBG $n=451$, RYGB $n=34$) versus a control group of well-matched obese patients managed conservatively. At 2 years, 72 % of diabetic subjects in the surgical group achieved remission of T2DM compared to 21 % in the medically treated arm. A recently published follow-up analysis from this study looking at glycaemic control 15 years after surgery shows that remission was sustained in the majority of patients who had short duration of diabetes (<3 years) and substantially declined in those with longer duration of disease at baseline [77]. It must be noted, however, that approximately 95 % of patients in the SOS study underwent gastric restrictive procedures rather than potentially more effective procedures such as RYGB or BPD.

Laparoscopic sleeve gastrectomy (LSG) has gained considerable popularity in recent years, owing to a relatively easy surgical procedure and a remarkable efficacy in inducing both weight loss and control of co-morbid disease. A systematic review by Gill et al. of 27 studies involving 673 patients (mean follow-up 13.1 months) who underwent sleeve gastrectomy has reported a overall T2DM resolution rate of 66.2 % in obese subjects and improved glycaemic control in 26.9 % [78]. A study specifically looking at 5-year durability of glycaemic control in diabetic patients undergoing bariatric surgery showed an overall recurrence of T2DM after initial remission in 19 % and that recurrence was associated with longer duration of T2DM [79]. Analysis by procedures showed that RYGB resulted in more durable glycaemic control compared to either SG or LAGB [79].

9.4.2 Surgery Versus Medical Therapy and Lifestyle Intervention

The efficacy of surgical vs medical treatment of T2DM in morbidly obese patients has been compared in several randomized controlled trials. In a study by Mingrone et al. [11] 60 patients aged 30–60 years, with duration of diabetes ≥5 years and a HbA1c level of 7.0 % or more were randomly assigned to receive conventional medical therapy or undergo either gastric bypass or biliopancreatic diversion. The primary end point of the study was the rate of diabetes remission at 2 years (defined as a fasting glucose level of <100 mg/dL [5.6 mmol/L] and a HbA1c level of <6.5 % in the absence of pharmacologic therapy). Diabetes remission occurred in no patients in the medical-therapy group versus 75 % in the gastric-bypass group and 95 % in the biliopancreatic-diversion group. A similar randomized clinical trial by Schauer et al. [12] (STAMPEDE Trial) used glycated haemoglobin level of 6.0 % or less (with or without diabetes medications) a 12 months after randomization as primary end point and compared intensive medical therapy and lifestyle modification vs surgical therapy by means of either RYGB or sleeve gastrectomy (LSG) in 150 patients with BMI 27–43 kg/m^2. The proportion of patients who reached the primary end point was 12 % in the medical-therapy group versus 42 % in the gastric-bypass group and 37 % in the sleeve-gastrectomy group. Significantly, all patients in the RYGB group who achieved the primary end point did so without any medication whereas patients in the sleeve-gastrectomy group required the use of one or more glucose-lowering drugs. A recent update of the STAMPEDE trial with 3-year follow-up data confirmed better glycaemic control and quality of life after surgery versus medical therapy and a greater reduction of diabetes medication usage after RYGB than after sleeve gastrectomy [34]. In the last 2 years, four other RCTs were published comparing RYGB [13], LAGB or both [31–33] versus medical therapy and lifestyle interventions. Consisting with previous trials, surgical treatment by any of these interventions resulted in better control of glycaemia and reduction of CV risk factors [13].

9.4.3 Surgical Control of Diabetes in Patients with BMI <35 kg/m^2

While the benefits of metabolic surgery in morbidly obese patients are clearly established, there is now increasing evidence for similar, salutary effects of gastrointestinal surgery on type 2 diabetes in patients with BMI <35 kg/m^2 using both traditional bariatric operations and novel GI procedures. Cohen and co-workers first used DJB to treat diabetes in low BMI patients with favourable short-term results [25]. De Paula et al. [80] have reported remission of diabetes in 65.2 % of patients with BMI 21–29 following laparoscopic ileal interposition associated to a duodenal bypass and sleeve gastrectomy. The long-term metabolic sequelae and safety of these novel procedures, however, remains to be evaluated and therefore they should still be considered experimental in humans.

The effect of traditional bariatric procedures in low-BMI patients has also been investigated in recent years.

Scopinaro and co-workers [81] reported on the effects of BPD on Type 2 DM in 30 patients (12 of whom on insulin preoperatively) with BMI 25–35 kg/m^2. BMI progressively decreased, stabilizing around 25 since the fourth month postoperatively. One year after BPD, mean HbA1c was 6.3 % ±0.8, with 25 patients (83 %) controlled (HbA1c ≤7 %) on free diet, without antidiabetic drugs, and the remaining showing improved glycaemic control.

Lee et al. [82] reported on the effect of loop gastric bypass, ("mini" – gastric bypass), for T2DM in a prospective study involving 44 patients with BMI <35 kg/m^2 (range 28.3–33.7 kg/m^2) versus 166 patients with BMI >35 kg/m^2 (4 years follow-up). In this study, 77 % of patients with BMI <35 kg/m^2 and 92 % of those with BMI >35 kg/m^2 achieved the American Diabetes Association target goals of HbA1C <7.0 %, LDL <100 mg/dL and triglycerides <150 mg/dL.

Demaria et al. [83] have reported more conservative albeit impressive figures for early postoperative outcomes of metabolic surgery to treat diabetes in 235 patients with BMI <35 kg/m^2 from sites participating in the ASMBS bariatric surgery center of excellence program in the USA. According the Bariatric Outcomes Longitudinal Database (BOLD), 55.2 % of patients after gastric bypass and 27.5 % of patients after gastric banding were reported to have discontinued medications to treat diabetes within 6–12 months of surgery for an overall medication cessation rate of 39.1 %.

The durability of diabetes control after RYGB in patients with BMI <35 kg/m^2 has been investigated by Cohen and co-workers in a recent studies published in *Diabetes Care*. The authors documented sustained >80 % remission 5-year postoperatively in 60 patients with T2DM and BMI 26–34 [84].

Patients with T2DM and BMI <35 kg/m^2 have also been included in several RCTs comparing surgery versus medical therapy. Dixon et al. [10] assigned 60 patients with BMI 30–40 kg/m^2 to receive conventional medical/behavioral therapy or LAGB plus conventional therapy. Two years after surgery, 73 % of post-LAGB patients achieved T2DM remission (defined as FBG <126 mg/dL and HbA1c <6.2 % on no diabetes medications), in contrast to only 13 % of the conventional-therapy group. In this study, remission of diabetes was predicted predominantly by greater weight loss in surgical patients at 2 years (20.7 vs. 1.7 %). A recent RCT from Australia also documented better diabetes control after LAGB than medical/lifestyle therapy in patients with BMI <30 kg/m^2.

Lee et al. [82] randomized 60 patients (BMI 25–35 kg/m^2, mean HbA1c level-10 %) to either RYGB or LSG; the remission rate for T2DM (defined as fasting plasma glucose levels less than 126 mg/dL in addition to HbA1c values less than 6.5 % without the use of oral hypoglycaemics or insulin) was 93 % for patients who underwent RYGB compared to 47 % for those who underwent sleeve gastrectomy. The STAMPEDE trial, compared advanced medical therapy and surgical therapy (RYGB or LSG) in 150 patients with BMI 27–43 kg/m^2 (of whom 34 % had BMI <35 kg/m^2) [12]. The 3-year postoperative follow-up analysis of this study recently published in the *New England Journal of Medicine* showed no differences in the effect of surgery between patients with BMI above or below 35 kg/m^2 [34].

9.4.3.1 Predictors of Diabetes Remission of T2DM

From a surgical perspective, the choice of procedure is an important determinant of outcome. There is an increasing gradient of efficacy from LAGB to RYGB and BPD. Although some observational studies have suggested similar remission rates after SG and RYGB [85], the recently published RCTs by Lee et al. [74] and Schauer et al. [12, 34] confirm the superior efficacy of RYGB. Although BPD appears to have the most profound effect on diabetes remission in both obese and non-obese patients, it is not widely favoured due to the greater surgical risk associated with it. Other factors that have been positively co-related with diabetes remission are percentage of excess weight loss (%EWL), younger age, lower pre-op HbA1c and shorter duration of diabetes (less than 5 years) [79]. Severity of diabetes, as judged by pre-operative insulin usage has also been noted to be a significant factor. Schauer et al. [86] have reported a diabetes remission rate of 97 % in diet controlled, 87 % in oral agent treated and 62 % in insulin treated subjects in their case series study. C-peptide >3 ng/mL has been identified as an important predictor of diabetes resolution after SG in non-morbidly obese diabetic subjects in one study [87]. In contrast to other published data; age, sex, baseline BMI, duration of diabetes and weight changes were not significant predictors of diabetes remission at 2 years or of improvement in glycaemia at 1 and 3 months in the recently published RCT by Mingrone et al. [11]. Future RCTs comparing medical versus surgical strategies for management of Type 2 DM will hopefully help clarify which factors best predict remission following surgery and guide patient selection particularly among the less obese.

9.4.3.2 Non-glycaemic Benefits of Metabolic Surgery

Several studies have demonstrated that the benefits of metabolic surgery extend beyond amelioration of hyperglycaemia and include improvement of other cardiovascular risk factors such as dyslipidaemia and hypertension. In addition, there is reduced cancer incidence in surgically treated obese females [88, 89]. The meta-analysis by Buchwald et al. [76] showed marked decrease in levels of total cholesterol, LDL cholesterol and triglycerides after bariatric procedures. Approximately 70 % of patients experienced an improvement in hyperlipidaemia, whereas hypertension improved or resolved in 79 % of patients. In the SOS study, the 2- and 10-year recovery rates from hypertriglyceridaemia, low levels of high-density lipoprotein cholesterol, hypertension and hyperuricaemia were more favourable in the surgery group than in the medically managed control group, whereas recovery from hypercholesterolaemia did not differ between the groups [90]. Furthermore, follow-up of participants in the SOS study after an average of 11 years found that bariatric surgery was associated with a 29 % reduction in all-cause mortality after adjusting for sex, age and risk factors in this severely obese group [35]. This survival benefit has previously also been reported by Adams et al. in a large retrospective cohort study [37] where 8,000 patients who had undergone gastric bypass surgery were compared for long-term mortality with age-, sex- and BMI-matched control subjects who had applied for driver's licences (Utah, USA). The analysis reported an adjusted long-term all-cause mortality reduction of 40 % in the surgical group, with specific mortality reductions in the operated group of 56 % for coronary artery disease, 92 % for diabetes and 60 % for cancer when compared with matched controls. Other studies have demonstrated major improvements in health-related quality of life following bariatric surgery using both generic and obesity-specific quality-of-life instruments.

9.4.3.3 Diabetes Surgery in the Treatment Algorithm for Type 2 Diabetes

The management of patients with obesity and T2DM is both complex and challenging. It is clearly evident from several experimental and observational studies and more recently from randomized controlled trials that diabetes surgery offers superior results both in terms of efficacy and durability of glycaemic control when compared to lifestyle modifications and pharmacotherapy. There is now also a significant body of evidence indicating that patients with BMI less than 35 kg/m^2 can also respond favourably to diabetes surgery in the short-term. The SOS study also shows that surgery can have a favourable influence on long-term complications of diabetes and mortality, although this needs to be confirmed in RCTs.

Given the level of clinical evidence, several organizations now recommend using surgery for the treatment of T2DM, especially in patients that do not adequately respond to conventional therapies or in presence of surgery-responsive co-morbidities (i.e. hypertension, dyslipidaemia) that increase CV risk. Accordingly, the International Diabetes Federation (IDF) recommends prioritization for bariatric surgery in morbidly obese patients (BMI >35 kg/m^2) with Type 2 diabetes and considers eligible for surgical treatment patients with BMI >30 kg/m^2 if HbA1c is higher than 7.5 % despite fully optimized conventional therapy, especially if weight is increasing, or in presence of other weight responsive co-morbidities not achieving targets on conventional therapies [14]. According to the IDF, in Asians and some other ethnicities of increased risk, BMI action points may be reduced by 2.5 kg/m^2 [14]. The American Diabetes Association recommends that bariatric surgery be considered as a treatment option for Type 2 diabetes when the patient's BMI exceeds 35 kg/m^2 [38]. At the time of this writing, the National Institute for Health and Care Excellence (NICE) in the UK has proposed a draft document to recommend surgical treatment of type 2 diabetes in all patients with BMI >30 kg/m^2 and diabetes duration <10 years.

9.5 Definition of "Metabolic" and "Diabetes Surgery": What's in a Name?

In spite of the rapidly increasing popularity, the concept and practice of metabolic and diabetes surgery have not been clearly defined. Buchwald and Varco first proposed the term *metabolic surgery* as "the operative manipulation of a normal organ or organ system to achieve a biological result for a potential health gain" [91]. Gastrectomies and vagotomies for peptic ulcer disease, portal diversion for glycogen storage disease and partial ileal bypass for hyperlipidaemia were cited as examples. More recently, the term metabolic surgery has been used instead to indicate a yet-investigational approach to non-obese diabetics or a set of novel experimental procedures such as ileal interposition and duodenal-jejunal bypass. The definitions above have historical interest but are not consistent with the principles that usually guide the definition of other surgical disciplines. In fact, surgical specialties are distinguished by the target organ-system (i.e. "digestive" or "GI surgery") or by the disease or disease-group that one intends to treat (i.e. endocrine surgery, surgical oncology etc). Organ-systems and disease groups are indeed defining aspects since they determine what specific set of technical and clinical skills the specialist surgeon needs to learn. Defining the exact meaning of diabetes/metabolic surgery and using the proper terminology is neither a mere semantic issue nor a mere academic exercise. A clear definition indeed is the first step to frame the boundaries of this emerging field and has important conceptual and practical ramifications.

We have suggested that *gastrointestinal metabolic surgery* should be defined and characterized by its intent to treat diabetes and obesity from the perspective of a metabolic illness as opposed to traditional bariatric surgery intended as a mere weight-reduction therapy [15]. The transition from bariatric to metabolic and diabetes surgery implies changes in every aspect of clinical practice, including the selection of surgical candidates, the prioritization of access to surgery, the definition of success of treatment, pre-operative diagnostics, post-operative outcome measures, follow-up and care team composition [15].

In fact, among patients who seek traditional bariatric surgery, females are over-represented and diabetes is less prevalent than expected for a severely obese population. Reported female/male ratio ranges between 3:1 and 4:1 and prevalence of diabetes is as low as 18–33 %. This reflects differences in the way individuals of different genders conceptualize the risks of obesity against the risks and benefits of surgery. Diabetes and other metabolic diseases instead are likely to be perceived equally as a medical problem by both genders and the focus on metabolic dysfunction rather than weight as the primary reason to seek surgical treatment may encourage more patients with long-standing disease, complex medical regimen or concerns about cardiovascular risk to seek surgical care.

We recently conducted a study [15] to compare demographics and peri-operative outcomes of two cohorts of patients undergoing surgery at two distinct surgical units within the same tertiary care medical center: the *Gastrointestinal Metabolic and Diabetes Surgery Center* whose model of clinical practice was shaped around the stated aim to surgically treat diabetes and metabolic disease and the section of *Bariatric Surgery*, a traditional

Table 9.1 Differences between bariatric and metabolic surgery

	Bariatric surgery	Metabolic surgery
Purpose	Weight loss	Glycaemic/metabolic control; CV risk reduction
Indication criteria	BMI centric	Uncontrolled type 2 diabetes, metabolic syndrome, NASH, Increased CV risk
Operations	Traditional (RYGB, SG, BPD, LAGB)	Traditional (RYGB, SG, BPD, LAGB) Investigational (DJB, IT endoscopic duodenal sleeve)
Measures of outcome	Weight loss (excess weight loss)	Glycaemic control, blood pressure, lipid control, CV risk reduction, weight loss
Presumed mechanisms of action	Restriction to food intake/malabsorption	Several, complex, neuroendocrine

Modified from Rubino and Cummings [92]
RYGB Roux-en-Y gastric bypass, *SG* sleeve gastrectomy, *BPD* biliopancreatic diversion, *LAGB* laparoscopic adjustable gastric banding, *DJB* duodenal jejunal bypass, *IT* ileal interposition

practice of weight loss surgery. Only patients with BMI levels within the accepted criteria for conventional bariatric surgery were included to rule out BMI as a confounding. The results showed that the patient population of metabolic surgery is characterized by older age, greater prevalence of male patients and significantly higher prevalence of all metabolic conditions examined, including type 2 diabetes, hypertension and dyslipidaemia. The severity of diabetes was greater in metabolic surgery patients as shown by higher fasting glycaemia, HBA1c and greater proportion of insulin users prior to surgery. At baseline, metabolic surgery patients also had a greater prevalence of established cardiovascular disease (i.e. ischaemic heart disease, congestive heart failure, cardiac arrhythmia) compared to bariatric surgery patents. Consistent with previous studies, the patient population in the bariatric surgery cohort was characterized by a preponderance of young female subjects with a relatively low prevalence of diabetes and cardiovascular disease.

The results of this study show that offering surgery to treat diabetes rather than as a mere weight-reduction therapy changes demographics and clinical characteristics of surgical candidates. This support consideration of metabolic/diabetes surgery as a novel practice distinct from traditional bariatric surgery. Based on these results we proposed a practical definition of *gastrointestinal metabolic surgery* (or metabolic surgery) as a broad surgical specialty where gastrointestinal operations are used with the primary intent to treat diabetes and metabolic disease. This definition is descriptive of the target organ-system (the GI tract) and of the disease-group (obesity, diabetes, metabolic syndrome), independent on type of procedures and patient's BMI. This definition is not based on the assumption of whether the site of surgery is normal or pathologic, yet it is consistent with the evidence that gastrointestinal operations engage mechanisms of action that are metabolic in nature.

According to such definition, standard procedures traditionally utilized in bariatric surgery (i.e. Roux-en-Y gastric bypass, sleeve gastrectomy, biliopancreatic diversion, gastric banding, etc) should be considered "metabolic" rather than "bariatric" surgery when used with the primary intent to treat metabolic illnesses even in morbidly obese patients (BMI >35). When the primary intent of surgery (or the reason why a patient is seeking surgical treatment) is specifically the treatment of diabetes, there are sufficient ramifications for clinical practice (impact on patients' expectations, need for specific outcome measures, involvement of appropriate multidisciplinary teams and support systems, etc.) to indicate the approach as "diabetes surgery". The name bariatric surgery should only be retained, in our opinion, for those cases where surgery is sought with the primary intent to address physical complications of excess weight. Table 9.1 shows differences between metabolic/diabetes surgery and bariatric surgery.

9.6 Diabetes Surgery: Current Priorities and Future Directions

The development of proper diabetes surgery implies a number of transformative changes to the model of care of traditional bariatric surgery. Traditional bariatric surgery practice in fact does not include accurate diagnostics measures of diabetes, evaluation of residual pancreatic function or careful screening for micro- and macrovascular complications of diabetes. Fasting insulin levels are not a mandatory routine test in most centers of excellence for bariatric surgery. This traditional practice is largely responsible for our current inability to accurately predict outcomes of bariatric surgery on diabetes based on preoperative patients' characteristics.

Appropriate therapeutic strategies should also be developed to optimize diabetes and metabolic control. For instance, preoperative medical/dietary interventions should be considered when appropriate to improve preoperative glycaemic control. Protocols for continuation of medical therapy after surgery should be tailored to complement mechanisms of action of specific operations, introducing the concept of "adjuvant" medical therapy after surgical or device-based gastrointestinal interventions.

Finally, development of appropriate disease-based criteria for selection of surgical candidates rather than mere "weight-centric" criteria should be implemented, including measures of risks-stratification, predicting factors of success and failure, lack of responsiveness to medical and lifestyle interventions.

Conclusion

The novel field of diabetes surgery has emerged from a surgical discipline initially focused primarily on weight loss. Surgery offers a unique opportunity for remission or improved control of type 2 diabetes and could potentiate traditional therapy by lifestyle and pharmaceutical interventions. It is envisaged that ongoing RCTs and future studies will help identify the best candidates for surgical treatment among the vast population of diabetic patients, including the less obese. Furthermore, mechanistic studies aimed at using gastrointestinal surgery to elucidate the role of the gut in glucose homeostasis may possibly uncover new targets and molecules for future less invasive therapeutic approaches of curative intent.

References

1. Rubino F, Marescaux J. The effect of duodenal-jejunal exclusion in a non-obese animal model of type 2 diabetes: a new perspective for an old disease. Ann Surg. 2004;239(1):1–11.
2. Rubino F, Gagner M. Potential of surgery for curing type 2 diabetes mellitus. Ann Surg. 2002;236(5):554–9.
3. Thaler JP, Cummings DE. Minireview: hormonal and metabolic mechanisms of diabetes remission after gastrointestinal surgery. Endocrinology. 2009;150(6):2518–25.
4. Pournaras DJ, Glicksman C, Vincent RP, Kuganolipava S, Alaghband-Zadeh J, Mahon D, Bekker JH, Ghatei MA, Bloom SR, Walters JR, Welbourn R, le Roux CW. The role of bile after Roux-en-Y gastric bypass in promoting weight loss and improving glycaemic control. Endocrinology. 2012;153:3613–9.
5. Liou AP, Paziuk M, Luevano Jr JM, Machineni S, Turnbaugh PJ, Kaplan LM. Conserved shifts in the gut microbiota due to gastric bypass reduce host weight and adiposity. Sci Transl Med. 2013;5(178):178ra41.
6. Breen DM, Rasmussen BA, Kokorovic A, Wang R, Cheung GW, Lam TK. Jejunal nutrient sensing is required for duodenal-jejunal bypass surgery to rapidly lower glucose concentrations in uncontrolled diabetes. Nat Med. 2012;18:950–5.
7. Saeidi N, Meoli L, Nestoridi E, Gupta NK, Kvas S, Kucharczyk J, Bonab AA, Fischman AJ, Yarmush ML, Stylopoulos N. Reprogramming of intestinal glucose metabolism and glycemic control in rats after gastric bypass. Science. 2013;341(6144):406–10.
8. Troy S, Soty M, Ribeiro L, Laval L, Migrenne S, Fioramonti X, Pillot B, Fauveau V, Aubert R, Viollet B, Foretz M, Leclerc J, Duchampt A, Zitoun C, Thorens B, Magnan C, Mithieux G, Andreelli F. Intestinal gluconeogenesis is a key factor for early metabolic changes after gastric bypass but not after gastric lap-band in mice. Cell Metab. 2008;8:201–11.
9. Jiao J, Bae EJ, Bandyopadhyay G, Oliver J, Marathe C, Chen M, Hsu JY, Chen Y, Tian H, Olefsky JM, Saberi M. Restoration of euglycemia after duodenal bypass surgery is reliant on central and peripheral inputs in Zucker fa/fa rats. Diabetes. 2013;62(4):1074–83. doi:10.2337/db12-068.
10. Dixon JB, O'Brien PE, Playfair J, Chapman L, Schachter LM, Skinner S, Proietto J, Bailey M, Anderson M. Adjustable gastric banding and conven-

tional therapy for type 2 diabetes: a randomized controlled trial. JAMA. 2008;299:316–23.
11. Mingrone G, Panunzi S, De Gaetano A, Guidone C, Iaconelli A, Leccesi L, Nanni G, Pomp A, Castagneto M, Ghirlanda G, Rubino F. Bariatric surgery versus conventional medical therapy for type 2 diabetes. N Engl J Med. 2012;366:1577–85.
12. Schauer PR, Kashyap SR, Wolski K, Brethauer SA, Kirwan JP, Pothier CE, Thomas S, Abood B, Nissen SE, Bhatt DL. Bariatric surgery versus intensive medical therapy in obese patients with diabetes. N Engl J Med. 2012;366:1567–76.
13. Ikramuddin S, Korner J, Lee WJ, Connett JE, Inabnet WB, Billington CJ, Thomas AJ, Leslie DB, Chong K, Jeffery RW, Ahmed L, Vella A, Chuang LM, Bessler M, Sarr MG, Swain JM, Laqua P, Jensen MD, Bantle JP. Roux-en-Y gastric bypass vs intensive medical management for the control of type 2 diabetes, hypertension, and hyperlipidemia: the Diabetes Surgery Study randomized clinical trial. JAMA. 2013;309(21):2240–9.
14. Dixon JB, Zimmet P, Alberti KG, Rubino F, on behalf of the International Diabetes Federation Taskforce on Epidemiology and Prevention. Bariatric surgery: an IDF statement for obese Type 2 diabetes. Diabet Med. 2011;28(6):628–42.
15. Rubino F, Shukla A, Pomp A, Moreira M, Ahn SM, Dakin G. Bariatric, metabolic and diabetes surgery: what's in a name? Ann Surg. 2014;259:117–22.
16. Leyton O. Diabetes and operation. A note on the effect of gastro-jejunostomy upon a case of mild diabetes mellitus with a low renal threshold. Lancet. 1925;206(5336):1162–3.
17. Friedman MN, Sancetta AJ, Magovern GJ. The amelioration of diabetes mellitus following subtotal gastrectomy. Surg Gynecol Obstet. 1955;100(2):201–4.
18. Angervall L, Dotevall G, Tillander H. Amelioration of diabetes mellitus following gastric resection. Acta Med Scand. 1961;169:743–8.
19. Ahmad U, Danowski TS, Nolan S, Stephan T, Sunder JH, Bahl VK. Remissions of diabetes mellitus after weight reduction by jejunoileal bypass. Diabetes Care. 1978;1(3):158–65.
20. Printen KJ, Blommers TJ, Scott D. The morbidly obese diabetic and gastric bypass. Am Surg. 1979;45(8):491–4.
21. Ackerman NB. Observations on the improvements in carbohydrate metabolism in diabetic and other morbidly obese patients after jejunoileal bypass. Surg Gynecol Obstet. 1981;152(5):581–6.
22. Pories WJ, Caro JF, Flickinger EG, Meelheim HD, Swanson MS. The control of diabetes mellitus (NIDDM) in the morbidly obese with the Greenville Gastric Bypass. Ann Surg. 1987;206(3):316–23.
23. Pories WJ, Swanson MS, MacDonald KG, Long SB, Morris PG, Brown BM, Barakat HA, de Ramon RA, Israel G, Dolezal JM. Who would have thought it? An operation proves to be the most effective therapy for adult-onset diabetes mellitus. Ann Surg. 1995;222: 339–50; discussion 350–2.
24. Scopinaro N, Adami GF, Marinari GM, Gianetta E, Traverso E, Friedman D, Camerini G, Baschieri G, Simonelli A. Biliopancreatic diversion. World J Surg. 1998;22(9):936–46.
25. Cohen RV, Schiavon CA, Pinheiro JS, Correa JL, Rubino F. Duodenal-jejunal bypass for the treatment of type 2 diabetes in patients with body mass index of 22-34 kg/m^2. Surg Obes Relat Dis. 2007;3:195–7.
26. Cohen RV, Pinheiro JC, Schiavon CA, Salles JE, Wajchenberg BL, Cummings DE. Effects of gastric bypass surgery in patients with type 2 diabetes and only mild obesity. Diabetes Care. 2012;35:1420–8.
27. Rubino R, Kaplan LM, Schauer PR, Cummings DE. The Diabetes Surgery Summit Consensus Conference: recommendations for the evaluation and use of gastrointestinal surgery to treat type 2 diabetes mellitus. Ann Surg. 2010;251:399–405.
28. Laferrere B, Teixeira J, McGinty J, Tran H, Egger JR, Colarusso A, Kovack B, Bawa B, Koshy N, Lee H, Yapp K, Olivan B. Effect of weight loss by gastric bypass surgery versus hypocaloric diet on glucose and incretin levels in patients with type 2 diabetes. J Clin Endocrinol Metab. 2008;93:2479–85.
29. Strader AD, Vahl TP, Jandacek RJ, Woods SC, D'Alessio DA, Seeley RJ. Weight loss through ileal transposition is accompanied by increased ileal hormone secretion and synthesis in rats. Am J Physiol Endocrinol Metab. 2005;288:E447–53.
30. Rubino F, Forgione A, Cummings DE, Vix M, Gnuli D, Mingrone G, Castagneto M, Marescaux J. The mechanism of diabetes control after gastrointestinal bypass surgery reveals a role of the proximal small intestine in the pathophysiology of type 2 diabetes. Ann Surg. 2006;244:741–9.
31. Halperin F, Ding SA, Simonson DC, Panosian J, Goebel-Fabbri A, Wewalka M, Hamdy O, Abrahamson M, Clancy K, Foster K, Lautz D, Vernon A, Goldfine AB. Roux-en-Y gastric bypass surgery or lifestyle with intensive medical management in patients with type 2 diabetes: feasibility and 1-year results of a randomized clinical trial. JAMA Surg. 2014;149(7):716–26. doi:10.1001/jamasurg.2014.514.
32. Courcoulas AP, Goodpaster BH, Eagleton JK, Belle SH, Kalarchian MA, Lang W, Toledo FG, Jakicic JM. Surgical vs medical treatments for type 2 diabetes mellitus: a randomized clinical trial. JAMA Surg. 2014;149(7):707–15. doi:10.1001/jamasurg.2014.467.
33. Wentworth JM, Playfair J, Laurie C, Ritchie ME, Brown WA, Burton P, Shaw JE, O'Brien PE. Multidisciplinary diabetes care with and without bariatric surgery in overweight people: a randomised controlled trial. Lancet Diabetes Endocrinol. 2014;2(7):545–52.
34. Schauer PR, Bhatt DL, Kirwan JP, Wolski K, Brethauer SA, Navaneethan SD, Aminian A, Pothier CE, Kim ES, Nissen SE, Kashyap SR, STAMPEDE Investigators. Bariatric surgery versus intensive medical therapy for diabetes–3-year outcomes. N Engl J Med. 2014;370(21):2002–13.
35. Sjöström L, Narbro K, Sjöström CD, et al.; Swedish Obese Subjects Study. Effects of bariatric surgery on mortality in Swedish obese subjects. N Engl J Med. 2007;357(8):741–52.

36. Sjostrom L, et al. Bariatric surgery and long-term cardiovascular events. JAMA. 2012;307:56–65.
37. Adams TD, Davidson LE, Litwin SE, et al. Health benefits of gastric bypass surgery after 6 years. JAMA. 2012;308(11):1122–31.
38. American Diabetes Association. Standards of medical care in diabetes--2009. Diabetes Care. 2009;32 Suppl 1:S13–61.
39. Bojsen-Møller KN, Dirksen C, Jørgensen NB, Jacobsen SH, Serup AK, Albers PH, Hansen DL, Worm D, Naver L, Kristiansen VB, Wojtaszewski JF, Kiens B, Holst JJ, Richter EA, Madsbad S. Early enhancements of hepatic and later of peripheral insulin sensitivity combined with increased postprandial insulin secretion contribute to improved glycemic control after Roux-en-Y gastric bypass. Diabetes. 2014;63:1725–37.
40. Salinari S, Bertuzzi A, Guidone C, Previti E, Rubino F, Mingrone G. Insulin sensitivity and secretion changes after gastric bypass in normotolerant and diabetic obese subjects. Ann Surg. 2013;257(3):462–8.
41. Dirksen C, Bojsen-Møller KN, Jørgensen NB, Jacobsen SH, Kristiansen VB, Naver LS, Hansen DL, Worm D, Holst JJ, Madsbad S. Exaggerated release and preserved insulinotropic action of glucagon-like peptide-1 underlie insulin hypersecretion in glucose-tolerant individuals after Roux-en-Y gastric bypass. Diabetologia. 2013;56(12):2679–87.
42. Kashyap SR, Bhatt DL, Wolski K, Watanabe RM, Abdul-Ghani M, Abood B, Pothier CE, Brethauer S, Nissen S, Gupta M, Kirwan JP, Schauer PR. Metabolic effects of bariatric surgery in patients with moderate obesity and type 2 diabetes: analysis of a randomized control trial comparing surgery with intensive medical treatment. Diabetes Care. 2013;36(8):2175–82.
43. Rubino F, Amiel SA. Is the gut the "sweet spot" for the treatment of diabetes? Diabetes. 2014;63(7):2225–8. doi:10.2337/db14-0402.
44. Service GJ, Thompson GB, Service FJ, Andrews JC, Collazo-Clavell ML, Lloyd RV. Hyperinsulinemic hypoglycemia with nesidioblastosis after gastric-bypass surgery. N Engl J Med. 2005;353(3):249–54.
45. Li Z, Zhang HY, Lv LX, Li DF, Dai JX, Sha O, Li WQ, Bai Y, Yuan L. Roux-en-Y gastric bypass promotes expression of PDX-1 and regeneration of beta-cells in Goto-Kakizaki rats. World J Gastroenterol. 2010;16(18):2244–51.
46. Speck M, Cho YM, Asadi A, Rubino F, Kieffer TJ. Duodenal-jejunal bypass protects GK rats from {beta}-cell loss and aggravation of hyperglycemia and increases enteroendocrine cells coexpressing GIP and GLP-1. Am J Physiol Endocrinol Metab. 2011;300(5):E923–32.
47. Lindqvist A, Spégel P, Ekelund M, Vaz EG, Pierzynowski S, Gomez M, Mulder H, Hedenbro J, Groop L, Wierup N. Gastric bypass improves ss-cell function and increases β-cell mass in a porcine model. Diabetes. 2014;63:1665–71.
48. Olszewski PK, Li D, Grace MK, Billington CJ, Kotz CM, Levine AS. Neural basis of orexigenic effects of ghrelin acting within lateral hypothalamus. Peptides. 2003;24(4):597–602. Epub 2003/07/16.
49. Langer FB, Reza Hoda MA, Bohdjalian A, Felberbauer FX, Zacherl J, Wenzl E, et al. Sleeve gastrectomy and gastric banding: effects on plasma ghrelin levels. Obes Surg. 2005;15(7):1024–9. Epub 2005/08/18.
50. DePaula AL, Macedo AL, Schraibman V, Mota BR, Vencio S. Hormonal evaluation following laparoscopic treatment of type 2 diabetes mellitus patients with BMI 20-34. Surg Endosc. 2009;23(8):1724–32. Epub 2008/10/03.
51. Ramon JM, Salvans S, Crous X, Puig S, Goday A, Benaiges D, et al. Effect of Roux-en-Y gastric bypass vs sleeve gastrectomy on glucose and gut hormones: a prospective randomised trial. J Gastrointest Surg Off J Soc Surg Aliment Tract. 2012;16(6):1116–22. Epub 2012/03/10.
52. Peterli R, Steinert RE, Woelnerhanssen B, Peters T, Christoffel-Courtin C, Gass M, et al. Metabolic and hormonal changes after laparoscopic Roux-en-Y gastric bypass and sleeve gastrectomy: a randomized, prospective trial. Obes Surg. 2012;22(5):740–8. Epub 2012/02/23.
53. Schindler K, Prager G, Ballaban T, Kretschmer S, Riener R, Buranyi B, et al. Impact of laparoscopic adjustable gastric banding on plasma ghrelin, eating behaviour and body weight. Eur J Clin Invest. 2004;34(8):549–54. Epub 2004/08/13.
54. Uzzan B, Catheline JM, Lagorce C, Airinei G, Bon C, Cohen R, et al. Expression of ghrelin in fundus is increased after gastric banding in morbidly obese patients. Obes Surg. 2007;17(9):1159–64. Epub 2007/12/13.
55. Nijhuis J, van Dielen FM, Buurman WA, Greve JW. Ghrelin, leptin and insulin levels after restrictive surgery: a 2-year follow-up study. Obes Surg. 2004; 14(6):783–7. Epub 2004/08/21.
56. Stoeckli R, Chanda R, Langer I, Keller U. Changes of body weight and plasma ghrelin levels after gastric banding and gastric bypass. Obes Res. 2004;12(2): 346–50. Epub 2004/02/26.
57. Batterham RL, Cowley MA, Small CJ, Herzog H, Cohen MA, Dakin CL, et al. Gut hormone PYY(3-36) physiologically inhibits food intake. Nature. 2002; 418(6898):650–4. Epub 2002/08/09.
58. Borg CM, le Roux CW, Ghatei MA, Bloom SR, Patel AG, Aylwin SJ. Progressive rise in gut hormone levels after Roux-en-Y gastric bypass suggests gut adaptation and explains altered satiety. Br J Surg. 2006;93(2): 210–5. Epub 2006/01/05.
59. Bose M, Machineni S, Olivan B, Teixeira J, McGinty JJ, Bawa B, et al. Superior appetite hormone profile after equivalent weight loss by gastric bypass compared to gastric banding. Obesity (Silver Spring). 2010;18(6):1085–91. Epub 2010/01/09.
60. Ochner CN, Gibson C, Shanik M, Goel V, Geliebter A. Changes in neurohormonal gut peptides following bariatric surgery. Int J Obes (2005). 2011;35(2):153–66. Epub 2010/07/14.
61. Tang-Christensen M, Vrang N, Larsen PJ. Glucagon-like peptide containing pathways in the regulation of feeding behaviour. Int J Obes Relat Metabol Disord J Int Assoc Study Obes. 2001;25 Suppl 5:S42–7. Epub 2002/02/13.

62. le Roux CW, Aylwin SJ, Batterham RL, Borg CM, Coyle F, Prasad V, et al. Gut hormone profiles following bariatric surgery favor an anorectic state, facilitate weight loss, and improve metabolic parameters. Ann Surg. 2006;243(1):108–14. Epub 2005/12/24.
63. Morinigo R, Moize V, Musri M, Lacy AM, Navarro S, Marin JL, et al. Glucagon-like peptide-1, peptide YY, hunger, and satiety after gastric bypass surgery in morbidly obese subjects. J Clin Endocrinol Metab. 2006;91(5):1735–40. Epub 2006/02/16.
64. Shak JR, Roper J, Perez-Perez GI, Tseng CH, Francois F, Gamagaris Z, et al. The effect of laparoscopic gastric banding surgery on plasma levels of appetite-control, insulinotropic, and digestive hormones. Obes Surg. 2008;18(9):1089–96. Epub 2008/04/15.
65. Cummings DE, Overduin J, Foster-Schubert KE, Carlson MJ. Role of the bypassed proximal intestine in the anti-diabetic effects of bariatric surgery. Surg Obes Relat Dis Off J Am Soc Bariatric Surg. 2007;3(2):109–15. Epub 2007/03/28.
66. Patel RT, Shukla AP, Ahn SM, Moreira M, Rubino F. Surgical control of obesity and diabetes: the role of intestinal vs. gastric mechanisms in the regulation of body weight and glucose homeostasis. Obesity (Silver Spring). 2014;22(1):159–69. Epub 2013/03/21.
67. Mokadem M, Zechner JF, Margolskee RF, Drucker DJ, Aguirre V. Effects of Roux-en-Y gastric bypass on energy and glucose homeostasis are preserved in two mouse models of functional glucagon-like peptide-1 deficiency. Mol Metabol. 2014;3(2):191–201. Epub 2014/03/19.
68. Jimenez A, Casamitjana R, Viaplana-Masclans J, Lacy A, Vidal J. GLP-1 action and glucose tolerance in subjects with remission of type 2 diabetes after gastric bypass surgery. Diabetes Care. 2013;36(7):2062–9. Epub 2013/01/30.
69. Rasmussen BA, Breen DM, Duca FA, Cote CD, Zadeh-Tahmasebi M, Filippi BM, et al. Jejunal leptin-PI3K signaling lowers glucose production. Cell Metab. 2014;19(1):155–61. Epub 2013/12/24.
70. Zhang Y, Lee FY, Barrera G, Lee H, Vales C, Gonzalez FJ, et al. Activation of the nuclear receptor FXR improves hyperglycemia and hyperlipidemia in diabetic mice. Proc Natl Acad Sci U S A. 2006;103(4):1006–11. Epub 2006/01/18.
71. Watanabe M, Houten SM, Mataki C, Christoffolete MA, Kim BW, Sato H, et al. Bile acids induce energy expenditure by promoting intracellular thyroid hormone activation. Nature. 2006;439(7075):484–9. Epub 2006/01/10.
72. Ryan KK, Tremaroli V, Clemmensen C, Kovatcheva-Datchary P, Myronovych A, Karns R, et al. FXR is a molecular target for the effects of vertical sleeve gastrectomy. Nature. 2014;509(7499):183–8. Epub 2014/03/29.
73. Sweeney TE, Morton JM. The human gut microbiome: a review of the effect of obesity and surgically induced weight loss. JAMA Surg. 2013;148(6):563–9. Epub 2013/04/11.
74. Lee WJ, Chong K, Ser KH, et al. Gastric bypass vs sleeve gastrectomy for type 2 diabetes mellitus: a randomized controlled trial. Arch Surg. 2011;146(2):143–8.
75. Salinari S, Debard C, Bertuzzi A, Durand C, Zimmet P, Vidal H, et al. Jejunal proteins secreted by db/db mice or insulin-resistant humans impair the insulin signaling and determine insulin resistance. PLoS One. 2013;8(2):e56258. Epub 2013/02/26.
76. Buchwald H, Avidor Y, Braunwald E, et al. Bariatric surgery: a systematic review and meta-analysis. JAMA. 2004;292(14):1724–37.
77. Sjöström L, Peltonen M, Jacobson P, Ahlin S, Andersson-Assarsson J, Anveden Å, Bouchard C, Carlsson B, Karason K, Lönroth H, Näslund I, Sjöström E, Taube M, Wedel H, Svensson PA, Sjöholm K, Carlsson LM. Association of bariatric surgery with long-term remission of type 2 diabetes and with microvascular and macrovascular complications. JAMA. 2014;311(22):2297–304. doi:10.1001/jama.2014.5988.
78. Gill RS, Birch DW, Shi X, Sharma AM, Karmali S. Sleeve gastrectomy and type 2 diabetes mellitus: a systematic review. Surg Obes Relat Dis. 2010;6(6):707–13.
79. Brethauer SA, Aminian A, Romero-Talamás H, Batayyah E, Mackey J, Kennedy L, Kashyap SR, Kirwan JP, Rogula T, Kroh M, Chand B, Schauer PR. Can diabetes be surgically cured? Long-term metabolic effects of bariatric surgery in obese patients with type 2 diabetes mellitus. Ann Surg. 2013; 258(4):628–36.doi:10.1097/SLA.0b013e3182a5034b; discussion 636–7.
80. DePaula AL, Macedo AL, Prudente AS, et al. Laparoscopic sleeve gastrectomy with ileal interposition ("neuroendocrine brake")—pilot study of a new operation. Surg Obes Relat Dis. 2006;2:464–6.
81. Scopinaro N, Adami GF, Papadia FS, et al. Effects of Biliopancreatic Diversion on Type 2 Diabetes in Patients With BMI 25 to 35. Ann Surg. 2011;253(4):699–703.
82. Lee WJ, Wang W, Lee YC. Effect of laparoscopic mini-gastric bypass for type 2 diabetes mellitus: comparison of BMI>35 and <35 kg/m^2. J Gastrointest Surg. 2008;12:945–52.
83. Demaria EJ, Winegar DA, Pate VW, Hutcher NE, Ponce J, Pories WJ. Early postoperative outcomes of metabolic surgery to treat diabetes from sites participating in the ASMBS bariatric surgery center of excellence program as reported in the Bariatric Outcomes Longitudinal Database. Ann Surg. 2010;252(3):559–66; discussion 566–7.
84. Cohen RV, Pinheiro JC, Schiavon CA, Salles JE, Wajchenberg BL, Cummings DE. Effects of gastric bypass surgery in patients with type 2 diabetes and only mild obesity. Diabetes Care. 2012;35(7):1420–8. doi:10.2337/dc11-2289.
85. Lakdawala MA, Bhasker A, Mulchandani D, Goel S, Jain S. Comparison between the results of laparoscopic sleeve gastrectomy and laparoscopic Roux-en-Y gastric bypass in the Indian population: a retrospective 1 year study. Obes Surg. 2010;20(1):1–6.
86. Schauer PR, Burguera B, Ikramuddin S, et al. Effect of laparoscopic Roux-en Y gastric bypass on type 2 diabetes mellitus. Ann Surg. 2003;238(4):467–84.

87. Lee WJ, Ser KH, Chong K, Lee YC, Chen SC, Tsou JJ, Chen JC, Chen CM. Laparoscopic sleeve gastrectomy for diabetes treatment in nonmorbidly obese patients: efficacy and change of insulin secretion. Surgery. 2010;147(5):664–9.
88. Sjostrom L, Gummesson A, Sjostrom CD, et al. Effects of bariatric surgery on cancer incidence in obese patients in Sweden (Swedish Obese Subjects Study): a prospective, controlled intervention trial. Lancet Oncol. 2009;10:653–62.
89. Ashrafian H, Ahmed K, Rowland SP, et al. Metabolic surgery and cancer: protective effects of bariatric procedures. Cancer. 2011;117(9):1788–99.
90. Sjöström L, Lindroos AK, Peltonen M, et al.; Swedish Obese Subjects Study Scientific Group. Lifestyle, diabetes, and cardiovascular risk factors 10 years after bariatric surgery. N Engl J Med. 351(26):2683–93.
91. Buchwald H, Varco RL. Metabolic surgery. New York: Grunne and Stratton; 1978.
92. Rubino F, Cummings DE. Surgery: The coming of age of metabolic surgery. Nature Rev Endo. 2012;8: 702–4. doi:10.1038/nrendo.2012.207.

The Role of Laparoscopy in Bariatric Surgery

10

Marcello Lucchese, Alessandro Sturiale,
Giovanni Quartararo, and Enrico Facchiano

In 1902, Georg Kelling (Dresden, Saxony) performed the first laparoscopic procedure in dogs, and in 1910, Hans Christian Jacobaeus (Sweden) reported the first laparoscopic operation in humans. In the ensuing several decades, numerous individuals refined and popularized the approach further for laparoscopy. The introduction of computer chip television camera was a seminal event in the field of laparoscopy. The first publication on diagnostic laparoscopy by Raoul Palmer, appeared in the early 1950s, followed by the publication of Frangenheim and Semm. Hans Lindermann and Kurt Semm practised CO_2 hysteroscopy during the mid-seventies. In 1981, Semm, from the Universitats Frauenklinik, Kiel, Germany, performed the first laparoscopic appendectomy. Following his lecture on laparoscopic appendectomy, the president of the German Surgical Society wrote to the Board of Directors of the German Gynecological Society suggesting suspension of Semm from medical practice. Subsequently, Semm submitted a paper on laparoscopic appendectomy to the *American Journal of Obstetrics and Gynecology*, which was rejected as unacceptable for publication on the ground that the technique reported on was "unethical". His paper was finally published in the *Journal of Endoscopy*. Prior to 1990, the only specialty performing laparoscopy on a widespread basis was gynecology, mostly for relatively short, simple procedures. Laparoscopy in general surgery began in 1985 with the first laparoscopic cholecystectomy performed by Erich Muhe and submitted to the Congress of the German Society of Surgery. The following year, Mouret presented the clip of his procedure at Dubois in Paris [1] and only afterwards it was also performed in the United States [2]. As result of these first experiences, laparoscopy spread widely—thanks to the innovation in the technological field too. This condition led to the application of the new approach to other surgical procedures, such as gastrointestinal and bariatric surgery, with variable success depending on the technique. In fact, 38 years after the first bariatric procedure, which was a jejuno-ileal bypass, performed to treat morbid obesity by Kremen in 1954 [3], Broadbent [4] and Catona [5], who placed a nonadjustable gastric band, performed the first laparoscopic bariatric surgery in 1992–1993. Belachew et al. and Forsell et al. were the first to perform a laparoscopic adjustable gastric banding. These laparoscopic roots of bariatric banding may explain the early

M. Lucchese (✉) • A. Sturiale • G. Quartararo
E. Facchiano
Department of Surgery, Bariatric and Metabolic Surgery Unit, Azienda Sanitaria Firenze, Santa Maria Nuova Hospital, Piazza Santa Maria Nuova, 1, Florence 50122, Italy
e-mail: mlucch@iol.it; a.sturialemd@gmail.com; giovanni.quartararo@gmail.com; enricofacchiano@yahoo.it

M. Lucchese, N. Scopinaro (eds.), *Minimally Invasive Bariatric and Metabolic Surgery: Principles and Technical Aspects*, DOI 10.1007/978-3-319-15356-8_10,

prevalence of laparoscopic adjustable gastric banding in Europe. In 1994, Wittgrove et al. performed the first laparoscopic gastric bypass in the United States, initiating preference for laparoscopic gastric bypass that has come to dominate the country's operative selection in the first decade of the twenty-first century. Also in 1994, Hess performed a laparoscopic vertical banded gastroplasty. In 1991, the National Institutes of Health Conference statement on gastrointestinal surgery for severe obesity stated that bariatric surgery is the only therapy which let the morbid obese patients to reach a stable and satisfactory weight loss [6]. Hence, bariatric surgery, which had a great expansion in the middle of 1900s, reached higher levels with the introduction of laparoscopy because it was proved to be safe and feasible. Nowadays, laparoscopy is considered the "gold standard" for the surgical treatment of morbid obesity. Many different types of operations can be performed: vertical banded gastroplasty (VBG), adjustable gastric banding (AGB), laparoscopic Roux-en-Y Gatric bypass (LRYGB), sleeve gastrectomy (SG), and biliopancreatic diversion (BPD). LRYGB is the procedure mostly performed [7]. It is demonstrated that a team of bariatric surgery recently built up is associated with a doubled or tripled complications rate due to the learning curve. In fact, the LRYGB is a challenging procedure because of visceral fat, liver size, and thickness of the abdominal wall. For this reason, the surgeon must be technically proficient. Some authors believe that a total number of procedures ranging from 75 to 120 are necessary to obtain a postoperative complications rate similar to that reported in literature. The American Society for Metabolic and Bariatric Surgery (ASMBS) asserts that to be a proficient surgeon it is needed to certify 100 bariatric procedures, whose half as first operator, with a good outcome, starting from the residency supervised by an experienced surgeon. This kind of skills standardization is not well established in the European countries where the achievement of such a training program is more difficult [8]. The difficulty for the training resident to perform LRYGB comes from the required advanced laparoscopic skills. To solve this limitation, a new training curriculum comprising five steps has been proposed:

- Knowledge-based learning about the procedures.
- Divide the process into tasks by identifying the most challenging parts.
- Laboratory environment training, identifying, and/or developing different training models.
- Transfer the acquired skills to the real environment showing the acquired technique.
- Granting privileges for operating room practices [7].

An evolution of laparoscopy is the application of a single-incision laparoscopy (SIL) in bariatric surgery. Several authors have reported their own experience showing that it is a feasible technique in groups of highly selected patients. The selection is based on the type of intervention which should be not complex and on body habitus. Patients with tall trunk are more difficult because of the distance between the epigastric zone and ombelicus that should be not more than 22–25 cm. The potential advantages include less postoperative pain, better cosmetic result, and satisfaction of the patient. Some authors report an increase of incisional hernia rate due to the longer fascial incision. Furthermore, these patients often undergo plastic surgery after the achievement and maintenance of ideal weight whereby the desired esthetic result is reached in a second phase [9].

The further innovation in the minimally invasive surgical techniques development led to the application of the robot in bariatric surgery, trying to overcome the limits of standard laparoscopy. The robotic approach is safe and feasible in all types of bariatric surgery with a postoperative complications rate, including anastomotic leakage, very low and only slightly different from the conventional laparoscopy [10]. Robotic bariatric surgery has a shorter learning curve; in fact, it is believed that 20 cases are enough to overcome the basic learning phase. The robot could be useful in patients with difficult anatomy or in cases of revisional surgery after restrictive procedures where the surgeon may find difficult dissection and reconstruction. At present time, there is no scientific evidence about the superiority of the robot-assisted technique on the conventional laparoscopy whereby the exact role of the robotic approach should be defined more precisely in larger studies, also evaluating the high costs [10, 11].

10.1 Preoperative Workup

It consists of all investigations that a morbid obese patient must preoperatively perform to establish whether the procedure chosen by the multidisciplinary equipe is safe and feasible.

- *Blood exams*: Routine preoperative blood exams including hormonal screening tests and to the lipid concentrations dosage.
- *Abdominal ultrasound*: The guidelines of the ASMBS suggest to perform the preoperative abdominal ultrasound only in patients with symptoms related to biliary disease and abnormal liver function tests. On the opposite, The Society of American Gastrointestinal and Endoscopic Surgeons in their guidelines of 2008 assess that it is appropriate to perform abdominal ultrasound as a preoperative screening. Ultrasound findings may be various as the fatty liver, gallstones, and hepatomegaly but their evidence does not add much value to the preoperative workup because it does not change the surgical choice. Hence, it may state that the performance of abdominal ultrasound is recommended as a preoperative screening only in symptomatic patients whereas the routinary use is not recommended [12].
- *Barium radiography*: Preoperative routine use is controversial. Angrisani assesses that this radiological examination is the standard procedure before gastric banding. Ghassemian does not consider it as part of his protocol for preoperative LRYGB whereas Bova argues that it is necessary only in patients with upper gastro-intestinal (UGI) pathology such as previous gastric surgery. However, the reported data are often not comparable because they describe different types of operations. For this reason, further prospectical studies are needed to establish if the preoperative radiological screening may be useful [13].
- *UGI endoscopy*: It is an essential tool in the preoperative workup because it allows to identify some pathological conditions such as *Helicobacter pylori*-related gastritis, ulcers, polyps, or tumors. The surgical treatment proposed to the patient may be delayed or modified according to the type of finding [14]. In case of polypoid lesions, LRYGB is contraindicated because it does not allow the periodic endoscopic exploration of the abandoned stomach. In case of gastritis or ulcerative lesions, the appropriate medical therapy is started and only after endoscopic demonstration of a complete resolution, surgery can be performed. In a recent study, the esophageal capsule endoscopy (ECE) was evaluated as an alternative to the standard esophago-gastro-duodenoscopy (EGD). The best advantage of this technique is the noninvasive approach thus reducing the cardiopulmonary complications rate, which is about 0.6 % and related to the conscious sedation. On the other hand, the main limit is the difficulty to evaluate the stomach and duodenum. Further studies are needed to determine and define the role of this method as a preoperative tool [15].
- *24-h pH monitoring*: It is the procedure that allows to diagnose gastro-esophageal reflux disease (GERD). It is more accurate if associated with impedentiometry. Some authors include this investigation in the preoperative workup of patients who have to undergo a SG. This attitude in based on the evidence that the SG seems to increase GERD symptoms [16], whereas LRYGB seems to improve them. However, the effects of SG on GERD remain controversial. The literature can be divided in two categories: those who show an increase of GERD prevalence after SG and those who demonstrate a reduction of GERD prevalence. The pathogenetic mechanisms proposed are different. The increase in GERD prevalence may be explained by lower esophageal sphincter (LES) hypotension, blunting of angle of His, decrease in gastric compliance and emptying, and decrease in plasma ghrelin. On the other hand, the reduction of GERD prevalence might be explained by decrease in abdominal obesity, decrease in

acid production and wall tension, increase in long-term gastric compliance and gastric emptying. Anyway, the studies supporting both categories are rather heterogeneous and difficult to compare each other because of different factors such as variable method of GERD evaluation, length of follow-up, and surgical technique. Hence, it cannot be certainly state to introduce this investigation in the preoperative workup [17]. It could be used only in symptomatic patients or with esophagitis [16]. It would be desirable to perform further studies where the preoperative and postoperative GERD is evaluated through a standardized technique such as the 24-h pH monitoring and analyzing the effects of the sleeve on GERD symptoms [17].

- *Esophageal manometry*: It is a technique that studies the esophageal motor activity. It must be included in the preoperative workup of all patients who undergo VLB because it is a valuable instrument to predict the outcome of these patients correlated to the long-term follow-up esophageal dilatation. There is only a small percentage of patients with normal preoperative manometry who develop postoperative GERD symptoms and esophageal dilatation due to the band fill being too tight. The treatment is to enlarge the band allowing the esophagus to recover in a few weeks. VLB has been shown to have beneficial effect on GERD symptoms, in fact, the symptoms disappear in the short-term follow-up with a normalization of the values of LES pressure and 24-h pH monitoring. This investigation may be useful even in the prognostic evaluation of GERD symptoms in patients who will undergo a SG. On the other hand, there is no scientific evidence to support the routinary use of this investigation in the preoperative workup for patients who will undergo an LRYGB [18].

10.2 Preoperative Weight Loss

Super obesity (BMI >50 kg/m^2) and super-super-obesity (BMI >60 kg/m^2) are associated with an increase in early and late morbidity and mortality if compared to patients with BMI <50 kg/m^2. In fact, the Longitudinal Assessment of Bariatric Surgery Consortium has recently demonstrated a high probability of adverse outcome in patients with BMI >55 kg/m^2 with an increase in the conversion rate, complications, and hospital stay [19]. Hence, this condition causes more anesthetic and surgical problems. The technical difficulties are due to the considerable thickness of the abdominal wall that hinders the movements of laparoscopic instruments, the massive presence of intra-abdominal adipose tissue with short mesentery and hepatomegaly with fragile liver [20]. The surgery of these patients is so challenging that the International Federation for the Surgery of Obesity and Metabolic Disorders suggests to avoid these patients during the first period of surgeon's practice [19]. Therefore, preoperative weight loss is used to reduce the conversion rate and improve the outcome [21]—thanks to the significant reduction of the volume of the liver left lobe and visceral adipose tissue.

The first attempt to gain preoperative weight loss is based on a conservative therapy such as the diet. In case of diet failure, the placement of an intragastric balloon is useful [20].

- *Diet*: It is demonstrated in literature that a preoperative very low calory diet (VLCD) followed for a period ranging from 3 to 6 weeks before the operation reduces the operative risk and improves the postoperative outcome These diets are usually based on industrial liquid preparations that are poorly accepted by the patients [22, 23]. The efficacy of preoperative VLCD based on homemade ingredients to achieve weight loss was recently reported. It is associated with a good patient's satisfaction, cost reduction, and few secondary effects such as nausea and diarrhea [22].
- *Intragastric balloon* (*IB*): It is widely demonstrated in literature that the positioning of the IB is not effective to obtain a permanent weight loss [19]. Although it could even reach a weight loss of 32 % of the excess weight at the time of the removal, which usually occurs 6 months after about 40-50 % of the patients regain the weight lost in 12 months [21].

Therefore, IB may be considered as a "bridge therapy" to surgery reducing operative time and overall risk of adverse outcome [19].

10.3 Operating Room

The operating room must be adequate to perform laparoscopic surgery. The total weight capacity of the operating table has to allow the placement of super-obese patient in anti-Trendelemburg position. The multidisciplinary equipe is fundamental during the operative time as much as in the preoperative evaluation. In fact, a group of well-trained nurses and anesthesiologist dedicated to follow the entire pathway of the patients from the preoperative investigations to intraoperative and postoperative management have the same importance of the surgeon for a good outcome.

10.4 Surgical Strategies

In the field of laparoscopic bariatric surgery, the surgeon has different options during the operation:

- *Laparoscopic access*: Many different methods of laparoscopic access are reported in literature. These include the closed technique, which has two options, and the open technique. The first variant of the closed technique is based on the insertion of the Verres needle into the peritoneal cavity, gas insufflations, insertion of the first trocar and then the introduction of the other trocars under direct view. The second variant, instead, consists in the introduction of an optical trocar into the peritoneal cavity followed by gas insufflation and subsequent insertion of the other trocars under visual control. The open technique is based on the opening of the peritoneal cavity, insertion of a blunt trocar, gas insufflation, and then introduction of the other trocars under optical control. The potential advantages of the latter technique are the prevention of vascular and visceral lesions, gas embolism, and preperitoneal insufflation. There is no consensus about the best approach. In a recent review, it has been observed that there are no differences between the open and closed technique about vascular and visceral lesions incidence, and that the open technique is associated with a reduction of failed entry. Among the closed technique, the use of optical trocar is the safest because Veress needle is associated with an increase of the incidence of failed entry, extraperitoneal insufflation, and omental lesions. These results may certainly be affected by the heterogeneity of the studies, whereby further randomized controlled trials are needed [24]. In morbidly obese patients, the optical trocar is generally used because it is demonstrated to be safe, effective, and a rapid technique. On the other hand, the open technique is time-consuming and more difficult because of the thickness of the abdominal wall and subcutaneous fat. The vascular damages are certainly more likely in case of midline trocar insertion because it is pushed directly against the spine and major vessels. For this reason, it is better to introduce the optical trocar into the left upper quadrant just below the ribs thus preventing the collapse of the abdominal wall on the viscera. It is the fundamental to understand the phases of the correct introduction through the abdominal wall to achieve a good safety level of the procedure [25]. However, some authors state that the midline insertion of the device appears to be a safe procedure [26].
- *Drain placement*: The placement of routine abdominal drainage during bariatric surgery is widely used and the basic purpose is the early detection of a leak so that it can be converted into a controlled fistula avoiding re-intervention. Several randomized trials and systematic reviews showed that the systematic use of abdominal drainage is associated with an increase of postoperative morbidity, costs, and length of hospital stay in different types of abdominal surgery. The placement of abdominal drainage alone is often not sufficient to make the diagnosis of anastomotic leak because neither the quantity nor the quality of the drainage allow to do certain diagnosis, whereby further investigations such as UGI contrast or CT scan are needed in clinically stable patients [27]. The drain does not

frequently allow a conservative treatment because it is placed near the gastro-jejunal anastomosis and it does not drain any jejuno-jejunal anastomotic leak. It has been observed that the drainage does not significantly reduce the incidence of re-interventions in patients with confirmed anastomotic leak; in fact, the post-re-intervention morbidity and mortality rate are similar to that of patients without drainage [28]. In some cases, even further radiological investigations fail to demonstrate the anastomotic leakage [29]. For these reasons, the clinical signs are the most sensitive marker to assess postoperative outcome. Laparoscopy significantly reduced the surgical insult, whereby the presence of one or more of persistent tachycardia, temperature higher than 38.5°C, reduced diuresis and poor control of abdominal pain, must alert the surgeon to perform investigations or reintervention [27, 30, 31]. The ASMBS states there is no high level of evidence to support the routine use of drainage to prevent GI leakage [32].

- *Intraoperative testing of anastomotic leakage*: It is a method that allows to evaluate the anastomotic integrity during the intervention in patients who undergo LRYGB. There are two options: the simplest procedure is the infusion of methylene blue through an orogastric tube. In this way it is possible to evaluate both the gastro-jejunal and jejuno-jejunal anastomosis. Some authors believe that this method has some drawbacks including the staining of the operative field in case of leak, making more difficult the further test after surgical repair, and the possible difficulty to blindly introduce the orogastric tube [33]. In our experience, the latter does not represent a difficulty because it is employed the same tube used to calibrate the gastric pouch and it is placed at peri-anastomotic level under optic control. The other reported method is the intraoperative endoscopy (IE) with hydro-pneumatic test. The advantages offered by this technique are the possibility of a direct visualization of the lumen and the anastomosis guiding the surgeon to identify the possible leak. It may be repeated after surgical repair without modifying its diagnostic accuracy and it even helps to identify bleeding sites and to test the anastomotic patency [28]. The availability of the endoscopist, as member of the multidisciplinary team, in the operating room to perform this procedure is fundamental. For this reason too, this type of surgery should be performed only in specialized centers. A possible complication of IE is related to an excessive air pressure during the procedure that may increase the risk of bleeding or leak, whereby it must be gently performed by skilled endoscopists. From the recent published studies, it may state that the intraoperative endoscopy is a safe and effective method to evaluate the patency of the gastro-jejunal anastomosis [33–35], but further randomized trials are needed to evaluate whether it is useful and cost-effective because the incidence of postoperative leaks in patients with intraoperative negative test is seldom reported.
- *Staple-line reinforcement* (*SLR*): Although the importance of staple-line reinforcement in bariatric surgery has been documented, its real advantage remains controversial. There are three options of reinforcement: oversewing the staple line, application of fibrin glue sealant, and incorporation of buttressing materials. The latter has been developed to increase the strength of the staple line by increasing the thickness of the wall. It is preloaded in the staple gun and incorporated into the staple line on firing. Many different products are available such as permanent and non-permanent bovine pericardial strips or synthetic bioadsorbable materials [36]. These types of staple-line reinforcement were used in both SG and LRYGB. The major postoperative complications after SG are the staple-line bleeding and the leakage which is the most life-threatening complication. It has an incidence of 2.7 % and occurs mainly in the highest part of the suture just below the gastro-esophageal junction. The pathophysiology of the leakage may be related to different factors such as reduced blood supply, mainly at the angle of His, stapler device failure, inadequate technique, postoperative high intragastric pressure due to gastroparesis.

The real advantages of the SLR for SG are not clear. Some authors believe that there are no differences in the outcome between the groups with and without SLR. This is in contrast with results of another meta-analysis, which demonstrates a reduction of leakage in SLR patients group. Another prospective randomized study, however, shows that there is no difference in the incidence of leaks or bleeding in the two groups, but a higher incidence of postoperative stenosis in the SLR group [37]. There is no evidence about the best practice regarding SLR in LRYGB too. Some authors report a reduction of bleeding with subsequently decrease of endo-clips application [38] and reduction of leak [39] if the bovine pericardial strips are used. A multicenter randomized trial, instead, report the preliminary results that fibrin glue does not have adverse effects, it is not time-consuming and may be effective to prevent leaks and internal hernias in morbidly obese patients [40].

- *Timing to perform cholecistectomy during bariatric surgery*: Most of the studies aim to establish the indications to perform a cholecystectomy in patients who undergo LRYGB or other bariatric procedures. There are three possible approaches: prophylactic, selective, or conventional cholecystectomy [41, 42]. The prophylactic cholecystectomy means to perform this intervention during LRYGB, regardless for the presence or absence of preoperative biliary stones. The reason for this approach is the evidence that the rapid postoperative weight loss is associated with an increase of the gallstone formation incidence if compared with the normal population. A percentage between 28 and 36 % of the patients after LRYGB develop stones within 3 years. The pathophysiology of this process lies in an increased hepatic secretion of cholesterol causing a cholesterol supersaturation of the bile [43]. The selective approach, instead, consists to perform cholecystectomy during LRYGB in asymptomatic patients with preoperative or intraoperative finding of cholelithiasis. This approach is based on the higher probability to have symptoms in patients with stones compared to those without stones. The conventional approach means to perform cholecystectomy during LRYGB only in patients with symptomatic stones according to the guidelines for the treatment of gallstone disease [42]. Another possible fourth approach is to delay the cholecystectomy after LRYGB only in patients who become symptomatic after weight loss. In this case, the intervention can be easier and has a lower perioperative morbidity [41]. Although the incidence of gallstones increases after bariatric surgery, only almost the 40 % of these patients become symptomatic [43, 44]. This finding could support the latter approach. For those patients who do not undergo simultaneous cholecystectomy, it has been shown that pharmacological prevention with ursodeoxycholic acid (UDCA) is effective in decreasing the biliary cholesterol saturation, but a low compliance to the therapy was also detected. Hence, although there are controversial opinions, it may be stated that a cholecystectomy performed during LRYGB is safe and feasible, usually using the same trocars, sometimes introducing the sixth. It is associated with an increased operative time and in some series increased hospitalization time without increasing the intervention-related complications rate [43]. The prophylactic approach seems to be an overtreatment because the risk of symptomatic gallstone disease requiring operation is low [44]. The selective approach reduces potential future gallstone-related morbidity, the need of readmission for further surgery thus reducing costs [41]. Instead, the conventional approach shows, regardless for the UDCA administration, that the majority of patients who develop stones remain asymptomatic, whereby they don't need surgical treatment. For this reason, the risks to perform a simultaneous cholecystectomy might be unwarranted [42].

10.5 Revisional Surgery

With the increase of the bariatric procedures worldwide, it has gradually emerged a new group of surgeries known as revisional surgery and the number of patients which require this type of operations is progressively raised. It consists of re-intervention in patients who have undergone previous bariatric surgery. The revisional surgery can be classified into two categories: conversion surgery that converts an initial procedure into another, such as converting an AGB into an LRYGB; and the return surgery that restores the initial anatomy of the patient [45]. There are several conditions requiring revisional surgery, such as intractable marginal ulcer, severe gastro-esophageal reflux, gastro-gastric fistula, severe nutritional or metabolic disorders, problems with the band including slippage, tubing leakage, esophageal motor problems, and at last inadequate weight loss or weight regain. Revisional bariatric surgery is complex and technically demanding. There are several publications showing that revisional laparoscopic surgery is safe and feasible without prejudicing the subsequent weight loss, but it should be performed in high-volume centers by experienced surgeons. The complication rate ranges from 0 to 39 % with a conversion rate between 0 and 47.6 %. The laparoscopic approach showed a progressive significant reduction of minor complications and it seems to be superior if compared to the open technique even if the primary procedure was performed in open way. However, the advantages of this surgery are greater than the risks in most of the patients [46] with perioperative outcomes very similar to those of primary procedures [47]. For these reasons, the evaluation of patients who have an inadequate weight loss or weight regain is complex and requires a multidisciplinary team. First, psychiatric and nutritional disorders must be excluded and then anatomical problems which can be treated endoscopically or surgically must be evaluated. In case of LRYGB as primary procedure, the main cause of inadequate weight loss or weight regain is the dilation of the gastric pouch or of the gastro-jejunal anastomosis. In this condition, the endoscopic procedures have conflicting results, but the introduction of new devices may change the future scenario. The surgical approach has the best results. On the other hand, in case of vomiting with feeding difficulties, the main cause can be an anastomotic stenosis that can be successfully treated by endoscopic treatment [45].

10.6 Laparoscopy Versus Open Technique

The introduction of the laparoscopy has widely proved its advantages over the open approach in various types of surgery. The same advantages are found in bariatric surgery with the difference that the morbid obese patients have more risks than non-obese patients for cardiopulmonary complications, infections, and wound-related complications [48, 49].

Advantages

- Reduction of the surgical insult with a consequent concentrations decrease of the mediators of the hypermetabolic stress response, such as catecholamines, cortisol, cytokines, and other acute-phase reactants. This condition determines a reduction in energy expenditure, pulmonary and renal workload, and myocardial O_2 demand that contributes to perioperative morbidity through unclear process, and a reduction of cell-mediated immunity impairment related to a fewer postoperative infections [48].
- Reduction of the postoperative ileum with a faster bowel function recovery and reduced hospitalization time [48].
- Reduction of pulmonary alterations that results in less reduction of oxygen saturation and total lung capacity, with fewer pulmonary complications [48].
- Reduction of wound-related complications such as seroma, hematoma, infection, dehiscence, and incisional hernias [48]. A recent meta-analysis showed a reduction of the risk of wound infection and incisional hernia, respectively, of 79 and 89 % compared to open surgery [49].
- Although the data are conflicting and in some cases difficult to compare each other, the rate of reinterventions, anastomotic leak, and all-cause mortality are similar to the open surgery. However, all-cause mortality is low in both type of surgery [49].
- The outcome of weight loss at 12 months was the same as that of the open surgery [49].
- Reduction of postoperative adhesions that makes less difficult further surgery.

- Best esthetic result even if its importance is limited because most of these patients undergo plastic surgery after stable weight loss.
- Reduction of the costs of postoperative complications management and shorter hospital stay.

Disadvantages

- Pneumoperitoneum has negative effects on the respiratory and cardiovascular systems [50]. Morbid obese patients have a baseline intrabdominal pressure approximately equal to 2–3 times that of a non-obese. The intraperitoneal introduction of CO_2 leads to a systemic absorption of CO_2, a reduction of cardiac preload due to venous compression reducing intraoperative urine output, a decrease of lung compliance, increase of airway pressure, and cardiac function impairment. The optimization of anesthesiologic procedures may minimize these adverse changes [51].
- Higher costs of surgical instruments, especially if disposable devices are used. It must be considered in relation to the cost of a longer hospitalization and more wound-related complications of open surgery.
- Learning curve longer than the open surgery [8].

References

1. Davis CJ, Filipi CJ. Principles of laparoscopic surgery: basic and advanced techniques. In: Arregui ME, Fitzgibbons RJ, McKernan JB, Reich H, editors. Principles of Laparoscopic surgery: basic and advanced techniques. 3rd ed. New York: Springer; 1995.
2. Reddick EJ, Olsen DO. Laparoscopic laser cholecystectomy. A comparison with mini-lap cholecystectomy. Surg Endosc. 1989;3(3):131–3.
3. Halverson JD, Wise L, Wazna MF, Ballinger WF. Jejunoileal bypass for morbid obesity. A critical appraisal. Am J Med. 1978;64(3):461–75.
4. Broadbent R, Tracey M, Harrington P. Laparoscopic gastric banding: a preliminary report. Obes Surg. 1993;3(1):63–7.
5. Catona A, Gossenberg M, La MA, Mussini G. Laparoscopic gastric banding: preliminary series. Obes Surg. 1993;3(2):207–9.
6. Gastrointestinal surgery for severe obesity: National Institutes of Health Consensus Development Conference Statement. Am J Clin Nutr. 1992;55(2 Suppl):615S–9S.
7. Zevin B, Aggarwal R, Grantcharov TP. Simulation-based training and learning curves in laparoscopic Roux-en-Y gastric bypass. Br J Surg. 2012;99(7):887–95.
8. Sanchez-Santos R, Estevez S, Tome C, Gonzalez S, Brox A, Nicolas R, et al. Training programs influence in the learning curve of laparoscopic gastric bypass for morbid obesity: a systematic review. Obes Surg. 2012;22(1):34–41.
9. Rogula T, Daigle C, Dua M, Shimizu H, Davis J, Lavryk O, et al. Laparoscopic bariatric surgery can be performed through a single incision: a comparative study. Obes Surg. 2014;24(7):1102–8.
10. Cirocchi R, Boselli C, Santoro A, Guarino S, Covarelli P, Renzi C, et al. Current status of robotic bariatric surgery: a systematic review. BMC Surg. 2013;13:53.
11. Buchs NC, Pugin F, Azagury DE, Huber O, Chassot G, Morel P. Robotic revisional bariatric surgery: a comparative study with laparoscopic and open surgery. Int J Med Robot. 2014;10(2):213–7.
12. Almazeedi S, Al-Sabah S, Alshammari D. Routine trans-abdominal ultrasonography before laparoscopic sleeve gastrectomy: the findings. Obes Surg. 2014; 24(3):397–9.
13. Sharaf RN, Weinshel EH, Bini EJ, Rosenberg J, Ren CJ. Radiologic assessment of the upper gastrointestinal tract: does it play an important preoperative role in bariatric surgery? Obes Surg. 2004;14(3):313–7.
14. Zeni TM, Frantzides CT, Mahr C, Denham EW, Meiselman M, Goldberg MJ, et al. Value of preoperative upper endoscopy in patients undergoing laparoscopic gastric bypass. Obes Surg. 2006;16(2):142–6.
15. Shah A, Boettcher E, Fahmy M, Savides T, Horgan S, Jacobsen GR, et al. Screening pre-bariatric surgery patients for esophageal disease with esophageal capsule endoscopy. World J Gastroenterol. 2013;19(37): 6188–92.
16. Braghetto I, Lanzarini E, Korn O, Valladares H, Molina JC, Henriquez A. Manometric changes of the lower esophageal sphincter after sleeve gastrectomy in obese patients. Obes Surg. 2010;20(3):357–62.
17. Laffin M, Chau J, Gill RS, Birch DW, Karmali S. Sleeve gastrectomy and gastroesophageal reflux disease. J Obes. 2013;2013:741097.
18. Klaus A, Weiss H. Is preoperative manometry in restrictive bariatric procedures necessary? Obes Surg. 2008;18(8):1039–42.
19. Zerrweck C, Maunoury V, Caiazzo R, Branche J, Dezfoulian G, Bulois P, et al. Preoperative weight loss with intragastric balloon decreases the risk of significant adverse outcomes of laparoscopic gastric bypass in super-super obese patients. Obes Surg. 2012;22(5):777–82.
20. Alfalah H, Philippe B, Ghazal F, Jany T, Arnalsteen L, Romon M, et al. Intragastric balloon for preoperative weight reduction in candidates for laparoscopic gastric bypass with massive obesity. Obes Surg. 2006;16(2):147–50.
21. Angrisani L, Lorenzo M, Borrelli V, Giuffre M, Fonderico C, Capece G. Is bariatric surgery necessary after intragastric balloon treatment? Obes Surg. 2006; 16(9):1135–7.

22. Gonzalez-Perez J, Sanchez-Leenheer S, Delgado AR, Gonzalez-Vargas L, Diaz-Zamudio M, Montejo G, et al. Clinical impact of a 6-week preoperative very low calorie diet on body weight and liver size in morbidly obese patients. Obes Surg. 2013;23(10):1624–31.
23. Fris RJ. Preoperative low energy diet diminishes liver size. Obes Surg. 2004;14(9):1165–70.
24. Ahmad G, O'Flynn H, Duffy JM, Phillips K, Watson A. Laparoscopic entry techniques. Cochrane Database Syst Rev. 2012;(2):CD006583.
25. Berch BR, Torquati A, Lutfi RE, Richards WO. Experience with the optical access trocar for safe and rapid entry in the performance of laparoscopic gastric bypass. Surg Endosc. 2006;20(8):1238–41.
26. Sabeti N, Tarnoff M, Kim J, Shikora S. Primary midline peritoneal access with optical trocar is safe and effective in morbidly obese patients. Surg Obes Relat Dis. 2009;5(5):610–4.
27. Kavuturu S, Rogers AM, Haluck RS. Routine drain placement in Roux-en-Y gastric bypass: an expanded retrospective comparative study of 755 patients and review of the literature. Obes Surg. 2012;22(1):177–81.
28. Lee S, Carmody B, Wolfe L, Demaria E, Kellum JM, Sugerman H, et al. Effect of location and speed of diagnosis on anastomotic leak outcomes in 3828 gastric bypass cases. J Gastrointest Surg. 2007;11(6):708–13.
29. Gonzalez R, Sarr MG, Smith CD, Baghai M, Kendrick M, Szomstein S, et al. Diagnosis and contemporary management of anastomotic leaks after gastric bypass for obesity. J Am Coll Surg. 2007;204(1):47–55.
30. Liscia G, Scaringi S, Facchiano E, Quartararo G, Lucchese M. The role of drainage after Roux-en-Y gastric bypass for morbid obesity: a systematic review. Surg Obes Relat Dis. 2014;10(1):171–6.
31. Quartararo G, Facchiano E, Scaringi S, Liscia G, Lucchese M. Upper gastrointestinal series after Roux-en-Y gastric bypass for morbid obesity: Effectiveness in leakage detection. A systematic review of the literature. Obes Surg. 2014;24(7):1096–101.
32. ASMBS Clinical Issues Committee. ASMBS guideline on the prevention and detection of gastrointestinal leak after gastric bypass including the role of imaging and surgical exploration. Surg Obes Relat Dis. 2009;5(3):293–6.
33. Alasfar F, Chand B. Intraoperative endoscopy for laparoscopic Roux-en-Y gastric bypass: leak test and beyond. Surg Laparosc Endosc Percutan Tech. 2010;20(6):424–7.
34. Cingi A, Yavuz Y. Intraoperative endoscopic assessment of the pouch and anastomosis during laparoscopic Roux-en-Y gastric bypass. Obes Surg. 2011; 21(10):1530–4.
35. Mohos E, Schmaldienst E, Richter D, Prager M. Examination of the efficacy and safety of intraoperative gastroscopic testing of the gastrojejunal anastomosis in laparoscopic Roux Y gastric bypass surgery. Obes Surg. 2011;21(10):1592–6.
36. Albanopoulos K, Alevizos L, Flessas J, Menenakos E, Stamou KM, Papailiou J, et al. Reinforcing the staple line during laparoscopic sleeve gastrectomy: prospective randomized clinical study comparing two different techniques. Preliminary results. Obes Surg. 2012;22(1):42–6.
37. Knapps J, Ghanem M, Clements J, Merchant AM. A systematic review of staple-line reinforcement in laparoscopic sleeve gastrectomy. JSLS. 2013;17(3):390–9.
38. Angrisani L, Lorenzo M, Borrelli V, Ciannella M, Bassi UA, Scarano P. The use of bovine pericardial strips on linear stapler to reduce extraluminal bleeding during laparoscopic gastric bypass: prospective randomized clinical trial. Obes Surg. 2004;14(9):1198–202.
39. Shikora SA. The use of staple-line reinforcement during laparoscopic gastric bypass. Obes Surg. 2004; 14(10):1313–20.
40. Silecchia G, Boru CE, Mouiel J, Rossi M, Anselmino M, Tacchino RM, et al. Clinical evaluation of fibrin glue in the prevention of anastomotic leak and internal hernia after laparoscopic gastric bypass: preliminary results of a prospective, randomized multicenter trial. Obes Surg. 2006;16(2):125–31.
41. Tucker ON, Fajnwaks P, Szomstein S, Rosenthal RJ. Is concomitant cholecystectomy necessary in obese patients undergoing laparoscopic gastric bypass surgery? Surg Endosc. 2008;22(11):2450–4.
42. Quesada BM, Kohan G, Roff HE, Canullan CM, Chiappetta Porras LT. Management of gallstones and gallbladder disease in patients undergoing gastric bypass. World J Gastroenterol. 2010;16(17):2075–9.
43. Hamad GG, Ikramuddin S, Gourash WF, Schauer PR. Elective cholecystectomy during laparoscopic Roux-en-Y gastric bypass: is it worth the wait? Obes Surg. 2003;13(1):76–81.
44. Taylor J, Leitman IM, Horowitz M. Is routine cholecystectomy necessary at the time of Roux-en-Y gastric bypass? Obes Surg. 2006;16(6):759–61.
45. Ferraz AA, de Siqueira LT, Nunes FE, de Araujo JGJ, Campos JM, de Barros-Correia TX, et al. Revision surgery for treatment of weight regain after Roux-en-Y gastric bypass. Obes Surg. 2014;24(1):2–8.
46. Shimizu H, Annaberdyev S, Motamarry I, Kroh M, Schauer PR, Brethauer SA. Revisional bariatric surgery for unsuccessful weight loss and complications. Obes Surg. 2013;23(11):1766–73.
47. Stefanidis D, Malireddy K, Kuwada T, Phillips R, Zoog E, Gersin KS. Revisional bariatric surgery: perioperative morbidity is determined by type of procedure. Surg Endosc. 2013;27(12):4504–10.
48. Schauer PR, Ikramuddin S. Laparoscopic surgery for morbid obesity. Surg Clin North Am. 2001;81(5): 1145–79.
49. Reoch J, Mottillo S, Shimony A, Filion KB, Christou NV, Joseph L, et al. Safety of laparoscopic vs open bariatric surgery: a systematic review and meta-analysis. Arch Surg. 2011;146(11):1314–22.
50. Nguyen NT, Wolfe BM. The physiologic effects of pneumoperitoneum in the morbidly obese. Ann Surg. 2005;241(2):219–26.
51. Gaszynski T, Szewczyk T. The influence of laparoscopic vs. open gastric bypass on hemodynamic function in morbidly obese patients during general anesthesia. Wideochir Inne Tech Malo Inwazyjne. 2014;9(1):83–8.

Anesthesia in Bariatric Surgery 11

Jay B. Brodsky

11.1 Preoperative Considerations

11.1.1 Preoperative History and Physical Examination

A thorough preoperative past medical history and physical examination are always important. Special attention should be directed at identifying potential intraoperative airway management problems. A high Mallampati score (III or IV), large neck circumference, poor dentition, limited mouth opening, and reduced range of head and neck motion should all be evaluated.

Besides the anatomic and mechanical problems often present, extreme obesity is associated with many potentially serious medical conditions (Table 11.1). Medical co-morbidities must be recognized, and when possible optimized before elective bariatric surgery. Of particular concern are patients with the metabolic syndrome (MetS). Although definitions of the constituents of MetS vary by degree, the presence of central or visceral obesity, dyslipidemia, hypertension, and diabetes or insulin resistance are always present (Table 11.2).

J.B. Brodsky, MD
Department of Anesthesiology, Perioperative and Pain Medicine, Stanford University School of Medicine, Stanford, CA 94305, USA
e-mail: Jbrodsky@stanford.edu

Most obese patients, especially younger ones without serious medical co-morbidities scheduled for elective bariatric procedures, do not require an expensive and complex preoperative workup [1]. A comprehensive metabolic panel, a chest radiograph, and perhaps an EKG in older patients are usually all that need to be routinely obtained. Any patient who has had previous bariatric surgery should be evaluated for metabolic changes that can include protein, vitamin, iron, and calcium deficiencies. Patients with MetS, with sleep-disordered breathing problems, and with other significant cardiovascular conditions are of special concern, and when present may indicate the need for further diagnostic evaluation and perhaps consultation with a cardiologist, endocrinologist, or sleep physician.

The most common sleep-disordered breathing condition is obstructive sleep apnea (OSA). Patients maintain a normal $PaCO_2$ during the day but have CO_2 retention, sleep disturbances, intermittent airway obstruction with hypoxemia, and cardiac arrhythmias at night. OSA is characterized by frequent episodes of apnea (>10 s cessation of airflow despite continuous respiratory effort against a closed airway) and hypopnea (50 % reduction in airflow or reduction associated with a decrease of oxyhemoglobin saturation (SpO_2) >4 %). OSA is very common in obesity and has been reported to be present in as many as 70 % of morbidly obese

M. Lucchese, N. Scopinaro (eds.), *Minimally Invasive Bariatric and Metabolic Surgery: Principles and Technical Aspects*, DOI 10.1007/978-3-319-15356-8_11,

Table 11.1 Pathophysiology and diseases associated with obesity

1. Cardiovascular system (a) Hypertension (both systemic and pulmonary) (b) Atherosclerosis and hyperlipidemia (c) Congestive heart failure (d) Coronary artery disease (e) Peripheral vascular disease and chronic venous insufficiency
2. Respiratory system (a) Dyspnea (restrictive lung disease) (b) Altered sleep disorders (obstructive sleep apnea, obesity hypoventilation syndrome) (c) Pulmonary embolism
3. Gastrointestinal system (a) Hepatic steatosis and abnormal liver function tests (b) Cholelithiasis (c) Abdominal, inguinal, and hiatal hernias (d) Higher incidence of gall bladder cancer (females) (e) Higher incidence of colon cancer (males)
4. Reproductive system (a) Female infertility, disrupted menstruation, and ovulation (b) Urinary incontinence (c) Gestational diabetes (d) Higher incidence of cervical, endometrial, ovarian, and breast cancer (e) Higher incidence of prostate cancer
5. Endocrine system (a) Type 2 diabetes mellitus (b) Disorders of plasma cortisol and growth hormone (c) Decreased levels of testosterone and increased levels of estradiol and estrogen in men
6. Musculoskeletal system (a) Osteoarthritis (hips, knees) (b) Hyperuricemia and gout (c) Rhabdomyolysis (d) Spinal column problems
7. Dermatologic system (a) Acanthosis nigricans (b) Fungal skin infections
8. Psychiatric (a) Depression (b) Low self-esteem (c) Impaired body image

Increasing obesity is associated with pathophysiologic changes in all organ systems and with many associated medical co-morbidities. These conditions should be sought during the preoperative evaluation and should be optimized before surgery when possible

Table 11.2 Metabolic Syndrome (MetS)

1. Abnormal glucose metabolism (must be present) (a) Diabetes mellitus (b) Impaired glucose tolerance (c) Impaired fasting glucose insulin resistance
Plus at least two of the following
2. Hypertension (blood pressure >140/90 mmHg)
3. Dyslipidemia: (d) Triglycerides ≥1.695 mmol l^{-1} (e) High-density lipoprotein cholesterol (i) ≤0.9 mmol l^{-1} (male) (ii) ≤1.0 mmol l^{-1} (female)
4. Central obesity: large waist; waist:hip ratio (iii) >0.90 (male) (iv) >0.85 (female)
5. Microalbuminuria (f) Urinary albumin excretion ratio ≥2 min^{-1} (g) Albumin:creatinine ratio 30 mg g^{-1}

Metabolic syndrome: World Health Organization (WHO) definition (1999)
Patients with the metabolic syndrome have a much greater incidence of serious medical problems than do patients of similar weight

(BMI > 40 kg/m^2) patients undergoing bariatric surgery [2]. OSA is associated with many potentially serious conditions including systemic and pulmonary hypertension, coronary artery disease, congestive heart failure, and stroke. Polysomnography (PSG) will give a definitive diagnosis of OSA; however, preoperative testing has not been shown to be cost effective or to actually improve operative outcomes in bariatric patients. In the absence of a PSG diagnosis, we use the STOP-BANG questionnaire to identify patients with OSA [3] (Table 11.3). Many of the anatomic and pathophysiologic consequences that are associated with OSA can be reduced or corrected by applying nasal continuous positive airway pressure (CPAP) or bi-level positive airway pressure (BiPAP) devices, but only if the treatment is instituted weeks or months before surgery. Unfortunately, many OSA patients do not use their prescribed CPAP masks. Those patients who do have their own devices should be instructed to bring them to the hospital on the day of surgery for use during their recovery.

Table 11.3 STOP-BANG Questionnaire for Identifying Patients with Obstructive Sleep Apnea (OSA)

*S*NORE:	Do you snore loudly? (snoring can be heard through closed door)
*T*IRED:	Do you feel tired, sleepy, fatigued, during daytime?
*O*BSERVED:	Has anyone seen you stop breathing during sleep?
BLOOD *P*RESSURE:	Do you have, or are you being treated, for high blood pressure?
*B*MI:	Is your BMI >35 kg/m^2?
*A*GE:	Are you older than 50?
*N*ECK CIRCUMFERENCE:	Is your neck circumference >40 cm?
*G*ENDER:	Are you a male?

Modified from: Chung and Elsaid [34]
This questionnaire is used to identify patients with OSA who have not undergone diagnostic polysomnography. If the answer to any three of these questions is "yes", then a presumptive diagnosis of OSA can be made. If the answer to five or more is "yes," a more "definitive" diagnosis of OSA can be made

11.1.2 Premedication

As a rule sedative premedication should be avoided, especially for patients with OSA. We occasionally give small amounts of an anxiolytic (e.g., midazolam) for very anxious patients. We usually continue most medications for chronic hypertension. The exception are angiotensin-converting enzyme (ACE) inhibitors (e.g., lisinopril, captopril, losartan), which are stopped for the day of surgery. These drugs can cause profound hypotension following induction of general anesthesia. The preoperative administration of a beta-blocker remains controversial, and it we do routinely use them.

MO patients were once considered at risk for gastric acid aspiration because of their increased intra-abdominal pressure and a high incidence of gastro-esophageal reflux disease (GERD). Recent studies and clinical experience have not demonstrated a need for routine aspiration prophylaxis. For patients with severe GERD and for those who have previously undergone gastric banding procedures, an H_2-receptor antagonist (e.g., ranitidine, famitidine) is given preoperatively.

Diabetic medications (e.g., insulin, oral hypoglycemics) are also withheld on the day of surgery. Prophylaxis, with an antibiotic against wound infection and with heparin to prevent deep venous thrombosis, is usually given at the surgeon's request. An anti-sialogogue (e.g., atropine, glycopyrrolate) can also be administered if a fiber-optic tracheal intubation is planned.

11.2 Intraoperative Considerations

11.2.1 Positioning

Extremely obese patients have a marked reduction in lung volume, which is further exaggerated when they lie flat. Once a patient is moved onto the operating room table, they should be positioned with pillows, blankets, or a commercial "elevation" device so that their head, upper body, and shoulders are in the *head elevated laryngoscopy position* (HELP). In this position the patient's ears should be level with their sternum. When compared to MO patients placed in the conventional "sniff" intubating position, HELP facilitates gas exchange while improving visual exposure during direct laryngoscopy (DL) [4].

The position of the operating room table influences the size of the surgical workspace in obese patients (BMI>35 kg/m^2) undergoing laparoscopy. In one study the operating room table was placed, in random order, in five different positions: (1) table horizontal with the legs flat, i.e., supine position, (2) table in 20° reverse Trendelenburg (RT) with the legs flat, (3) table in 20° RT with the legs flexed 45° upward at the hips, i.e., beach chair position, (4) table horizontal with the legs flexed 45° upward at the hips, and (5) table in 20° Trendelenburg with the legs flat. This study found that the mean inflated intra-abdominal volume in the supine position was about 3.2 l, and that volume increased by 900 ml in both the Trendelenburg position or when the legs were flexed at the hips with RT. Intra-abdominal volume decreased by 230 ml in the RT position. The conclusion was that the Trendelenburg position was best for lower abdominal surgery, and RT combined with leg flexion at the hips gave the largest workspace for upper abdominal surgery [5]. They noted that although the Trendelenburg position increased intra-abdominal space, it should not be used during bariatric surgery because ventilation of the MO patient could be significantly compromised in this position.

All pressure points must be carefully padded to prevent pressure sores, neurologic injury, and rhabdomyolysis (RML), each of which occurs more frequently in obese surgical patients. The patient's neck, arms, and legs should also be supported to avoid stretch injuries and subsequent peripheral nerve damage.

11.2.2 Physiologic Monitoring

Standard physiologic monitors (EKG, noninvasive blood pressure cuff, pulse oximetry, end-tidal capnography, and temperature probe) are always applied.

An indwelling urinary catheter is important in order to monitor urine output. There is normally a transient decrease in urine production during laparoscopy, with return of normal kidney function following release of the pneumo-peritoneum.

An arterial line is usually unnecessary for continuous blood pressure monitoring, except in patients with significant hypertension or other cardiovascular conditions. When intraoperative blood tests are planned, an indwelling arterial line allows frequent sampling for blood gas analysis and for intermittent serum glucose monitoring. Central venous or pulmonary artery lines and trans-esophageal echocardiography (TEE) are seldom indicated, except in patients with significant cardiopulmonary disease or to guide fluid resuscitation. A central venous line may be necessary when peripheral venous access is limited. Ultrasonography greatly increases the success rate of internal jugular vein cannulation in obese patients.

A nerve stimulator is very important to assess the degree of neuromuscular blockade. Many anesthesiologists routinely use an electroencephalography (EEG) depth of anesthesia monitor, especially to titrate down the concentration of inhalational and intravenous anesthetics toward the end of surgery prior to emergence [6].

The anesthesiologist is responsible for proper placement of gastric tubes, used to decompress the stomach, to size the gastric pouch, and to test for anastomotic leaks. Any foreign body in the esophagus (gastric tube, temperature probe, TEE probe) must be completely withdrawn before the gastric pouch is stapled.

11.2.3 Fluid Management

Intraoperative fluid requirements in obese patients are usually greater than for normal-weight patients undergoing similar laparoscopic procedures. Obese patients receiving several liters of intravenous crystalloid had a faster recovery and fewer complications after laparoscopic cholecystectomy than those with restrictive fluid replacement [7]. There are few studies of fluid replacement in MO patients. Liberal amounts of intra-operative intravenous fluid may reduce the incidence of postoperative nausea and vomiting (PONV) in bariatric patients [8]. Generous amounts of intravenous fluid should also be given intraoperatively to reduce the risk of RML and postoperative renal failure [9].

11.2.4 Temperature Maintenance

All anesthetized patients lose heat and become poikilothermic during surgery. Even though adipose tissue is a thermal insulator, heat loss is increased during laparoscopy in obese patients due to the cool, dry CO_2 that is used for the pneumo-peritoneum and when cold irrigating fluids are used. Forced-air heating blankets are always applied, and warmed intravenous and irrigating fluid are occasionally needed. Attempts to minimize heat loss using heated and humidified gas for the pneumo-peritoneum have not been successful [10].

11.3 Anesthetic Drug Administration

11.3.1 Pharmacologic Principles

Increases in cardiac output (CO), lean body weight (LBW), adipose tissue, extracellular fluid volume, liver and kidney abnormalities, and changes in plasma protein binding all occur with increasing obesity. Each of these parameters can alter the pharmacology of the agents used during anesthesia. Drug dosing based on actual or total body weight (TBW) is valid for normal-weight patients, but must be strictly avoided in obese patients.

LBW (muscles, bones, tendons, ligaments, body water) is equal to TBW minus the weight of body fat. In normal males, LBW is about 80 % TBW and in normal females 75 % of TBW. There is an overall increase in LBW with obesity, mainly due to an increase in total body water. However, whereas adipose tissue increases proportionally with increasing weight, the percentage of lean body tissue per kilogram of TBW decreases. Since metabolic activity in the body mainly occurs in lean tissues, LBW is a more practical scalar for drug dosing in every patient, but especially those with extreme obesity. As a general guideline for MO patients, simply adding 20–30 % to the patient's ideal body weight (IBW) will give a value for LBW that can be used for dosing drugs. IBW, for both men and women, can be estimated by multiplying patient's height in meters squared by 22 [11].

11.3.2 Intravenous Drugs

The dosing of lipid soluble intravenous anesthetic induction agents (thiopental, propofol) should be based on LBW [12]. Anesthetic induction and maintenance using total intravenous anesthesia (TIVA) with target-controlled infusions (TCI) have improved the accuracy of drug delivery for normal-weight patients. However, due to the lack of pharmacokinetic/pharmacodynamic parameters specific to the MO population, the algorithms used by TCI devices are derived from normal subjects and these formulae can result in inappropriate overdosing of heavier patients. TBW is capped at 150 kg in some models, but TCI infusions in bariatic patients are almost always inaccurate and can be potentially dangerous [13]. Intraoperative drug dosing is best guided by monitoring clinical end points such as heart rate and blood pressure, degree of sedation, and degree of neuromuscular blockade.

We prefer using succinylcholine for muscle relaxation for laryngoscopy and tracheal intubation because of its rapid onset and its short duration of action. Pseudocholinesterase levels and extracellular fluid space both increase in obesity, and unlike other drugs the dose of succinylcholine in obese patients is based on actual or TBW (1.0 mg/kg), which reflects these changes [14]. Rocuronium can also be used for DL and tracheal intubation if the reversal agent sugammadex is available. Sugammadex can immediately reverse paralysis by rocuronium or vecuronium if and when airway intubation difficulties are encountered. At this time sugammadex is not released for clinical use in the United States. For maintenance of muscle paralysis, there appears to be no advantage between any of the nondepolarizing muscle relaxants (e.g., atracurium, vecuronium, rocuronium) in bariatric patients. The initial dose of these neuromuscular agents should be based on IBW or LBW and the degree of motor blockade during surgery carefully monitored with a nerve stimulator. Paralysis must be completely reversed before the patient's trachea is extubated.

Opioids, but especially long-acting agents (e.g., morphine, hydromorphone, demerol) should be kept to a minimum due to their respiratory depressive effects. We use an intravenous infusion of the ultrashort acting opioid remifentanil during bariatric surgery to supplement inhalational anesthesia. Toward the completion of the procedure, usually at the time the trocars are removed and after the wounds are infiltrated with local anesthetic, we discontinue the inhalational agent but continue the remifentanil. Once surgery is complete, the remifentanil infusion is stopped. The patient will usually emerge from anesthesia and be fully awake within 2–3 min.

11.3.3 Choice of Inhalational Anesthetic

Desflurane is the least lipid soluble inhaled anesthetic, and some have recommended its use for obese patients based on the belief that slower release from fat of the more lipid soluble anesthetics (isoflurane, sevoflurane) will prolong emergence from anesthesia [15]. Although lower blood flow to adipose tissue may limit the initial delivery of volatile agents to fat, anesthetic concentrations in the highly perfused brain and lungs rapidly decrease once any agent is discontinued. In MO patients, there are no significant *clinical* differences in recovery time with any of the inhalational anesthetics [16].

11.4 Airway and Ventilatory Management

11.4.1 Securing the Airway

Ventilation by bag and mask can be difficult in obese patients due to their heavy chest wall and reduced pulmonary compliance. The presence of a high Mallampati score (III or IV) and OSA with upper airway obstruction are additional risk factors for difficulty with mask ventilation [17]. Besides the potential of hypoventilation during ineffective mask ventilation, gastric insufflation can occur which will increase the risk of regurgitation and pulmonary aspiration. For effective mask/bag ventilation two people are often needed, one to apply and maintain a tight mask fit while keeping the airway open and one to bag-ventilate the patient.

Despite the popularity of supra-glottic airways for all types of surgery including laparoscopy, these devices should be avoided in MO patients. An endotracheal tube protects against acid aspiration, and allows for controlled or assisted positive-pressure ventilation. A major audit of airway complications during and after general anesthesia recently reported a several-fold increased risk of pulmonary problems, especially acid aspiration, in obese patients anesthetized with a laryngeal mask airway (LMA) instead of an endotracheal tube [18]. The UK Society of Bariatric Anaesthetists recommended that an endotracheal tube always be the *default airway* in obese surgical patients [19].

MO patients have limited oxygen stores due to their reduced lung volume. Their hemoglobin will desaturate rapidly once they are made apneic for tracheal intubation. A secure airway must be established quickly. The *safe apnea period* (SAP), i.e., the time from onset of paralysis to a S_pO_2 of 90–92 %, is only about 2–3 min in MO patients compared to 8–10 min in a normal-weight patient [20]. To "unload" the diaphragm and maximize functional residual capacity, the OR table should be placed in a 20°–30° RT position before induction of anesthesia [21]. Application of positive-end expiratory pressure and/or noninvasive positive-pressure ventilation during pre-oxygenation prior to intubation decreases atelectasis and increases the SAP in MO patients.

11.4.2 Tracheal Intubation

A high Mallampati airway score (III or IV) combined with large neck circumference (>60 cm) are the most reliable predictors for potential difficulty with conventional DL [22]. Increasing BMI itself *is not* a risk factor for failed tracheal intubation. The most important strategy for success with DL is to pre-oxygenate the patient until their end-tidal oxygen concentration is >90 %, while placing the patient in the HELP (which significantly improves view with direct laryngoscopy), and tilting the OR table to RT (which increases SAP) (Fig. 11.1). A longer SAP provides the laryngoscopist with additional time to secure the airway before hypoxemia develops. An assistant, who is experienced with airway management, should always be immediately available to help.

If difficulty with intubation is encountered, an LMA can serve as a temporary *bridge* until an endotracheal tube can be successfully placed [23]. Intubation aids, including a short laryngoscope handle and different laryngoscope blades, a gum elastic bougie, a video-laryngoscope, and equipment for emergency crico-thyrotomy

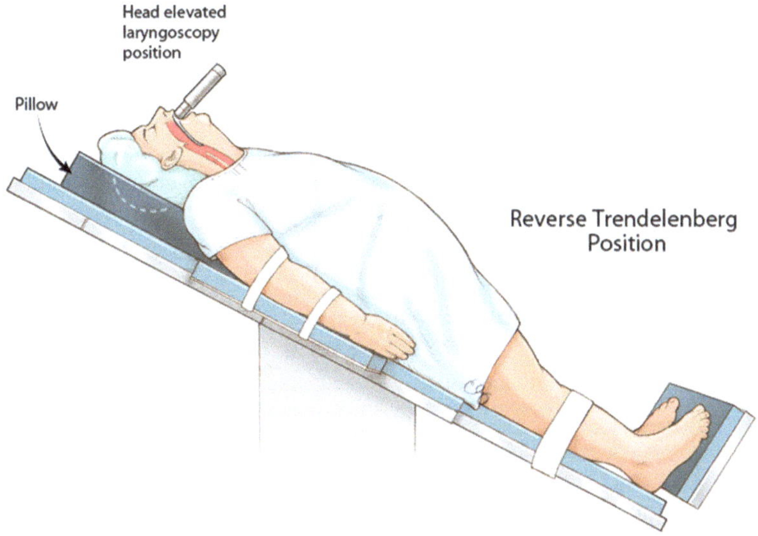

Fig. 11.1 The ideal position for induction of general anesthesia in a morbidly obese patient is shown. The patient should be positioned with pillows, blankets, and/or elevation devices so that the head, upper body, and shoulders raised so that an imaginary horizontal line can connect the patient's ears with their sternum, the *head elevated laryngoscopy position* (HELP). The operating room table should be tilted 20°–30° in reverse Trendelenburg (RT). HELP improves visual exposure during direct laryngoscopy, while RT maximizes lung volumes increasing the *safe apnea period.*

and trans-tracheal jet ventilation, should always be available.

Historically, an *awake* fiber-optic bronchoscopy has been used for MO patients when a difficult intubation was anticipated. Video-laryngoscopes have generally replaced the bronchoscope in anticipated situations, and also when unanticipated difficulty is encountered during conventional DL [24]. In some institutions, a video-laryngoscope, rather than direct rigid laryngoscopy, is now used for the first intubation attempt for all MO patients.

11.4.3 Mechanical Ventilation

MO patients should never be allowed to breathe spontaneously during laparoscopy, so ventilation should always be controlled during bariatric surgery. Following successful intubation, we mechanically ventilate our patients with a FiO_2 of 0.5–1.0 and a tidal volume of 10 ml/kg (IBW). Even smaller tidal volumes and/or pressure-controlled ventilation have been recommended to minimize peak airway pressure and potential lung injury, but there is no evidence that these practices are actually beneficial [25].

Peak ventilatory pressure increases with the laparoscopic pneumo-peritoneum, and lowering tidal volume even further, increasing respiratory rate, and adding positive end-expiratory pressure (PEEP) and/or alveolar recruitment maneuvers can maintain satisfactory oxygenation and help maximize the surgical workspace [26]. However, end-tidal CO_2 levels, which normally increase at the start of the pneumo-peritoneum will increase even further during small tidal volume ventilation, and this will result in *permissive hypercapnia* and respiratory acidosis.

The pneumo-peritoneum can cause cephalad displacement of the diaphragm causing the tip of the endotracheal tube to enter the right bronchus. Tube displacement during laparoscopy should always be considered in the differential diagnosis of hypoxemia and marked increase in peak inspiratory pressure during surgery.

11.5 Postoperative Considerations

11.5.1 Admission to the PACU

As with tracheal intubation at the start of the case, careful attention to the airway is also essential during emergence from anesthesia. The vast majority of bariatric patients can have their endotracheal tube removed in the operating room immediately following the completion of surgery. If hemodynamically stable, the airway should be extubated with the patient's head and upper body elevated. The patient should then be transferred to the PACU and recovered in the same position. Postoperative mechanical ventilation is seldom needed, and ICU admission is rare following laparoscopic surgery.

11.5.2 Management of OSA

For patients with severe OSA, we insert a nasal trumpet prior to tracheal extubation in order to avoid upper airway obstruction immediately following removal of the endotracheal tube. Patients who use nasal CPAP or BiPAP at home should bring their devices to the hospital to be used in the PACU if there is any sign of airway obstruction. There is no evidence that CPAP causes anastomotic leaks from a distended gastric pouch following bariatric surgery [27]. A commercially available Boussignac mask helps maintain satisfactory S_pO_2 levels in patients who do not have their own CPAP equipment [28].

11.5.3 Postoperative Nausea and Vomiting

Obesity is not a risk factor for PONV. However, many patients undergoing bariatric procedures do have multiple risk factors (e.g., female, receiving opioids, emetogenic surgery). We always start multimodal drug prophylaxis for PONV during the procedure. Dexamethasone (4–8 mg) is a very effective antiemetic agent, and it is routinely included in our therapeutic regimen, unless the patient has poorly controlled diabetes. A 5-HT_3 antagonist (e.g., odonsatron, granisitron) is also given during surgery. Administering several different antiemetic agents can reduce, but not eliminate the development of PONV. Liberal amounts of intravenous crystalloid fluid replacement may also help reduce the incidence of PONV after laparoscopy.

11.5.4 Postoperative Analgesia

At the completion of the laparoscopic procedure, the surgeon infiltrates local anesthetic into the trocar sites. Incisional wound pain in the immediate recovery period should be less than would be expected after a laparotomy. However, many patients do complain of mild to moderate general discomfort, probably from peritoneal irritation and/or distention from the pneumo-peritoneum. Opioid analgesia should be kept to a minimum and use of non-opioid adjuncts should be instituted early. Alpha-2 agonists (e.g., clonidine, dexmedetomidine) reduce analgesic requirements with no respiratory depressant effects, and can be used as an alternative or as a supplement to opioids [29]. Nonsteroidal anti-inflammatory (NSAIDs) drugs are helpful initially, but should be discontinued within a day or two to avoid the potential complication of gastric ulceration. Additional analgesic strategies include low-dose ketamine, intravenous lidocaine or acetaminophen, and/or continuous infusion of local anesthetics, either intraperitoneally or at the wound sites [30]. The goal of any of multimodal analgesic technique is to reduce or completely eliminate the use of opioids. Small doses of short-acting opioids (fentanyl) are used for intravenous patient-controlled analgesia (PCA). A baseline opioid infusion should be avoided in bariatric patients, and the fentanyl administered only as needed by patient control.

11.5.5 Complications

Thrombo-embolism can present in the PACU and is a major cause of postoperative mortality. MO patients are at risk for venous thrombosis because of their greater blood volume, relative polycythemia, high fatty acid levels, hyper-cholesterolemia and diabetes. Preoperative anticoagulation is always indicated and a vena caval umbrella is sometimes placed in older and very high-risk patients. Early ambulation must be encouraged. To achieve this, the anesthetic technique should allow the patient to recover quickly and be able to get out of bed on the same day shortly after surgery. Many bariatric procedures, including gastric banding and gastric bypass operations, are currently performed in out-patient ambulatory surgical centers. The most common presentation of a pulmonary embolism in the PACU is tachycardia, hypertension, and hypoxemia. Patients can also experience increased anxiety, dyspnea, and a "feeling of doom." These signs and symptoms are similar to those occurring with an anastomotic leak, so the latter must be considered in the differential diagnosis.

During long-duration surgery, especially in super-obese (BMI >50 kg/m^2) male patients with diabetes and peripheral vascular disease, muscle tissue can experience pressure injury. The resulting RML can be present immediately after surgery in the PACU. The patient may complain of tender or weak muscles, usually in the dependent buttock, hip, and shoulder areas. Dark "tea" colored urine, due to myoglobin in the urine, may also be present. If unrecognized or untreated, RML can proceed to severe electrolyte disturbances with hyperkalemia, hypocalcemia, cardiac dysrhythmias, and even cardiac arrest. Late complications of RML include renal failure and disseminated intravascular coagulation. The primary diagnostic indicator of RML is an elevation of serum creatine phosphokinase (CPK) levels, which can be present in as many as 25 % of bariatric surgical patients. A CPK value five times greater than normal (1,000 IU/l) is diagnostic of RML, but renal problems from myoglobinuria usually do not occur until CPK levels are significantly higher (>5,000 IU/l) [31]. Early diagnosis of RML leads to earlier treatment and a better prognosis. Diuresis with large amounts of intravenous fluids is the mainstay of treatment.

Conclusion

The incidence of obesity in the population is rising throughout the world, and increasing numbers of obese patients are presenting for weight-loss procedures. Absolute weight, per se, does not increase anesthetic risk for these patients. There are no differences in outcomes between MO and super-MO patients undergoing bariatric operations under similar anesthetic management [32]. Fast-track laparoscopic bariatric surgery can be safely performed, even in the outpatient setting, as long as the anesthesiologist is aware of the special needs of obese patients and is prepared to meet those challenges [33].

References

1. Schumann R, Jones SN, Cooper B, et al. Update on best practice recommendations for anesthetic perioperative care and pain management in weight loss surgery, 2004–2007. Obesity (Silver Spring). 2009;17:889–94.
2. Frey WC, Pilcher J. Obstructive sleep-related breathing disorders in patients evaluated for bariatric surgery. Obes Surg. 2003;13:676–83.
3. Chung F, Yang Y, Liao P. Predictive performance of the STOP-Bang score for identifying obstructive sleep apnea in obese patients. Obes Surg. 2013;23:2050–7.
4. Collins JS, Lemmens HJM, Brodsky JB, et al. Laryngoscopy and morbid obesity: a comparison of the "sniff" and "ramped" positions. Obes Surg. 2004;14:1171–5.
5. Mulier JP, Dillemans B, Van Cauwenberge S. Impact of the patient's body position on the intraabdominal workspace during laparoscopic surgery. Surg Endosc. 2010;24:1398–402.
6. Arain SR, Barth CD, Shankar H, et al. Choice of volatile anesthetic for the morbidly obese patient: sevoflurane or desflurane. J Clin Anesth. 2005;17:413–9.
7. Holte K, Klarskov B, Christensen DS, et al. Liberal versus restrictive fluid administration to improve recovery after laparoscopic cholecystectomy: a randomized, double-blind study. Ann Surg. 2004;240:892–9.
8. Schuster R, Alami RS, Curet MJ, et al. Intra-operative fluid volume influences postoperative nausea and vomiting after laparoscopic gastric bypass surgery. Obes Surg. 2006;16:848–51.
9. Wool DB, Lemmens HJ, Brodsky JB, et al. Intraoperative fluid replacement and postoperative creatine phosphokinase levels in laparoscopic bariatric patients. Obes Surg. 2010;20:698–701.

10. Davis SS, Mikami DJ, Newlin M, et al. Heating and humidifying of carbon dioxide during pneumoperitoneum is not indicated: a prospective randomized trial. Surg Endosc. 2006;20:153–8.
11. Lemmens HJ, Brodsky JB, Bernstein DP. Estimating ideal body weight – a new formula. Obes Surg. 2005;15:1082–3.
12. Ingrande J, Brodsky JB, Lemmens HJ. Lean body weight scalar for the anesthetic induction dose of propofol in morbidly obese subjects. Anesth Analg. 2011;113:57–62.
13. Ingrande J, Lemmens HJ. Dose adjustment of anaesthetics in the morbidly obese. Br J Anaesth. 2010;105 Suppl 1:i16–23.
14. Lemmens HJ, Brodsky JB. The dose of succinylcholine in morbid obesity. Anesth Analg. 2006;102:438–42.
15. Brodsky JB, Lemmens HJ, Saidman LJ. Obesity, surgery, and inhalation anesthetics – is there a "drug of choice"? Obes Surg. 2006;16:734.
16. Schumann R. Anaesthesia for bariatric surgery. Best Pract Res Clin Anaesthesiol. 2011;25:83–93.
17. Kheterpal S, Martin L, Shanks AM, et al. Prediction and outcomes of impossible mask ventilation: a review of 50,000 anesthetics. Anesthesiology. 2009;110:891–7.
18. Cook TM, Woodall N, Frerk C. Major complications of airway management in the UK: results of the Fourth National Audit Project of the Royal College of Anaesthetists and the Difficult Airway Society. Part 1: anaesthesia. Br J Anaesth. 2011;106:617–31.
19. Nightingale CE, Cousins J, Fox WT, et al. Comment on Fourth National Audit Project from the Society of Bariatric Anaesthetists. Br J Anaesth. 2011;107:272–3.
20. Jense HG, Dubin SA, Silverstein PI, et al. Effect of obesity on safe duration of apnea in anesthetized humans. Anesth Analg. 1991;72:89–93.
21. Boyce JR, Ness T, Castroman P, et al. A preliminary study of the optimal anesthesia positioning for the morbidly obese patient. Obes Surg. 2003;13:4–9.
22. Brodsky JB, Lemmens HJ, Brock-Utne JG, et al. Morbid obesity and tracheal intubation. Anesth Analg. 2003;94:732–6.
23. Keller C, Brimacombe J, Kleinsasser A, et al. The Laryngeal Mask Airway ProSeal(TM) as a temporary ventilatory device in grossly and morbidly obese patients before laryngoscope-guided tracheal intubation. Anesth Analg. 2002;94:737–40.
24. Marrel J, Blanc C, Frascarolo P, et al. Videolaryngoscopy improves intubation condition in morbidly obese patients. Eur J Anaesthesiol. 2007;24:1045–9.
25. Aldenkortt M, Lysakowski C, Elia N, et al. Ventilation strategies in obese patients undergoing surgery: a quantitative systematic review and meta-analysis. Br J Anaesth. 2012;109:493–502.
26. Talab HF, Zabani IA, Abdelrahman HS, et al. Intraoperative ventilatory strategies for prevention of pulmonary atelectasis in obese patients undergoing laparoscopic bariatric surgery. Anesth Analg. 2009;109:1511–6.
27. Weingarten TN, Kendrick ML, Swain JM, et al. Effects of CPAP on gastric pouch pressure after bariatric surgery. Obes Surg. 2011;21:1900–5.
28. Wong DT, Adly E, Ip HY, et al. A comparison between the Boussignac™ continuous positive airway pressure mask and the venturi mask in terms of improvement in the PaO2/F(I)O2 ratio in morbidly obese patients undergoing bariatric surgery: a randomized controlled trial. Can J Anaesth. 2011;58:532–9.
29. Tufanogullari B, White PF, Peixoto MP, et al. Dexmedetomidine infusion during laparoscopic bariatric surgery: the effect on recovery outcome variables. Anesth Analg. 2008;106:1741–8.
30. Iyer CP, Robertson BD, Lenkovsky F, et al. Gastric bypass and On-Q pump: effectiveness of Soaker Catheter system on recovery of bariatric surgery patients. Surg Obes Relat Dis. 2010;6:181–4.
31. Chakravartty S, Sarma DR, Patel AG. Rhabdomyolysis in bariatric surgery: a systematic review. Obes Surg. 2013;23:1333–40.
32. Leykin Y, Pellis T, Del Mestro E, et al. Perioperative management of 195 consecutive bariatric patients. Eur J Anaesthesiol. 2008;25:168–70.
33. Elliot JA, Patel VM, Kirresh A, et al. Fast-track laparoscopic bariatric surgery: a systematic review. Updates Surg. 2013;65:85–94.
34. Chung F, Elsaid H. Screening for obstructive sleep apnea before surgery: why is it important? Curr Opin Anaesthesiol. 2009;22:405–11.

12 Fast-Track in Bariatric Surgery: Safety, Quality, Teaching Aspects, Logistics and Cost-Efficacy in 8,000 Consecutive Cases

Hjortur Gislason, H.J. Jacobsen, A. Bergland, E. Aghajani, B.J. Nergard, B.G. Leifsson, and J. Hedenbro

12.1 Introduction

In the last decades, there has been continuous development in surgical and anaesthesia techniques with a shift towards less invasive and less traumatic treatment. Many of the standard modalities in abdominal surgery like routine use of nasogastric tubes, drains and urine catheters have been shown to be unnecessary or even harmful. Minimally invasive surgery and, especially, the use of laparoscopic technique have been proved as safe and associated with enhanced recovery. The term "fast-track surgery" originally described by Kehlet [1] dealt primarily with patients' pain and length of hospital stay. The term now refers to a multimodal package of techniques, which aim to decrease post-surgical organ dysfunction, improve post-operative recovery and reduce complications. This includes enhanced recovery after surgery (ERAS); ERAS protocols are aimed at improving surgical recovery and implement several evidence-based perioperative care interventions [2, 3]. Another and no less important issue for patient safety is the teaching and training aspects of new surgeons as well as of the whole surgical team [4–8]. The use of short-acting opioids and lower dose of propofol only in the induction of anaesthesia are useful to ensure quicker emergence from anaesthesia [9, 10]. Results can be improved by making a medical audit and standardizing all aspects of the treatment process. Continuously entering own data to a database increases awareness of the results.

In times of limited economic resources, most countries have a limited health budget but a large number of patients needing our treatment [11–16]. It is our obligation to secure a good use of these resources by treating as many patients as possible for a low cost and with high quality.

Good logistics are also a key element in order to streamline the work and secure maximal use of the resources, improve patient quality and obtain good long-term results. Economical awareness is especially important and easily incorporated in the treatment process without compromising patient safety and quality.

H. Gislason (✉) • H.J. Jacobsen • E. Aghajani
B.J. Nergard • B.G. Leifsson
Department of Surgery, Aleris Hospital,
Aleris Obesity, Fredrik-Stangs gate 11-13,
Oslo 0264, Norway

Aleris Obesity Skåne, Skåne, Sweden
e-mail: hjortur.gislason@aleris.no

A. Bergland
Department of Anaesthesia, Aleris Hospital,
Aleris Obesity, Fredrik-Stangs gate 11-13,
Oslo 0264, Norway

Aleris Obesity Skåne, Skåne, Sweden

J. Hedenbro
Department of Surgery, Aleris Hospital,
Aleris Obesity, Fredrik-Stangs gate 11-13,
Oslo 0264, Norway

Aleris Obesity Skåne, Lund-Kristianstad, Sweden

M. Lucchese, N. Scopinaro (eds.), *Minimally Invasive Bariatric and Metabolic Surgery: Principles and Technical Aspects*, DOI 10.1007/978-3-319-15356-8_12,

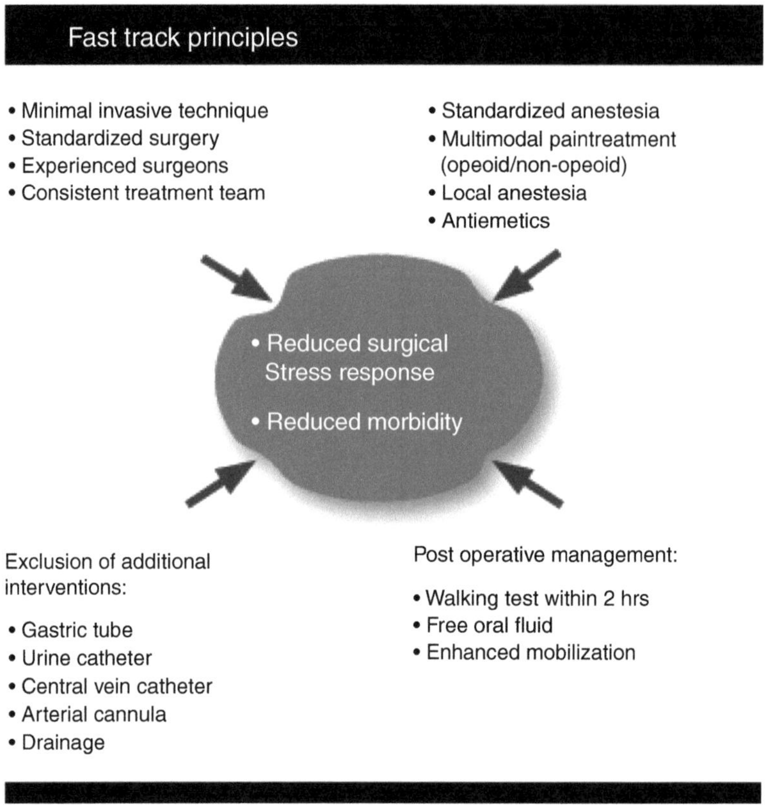

Fig. 12.1 Factors involved in ERAS/fast-track surgery (From Jacobsen et al. [17], with permission)

Outcome of treatment is measured by hospital stay, rate of readmissions and complications, economical aspects and long-term results on weight and comorbidity.

12.2 Our Practical Implementation

Experienced surgeons, well beyond their learning curves, initiated a high-volume bariatric surgery programme in 2005. Clinical pathways were established and time recordings from all parts of the treatment as well as clinical outcome were prospectively registered. With time, we have implemented our approach to four different hospitals. In order to provide good-quality treatment for high volumes of patients, a separate department was deemed necessary, so that no interference occurred from the emergency room patients or other type of surgery. The nursing staffs were offered good conditions in order to avoid shifts in personnel.

We present a cohort study with 8,000 consecutive LRYGB using a standardized programme for bariatric surgery based on "fast-track" methodology with focus on quality, cost-efficiency and training of new bariatric surgeons.

12.3 Materials and Methods

Aleris Hospital in Oslo, Norway, and Aleris Obesity Skåne, Sweden, are two surgical private practice units specializing in bariatric surgery. The treatment protocol was started and developed in Oslo in 2005–2008 [10, 17]. Evidence-based elements of "fast-track" surgery with minimal invasive technique were implemented in the programme from the beginning (Fig. 12.1). Both units used the same treatment protocol and a joint database, and all operations were performed in a standardized manner using the same rotating team of surgeons. All 8,000 consecutive LRYGBs performed in the two hospitals between September 2005 and February 2014 were included in the study. Indications for surgery were the same as those generally accepted as good standard

Table 12.1 Enhanced recovery after surgery (ERAS) protocol

Pre-operative preparation	Screening by phone: criteria for surgery? Medical records collected A 1-day course on education and information by the multidisciplinary team Initiation of patient contribution: physical activities, diet, stop smoking
Day of operation	Clear oral fluid up to 2 h before surgery, no solid food for 8 h Shower with antiseptic sponge 2 h before surgery, empty urinary bladder Single-dose cefuroxime (1.5 g iv) or 800 mg Bactrim® orally 2 h before surgery No thrombosis prophylactics unless history of thrombo-embolic diseases, or APC resistance in family history
During operation	8 mg i.v. dexamethasone at induction of anaesthesia Standardized anaesthesia Local anaesthetics in wounds
In the recovery room	Observation (telemetry, oxygen saturation), pain medication and antiemetics when needed Free oral fluid (amount recorded) Walking test (20 m) after 2 h and arrival to the ward
At the ward – day of surgery	Standard multimodal analgesia and anti-emetic Intensive mobilization; out of bed every h, using the PEP whistle, "keep the patient busy" 5,000 IU low molecular heparin 6 h after surgery If tachycardia, more pain than expected or not getting out of bed the surgeon notified
Day after surgery	Shower and changing the bandages Group meeting with the dietician (liquid and pure diet for 5 weeks) Going through pre-operative blood test and administering the supplements Discharge meeting with the surgeon emphasizing "early sign of complication" and the importance of early contact by phone Patients living within 90 min from hospital discharged home, the others to the neighbouring hotel for 1–4 days
After discharge	Phone call 1 and 7 days and 3 weeks after discharge Self-administration of low molecular heparin s.c. for 10 days Omeprazole 40 mg daily for 3 months

for bariatric surgery in the European Guidelines [18].

12.4 Pre-operative Preparation and Organization

At first contact, a screening phone call is made providing medical history, and the previous medical records are collected. The patients attended a mandatory full-day course with information and education in group sessions held by a surgeon, anaesthesiologist, nurse, dietician and physiotherapist. The patient was fully informed about the fast-track set-up and what will happen on the day of surgery. Weight loss of 5 % and change in lifestyle and eating habits were strongly encouraged prior to surgery. At the end of the day of the first visit, patients were evaluated for indication for surgery, type of operation was decided and day of surgery was scheduled, usually 5–6 weeks later (Table 12.1).

We developed a "length of hospital stay prediction system" based on comorbidity, BMI, psychosocial status and distance of residence from the hospital [17]. The ambition was to close the ward during most weekends, and this was facilitated by identifying and scheduling patients with anticipated longer hospital stay to the beginning of the week. Initially, patients were offered 3-day post-operative hospital care, but in 2008 this was reduced to 2 days and in 2009 patients were planned to be discharged on the first post-operative day. Patients living more than 1 hour of transport from the hospital were encouraged to stay near the hospital until 5 days after surgery.

The ward and one operating theatre were booked for 4 days at a time; the frequency of "bariatric weeks" depended on the number of patients cleared for surgery. The ward is usually closed on Friday evenings but remained open during the weekend only due to emergency cases or prolonged hospital stay.

12.5 Logistics and Fast-Track Principles

Medical audit for the patient flow was made. All elements of the treatment procedures before, during and after surgery were thoroughly standardized. The team in the operating theatre consisted of two surgeons, one senior bariatric surgeon and the other a surgeon skilled in laparoscopy but in training for bariatric surgery. There were also two operating nurses, one anaesthesiologist and one anaesthetist nurse. The time recordings were continuously registered in a database. The whole treatment was based on teamwork and all co-workers were primed on their role to get a streamlined logistics and avoid unnecessary waiting. An important principle at the operating theatre was "parallel working", many staff members working with the patient at the same time, washing and covering abdomen before the patient was intubated, reflecting the fact that the "busy time in the process is the turnover-time".

Standardization of the procedure makes the surgery safer, as it is performed precisely the same way by all surgeons of the team. Most authors agree that the experience and skill of the individual surgeon is the most important single factor for patient safety and good outcome [4–8]. Thus, training programmes for new surgeons are of great importance in order to avoid painful learning curves. Technical training in intracorporeal suturing and use of staplers needs numerous repetitions under guidance (Table 12.2).

All the instruments used for each operation were pre-packed into three standardized packages. One package contained the reusable surgical tools, packed and sterilized at our hospital. The other two packages were custom made for our purposes by surgical tools suppliers: one containing staplers and troacars (Ethicon Endo-Surgery or Covidien) and the other containing all other single-use items for one operation (Mölnlycke Health Care AB, Gothenburg, Sweden).

Table 12.2 Safe surgery, teaching aspects and quality control

All members of the team	Continuous medical education of all staff Standardization Research and development projects for all categories
Surgeon	Two surgeons procedure
Five-step training programme for new surgeon	1. Assisting in 50 operations 2. Starting operation and operating for 45 min with strict hands-on guidance (two of six operations that day) 3. When technically sufficient and good progression within 45 min, the trainee is allowed to complete the operation, but not exceeding 60 min 4. The trainee is performing 100 more operations still with hands-on guidance 5. The trainee becomes expert surgeon and starts performing surgery with a trainee
Early sign of complication	Immediate re-operation
Recordings of operation	If complication within 30 days, video recording of the operation examined in order to learn and improve
Continuous database recordings	Individual surgeon's complication rate can be followed

12.6 Surgical Procedure

The surgical procedure was meticulously standardized and the time used for different parts of the operation was recorded (Fig. 12.2). The purpose was to enhance technical improvements and shorten the surgical time. This also helps the anaesthesiologist to monitor the anaesthesia according to the progress of the surgery and to time the termination of the anaesthesia.

The surgical procedure has been described in detail previously [17, 19]. The patient was placed in a supine, split-leg, reversed Trendelenburg position. Five ports were used: two 5-mm and two 12-mm ports for instruments and one 10-mm port for the camera. A 45° scope and intra-abdominal pressure at 18 mmHg were used.

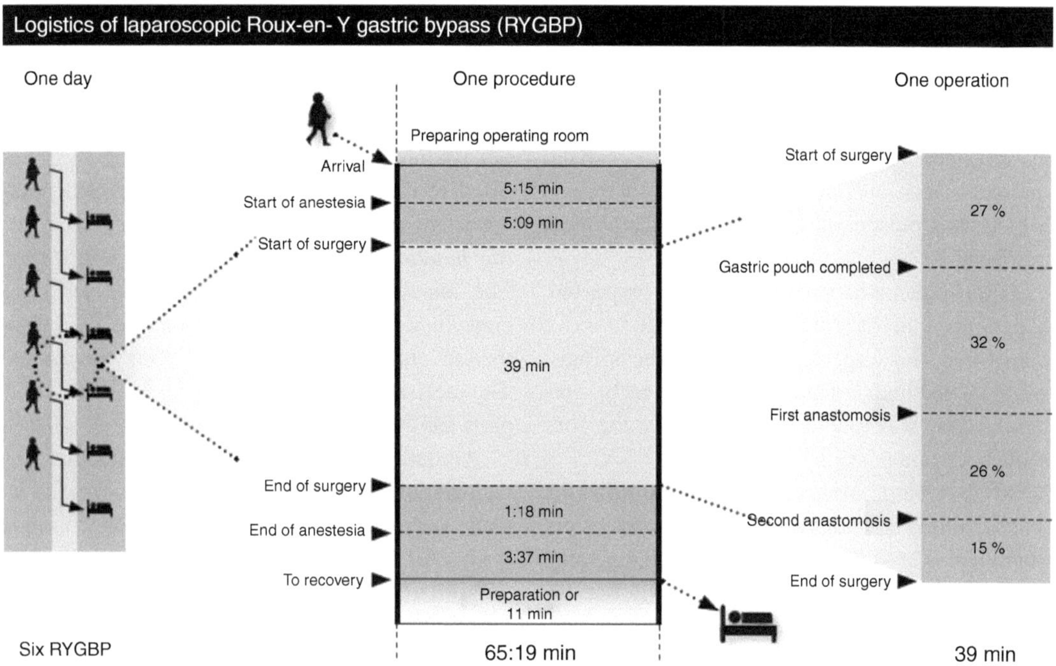

Fig. 12.2 Logistic of the treatment process from when a patient walks into the operating theatre until next patient arrives for 261 patients operated during second half of 2010. Non-operative time is mean time (minutes: seconds). The operating time is referred as median (From Jacobsen et al. [17], with permission)

In brief, a small gastric pouch (15 ml) was created with the bowel in an antecolic and antegastric position. The gastroenteric (GE) anastomosis and the enteroenteric (EE) anastomosis were stapled linearly and the staple holes handsewn. The bowel was approximated to the gastric pouch as an omega loop, subsequently divided by stapling between the two anastomoses. The last step was to test the integrity of the GE anastomosis by inflation with methylene blue–dyed saline via a nasogastric tube. The nasogastric tube was inserted and removed during the period of anaesthesia. Until June 2010, LRYGBs were performed without closing the mesenteric defects, but since July 2010 the mesenteric defects were stapled as described previously [20].

During the period from 2007 to 2013, five skilled laparoscopic surgeons went through a specific training programme in bariatric surgery. In order to minimize the negative consequences of the learning curve, the training programme was strictly organized in five steps as shown in Table 12.2.

12.7 Anaesthesia

The patient walked into the OR after receiving a peripheral venous cannula and IV antibiotic prophylaxis with single dose of cefuroxim 1.5 g. The anaesthetic method has been described in detail [10, 17]. In brief, induction of anaesthesia was performed in semi-reversed Trendelenburg position, using fentanyl and target controlled infusion of propofol and remifentanyl based on the patient's ideal weight. Muscle relaxation was facilitated with a small dose of vecuronium. After tracheal intubation, propofol was substituted with desflurane to ensure rapid recovery from anaesthesia after the surgery.

12.8 Post-operative Care (Table 12.1)

The patients were observed post-operatively and monitored at the recovery unit for approximately 2 h. Within the first 2 h, the patients were mobilized out of bed and were allowed to drink freely. The patients were encouraged to drink at least 1 L of water until the next day.

Post-operative pain was controlled with paracetamol, parecoxib and oxycodone at fixed intervals. Post-operatively, 1,000 mL Ringer's acetate was prescribed as IV fluid until the next morning.

If the patient had more pain than expected, experienced tachycardia or was not able to move out of bed, the surgeon and/or anaesthesiologist were consulted. Threshold for early re-laparoscopy was low in order to reduce the consequences of a possible complication.

At the ward, observation and mobilization were continued. Patients were instructed to get out of bed at least once every hour, drinking small sips and blowing the PEP whistle. Early the day after surgery patients took a shower and got new bandages. They also attended a group meeting with the dietician to discuss fluid and pureed food, and with the surgeon for instruction about possible complications and how to react. After discharge the patients had open access for readmission to the hospital and were carefully instructed to contact the ward or surgeon in case of any adverse events. The patient also had the telephone numbers of the surgeon on call at any time, of the ward and the outpatient clinic.

A questionnaire was sent to all the patients 4 weeks after surgery in order to evaluate patient satisfaction. This questionnaire consisted of questions about the patient's perception of the different parts of the treatment process.

12.9 Follow-Up Routines

Our patients also entered a 5-year interdisciplinary follow-up programme. This includes lifestyle courses consisting of a group of 16–18 patients at 3 months, 1 and 3 years. Metabolic follow-up is done twice a year in the first 3 years and then once a year, most often in co-operation with their general practitioner. Abdominal problems that could be related to the obesity surgery are a part of the treatment package and taken care of by the surgeons of the team.

12.10 Data Collection and Statistics

Data were prospectively collected and registered in our database (FileMaker 11), which is a part of our routine patient record system. The surgeons filled in data regarding the operation and post-operative care, as well as primary data concerning patient characteristics and discharge status. The anaesthesia personnel registered the time consumption for different tasks in the operation theatre and turnover time between operations. The theatre procedure was divided in six different parts for this purpose (Fig. 12.2).

All data regarding weight loss, metabolic status and post-operative changes in comorbidity as well as complications were registered continuously. All patient contacts with personnel from the obesity team were recorded and relevant information registered in the database. All patients operated in Sweden had their data entered into the database of the Scandinavian Obesity Surgery Registry (SOReg) that covers >98 % of bariatric surgery in Sweden. This enabled us to make frequent comparisons with other specialist centres.

Proportions are referred to as numbers (%). All continuous data are presented as median (range) unless otherwise stated. Differences were estimated by Student's *t* test, with a p-value <0.05 being regarded as significant. Weight loss was expressed as percentage excess BMI loss (%EBMIL).

12.11 Results

During the period September 2005–February 2014, 8,000 patients were admitted at our units for bariatric surgery. Primary LRYGB was performed successfully in all cases and no conversions to open surgery were needed. In 97.8 % of the patients, the data collection was complete. Eighty-one patients (1 %) were lost from our follow-up system with no data available at 1 month or more after surgery; 7,639 (95.5 %) were primary operations and 359 (4.5 %) operations were revisional procedures, where most of the latter had previously undergone open VBG or gastric banding; 78 % were females, with median age 41.9 years (17–77) and mean BMI 42.8 (28.7–81.1).

12.12 Complications

Total complications rate (<30 days) was 2.3 %; 126 patients (1.6 %) had reoperation within 30 days. Of these, 69 (0.9 %) had gastrointestinal leakage, 50 (0.63 %) were re-operated and 19 were conservatively treated. Fifty-nine patients (0.7 %) had clinically significant bleeding, defined as bleeding requiring either re-operation, blood transfusion, endoscopic intervention or haemoglobin <8.5 g/100 mL. Twenty-seven (0.34 %) of these patients had an early re-operation; two (0.03 %) had endoscopic treatment. Seventeen (0.21 %) received blood transfusions only, and 13 patients were observed without any intervention.

Twenty-eight patients (0.35 %) were re-operated due to bowel obstruction. There were 21 negative laparoscopies (0.3 %). Thus, 21 (16.7 %) of the 126 reoperations failed to demonstrate any suspected complication.

Nine patients (0.1 %) were admitted to the intensive care unit (ICU) with serious complications. Three of those patients died; two due to severe peritonitis due to late leakage that manifested itself on the fifth and on the seventh post-operative day, respectively. One patient died due to aspiration at intubation secondary to bowel obstruction. Thus, the mortality rate within 30 days was 0.04 % (3/8,000).

12.13 Fast-Track Principles (Table 12.3)

Time consumption in all parts of the procedure was gradually reduced from 102 min in 2005–2007 to 49 min in 2011–2013 ($p<0.001$). This includes non-surgical time consumption in the operation theatre was reduced from 43 min in 2005–2006 to 13 min in 2011–2013 ($p<0.001$). The surgical time was reduced from median 59 (40–96) to 36 (22–144) min in the same period ($p<0.001$) and the turnover time from 13 to 7 min ($p<0.001$).

Figure 12.2 illustrates the logistics and time consumption during all stages of the operation including the turnover time between operations during the second half of 2010 (261 procedures).

The median hospital stay was 1.7 (1–110) days for the total patient material. From 2005 to 2007 compared to 2011–2013, the hospital stay was reduced from 3.1 (2–110) to 1.3 (1–13) days

Table 12.3 Results and progression in the fast-track programme

			First part of study period 2005–2007 $N=425$	Last part of study period 2011–2013 $N=4618$	
Logistics	One procedure (minutes)	Total time	102	49	($p<0.001$)
		Operation time	59 (40–96)	36 (22–144)	($p<0.001$)
		Non-operation time	43	13	($p<0.001$)
	Time between procedures		13	7	($p=0.04$)
Economics		Number of patients operated from 8 am to 4 pm	3.7 (2–5)	7.3 (5–8)	100 % increase in production with 7 % increase in staff
ERAS		Complication rate (<30 days)	1.4 %	2.6 %	($p=0.20$). Include five learning curves
ERAS		Readmission rate (days)	1.3 %	2.6 %	($p=0.20$)
ERAS		Hospital stay (days)	3.1 (2–110)	1.3 (1–56)	($p<0.001$)

Table 12.4 Factors to ascertain economy

1. Well-organized teamwork – logistics
2. Risk and discharge classification of patients
3. High volume of patients and the ward closed at most weekends
4. Surgical procedure without excessive use of staplers, use of multiple use instruments
5. Short hospital stay
6. Low readmission and complication rate

($p<0.001$) (Table 12.3). A total of 160 (2.0 %) patients were readmitted during the first 30 days, most often because of dehydration or constipation.

The average excess BMI loss after 18 months was 81, and 73.1 % at the observed median follow-up time of 43 months (range 4–96) after surgery.

Data on hospital satisfaction were obtained from 706 patients during 2008–2010. The evaluation showed that 95 % of the respondents were well or very well satisfied (score 5 or 6 on a scale of 1–6) with the treatment and stay at the ward. Further, 99 % expressed that they would recommend our facility to others for the same treatment.

The cost to keep the ward open for 5 days was approximately 31.000 EUR (250.000 NOK) and for the weekends 12.500 EUR (100.000 NOK). Personnel costs represent almost half of the total cost. Out of 83 treatment weeks in our two units, wards were closed during weekends in 62 (75 %). In 2007, nine nurses were required per ward to cover day, evening and night shift. From 2010 this number was increased to ten nurses and remained constant. In comparison with 2007, in 2010 we treated 100 % more patients with only 7 % increase of personnel on the wards, and no change in personnel in the operating theatres. Table 12.4 outlines the distribution of the cost of the treatment process other than salaries.

During the study period five surgeons were educated in bariatric surgery. After assisting on 50 operations, trainees were successively allowed to perform more parts of the surgery (Table 12.2). In 2010, they performed 427 cases as chief surgeons with only 11 (2.6 %) major complications, 5 (1.2 %) of which required re-operation. The surgical time for the five trainees for the first and last 100 complete operations decreased from median 60 to median 43 min ($p<0.001$).

In Table 12.3, the main results of the fast-track programme are summarized.

12.14 Discussion

By implementing a fast-track protocol with continuous recording and analysis of results, we have been able to improve our results step by step.

We have managed to double the volume of patients treated with relatively small increases in total hospital costs, perfoming 1,600–1,900 bypasses per year with the same staff during the last 4 years at the two units. Time consumption for the total procedure was reduced from 102 min to 49 min ($p<0.001$), comparing the first and last 3 years. With only 7 min turnover time between the patients, total time for one patient has been reduced to 56 min, enabling us to perform 6–8 operations in a single operating theatre during ordinary daytime.

We were able to keep the complication rate more or less constantly low throughout this 8-year period, but at the same time five surgeons were trained into fully qualified senior bariatric surgeons. By using ERAS protocols, we were gradually able to reduce scheduled hospital stay from 3 to 1 day, without increasing the readmissions significantly (constant around 2 %).

We used pre-operative ASA score to guide patient selection; patients with an ASA score greater than 3 were not included in the fast-track protocol. However, only very few patients scoring ASA 4 were excluded. We found, as others have shown, that pre-operative education and preparation of patients are vital steps in order to secure successful fast-track programme [9, 21]. Patient demographics in our study are comparable with other European studies, both regarding BMI and comorbidities [7, 22, 23].

Our early complication rate at 2.3 % is acceptable and comparable with good results from other high-volume units [7, 22–24]. A protocol for enhanced recovery makes the post-operative management easier. Our re-operations rate was 1.6 %, but some of the leaks and bleedings could probably have been treated conservatively. However, by performing an early re-operation, usually without prior radiological examination, prolonged hospital stay can be avoided. Also, due to an aggressive attitude to early re-operation, only nine patients (0.1 %) needed ward in the ICU. Still, three of these patients died (0.04 %), two due to late leakage and delay in treatment. In order to prevent such deleterious outcome, thorough information to the patient is very important. In case of acute adverse events, hospital ward or surgeon on call should be contacted immediately and early readmission and treatment secured.

In many hospitals, long delays between operations, i.e. turnover time, is a barrier, keeping the production at a low volume. Our time recording system was an important control tool in order to increase and maintain a high efficacy in our clinic. Issues that created delays in our logistics were identified and corrected at early stages. In our setting, the surgeons were highly involved in the turnover process by getting the next patient ready for operation.

We found our education programme for new bariatric surgeons to be useful. In our fast-track system, the surgery should not take more than 1 hour. In order to measure the trainee's progression, we found it useful to record the four different parts of the operation (Fig. 12.2). The operating time for our five trainees declined significantly from their first to their last 100 cases ($p<0.001$). Further, the complication rate was not increased during their learning curves.

Recently, many studies have demonstrated that multimodal evidence-based care within the fast-track methodology and implementation of clinical pathways significantly enhances post-operative recovery and reduces morbidity. It should therefore be more widely adopted [7, 9, 22–25]. Our study supports this conclusion. We found no need for traditional surgical approaches such as the use of post-operative nasogastric tubes, abdominal drainage, perioperative bowel clearance or enforced bed rest. On the contrary, by mobilizing our patients within 2 h, using no urine catheter and allowing them to drink fluids freely, we were able to reduce the use of intravenous fluids and we have noticed considerable reduction in the use of pain and anti-emetic medication. Arterial cannulas for intra-operative blood pressure recordings or central vein catheters were rarely used.

The hospital stay in our study was reduced throughout the study period and mean hospital stay was 1.7 days. Several studies have evaluated ERAS protocols in bariatric surgery and demonstrated similar reductions in post-operative hospital stay without increase in perioperative morbidity [10, 17, 26–28].

We had a high follow-up rate (98.6 %) on weight loss and early and serious complications. The average excess BMI loss was 73.1 % observed median 43 months (range 4–96) after surgery. This is acceptable but long-term data are still not available.

Salaries for the physicians and staff represent 49 % of our total costs. Only a fraction of these costs are volume dependent. High production volume, as in our centre, is therefore cost effective. From 2007 to 2010, we managed to double the number of procedures per bariatric surgical week, by increasing the staff of ward nurses by only 7 % and without increasing the staff at the operating theatre. We also find our "discharge classification" to be a useful logistics tool for increasing the likelihood of being able to close the ward in most (75 %) of the weekends. Of costs other than salaries, stapler devices make up a very significant part (Fig. 12.3). It is therefore crucial to optimize their use, e.g. with reusable instruments.

In order to spread knowledge of our methods, we have had numerous courses demonstrating our fast-track model for colleagues from other countries, and we organize an annual meeting dedicated to bariatric surgery. This kind of approach and experience may also be transferred to other types of standardized surgery.

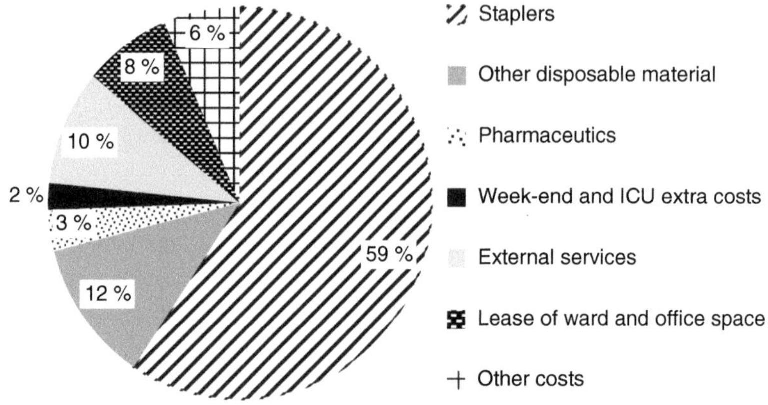

Fig. 12.3 Pie chart of distribution of costs other than salaries. Analysis of one full fiscal year at one centre

Conclusion

By establishing a dedicated treatment team, implementing fast-track methodology and following closely our results, we were able to increase the production volumes, reduce costs, and at the same time train new bariatric surgeons without new learning curves and without compromising the safety or quality for the patients.

Conflict of Interest All contributing authors declare that they have no conflicts of interest.

References

1. Kehlet H, Wilmore DW. Multimodal strategies to improve surgical outcome. Am J Surg. 2002;183(6):630–41.
2. Varadhan KK, Neal KR, Dejong CHC, et al. The enhanced recovery after surgery (ERAS) pathway for patients undergoing major elective open colorectal surgery: a meta-analyssis of randomized controlled trials. Clin Nutr. 2010;29:434–40.
3. Spanjersberg WR, Reurings J, Keus F, et al. Fast track surgery versus conventional recovery strategies for colorectal surgery. Cochrane Database Syst Rev. 2011;(2):CD007635.
4. Lublin M, Lyass S, Lahmann B, et al. Leveling the learning curve for laparoscopic bariatric surgery. Surg Endosc. 2005;19(6):845–8.
5. Ali MR, Tichansky DS, Kothari SN, et al. Validation that a 1-year fellowship in minimally invasive and bariatric surgery can eliminate the learning curve for laparoscopic gastric bypass. Surg Endosc. 2010;24(1):138–44.
6. Shikora SA, Kim JJ, Tarnoff ME, et al. Laparoscopic Roux-en-Y gastric bypass: results and learning curve of a high-volume academic program. Arch Surg. 2005;140(4):362–7.
7. Sommer T, Larsen JF, Raundahl U. Eliminating learning curve- related morbidity in fast track laparoscopic Roux-en-Y gastric bypass. J Laparoendosc Adv Surg Tech A. 2011;21(4):307–12.
8. Ballantyne GH, Ewing D, Capella RF, et al. The learning curve measured by operating times for laparoscopic and open gastric bypass: roles of surgeon's experience, institutional experience, body mass index and fellowship training. Obes Surg. 2005;15(2):172–82.
9. Kehlet H, Wilmore DW. Evidence-based surgical care and the evolution of fast-track surgery. Ann Surg. 2008;248(2):189–98.
10. Bergland A, Gislason H, Raeder J. Fast-track surgery for bariatric laparoscopic gastric bypass with focus on anaesthesia and peri- operative care. Experience with 500 cases. Acta Anaesthesiol Scand. 2008;52(10):1394–9.
11. Buchwald H, Oien DM. Metabolic/bariatric surgery worldwide 2008. Obes Surg. 2009;19(12):1605–11.
12. Ashrafian H. Bariatric surgery: can we afford to do it or deny doing it? Frontline Gastroenterol. 2011;2:82–9.
13. Anselmino M, Bammer T, Fernandez Cebrian JM, et al. Cost- effectiveness and budget impact of obesity surgery in patients with type 2 diabetes in three European countries (II). Obes Surg. 2009;19(11):1542–9.
14. Mullen DM, Marr TJ. Longitudinal cost experience for gastric bypass patients. Surg Obes Relat Dis. 2010;6(3):243–8.
15. Powers KA, Rehrig ST, Jones DB. Financial impact of obesity and bariatric surgery. Med Clin North Am. 2007;91(3):321–38. ix. 5.
16. Keating CL, Dixon JB, Moodie ML, et al. Cost-effectiveness of surgically induced weight loss for the management of type 2 diabetes: modeled lifetime analysis. Diabetes Care. 2009;32(4):567–74. 6.

17. Jacobsen HJ, Bergland A, Raeder J, Gislason HG. High-volume bariatric surgery in a single center: safety, quality, cost-efficacy and teaching aspects in 2,000 consecutive cases. Obes Surg. 2012;22(1):158–66.
18. Fried M, Hainer V, Basdevant A, et al. Interdisciplinary European guidelines on surgery of severe obesity. Obes Facts. 2008;1(1):52–9.
19. Leifsson BG, Gislason HG. Laparoscopic Roux-en-Y gastric bypass with 2-metre long biliopancreatic limb for morbid obesity: technique and experience with the first 150 patients. Obes Surg. 2005;15(1):35–42.
20. Aghajani E, Jacobsen H, Nergaard BJ, et al. Internal hernia after gastric bypass: a new and simplified technique for laparoscopic primary closure of the mesenteric defects. J Gastrointest Surg. 2012;16:641–5.
21. Delaney CP, Fazio VW, Senagore AJ, et al. "Fast track" postoperative management protocol for patients with high co-morbidity undergoing complex abdominal and pelvic colorectal surgery. Br J Surg. 2001; 88:1533–8.
22. Birkmeyer NJ, Dimick JB, Share D, et al. Hospital complication rates with bariatric surgery in Michigan. JAMA. 2010;304(4):435–42.
23. Dillemans B, Sakran N, Van CS, et al. Standardization of the fully stapled laparoscopic Roux-en-Y gastric bypass for obesity reduces early immediate postoperative morbidity and mortality: a single center study on 2606 patients. Obes Surg. 2009;19(10):1355–64.
24. Agaba EA, Shamseddeen H, Gentles CV, et al. Laparoscopic vs open gastric bypass in the management of morbid obesity: a 7- year retrospective study of 1,364 patients from a single center. Obes Surg. 2008;18(11):1359–63.
25. Lemmens L, van Zelm R, Borel RI, et al. Clinical and organizational content of clinical pathways for digestive surgery: a systematic review. Dig Surg. 2009; 26(2):91–9.
26. Bamgbade OA, Adeogun BO, Abbas K. Fast-track laparoscopic gastric bypass surgery: outcomes and lessons from bariatric surgery service in the United Kingdom. Obes Surg. 2012;22:398–402.
27. Geubbels N, Bruin SC, Acherman YIZ, et al. Fast track care for gastric bypass patients decreases length of stay without increasing complications in an unselected patient cohort. Obes Surg. 2014;24(3): 390–6.
28. Lemanu DP, Singh PP, Berridge K, et al. Randomized clinical trial of enhanced recovery versus standard care after laparoscopic sleeve gastrectomy. Br J Surg. 2013;100:482–9.

Part III

Surgical Treatment

13 Indications for Bariatric Surgery

Marcello Lucchese, Giovanni Quartararo,
Lucia Godini, Alessandro Sturiale,
and Enrico Facchiano

13.1 Introduction

Early bariatric surgeries took place in the 1950s and initially consisted of the intestinal bypass procedure, aimed to induce an iatrogenic malabsorption resulting in weight loss.

In 1991 the National Institute of Health proposed the first guidelines for the practice of bariatric surgery, eventually creating new guidelines expanding indications and procedures [1].

Indications for bariatric surgery have been analysed and accepted by different scientific societies over years, including the last revision published by the European Chapter of International Federation for the Surgery of Obesity in 2014 [2].

On the other hand, there are no precise recommendations concerning the type of procedure based on patient characteristics. This choice seems to be related to surgeon experience more than anything else, since there is a wide disparity in the proportions of different types of operations performed between centres and countries [3].

M. Lucchese (✉) • G. Quartararo
A. Sturiale • E. Facchiano
Department of Surgery, Bariatric and Metabolic Surgery Unit, Azienda Sanitaria Firenze, Santa Maria Nuova Hospital, Piazza Santa Maria Nuova, 1, Florence 50122, Italy
e-mail: mlucch@iol.it; giovanni.quartararo@gmail.com; a.sturialemd@gmail.com; enricofacchiano@yahoo.it

Lucia Godini
Department of Neuroscience, Psychology, Drug Research and Child Health, University of Florence, Largo Brambilla, 3, Florence 50134, Italy

13.2 Actual Indications

Bariatric surgery is indicated in patient in the age from 18 to 60 years having:

1. BMI $\geq$40 kg/m^2
2. BMI $\geq$35 kg/m^2 with co-morbidities that can improve with weight loss (diabetes, hypertension, OSAS, severe joint disease, severe psychological problems secondary to obesity, etc.) [2]

13.3 Type 2 Diabetes

Bariatric surgery in these years took an important role in diabetes treatment. Medical therapeutic options targeting primarily glucose control, in fact, have very limited success in controlling blood glucose levels amongst the severely obese, with many of these patients not achieving targets [4].

Bariatric surgery has demonstrated to be effective in long-term control of type 2 diabetes.

RYGBP seems to be the best operation when obesity is associated with type 2 diabetes, even though some studies have shown that even pure restrictive procedures can be effective [5].

M. Lucchese, N. Scopinaro (eds.), *Minimally Invasive Bariatric and Metabolic Surgery: Principles and Technical Aspects*, DOI 10.1007/978-3-319-15356-8_13,

The problem of long-term recovery from type 2 diabetes after bariatric surgery has been extensively treated elsewhere in this volume.

13.4 Young Obese

Bariatric surgery in adolescents and child can be actually considered only in specialised centres and after a careful multidisciplinary evaluation [2].

According to the recent update of the ASMBS paediatric committee best practice guidelines, the selection criteria for adolescents being considered for a bariatric procedure should include a BMI of >35 kg/m^2 with major co-morbidities (i.e. type 2 diabetes mellitus, moderate-to-severe sleep apnoea, pseudotumour cerebri or severe NASH) or a BMI >40 kg/m^2 with other co-morbidities (e.g. hypertension, insulin resistance, glucose intolerance, substantially impaired quality of life or activities of daily living, dyslipidemia, sleep apnoea with apnoea–hypopnea index >5) [6, 7].

An adolescent with severe obesity bariatric surgery can be considered if he/she:

1. Has a BMI >40 kg/m^2 (or 99.5th percentile for respective age) and at least one co-morbidity
2. Has followed at least 6 months of organised weight-reducing attempts in a specialised centre
3. Shows skeletal and developmental maturity
4. Is capable to commit to comprehensive medical and psychological follow-up
5. Is willing to participate in a post-operative multidisciplinary treatment programme in a unit with specialist paediatric support (nursing, anaesthesia, psychology, post-operative care)

For what concerns European guidelines, recently the Interdisciplinary European Guidelines on Metabolic and Bariatric Surgery have been published on behalf of IFSO-EC and EASO [2], and we report their considerations:

It is also underlined that bariatric surgery can be considered in genetic syndromes, such as Prader–Willi syndrome, only after careful consideration of an expert medical, paediatric and surgical team [2, 8, 9].

In adolescent patients, the RYGB ensures the best weight maintenance but it requires an adherence to the follow-up, such a commitment is not always guaranteed in such subjects [10]. On the other hand, SG procedure seems to prove to be a viable option for the treatment of adolescent obesity, achieving both weight loss variations and resolution of co-morbidities comparable to the RYGB procedure without malabsorptive risks [2].

Despite single differences in recommendations guidelines, we can conclude that bariatric surgery in adolescents and children should be performed only in centres of excellence with extensive experience in bariatric surgery for adults. A multidisciplinary approach to these patients, including paediatric specialists, is mandatory.

13.5 Elderly Obese

In the elderly obese (>65yy), bariatric surgery did not necessarily show to be effective in significantly prolonging the average mean of life [2, 11].

Benefits of bariatric surgery in the senior obese patient are still being evaluated. Even if postoperative risks in the over 60 obese are potentially higher, the advantages of recovered mobility, the increased independence and the improved control of co-morbidity may lead to a better quality of life [12, 13].

The proof of favourable risk–benefit of bariatric surgery in elderly is lacking so far. Several recent studies proposed sleeve gastrectomy as the procedure of choice in elderly obese since it could obtain advantage in terms of quality of life from weight loss for the low complication rate and the absence of malabsorptive component [14].

Age seems to be a prognostic factor for weight loss and co-morbidities remission as well the degree of obesity, patient motivation and the presence of uncompensated binge-eating disorder. Further studies are needed to identify predictive factors of outcome after bariatric surgery, in particular regarding physical activity and psychiatric disorders [15, 16]. The identification of predictive factors of success will help to develop interventions targeting specific needs of patients.

As for young obese, in the elderly obese patients, an accurate multidisciplinary evaluation is mandatory in order to evaluate the risk–benefit ratio before possible bariatric surgery.

13.6 Novel Indications

In the last decade, we are assisting to a novel dynamic revaluation of the historical selection criteria for bariatric surgery. This is not just for the higher incidence of obesity worldwide but for the evidence of new obesity-related pathological conditions and co-morbidities.

The necessity of evaluating new obesity-related metabolic disorders that may potentially beneficiate of a surgically induced weight loss is getting evidence in literature.

13.6.1 Hypogonadism

Hypogonadism and sub-fertility can be frequently associated to obesity and metabolic syndrome. Hypogonadal state has demonstrated to induce a worsening of co-morbidities such as cardiovascular disorders and type II diabetes [17]. In particular the correlation between testosterone low level and peripheral insulin resistance could lead to presume an important role of testosterone on the glycaemic metabolic improvement after bariatric surgery [18, 19]. As recently reported in literature, alterations in sex hormones, testosterone in male obese patients, can improve drastically after weight [15, 18, 20, 21]. Obviously, treatment of impaired fertility and poor sexual life in obese patients will result in implementation of overall health and quality of life.

In a recent meta-analysis, it has been demonstrated that body weight loss significantly increases testosterone levels in obese patients. Moreover, testosterone recovery seems to be directly correlated with the weight loss. Testosterone rise induced by lifestyle interventions was only modest, probably reflecting the relatively modest results of the targeted diet and physical activity on body weight loss. The testosterone increase would be more important after surgical-induced weight loss (9.8 % with diet vs. 32 % with surgery) [20].

As a matter of fact, male hypogonadism could represent a new co-morbidity to consider when evaluating patients for bariatric surgery, and so it could become a new possible criterion for patients with BMI $\geq$35 [19].

More studies, based on randomised trials, are needed to confirm the role of testosterone of glycaemic metabolic control after bariatric surgery.

13.6.2 NALFD

Morbid obesity is strongly associated with nonalcoholic fatty liver disease (NAFLD), which is one of the most common causes of chronic liver disease worldwide [22].

NAFLD includes a broad spectrum of liver tissue alterations, which range from steatosis (pure fatty liver) through nonalcoholic steatohepatitis (NASH) to fibrosis, cirrhosis and liver failure. In the severely obese, the fatty liver and its stages often have progressed to NASH or cirrhosis even before contemplating therapy [23].

Weight loss should be a primary therapy for NAFLD. However, evidence supporting intentional weight loss as a therapy for NAFLD is limited [24].

Since insulin resistance causes abnormal deposition of triglycerides in the liver, the link between metabolic syndrome and NALFD is clear. By the way bariatric surgery could improve NALFD, ameliorating also other factors like weight loss, inflammation, dyslipidaemia and intestinal hormones. These are the reasons bariatric surgery has to be considered a potential treatment of NALFD [22, 25].

The NAFLD guideline does not formally recommend bariatric surgery for the treatment of NASH because beyond potential benefits, there is an important lack of scientific evidence that could demonstrate any recommendation to support or reject bariatric surgery to treat NASH patients [26, 27].

On the other hand, it is important to note that bariatric surgery is not contraindicated in NASH patients without cirrhosis [28, 29].

The promising results in literature about metabolic surgical treatment of liver steatosis should encourage to design new randomised clinical trials in order to assess the therapeutic effect of bariatric surgery with long follow-up periods.

13.6.3 Class I Obesity

Class I obesity (BMI >30<35 kg/m^2) has been demonstrated to have a co-morbidity burden, in particular type II diabetes, similar than class II or III obesity; even class I obesity is associated with lower mortality rate than higher obesity class [30].

In the Consensus Conference Statement on Bariatric Surgery for morbid obesity published 10 years ago, Buchwald already proposed the possibility in extending the benefits of bariatric surgery to patients with class I obesity who have a condition that can be cured or markedly improved by substantial and sustained weight loss [31]. Since 2004 a considerable number of trials, meta-analysis and observational studies have been published about possible extension of the NIH recommendation of 1991 [1, 32–34].

In 2009 the American Diabetes Association considered the current evidence insufficient to recommend surgery to BMI >30 with type II diabetes. Recently the International Diabetes Federation suggested that patients with type II diabetes with class I obesity could be candidate to surgery if they fall in the same metabolic and clinical conditions warranting prioritisation in the 35–40 BMI class [4].

Recently ASMBS stated that the BMI alone is a poor index of adiposity and risk. Underlining the limitation of the 35 BMI cut-off, the ASMBS concluded that bariatric surgery shouldn't be denied to patient with BMI >30<35 kg/m^2 or >27.5 kg/m^2 for at-risk ethnicities who do not achieve substantial and durable weight and co-morbidity improvement [35, 36].

In conclusion, as clearly stated in the recent position statement of IFSO, the access to bariatric surgery should not be denied to patient with class I obesity associated with significant obesity-related co-morbidities simply on the basis of BMI level [37].

13.7 Contraindications for Bariatric Surgery

Mean contraindications are regarding psychiatric (not stabilised) disorders, behavioural eating disorders (such as bulimia and binge-eating disorder), addictions (alcoholism, toxicomania) and uncontrolled progressive severe chronic disease

1. Absence of a period of identifiable medical management
2. Patient who is unable to participate in prolonged medical follow-up
3. Non-stabilised psychotic disorders, severe depression and personality and eating disorders, unless specifically advised by a psychiatrist experienced in obesity
4. Alcohol abuse and/or drug dependencies
5. Diseases threatening life in the short term
6. Patients who are unable to care for themselves and have no long-term family or social support that will warrant such care

Specific exclusion criteria for bariatric surgery in the treatment of T2DM are as follows:

1. Secondary diabetes
2. Antibodies positive (anti-GAD or ICA) or C-peptide <1 ng/ml or unresponsive to mixed meal challenge

(cancer, cirrhosis, inflammatory bowel disease, etc.).

Here we report the schematic contraindications to bariatric surgery of the *Interdisciplinary European Guidelines on Metabolic and Bariatric Surgery* [2].

Fried et al. [2]

13.8 Co-morbidities That Could Influence the Choice of Bariatric Procedure

13.8.1 GERD

Gastroesophageal reflux disease (GERD) is one most common disease worldwide. Obesity has demonstrated to increase the severity and the incidence of GERD due to several factors such as augmented intra-abdominal pressure, increased hiatal hernia incidence, oesophageal dismotility disorders and lower oesophageal sphincter decreased pressure [38, 39]. Roux-en-Y gastric bypass (RYGB) is considered an anti-reflux system, and there is accordance in literature about GERD remission after RYGB. In fact RYGB has been proposed by many authors as a good choice for redo surgery in case of failed anti-reflux operations [40–42].

Studies in literature are inconsisted regarding the possible effect of laparoscopic adjustable gastric banding (LAGB) or laparoscopic sleeve gastrectomy (LSG) on patients with preoperative existing GERD. There is not a clear evidence of worsening of GERD after LAGB because of the difficulty of distinguishing recurrent GERD and symptoms indicating a complication of the banding [43, 44].

Some series demonstrated an initial GERD remission after surgery probably due to the weight loss, reduced intra-gastric pressure and reduced number of transient lower oesophageal relaxation (TLESR) after LAGB. However, a significant worsening of reflux symptoms and de novo esophagitis has been demonstrated during long-term follow-up [38, 45]. Outcomes in terms of GERD after LSG are contradictory [46].

Symptomatic GERD complicates sleeve gastrectomy up to 25 % of cases according to the literature [47, 48].

In fact despite the initial high incidence of de novo GERD symptoms or worsening of GERD after LSG, many studies demonstrate a decrease of GERD on long-term follow-up. Possible causes are the weight loss and the "Angle of His" restorations [38, 49, 50].

Some technical precautions could avoid the worsening of GERD or creation of de novo GERD symptoms after LSG: avoiding large pouch, strictures that could decreased the acid clearance, the lesion of lower oesophageal sphincter and antrum narrowing [38, 49, 50].

The presence of GERD symptoms could be actually considered only a relative contraindication to sleeve gastrectomy and gastric banding in morbidly obese patients [51, 52].

Even in the absence of large RCT, RYGBP could be the procedure of choice in case of symptomatic GERD [14, 43] As suggested by many authors, a preoperative oesophageal manometry and pH-metry should be performed in patients candidate to LSG [38, 39].

Further prospective studies are needed to clarify the role of GERD in the selection for bariatric operations.

13.8.2 Osteoporosis

Several studies demonstrate a significant worsening of bone density after bariatric surgery, in particular in postmenopausal women.

As calcium absorption happens in the duodenum and proximal jejunum, performing procedures with the bypass of duodenum or with a malabsorptive component in patients with preexisting osteoporosis could not be recommended [53, 54].

13.8.3 Familiarity for Upper GI Cancer

In these cases, preoperative endoscopy is mandatory. In case of direct familiarity with upper GI cancer, procedures that consist of the exclusion of part of the stomach are not recommended. If LAGB or SG is not suitable for a patient with upper GI cancer familiarity, it is possible to perform RYGBP with subtotal gastrectomy [55, 56].

13.8.4 Suspected Low Adherence to the Follow-Up

In case of high suspicion of low adherence to the follow-up after bariatric surgery, a SG should be recommended, avoiding the procedures that can require a strict follow-up (malabsorptive or LAGB) [14, 57, 58]. However, the exclusion of these patients from bariatric surgery programmes should be evaluated.

13.8.5 Systemic Disease Requiring Chronic Drug Somministration (IBD, Neurological Syndromes, Transplant Patient, IRC)

When a morbid obese patient is affected by systemic diseases, it should be recommended to perform a pure restrictive procedure [3, 59, 60].

13.8.6 Type I Diabetes

There isn't too much literature about obesity surgery and type I diabetes. After bariatric surgery, patients with type I diabetes demonstrate a significant improvement in terms of quality of life, with an improvement of glycaemic control and reduction of overall doses of insulin.

In case of malabsorptive procedure, there are risks of impaired or inadequate drugs absorption; this is why a restrictive procedure should be performed. On the other hand, it should be considered that the bypass of duodenum and proximal part of jejunum represents weight-independent factor of insulin sensibilisation [14, 61, 62].

13.9 Psychological and Psychiatric Aspects in the Choice of the Type of Bariatric Surgery

Patients candidate for bariatric surgery show frequently high rates of current and lifetime psychiatric axis I pathologies, with rates of up to 70 %. Mood disorders, anxiety disorders and binge-eating disorder (BED) are the most prevalent psychiatric diseases found in these patients [63]. Pre-bariatric surgery individuals display also several other bad eating habits such as sweet eating, snack eating, food craving and nighttime eating and have significantly increased odds of alcohol use and personality disorders [64] and lower levels of self-esteem and quality of life [65].

Although the presence of depression, anxiety and eating pathologies has been demonstrated in candidates for bariatric surgery, its impact on the short- and long-term weight loss outcome is still unclear [63].

Some studies support no influence of pre-surgical co-morbidity on post-operative weight loss [66, 67], whereas others show a negative impact of preoperative depression, phobic anxiety, interpersonal sensitivity and binge eating (BE) [68–71] with a higher risk for poorer post-surgery outcome and increased rates of complications. Legembauer et al. [71] found that in bariatric surgery patients, depressive disorders at baseline and within one's lifetime represented a negative predictive value for the percentage of BMI lost in the long term, 4 years after the operation. Brolin et al. [72] assessed different eating patterns and weight loss after bariatric surgery and found that the snack-eating patients had lesser weight loss and that Roux-en-Y gastric bypass (RYGBP) patients are not in the habit of consuming sweets [72].

A multidisciplinary approach has been recommended by the major national and international bariatric surgical societies (Società Italiana di Chirurgia dell'Obesità (SICOB), American Society for Metabolic and Bariatric Surgery (ASMBS)) to investigate psychiatric disorders and/or abnormal psychological profiles, patient motivation and post-operative management. A multidisciplinary treatment, where psychological support, physical education and diet are available, allows a decrease of preoperative weight surgical risks and improves postoperative adherence to a long-term follow-up programmes [73].

To date, no indications are available for the choice of a specific surgery procedure, on the basis of the pathological eating behaviour assessed before the operation.

A study reported that the laparoscopic adjustable gastric band (LAGB) was less successful in patients with binge-eating disorder or sweet-eating behaviour [74]. Bad eating habits such as sweet eating, binge eating and nighttime eating are often present before bariatric surgery. They may persist after surgery and unfortunately are hidden by patients [75, 76]. These findings suggest that subjects with a pathological eating behaviour might be candidates for a different bariatric procedure different from LAGB [74].

According this, another research sustained that, considering the mechanisms of action of LAGB and Roux-en-Y gastric bypass (RYBP), the second one could be a better choice than gastric banding for patients with poor control over their eating [77].

13.9.1 Psychological Profile After the Surgery

After the weight loss surgery, affective disorders, anxiety, eating behaviours and other symptoms of psychopathology seem to decrease significantly in most individuals. Researchers found that after the surgery, patients substantially display changed eating behaviour and meal patterns, achieving a relevant weight loss [57] A recent study has investigated three different bariatric surgery procedures, LAGB, RYGB and BPD (bilio-pancreatic diversion), comparing the different outcomes in terms of weight loss efficacy and psychological effects [78]. The results have showed that all the three types of operation significantly improved psychopathology and eating disordered behaviours [78].

Unfortunately, psychological conditions appear to improve in most, although not in all, individuals. Despite some findings supporting that BE behaviour is stricken out by gastric restrictive surgeries, many patients keep on, even if less seriously, to have maladaptive and psychologically distressing eating patterns post-surgery [79]. In patients continuing to have BE and BED after the surgery, weight loss outcomes are worse compared with individuals who never had these behaviours or who were remitted [79].

This position was confirmed by another research, reporting that the post-operative loss of control over eating (LOC) appeared to obstruct the rate of weight loss, especially as the time since the surgery passed. For this, post-operative LOC over eating may represent a useful index of limited post-surgical improvements and a clinical focus in post-surgical care [80]. Supervising pathological eating patterns soon after the surgery and for several years thereafter, particularly amongst those who engaged in BE prior to surgery, may help to detect patients who can benefit from additional treatment for their binge eating [81].

Drug treatment post-surgery and, in addition, non-pharmacological cognitive–behavioural treatments for BE and BED, in individual or group context, represent valid alternatives [79]. They have demonstrated positive results in the treatment of BE and should be accounted for bariatric surgery candidates to improve the outcomes [82].

These data suggest the importance to identify individuals at high risk to develop or to maintain psychiatric symptoms after the surgery and to follow them post-operatively driving them step by step to the therapeutic approach. The cooperation amongst the specialists, with the aim to develop appropriate interventions, facilitates the weight loss outcomes and a long-term successful management of the patient in the most profitable timing [83].

Conclusion

When we perform a bariatric surgical procedure, we create an experimental model that is permitting to discover year by year new pathways of research [84].

Weight loss is just one of the outcomes of such surgery that clearly provide metabolic changes that cannot be completely explained by the weight loss by itself. This is why nowadays, the concept of obesity surgery has been changed appropriately in metabolic surgery.

Indications and so preoperative evaluation are on the basis for a safe and better outcome after bariatric surgery. In fact bariatric surgery has been demonstrated to be cost-effective for national healthcare systems only if a accurate selection and evaluation of the patients have been performed. This is why a multidisciplinary team for preoperative evaluation in bariatric surgery is mandatory.

To date there are no data in the literature that allow predicting the chances of success according to the type of operation and patient characteristics.

Publications of new RCT are needed, and they would permit in the future to create evidence-based guidelines and the indications for each type of operation to improve the outcomes.

References

1. NIH conference. Gastrointestinal surgery for severe obesity. Consensus Development Conference Panel. Ann Intern Med. 1991;115(12):956–61.
2. Fried M, Yumuk V, Oppert JM, Scopinaro N, Torres A, Weiner R, et al. Interdisciplinary European guidelines on metabolic and bariatric surgery. Obes Surg. 2014;24(1):42–55.
3. Msika S, Castel B. Present indications for surgical treatment of morbid obesity: how to choose the best operation? J Visc Surg. 2010;147(5 Suppl):e47–51.
4. Dixon JB, Zimmet P, Alberti KG, Rubino F. Bariatric surgery: an IDF statement for obese Type 2 diabetes. Diabet Med. 2011;28(6):628–42.
5. Himpens J, Dapri G, Cadiere GB. A prospective randomized study between laparoscopic gastric banding and laparoscopic isolated sleeve gastrectomy: results after 1 and 3 years. Obes Surg. 2006;16(11):1450–6.
6. Michalsky M, Reichard K, Inge T, Pratt J, Lenders C. ASMBS pediatric committee best practice guidelines. Surg Obes Relat Dis. 2012;8(1):1–7.
7. Pratt JS, Lenders CM, Dionne EA, Hoppin AG, Hsu GL, Inge TH, et al. Best practice updates for pediatric/adolescent weight loss surgery. Obesity (Silver Spring). 2009;17(5):901–10.
8. Apovian CM, Baker C, Ludwig DS, Hoppin AG, Hsu G, Lenders C, et al. Best practice guidelines in pediatric/adolescent weight loss surgery. Obes Res. 2005;13(2):274–82.
9. Inge TH, Krebs NF, Garcia VF, Skelton JA, Guice KS, Strauss RS, et al. Bariatric surgery for severely overweight adolescents: concerns and recommendations. Pediatrics. 2004;114(1):217–23.
10. Olbers T, Gronowitz E, Werling M, Marlid S, Flodmark CE, Peltonen M, et al. Two-year outcome of laparoscopic Roux-en-Y gastric bypass in adolescents with severe obesity: results from a Swedish Nationwide Study (AMOS). Int J Obes (Lond). 2005;36(11):1388–95.
11. Sjostrom L, Narbro K, Sjostrom CD, Karason K, Larsson B, Wedel H, et al. Effects of bariatric surgery on mortality in Swedish obese subjects. N Engl J Med. 2007;357(8):741–52.
12. Dorman RB, Abraham AA, Al-Refaie WB, Parsons HM, Ikramuddin S, Habermann EB. Bariatric surgery outcomes in the elderly: an ACS NSQIP study. J Gastrointest Surg. 2012;16(1):35–44; discussion 44.
13. Giordano S, Victorzon M. Laparoscopic Roux-en-Y gastric bypass is effective and safe in over 55-year-old patients: a comparative analysis. World J Surg. 2014;38(5):1121–6.
14. Lannoo M, Dillemans B. Laparoscopy for primary and secondary bariatric procedures. Best Pract Res Clin Gastroenterol. 2014;28(1):159–73.
15. Facchiano E, Scaringi S, Veltri M, Samavat J, Maggi M, Forti G, et al. Age as a predictive factor of testosterone improvement in male patients after bariatric surgery: preliminary results of a monocentric prospective study. Obes Surg. 2013;23(2):167–72.
16. Scozzari G, Passera R, Benvenga R, Toppino M, Morino M. Age as a long-term prognostic factor in bariatric surgery. Ann Surg. 2012;256(5):724–8; discussion 728–9.
17. Wu FC, Tajar A, Pye SR, Silman AJ, Finn JD, O'Neill TW, et al. Hypothalamic-pituitary-testicular axis disruptions in older men are differentially linked to age and modifiable risk factors: the European Male Aging Study. J Clin Endocrinol Metab. 2008;93(7):2737–45.
18. Hammoud AO, Gibson M, Peterson CM, Meikle AW, Carrell DT. Impact of male obesity on infertility: a critical review of the current literature. Fertil Steril. 2008;90(4):897–904.
19. Lucchese M, Maggi M. Hypogonadism as a new comorbidity in male patient's selection for bariatric surgery: towards an extended concept of metabolic surgery? Obes Surg. 2013;23(12):2018–9.

20. Corona G, Rastrelli G, Monami M, Saad F, Luconi M, Lucchese M, et al. Body weight loss reverts obesity-associated hypogonadotropic hypogonadism: a systematic review and meta-analysis. Eur J Endocrinol. 2013;168(6):829–43.
21. Rao SR, Kini S, Tamler R. Sex hormones and bariatric surgery in men. Gend Med. 2011;8(5):300–11.
22. Hafeez S, Ahmed MH. Bariatric surgery as potential treatment for nonalcoholic fatty liver disease: a future treatment by choice or by chance? J Obes. 2013;2013:839275.
23. Shaffer EA. Bariatric surgery: a promising solution for nonalcoholic steatohepatitis in the very obese. J Clin Gastroenterol. 2006;40 Suppl 1:S44–50.
24. Dixon JB. Surgical management of obesity in patients with morbid obesity and nonalcoholic fatty liver disease. Clin Liver Dis. 2014;18(1):129–46.
25. Losekann A, Weston AC, Carli LA, Espindola MB, Pioner SR, Coral GP. Nonalcoholic fatty liver disease in severe obese patients, subjected to bariatric surgery. Arq Gastroenterol. 2013;50(4):285–9.
26. Chalasani N, Younossi Z, Lavine JE, Diehl AM, Brunt EM, Cusi K, et al. The diagnosis and management of non-alcoholic fatty liver disease: practice Guideline by the American Association for the Study of Liver Diseases, American College of Gastroenterology, and the American Gastroenterological Association. Hepatology (Baltimore, Md). 2012;55(6):2005–23.
27. Chavez-Tapia NC, Tellez-Avila FI, Barrientos-Gutierrez T, Mendez-Sanchez N, Lizardi-Cervera J, Uribe M. Bariatric surgery for non-alcoholic steatohepatitis in obese patients. Cochrane Database Syst Rev. 2010;(1):CD007340.
28. Vargas V, Allende H, Lecube A, Salcedo MT, Baena-Fustegueras JA, Fort JM, et al. Surgically induced weight loss by gastric bypass improves non alcoholic fatty liver disease in morbid obese patients. World J Hepatol. 2014;4(12):382–8.
29. Younossi ZM, Reyes MJ, Mishra A, Mehta R, Henry L. Systematic review with meta-analysis: non-alcoholic steatohepatitis – a case for personalised treatment based on pathogenic targets. Aliment Pharmacol Ther. 2014;39(1):3–14.
30. Flegal KM, Kit BK, Orpana H, Graubard BI. Association of all-cause mortality with overweight and obesity using standard body mass index categories: a systematic review and meta-analysis. JAMA. 2013;309(1):71–82.
31. Buchwald H. Consensus conference statement bariatric surgery for morbid obesity: health implications for patients, health professionals, and third-party payers. Surg Obes Relat Dis. 2005;1(3):371–81.
32. Ikramuddin S, Korner J, Lee WJ, Connett JE, Inabnet WB, Billington CJ, et al. Roux-en-Y gastric bypass vs intensive medical management for the control of type 2 diabetes, hypertension, and hyperlipidemia: the Diabetes Surgery Study randomized clinical trial. JAMA. 2013;309(21):2240–9.
33. Lee WJ, Chong K, Ser KH, Lee YC, Chen SC, Chen JC, et al. Gastric bypass vs sleeve gastrectomy for type 2 diabetes mellitus: a randomized controlled trial. Arch Surg. 2011;146(2):143–8.
34. Schauer PR, Kashyap SR, Wolski K, Brethauer SA, Kirwan JP, Pothier CE, et al. Bariatric surgery versus intensive medical therapy in obese patients with diabetes. N Engl J Med. 2012;366(17):1567–76.
35. ASMBS Clinical Issues Committee. Bariatric surgery in class I obesity (body mass index 30–35 kg/m(2)). Surg Obes Relat Dis. 2013;9;e1–e10.
36. Committee ACI. Bariatric surgery in class I obesity (body mass index 30–35 kg/m(2)). Surg Obes Relat Dis. 2013;9(1):e1–10.
37. Busetto L, Dixon J, De Luca M, Shikora S, Pories W, Angrisani L. Bariatric surgery in class I obesity: a Position Statement from the International Federation for the Surgery of Obesity and Metabolic Disorders (IFSO). Obes Surg. 2014;24(4):487–519.
38. El-Hadi M, Birch DW, Gill RS, Karmali S. The effect of bariatric surgery on gastroesophageal reflux disease. Can J Surg. 2014;57(2):139–44.
39. DuPree CE, Blair K, Steele SR, Martin MJ. Laparoscopic sleeve gastrectomy in patients with preexisting gastroesophageal reflux disease: a national analysis. JAMA Surg. 2014;149(4):328–34.
40. Patterson EJ, Davis DG, Khajanchee Y, Swanstrom LL. Comparison of objective outcomes following laparoscopic Nissen fundoplication versus laparoscopic gastric bypass in the morbidly obese with heartburn. Surg Endosc. 2003;17(10):1561–5.
41. Raftopoulos I, Awais O, Courcoulas AP, Luketich JD. Laparoscopic gastric bypass after antireflux surgery for the treatment of gastroesophageal reflux in morbidly obese patients: initial experience. Obes Surg. 2004;14(10):1373–80.
42. Zainabadi K, Courcoulas AP, Awais O, Raftopoulos I. Laparoscopic revision of Nissen fundoplication to Roux-en-Y gastric bypass in morbidly obese patients. Surg Endosc. 2008;22(12):2737–40.
43. Caiazzo R, Pattou F. Adjustable gastric banding, sleeve gastrectomy or gastric bypass. Can evidence-based medicine help us to choose? J Visc Surg. 2013;150(2):85–95.
44. de Jong JR, van Ramshorst B, Timmer R, Gooszen HG, Smout AJ. The influence of laparoscopic adjustable gastric banding on gastroesophageal reflux. Obes Surg. 2004;14(3):399–406.
45. Woodman G, Cywes R, Billy H, Montgomery K, Cornell C, Okerson T. Effect of adjustable gastric banding on changes in gastroesophageal reflux disease (GERD) and quality of life. Curr Med Res Opin. 2012;28(4):581–9.
46. Burgerhart JS, Schotborgh CA, Schoon EJ, Smulders JF, van de Meeberg PC, Siersema PD, et al. Effect of sleeve gastrectomy on gastroesophageal reflux. Obes Surg. 2014;24:1436–41.
47. Deitel M, Gagner M, Erickson AL, Crosby RD. Third International Summit: Current status of sleeve gastrectomy. Surg Obes Relat Dis. 2011;7(6):749–59.

48. Petersen WV, Schneider JH. Functional importance of laparoscopic sleeve gastrectomy for the lower esophageal sphincter in patients with morbid obesity. Obes Surg. 2012;22(6):949.
49. Chiu S, Birch DW, Shi X, Sharma AM, Karmali S. Effect of sleeve gastrectomy on gastroesophageal reflux disease: a systematic review. Surg Obes Relat Dis. 2011;7(4):510–5.
50. Howard DD, Caban AM, Cendan JC, Ben-David K. Gastroesophageal reflux after sleeve gastrectomy in morbidly obese patients. Surg Obes Relat Dis. 2011;7(6):709–13.
51. Sharma A, Aggarwal S, Ahuja V, Bal C. Evaluation of gastroesophageal reflux before and after sleeve gastrectomy using symptom scoring, scintigraphy, and endoscopy. Surg Obes Relat Dis. 2014;10:600–5.
52. Tutuian R. Effects of bariatric surgery on gastroesophageal reflux. Curr Opin Gastroenterol. 2014;30(4):434–8.
53. Carrasco F, Basfi-Fer K, Rojas P, Valencia A, Csendes A, Codoceo J, et al. Changes in bone mineral density after sleeve gastrectomy or gastric bypass: relationships with variations in vitamin d, ghrelin, and adiponectin levels. Obes Surg. 2014;24(6):877–84.
54. Vilarrasa N, de Gordejuela AG, Gomez-Vaquero C, Pujol J, Elio I, San Jose P, et al. Effect of bariatric surgery on bone mineral density: comparison of gastric bypass and sleeve gastrectomy. Obes Surg. 2013;23(12):2086–91.
55. Madan AK, Lanier BJ, Tichansky DS, Ternovits CA. Laparoscopic Roux-en-Y gastric bypass with subtotal gastrectomy. Obes Surg. 2005;15(9):1332–5.
56. Voellinger DC, Inabnet WB. Laparoscopic Roux-en-Y gastric bypass with remnant gastrectomy for focal intestinal metaplasia of the gastric antrum. Obes Surg. 2002;12(5):695–8.
57. Facchiano E, Scaringi S, Quartararo G, Alpigiano G, Liscia G, Pavoni V, et al. Do preoperative eating behaviors influence weight loss after biliopancreatic diversion? Obes Surg. 2013;23(12):2080–5.
58. Won EJ, Tran TT, Rigby A, Rogers AM. A comparative study of three-year weight loss and outcomes after laparoscopic gastric bypass in patients with “yellow light” psychological clearance. Obes Surg. 2014;24(7):1117–9.
59. Marszalek R, Ziemianski P, Lisik W, Wierzbicki Z, Domienik-Karlowicz J, Trzebicki J, et al. Bariatric surgery as a bridge for kidney transplantation in obese subjects. Case report. Ann Transplant. 2012;17(1):108–12.
60. Sauerland S, Angrisani L, Belachew M, Chevallier JM, Favretti F, Finer N, et al. Obesity surgery: evidence-based guidelines of the European Association for Endoscopic Surgery (EAES). Surg Endosc. 2005;19(2):200–21.
61. Raab H, Weiner RA, Frenken M, Rett K, Weiner S. Obesity and metabolic surgery in type 1 diabetes mellitus. Nutr Hosp. 2013;28 Suppl 2:31–4.
62. Salinari S, Carr RD, Guidone C, Bertuzzi A, Cercone S, Riccioni ME, et al. Nutrient infusion bypassing duodenum-jejunum improves insulin sensitivity in glucose-tolerant and diabetic obese subjects. Am J Physiol Endocrinol Metab. 2013;305(1):E59–66.
63. de Zwaan M, Enderle J, Wagner S, Muhlhans B, Ditzen B, Gefeller O, et al. Anxiety and depression in bariatric surgery patients: a prospective, follow-up study using structured clinical interviews. J Affect Disord. 2011;133(1–2):61–8.
64. Petry NM, Barry D, Pietrzak RH, Wagner JA. Overweight and obesity are associated with psychiatric disorders: results from the National Epidemiologic Survey on Alcohol and Related Conditions. Psychosom Med. 2008;70(3):288–97.
65. Abiles V, Rodriguez-Ruiz S, Abiles J, Mellado C, Garcia A, Perez de la Cruz A, et al. Psychological characteristics of morbidly obese candidates for bariatric surgery. Obes Surg. 2010;20(2):161–7.
66. Hayden MJ, Murphy KD, Brown WA, O’Brien PE. Axis I disorders in adjustable gastric band patients: the relationship between psychopathology and weight loss. Obes Surg. 2014;24:1469–75.
67. Powers PS, Rosemurgy A, Boyd F, Perez A. Outcome of gastric restriction procedures: weight, psychiatric diagnoses, and satisfaction. Obes Surg. 1997;7(6):471–7.
68. Brunault P, Jacobi D, Miknius V, Bourbao-Tournois C, Huten N, Gaillard P, et al. High preoperative depression, phobic anxiety, and binge eating scores and low medium-term weight loss in sleeve gastrectomy obese patients: a preliminary cohort study. Psychosomatics. 2012;53(4):363–70.
69. Kalarchian MA, Marcus MD, Levine MD, Soulakova JN, Courcoulas AP, Wisinski MS. Relationship of psychiatric disorders to 6-month outcomes after gastric bypass. Surg Obes Relat Dis. 2008;4(4):544–9.
70. Legenbauer T, De Zwaan M, Benecke A, Muhlhans B, Petrak F, Herpertz S. Depression and anxiety: their predictive function for weight loss in obese individuals. Obes Facts. 2009;2(4):227–34.
71. Legenbauer T, Petrak F, de Zwaan M, Herpertz S. Influence of depressive and eating disorders on short- and long-term course of weight after surgical and nonsurgical weight loss treatment. Compr Psychiatry. 2011;52(3):301–11.
72. Brolin RE, Robertson LB, Kenler HA, Cody RP. Weight loss and dietary intake after vertical banded gastroplasty and Roux-en-Y gastric bypass. Ann Surg. 1994;220(6):782–90.
73. Nguyen N, Champion JK, Ponce J, Quebbemann B, Patterson E, Pham B, et al. A review of unmet needs in obesity management. Obes Surg. 2012;22(6):956–66.
74. Wolnerhanssen BK, Peters T, Kern B, Schotzau A, Ackermann C, von Flue M, et al. Predictors of outcome in treatment of morbid obesity by laparoscopic adjustable gastric banding: results of a prospective study of 380 patients. Surg Obes Relat Dis. 2008;4(4):500–6.
75. Horchner R, Tuinebreijer W, Kelder H. Eating patterns in morbidly obese patients before and after a gastric restrictive operation. Obes Surg. 2002;12(1):108–12.

76. Nugent C, Bai C, Elariny H, Gopalakrishnan P, Quigley C, Garone Jr M, et al. Metabolic syndrome after laparoscopic bariatric surgery. Obes Surg. 2008;18(10):1278–86.
77. Apovian CM, Huskey KW, Chiodi S, Hess DT, Schneider BE, Blackburn GL, et al. Patient factors associated with undergoing laparoscopic adjustable gastric banding vs Roux-en-Y gastric bypass for weight loss. J Am Coll Surg. 2013;217(6): 1118–25.
78. Castellini G, Godini L, Amedei SG, Faravelli C, Lucchese M, Ricca V. Psychological effects and outcome predictors of three bariatric surgery interventions: a 1-year follow-up study. Eat Weight Disord. 2014;19(2):217–24.
79. Niego SH, Kofman MD, Weiss JJ, Geliebter A. Binge eating in the bariatric surgery population: a review of the literature. Int J Eat Disord. 2007;40(4):349–59.
80. White MA, Kalarchian MA, Masheb RM, Marcus MD, Grilo CM. Loss of control over eating predicts outcomes in bariatric surgery patients: a prospective, 24-month follow-up study. J Clin Psychiatry. 2010;71(2):175–84.
81. Busetto L, Segato G, De Luca M, De Marchi F, Foletto M, Vianello M, et al. Weight loss and postoperative complications in morbidly obese patients with binge eating disorder treated by laparoscopic adjustable gastric banding. Obes Surg. 2005;15(2):195–201.
82. Vaidya V. Psychosocial aspects of obesity. Adv Psychosom Med. 2006;27:73–85.
83. Meany G, Conceicao E, Mitchell JE. Binge eating, binge eating disorder and loss of control eating: effects on weight outcomes after bariatric surgery. Eur Eat Disord Rev. 2014;22(2):87–91.
84. Pattou F. Bariatric surgery in 2010: towards a metabolic surgery. J Visc Surg. 2010;147(5 Suppl):e1–3.

Endoscopic Treatment: Intragastric Balloon

14

Alfredo Genco, Roberta Maselli, Massimiliano Cipriano, Emanuele Soricelli, Giovanni Casella, and Adriano Redler

14.1 Introduction

At the present time there is no medical cure for obesity and, despite the numerous dietary treatments, the natural course of the disease is characterized by an ongoing, sometimes unstoppable, weight gain. There are now one billion overweight or obese persons worldwide. The indications inherent to surgical treatment are far from acceptable to patients. Bariatric surgery has been shown to lead to a greater incidence of intra- and post-operative complications, directly correlated to the numerous diseases resulting from obesity [1]. Only some of these patients, however, express the desire or are able to undergo a surgical operation. In this context, the intragastric balloon can play a very clear role in interrupting the ongoing and inexorable weight gain in patients with first-degree obesity and in achieving positive control or resolution or improving of the relevant comorbidities. In super-obese patients, where there are numerous comorbidities, the weight loss obtained with the BIB® represents, on the other hand, a chance to reduce the surgical and anaesthesiologic complications deriving from bariatric surgery.

In 1986, Pasulka et al. demonstrated how a small preoperative weight loss (10–20 %) reduced surgical complications [2] resulting from bariatric surgery. Consequently, over the last few years, the interest of operating in the sector has turned to devices able to help patients to maintain diet programmes, making diet more 'aggressive' and effective, and thus leading to greater control of the comorbidities in view of radical surgical treatment.

One of these remedies is the intragastric balloon.

The first intragastric balloon was launched in the market 30 years ago. From that date, several intragastric prosthesis have been presented and used worldwide. The concept first saw the light in 1921 when Davies observed that patients with *bezoars* (partially digested agglomerates of hairs or vegetable fibres), often complained of postprandial fullness, nausea and vomiting. This led to the idea of contriving a device that would imitate an intragastric bezoar by partially filling the stomach [3].

All the balloons used in the past showed poor results and complications but with the introduction of the BioEnterics® Intragastric Balloon (BIB®, Allergan Inc., Irvine, CA, USA), a new chapter in the history of intragastric balloons is being written (Fig. 14.1).

A. Genco (✉) • R. Maselli • M. Cipriano
E. Soricelli • G. Casella • A. Redler
Department of Surgical Sciences,
Sapienza, University of Rome,
Viale del Policlinico 155, Rome 00161, Italy
e-mail: Alfredo.genco@uniroma1.it; roberta.maselli.md@gmail.colm; maxcip76@gmail.com; lelesori@hotmail.com; giovanni.casella@uniroma.it; adriano.redler@uniroma1.it

M. Lucchese, N. Scopinaro (eds.), *Minimally Invasive Bariatric and Metabolic Surgery: Principles and Technical Aspects*, DOI 10.1007/978-3-319-15356-8_14,

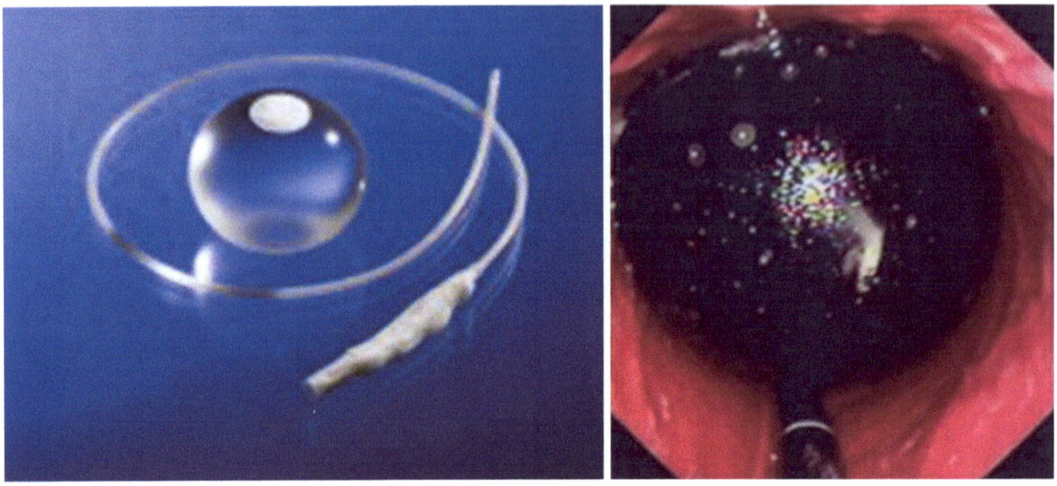

Fig. 14.1 BIB intragastric balloon (BIB®, Allergan Inc., Irvine, CA, USA) (*left*); device placed in the stomach (*right*)

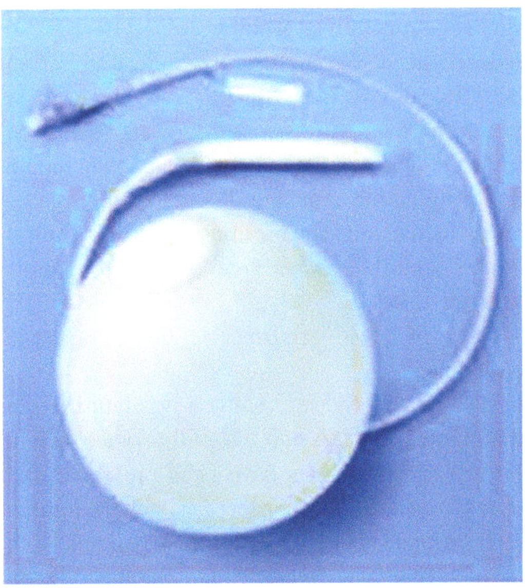

Fig. 14.2 Heliosphere intragastric ballooon (Helioscopie, Vienne, France)

On the market there are, nowadays, other types of intragastric balloons, including the 'Heliosphere bag' (Helioscopie, Vienne, France) [4], a balloon filled with air and inducing a minor discomfort compared to that induced by liquid-filled balloon, which has been proved to be effective in treating short-term obesity (Fig. 14.2).

It should also be mentioned the Endogast (Adjustable Totally Implantable Intragastric Prosthesis,ATIIP) (Districlass Medical, France), placed by a combined endoscopic surgical procedure, filled with air and attached to the abdominal wall [5]. It is currently used in few centres (Fig. 14.3).

The Obalon® Gastric Balloon (OBG) (ObalonTherapeutics, Inc., San Diego, CA, USA) is a non-surgical and fully repeatable and reversible weight loss device. Compared with other commercially available intragastric balloons, the Obalon is totally swallowable and does not need endoscopy for its placement. Up to three devices can be placed together [6] (Fig. 14.4).

14.2 Intragastric Balloon: Mechanism of Action

The efficacy of the device in inducing weight loss is due not to a placebo effect but to the characteristics which make it effective 'in itself'. How it actually works chiefly depends on its characteristics:

- *Its weight* (if it is filled with liquid), which stimulates the baroceptors at the gastric wall level. These, through the brain–gut axis, stimulate the satiety centre located at hypothalamic level.
- *Delayed gastric emptying*: an ultrasonographic study highlighted the fact that in patients with-

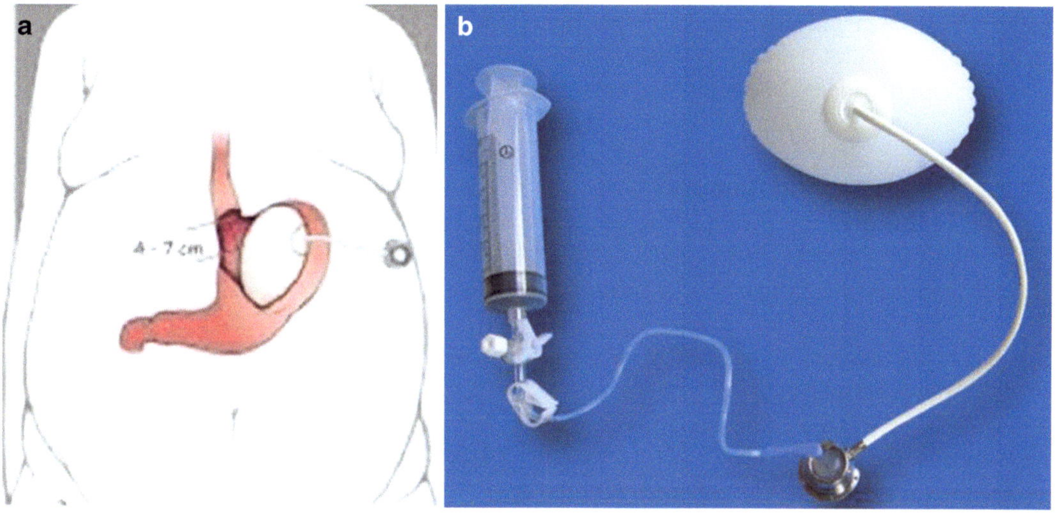

Fig. 14.3 Endogast (Adjustable Totally Implanted Intragastric Prosthesis, ATIIP) (Districlass Medical, France). (**a**) Schematic illustration of the device, (**b**) the device

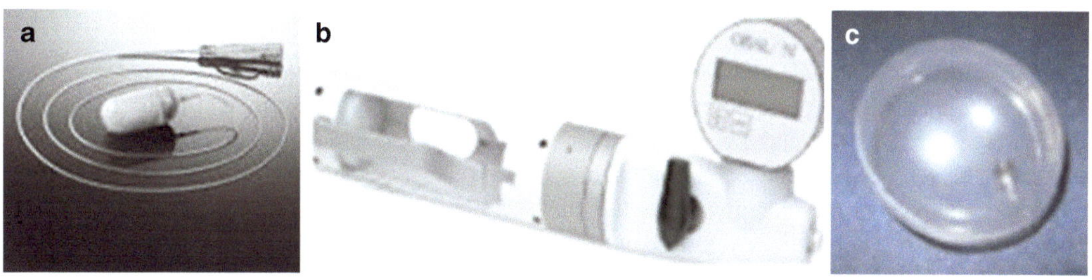

Fig. 14.4 The Obalon® Gastric Balloon (ObalonTherapeutics, Inc., San Diego, CA, USA) as it appears deflated (**a**), (**b**) the inflation system gauge to remotely inflate the device, (**c**) inflated device

out the balloon, food could already be visualized in the antrum 32 min after the consumption of a solid meal. Thirty days after BIB® placement in the same patients, this study visualized food after 300 min.

- Reduction of the unoccupied gastric volume by about 750 cm^3 due to the presence of the device.
- *Discomfort*: the overall disorders (nausea, precocious sense of satiety, vomiting, epigastric pain) suffered during the first 24–30 h post-placement and if the patient fails to adhere to the prescribed dietary regime.
- *Hormonal mechanisms*: during treatment with the BIB® in the first 3 months a significant increase in the plasmatic ghrelin levels was observed, followed by a gradual reduction until the basal levels reached after removal.

14.2.1 Indications

The balloon system is indicated for temporary use associated with a specific diet treatment in patients with a history of obesity (at least 5 years), after numerous failures of the dietary treatment only.

The balloon is indicated in patients with:

- <35 BMI with obese-related comorbidities whose resolution or improvement requires mandatory weight loss

- >35 BMI, as a pre-surgery role in patients with comorbidities, before any other type of surgery, or in patients who refuse surgery

14.2.2 Placement and Removal Technique

Balloon placement and removal can be performed in conscious sedation with diazepam or midazolam, in unconscious sedation with propofol or with orotracheal intubation. Before placement, a diagnostic oesophago-gastro-duodenoscopy is performed.

The BIB balloon is then positioned with the valve under the cardia and is filled, under endoscopic vision, with 500–700 ml of physiological solution and 10 ml vital staining solution (methylene blue). The connection catheter is removed and the valve checked for possible leaks. The mean duration of the procedure is 12 min. Balloon removal is carried out after 6 months. The removal procedure should be preceded by a 72-h, no-'roughage' diet and by a 24-h semi-liquid diet. The procedure foresees a gastroscopy to see the balloon and subsequently deflate it with a specific device. The BIB® is removed with a dedicated 'grasper' when completely deflated. Stomach observation is necessary to exclude possible mucosal lesions.

The Endogast is placed by a combined endoscopic surgical procedure, filled with air and attached to the abdominal wall. The device is connected to a subcutaneous system to adjust the volume of air.

For the Obalon, the patient swallows a capsule attached to a micro-catheter (the balloon is inside this gelatin capsule). Once in the stomach, verified by fluoroscopy and by the inflation system gauge, the balloon is remotely inflated with gas (nitrogen). After the inflation the micro-catheter is detached and removed, leaving the balloon in the stomach.

After a 3-month treatment period, all the balloons are retrieved by an upper GI endoscopy, using standard, commercially available endoscopic tools.

14.2.3 Post-placement Pharmacological Treatment

Due to the secondary effects deriving from the presence of the balloon (nausea, regurgitation or vomiting, cramp-like epigastric pains) and from the almost total impossibility of eating during the first 24–36 h, all patients must receive support treatment consisting in the infusion of electrolytic solutions, proton pump inhibitors, antispasmodic and antiemetic drugs.

14.2.4 Discharge

Before discharge the patient is made aware of the importance of optimum hydration and of ongoing urine checks (if methylene blue has been used), in order to diagnose in time the premature rupture of the balloon or a possible valve leak in a case a BIB has been placed.

On the first day, the patient receives a liquid diet only. From the second and up to the sixth or seventh day, a semi-liquid diet is followed.

14.2.5 Follow-Up

The dietetic regime from the seventh day is a daily intake of 1,000–1,200 kcal consumed over three main meals and two snacks. This dietetic regime is maintained until removal of the device. When there are signs (e.g. blue urine for the BIB) or symptoms indicating a possible complication, an immediate clinical evaluation of the patient is essential. Decubital ulcers or gastrectasia indicates the need to remove the balloon.

All the patients are informed of the increased chance of balloon rupture if it remains in the gastric cavity for longer than the prescribed period.

At the end of the treatment, the device will, in any case, be removed. The following alternatives are then evaluated: (a) starting the patient of on a 'maintenance' diet programme; (b) subjecting him/her to the consensual placement of a second balloon (multiple treatment); or (c) performing the previously planned bariatric surgery.

14.3 Results

14.3.1 Early Secondary Effects

In our experience with the BIB, the secondary post-placement effects were the following: nausea for 24–36 h in 87 % of the patients; vomiting (a mean two episodes) in 51 %; slight epigastralgia in 61 %, regressed with antispasmodic drugs; increased intestinal meteorism in 36 %; diarrhea (5–6 episodes/day) in 5 %; and halitosis in 12 % .

For the Heliosphere, nausea and vomit were present in 7.4 % of the patients during the first week.

14.3.2 Weight Loss

From March 1998 to May 2013, our case histories recorded 1,596 placements of BIB® in 1,503 patients (461 males/842 females). The mean age was 36.5 (19–69); mean BMI 38.9 (27.7–56.5); mean EW percentage 59.2 (34–117.6). At the end of the treatment, the patients presented BMI 31.8, EWL 34.4 %. These results can be superimposed on those reported by the Italian LAP-BAND® and BIB® group (GILB) relevant to 2,515 cases with a mean weight loss of 9.0 BMI and 33.9 % EWL21. Other important results derive from our study which compares weight loss achieved by BIB® versus a diet therapy at 6 months, when the balloon was removed, and at 18 months and 12 months after BIB® removal. The experimental group (BIB®+diet) consisted in 122 obese patients with mean BMI 41.8±6.8; the control group (diet alone) comprised 128 patients with mean BMI 42.0±6. Weight loss was significantly higher in patients treated with BIB® when compared to the group of patients treated by diet alone (weight loss 16.2 vs 6.6 kg, BMI decrease 5.7 vs 2.5 kg/m^2) at 6 months. The difference persisted to a lesser degree but was still significant at follow-up (12 months); both groups showing a tendency to regain weight at the follow-up after the treatment: in the BIB® group the average weight loss from baseline was reduced to 11.2 kg and the BMI loss to 3.5 kg/m^2, while in the diet control group, weight loss from baseline was 5.5 kg and BMI loss was 2.0 kg/m^2. These results demonstrate that intragastric balloon combined with dietary instructions induces significantly higher weight loss than simple dietary therapy in the first 6 months of treatment and persists at 12 months of follow-up [7].

Regarding the Heliosphere treatment, in a recent published study of 84 patients, the efficacy in terms of EWL was 33.2 % at 6 months. The only study existing at the moment on the Endogast is a report on 57 patients who reached an EWL of 39.2 % at 1-year follow-up.

To our knowledge only a pilot feasibility study has been published on the Obalon results [6], showing a significant weight loss induced by the balloon.

14.3.3 Long-Term Results

It is difficult to consider the long-term efficacy of a device such as the intragastric balloon, created for temporary treatment. In almost all morbid obese patients, the weight loss is followed by subsequent weight regain. Several authors have reported a successful weight loss in the short time, but only few studies have investigated the long-term results after removal.

In our experience from March 1998 to July 2006 (613 patients), we selected those having at least a 48-month post-removal follow-up ($n=145$). We excluded patients who had undergone bariatric surgery after BIB® removal ($n=52$) and who had a sequential BIB® placement or other non-surgical weight loss treatment ($n=30$). The remaining patients ($n=45$) were contacted and submitted to clinical evaluation.

Excess weight loss (EWL) ≥25 % when the BIB® was removed was considered a success 69% of patients lost ≥25 % (range 25.0–69.0) of their EW on balloon removal and were classified as 'successes', while 15 patients (31 %) lost from 0 to 21.0 % of their EW and were categorized as 'failures'. At 60 months follow-up (60 months±21.47; range 48–96), 30 % (9/30) of the 'success' group had an EWL percentage of

≥25 and were categorized as 'long-term successes', whereas 70 % (21/30) of them had an EWL percentage of <25 and were categorized as 'long-term failures'. To individualize possible predictive factors in long-term success, we evaluated the association between follow-up results and three factors: initial BMI (<35, 35–40, 40–50, >50), pre-BIB® age (>35 years, <35 years) and sex (male/female). A statistical analysis was done on the investigated predictive factors that have confirmed the associations: female gender, age <35 years and initial BMI from 35 to 40 are long-term success predictive factors. The results of this study confirm the safety and the short-term efficacy of the BIB®: at 6 months about 70 % of the treated patients lost at least 25 % of their excess weight. At 60 months follow-up 30 % of the patients were able to control their weight loss and had at least 25 % of their EWL percentage. These results indicate a possible role for BIB® in the long-term weight loss control.

14.3.4 Multiple Treatment

The m*ultiple treatment* consists of placing two intragastric balloons one after the other, respecting an interval of at least 30 days between the removal and the second balloon placement generally in patients refusing surgery. The reason underlying the delay of at least 1 month is the need to allow the patient to 'get the feel' of the balloon again. This is probably due to the saturation of the gastric receptors which 'adapt' to the presence of the intragastric prosthesis. We evaluated 83 patients with BMI >40, good candidates for surgery but refusing it, in a clinical treatment involving multiple intragastric balloon placement [8]. After removing the first balloon, a second balloon was placed when the patients had regained ≥50 % of the weight loss achieved with the previous balloon. Weight, comorbidities parameters and quality of life test were recorded until a follow-up of 72 months. All the patients experienced a second balloon placement; 22.2 % were placed a third device and only one patient received the fourth. At 76 months follow-up mean BMI was 37.6 kg/m^2 ($p<0.001$) and weight cycling periods were observed. Significant difference was recorded in the presence of comorbidities at baseline (80 % of the patients) and follow-up (30 %) ($p=0.02$). Quality of life test in the follow-up showed better scores than those at baseline ($p<0.001$). These results demonstrate that, although the weight cycling, in patients refusing surgery, multiple intragastric balloons are the recommended treatment, allowing the patients to achieve a good weight loss, a better control of comorbidities and better quality of life than baseline.

14.3.5 Preoperative Strategy: Sequential Treatment

In our series, the rapid weight loss induced by the BIB® drastically affects the progression of obesity-related diseases, thus determining the suspension or reduction of the pharmacological therapy. The dyslipidemic values improve in 58 %; there is significant control in hypertension in 38 %. In 61 % joint diseases improved, including pain regression, and in 80 % the rapid weight loss led to the prompt improvement of respiratory function and sleeping difficulties with the disappearance of apnoea (breath-holding) attacks. After BIB® treatment the apnoea index ranged from 33 to 5 episodes/h. Furthermore, weight loss induced by the intragastric balloon, as demonstrated by various studies in the literature, led to a significant reduction in intestinal fat and liver volume. The role and importance of the pre-surgery use of the intragastric balloon is also clearly shown in Busetto's study [9] where the pre-LAP-BAND® treatment together with BIB® induces a weight loss that shortens operating time and reduces the intraoperative complications, the conversion rate for patients subsequently subjected to gastric banding and hospital stay when compared with patients submitted directly to LAP-BAND®.

In conclusion, the findings of the Italian LAP-BAND® and BIB® (GILB group), in a study on 2,515 patients, indicate that the use of the intragastric balloon induced a normalization of the comorbidities in 44.3 % and a marked improvement in 44.8 %. In only 10.9 % of the cases did the comorbidities show no positive effects whatever from the treatment [10].

The use of the intragastric balloon is defined as 'sequential treatment' before any surgical treatment, whether bariatric or not, aimed at improving comorbidities in order to reduce surgical and anaesthesiologic complications deriving from such surgery [11, 12]. It is evident that such changes are related to the weight loss and not to the use of the BIB® per se. In any case, it has been demonstrated that the weight loss obtained with the balloon is greater than the reduction achieved by dieting alone.

14.4 Complications

14.4.1 Minor Complications

In the Italian BIB® experience of 3,252 patients, the incidence of minor complications was 2.1 % (71 patients). The intragastric balloon was removed due to intolerance in 13 patients (0.39 %). These patients decided to have it removed because they found the symptoms intolerable. Breakage of the device occurred in 19 patients (0.58 %) and, except in two cases, always after the period advised by the company (6 months). Oesophagitis diagnosed after removal of the BIB® occurred in 39 patients (1.2 %), probably due to the discontinuous use of the proton pump inhibitors.

Among the Endogast complications should be mentioned subcutaneous infections (12.2 %) and the port erosion (5.2 %).

14.4.2 Major Complications

In the same series, the overall major complication was seen in 32/3,252 (0.9 %) patients (10). In 19 (0.58 %) patients, the device caused a typical case of gastric obstruction which totally blocked gastric emptying. This condition was resolved with medical treatment in three cases by inserting a nasogastric tube for 24–48 h, but in 16 cases this proved to be ineffective and removal of the BIB® was required. Another complication is gastric ulceration, occurred in 0.15 % (five patients). Gastric perforation, the most frightening complication, occurred in five patients (0.15 %). Four of the latter had already undergone surgery: three at gastric level (fundoplication according to Nissen, a vertical gastroplasty complicated by fistula, gastric banding removed because of intragastric migration) and one due to prior, thoracic–abdominal trauma. In three patients, this complication was treated and solved by surgical means. Two other patients died: one during surgery and the other during diagnostic tests.

The authors report two spontaneous desufflation (1.2 %) requiring surgical removal in the Heliosphere treatment.

14.5 Discussion and Conclusion

Our experience, and the literature illustrated here, indicates that the intragastric BIB® is a totally different prosthesis from that used in the 1980s because, over a short term, it is a safe and effective device. Even though the incidence of major complications is <1 %, its use solely for cosmetic purposes is not at the moment advisable, and because four of the five perforations occurred in patients with previous gastric surgery, the contraindication of this factor is absolute.

The placement and removal procedures are easy, both for gastroenterologists and for surgeons who perform endoscopies. Physicians must, however, take great care to follow up their patients very closely, particularly in the first 7 days after placement. Only an attentive and rigorous follow-up permits the timely diagnosis and appropriate treatment of the dangerous complications which could arise in this first phase: gastric ischaemic ulcer, with subsequent perforation (4/5 occurred during the first 5 days after placement, GILB data) and dehydration.

In patients suffering from morbid obesity, incapable of keeping to any diet and who are candidates for bariatric or other types of surgery, the intragastric balloon is the only non-surgical procedure able to induce a rapid and consistent weight loss which positively affects all the obesity related comorbidities and reduces the risks of surgery and anaesthesia.

The ongoing trend relate to the use of the device points to sequential treatment, that is, before and in preparation for surgery. The unexpected results deriving from the evaluation of our experience in patients with 5-year follow-up lead us to think that the BIB® will be able to play an important role in the prevention of super-obesity, so little discussed even by the experts in this field.

Use of the intragastric balloon in adolescent and paediatric patients is another possible and important field. To be truthful, however, there is not enough scientific evidence at the moment to support verified affirmations.

At the present time, there is no medical cure for obesity and, despite the numerous dietary treatments, the natural course of the disease is characterized by an ongoing, sometimes unstoppable, weight gain. There are now one billion overweight or obese persons worldwide. Only some of these patients, however, express the desire or are able to undergo a surgical operation. In this context, the intragastric balloon can play a very clear role in interrupting the ongoing and inexorable weight gain in patients with first-degree obesity and in achieving positive control or resolution or improving of the relevant comorbidities. In super-obese patients, where there are numerous comorbidities, the weight loss obtained with the BIB® represents, on the other hand, a chance to reduce the surgical and anaesthesiologic complications deriving from bariatric surgery.

References

1. Ogunnaike BO, Jones SB, Jones DB, et al. Anesthetic considerations for bariatric surgery. Anesth Analg. 2002;95:1793–805.
2. Pasulka PS, Bistrian BR, Benotti PN, et al. The risks of surgery in obese patients. Ann Intern Med. 1986;104:540–6.
3. Lindor KD, Hughes Jr RW, Ilstrup DM, et al. Intragastric balloons in comparison with standard therapy for obesity — a randomized, double-blind trial. Mayo Clin Proc. 1987;62(11):992–6.
4. Lecumberri E, Krekshi W, Matía P, et al. Effectiveness and safety of air-filled balloon Heliosphere BAG® in 82 consecutive obese patients. Obes Surg. 2011;21(10):1508–12.
5. Gaggiotti G, Tack J, Garrido Jr AB, et al. Adjustable totally implantable intragastric prosthesis (ATIIP)-Endogast for treatment of morbid obesity: one-year follow-up of a multicenter prospective clinical survey. Obes Surg. 2007;17(7):949–56.
6. Mion F, Ibrahim M, Marjoux S, Ponchon T, Dugardeyn S, Roman S, Deviere J. Swallowable Obalon® gastric balloons as an aid for weight loss: a pilot feasibility study. Obes Surg. 2013;23(5):730–3.
7. Genco A, Balducci S, Bacci V, et al. Intragastric balloon or diet alone? A retrospective evaluation. Obes Surg. 2008;18(8):989–92.
8. Genco A, Maselli R, Cipriano M, et al. Long-term multiple intragastric balloon treatment: a new strategy to treat morbid obese patients refusing surgery. Prospective 6-year follow-up study. Surg Obes Relat Dis. 2014;10(2):307–11.
9. Busetto L, Segato G, De Luca M, et al. Preoperative weight loss by intragastric balloon in super-obese patients treated with laparoscopic gastric banding: a case–control study. Obes Surg. 2004;14(5):671–6.
10. Genco A, Bruni T, Doldi SB, et al. Bioenterics intragastric balloon: the Italian experience with 2,515 patients. Obes Surg. 2005;15:1161–4.
11. Weiner R, Gutberlet H, Bockhorn H. Preparation of extremely obese patients for laparoscopic gastric banding by gastric balloon therapy. Obes Surg. 1999;9:261–4.
12. Genco A, Lorenzo M, Baglio G, et al. Does the intragrastric balloon have a predictive role in subsequent LAP-BAND surgery? Italian multicenter study results at 5-years follow-up. Surg Obes Relat Dis 2014;10(3):474–8.

15 Endoscopic Treatment: New Technologies

Nicola Di Lorenzo and Francesco Maria Carrano

Minimally invasive surgery (MIS) is the gold standard in bariatric patients providing a reduced complication rate and post-operative recovery length, compared to "open" techniques.

The trend to minimal invasiveness is continuously evolving, including complex procedures performed by endolumenal approaches using innovative technologies.

Although in experimental settings many devices and techniques have been tested with the aim of reproducing the results of conventional surgical treatment, only a few of them have reached the clinical field after passing both safety and efficacy tests.

This chapter describes currently available innovative devices for obesity treatment, for which only limited data is currently available. Nevertheless, the trend towards endolumenal approaches, for most abdominal pathologies, is in our opinion, unavoidable.

N. Di Lorenzo (✉) • F.M. Carrano
Department of Experimental Medicine and Surgery,
Università di Roma Tor Vergata,
V..le Oxford 81, Rome 00133, Italy
e-mail: Nicola.di.lorenzo@uniroma2.it;
carranofm@gmail.com

15.1 Electrical Pacing

15.1.1 Introduction

Electrical pacing is a modern method based on the use of electrical stimuli to obtain weight reduction on obese patients, while preserving normal GI anatomy. Two main approaches are considered for clinical application: gastric pacing and intra-abdominal vagal blocking.

The concept of selective autonomic activation by electrical pacing to treat obesity was introduced by V. Cigaina (1996) [1] and recently reintroduced as Implantable Gastric Stimulator® (IGS® –Transcend®), a gastric pacemaker which stimulates the vagal innervation of the stomach through a lead wire [2]. The lead is implanted by laparoscopy on the lesser curvature, 6 cm from the pylorus, and distally fixed with clips to impede dislodgement. A pace generator is connected to the lead, placed on the fascia and then fixed with sutures. During operation, the gastric mucosa is monitored by gastroscopy to exclude inadvertent needle perforation into the gastric lumen [3].

Preliminary studies were encouraging, with %EWL around 10–21 at 12 months [4] however revealed poor results compared to placebo in more recent and wide SHAPE Trial [5].

M. Lucchese, N. Scopinaro (eds.), *Minimally Invasive Bariatric and Metabolic Surgery: Principles and Technical Aspects*, DOI 10.1007/978-3-319-15356-8_15,

15.1.2 From Pacing to Modulation

The concept of pacing then evolved to that of modulation where three new devices were tested: the Diamond System®, the Abiliti System® and the VBLOC® therapy.

15.1.2.1 Diamond System

The Diamond®(MetaCure) is a meal-activated implantable system that delivers gastric contractility modulation (GCM) signals that are synchronized with the intrinsic electrical activity of the stomach and show to enhance the force of antral contractions, increasing afferent signalling in the vagus nerve without interfering with the intrinsic gastric electrical rhythm [6].

Implant procedure is performed by laparoscopy and controlled by intraoperative gastroscopy. Three bipolar leads are implanted in the stomach muscular layers, and then connected to an implantable pulse generator located in a subcutaneous pocket sited in the left anterior abdominal wall [7].

Although limited by the relatively small numerical dimension, results from first trials appear encouraging and show lipidic profile improvements, sustained decrease of blood pressure levels from 124 ± 12 to 112 ± 10 mmHg at 6 months, sustained weight loss [7] and EWL of 30.5 ± 8.5 % at 1 year [8, 9] with minor adverse events.

15.1.2.2 Abiliti System

The Abiliti System® (IntraPace) includes a laparoscopically implanted device composed of a transgastric sensor which detects food intakes and triggers the stimulator, placed on the lesser curvature of the stomach, to deliver a tailored gastric stimulation which should result in early satiety. Differently from the previously cited devices, the Abiliti System® constantly records physical activity, using a 3D accelerometer embedded in the implanted device. Patients can download all data through a personal website and adjust diet and physical activity accordingly.

Preliminary results of 25 patients from a multi-centre ongoing clinical trial conducted in Germany suggest its safety and effectiveness. The mean %EWL resulting from this trial was 17.1 ± 8.9 at 3 months, 23.9 ± 11.9 at 6 months and 30.0 ± 17.1 at 12 months [10].

15.1.2.3 VBLOC Therapy

The VBLOC® vagal blocking therapy, based on a different principle, induces an intermittent intra-abdominal vagal block using high-frequency electrical currents by two electrodes positioned laparoscopically on the anterior and posterior vagal trunks near the oesophagogastric junction (EGJ). The neuroregulator with a rechargeable battery is placed subcutaneously.

Several clinical and experimental observations hypothesized intermittent vagal blockade (IVB) to be an important factor for achieving and maintaining clinical benefits [11–13]. According to various clinical trials, the procedure is safe; results in terms of %EWL around 25 are being further investigated. Post-study analysis also suggests that IVB has a positive effect on arterial hypertension since the very first days of use. Patient's selection may play a key role, since lower BMI patients seem to respond better to VBLOC therapy. Metabolic implications also emerged in a recent trial by Shikora et al., as HbA1c was reduced at all time periods from a baseline of 7.8 ± 0.2 % (mean ± SEM), mean % HbA1c reduction at 12 months was 1.0 ± 0.2 %. FPG was also reduced at all time periods from a baseline of 151 ± 7 mg/dL. Mean FPG reduction at 12 months was 28 ± 8 mg/dL [14].

15.2 Endoscopic Aspiration Therapy

Derived from percutaneous endoscopic gastrostomy (PEG) tube technology, endoscopic aspiration therapy (EAT) represents a new way, although controversial, to induce weight loss by aspirating a portion of ingested meals from the stomach; thanks to the AspireAssist Aspiration Therapy System (Aspire Bariatrics) which is composed of:

(a) An all-silicon A-Tube with holes in the intragastric portion to allow aspiration of gastric contents;

(b) A valved Skin-Port to prevent gastric leakage, connected to the extra-gastric portion of the A-Tube;
(c) A connector to open the Skin-Port valve with an embedded safety device (consisting of a "counter" that tracks the number of times the connector is attached to the Skin-Port until it reaches 115 aspiration cycles when it locks the connector, so the Skin-Port cannot be accessed for aspiration and the patient must return to hospital to obtain a new connector to continue aspiration therapy);
(d) A "companion" device, which is a siphon that allows two-way flow of fluids thus permitting stomach draining while infusing water in the stomach. Approximately 30 % of ingested calories are removed by aspiration according to currently available data;
(e) A 600 mL soft reservoir that allows subjects to flush tap water into the stomach to facilitate aspiration;
(f) A drain tube to dispose the aspirated content into the toilet.

The gastrostomy procedure is the standard one and the A-Tube is inserted by pulling technique under antibiotic. Ten to 14 days after the A-Tube placement – this is shortened within 1 cm of the abdominal wall and then attached to the Skin-Port. The whole device is ready for use.

Twenty minutes after meals containing more than 200 kcal, patients are required to perform aspiration. They flush food particles out through the A-Tube by infusing water into the stomach from the reservoir in 150–200 mL increments and then reversing the flow by lowering the lever on the companion device to allow contents to drain out of the stomach. This process can be repeated several times, until food particles are no longer seen in the aspirate. The whole aspiration sequence takes 5–15 min, depending on the meal size. Patients should receive PPI treatment and potassium chloride supplements to reduce acid loss and potential potassium depletion [15].

This technique is controversial and, until April 2014, independent scientific papers on the outcomes of this technique are not yet available.

15.3 Endoluminal Treatment

The concept of endoluminal treatment includes many different devices and techniques.

15.3.1 Restrictive Procedures

The advantage of an endoluminal procedure to treat MO is the reversibility and possibility to undergo surgery as RYGB, in case of unsatisfactory weight loss [16].

The new trend of minimal invasiveness MO treatment has lead major biomedical companies to develop at least one endoscopic suturing device to perform sutures or plication inside the stomach cavity (see Table 15.1). Only some devices have been clinically introduced successfully and this chapter will focus on them.

Some endoscopic suturing devices (ESDs) were primarily developed, years ago, for endoluminal treatment of gastroesophageal reflux disease (GERD). Being capable of applying a partial thickness suture on the EGJ, their previous goal was to create a fold at the EGJ to reduce reflux. Results have been controversial and largely debated [17].

Table 15.1 Endoscopic suturing devices

TOGa system® (Satiety Inc.)	*Incisionless Operating Platform*® (USGI Medical)	*Endoscopic suturing device* (Wilson-Cook Medical)
Stomaphyx® (EndoGastric Solutions)	*Anubis* (Storz)	*SafeStitch* (SafeStitch Medical, Inc.)
Endo-Cinch and *RESTORe Suturing System*™ (C.R. Bard Inc.)	*Spider* (Transenterix)	*NDO plicator*® (NDO Surgical, Inc.)
TERIS (Barosense Inc.)	*Endosamurai* (Olympus)	*Overstitch* (Apollo Endosurgery, Inc.)
Spiderman (Ethicon Johnson & Johnson)	*DDES – Direct Drive Endoscopic system* (Bard, Inc.)	

They have been recently reintroduced in bariatric surgery to produce a gastric plication of stomach layers (mucosal and submucosal) with the aim of reducing gastric volume, and then performing a trans-oral gastroplasty.

The first reported device used was the EndoCinch Suturing System® (Davol Inc.). It is inserted over a standard endoscope and fires a straight threaded needle through a tissue fold obtained by suction. A series of sutures can be placed in two rows in a full thickness manner [18, 19].

In 2008, Fogel et al. reported a series of 64 obese patients treated by means of an endoscopic vertical gastroplasty with a 1-year follow-up. They registered a significant reduction in BMI at 12 months (mean BMI 39.9 ± 5.1 kg/m^2 vs 30.6 ± 4.7 kg/m^2) and %EWL of 21.1 ± 6.2, 39.6 ± 11.3 and 58.1 ± 19.9 at 1, 3 and 12 months, respectively, comparable with the control group treated by mean of LRYGB [20]. Fogel's excellent results have not been achieved in other published trials.

15.3.1.1 TOGA System

Promising results have been reported for a series of patients treated by means of TOGA system (Satiety Inc.), used to create a stapled restrictive pouch along the lesser curvature of the stomach [16].

The TOGA system has two disposable stapling devices: the TOGA Sleeve Stapler and the TOGA Restrictor. The first is used to create a vertical sleeve along the lesser curvature of the stomach, approximately 8 cm in length and 2 cm in diameter. The second is used to reduce the sleeve outlet size by creating folds at the distal end of the pouch created [21].

The procedure consists in the introduction of a 60-French bougie through the mouth and oesophagus over a guide wire, to dilate and test for any resistance. The TOGA Sleeve Stapler is then introduced over the guide wire and a small endoscope is routed through a channel in the device. Once the stomach cavity is reached, a septum with attached retraction wire spreads and orients the stomach tissue, while suction is applied from the vacuum pods included in the device. Three rows of titanium staples are usually delivered to create a staple line that connects the anterior and posterior stomach, beginning 1 cm proximal to the Z line and extending distally 4.5 cm, parallel to the lesser curvature [22]. According to the latest method tested, a second staple line is added distally. The result of this procedure is a small, restrictive pouch along the lesser gastric curvature [21].

The first human multicentre study in 2007 enrolled 21 patients and reported good results in terms of safety (no serious adverse events occurred) and EWL of 16.2 %, 22.6 % and 24.4 %, respectively, at 1, 3 and 6 months. However, this first study showed a possible flaw of the procedure, since gaps in the staple line were evident in 13 of the 21 patients. At that time, only one staple line was created [23]. Following this first trial, an Italian study analyzed the effects of TOGA on insulin sensitivity and secretion on a series of nine patients. Insulinemia was significantly reduced at fast and at 120′ after OGTT, as well as the insuline secretion rate (from 235.05 ± 27.50 to 124.77 ± 14.50 nmol/min/m^2) while insulin sensitivity increased (from 348.45 ± 20.08 to 421.18 ± 20.84 mL/min/m^2). Total insulin secretion rate was demonstrated to correlate with weight, fat mass and BMI [22]. A second prospective, multicentre, single-arm trial with a 1-year outcome ended in 2011 and involved 53 patients. A second staple line was added distally, to prevent possible gaps. Nevertheless, 7 patients had a gap on the proximal part of the staple line, 16 had gaps between staple lines and 2 had a combination of gap types; this replicates the same complication of Masons's gastroplasty which lead to the McLean modified technique. Gap presence negatively correlates with procedure efficacy, remaining an unsolved problem of the TOGA procedure, since no special treatments or salvage techniques are currently available. Patients with no or small gaps (<15 mm) had a responder rate of 87.5 % whereas patients with large gaps (>15 mm) had a rate of 45.5 %. There were only mild side effects related to the procedures, such as nausea, vomiting, abdominal pain, throat pain and dysphagia, which resolved within 1 week. After the post-procedural routine radiographic control, one patient was diagnosed with asymptomatic pneumoperitoneum, which resolved without further complication. This second TOGA trial confirmed the promising results of the first, showing a %EWL of 29.3 ± 11.6 % at 3 months, 36.8 ± 15.7 % at 6 months and 38.7 ± 17.1 % at 12 months. Improvements in the metabolic profile were also reported: HbA1c levels decreased from 7.0 % at baseline to 5.7 % at 12 months for nine diabetic patients. HbA1c levels decreased from 5.9 % at baseline to 5.4 % at 12 months for all others. Triglyceride levels decreased from 142.9 mg/dL at baseline to 98.0 mg/dL at 12 months [21].

15.3.1.2 RESTORe Suturing System

The RESTORe Suturing System™ is a new generation suturing device by Bard Inc., characterized by single-intubation, multistitch capability and designed to place sutures through the muscular wall of the stomach and approximate gastric tissue. The suturing system is activated by depressing a plunger on the top of the device. When activated, the system deploys a 3-0 polypropylene suture through the tissue in the suction chamber and deposits the suture tag in the end of the capsule [24].

The results of a very first trial have been presented at the XVI World congress of the IFSO 2011 by P. Schauer after 12 months of follow-up. Eighteen subjects with a BMI 30–45 kg/m^2 (mean 38.6 kg/m^2) underwent a gastric volume reduction procedure, each patient required four to eight plications (mean 6), and the average procedure time was 125 min. No serious or significant procedure-related complications have been observed. They report a EWL >30 % for half of the patients and an EWL 30.5 ± 16.8 % for subjects with a BMI between 30 and 35 (TRIM trial investigators, personal communication). The RESTORe is currently being evaluated in the TRIM (Transoral Gastric Volume Reduction as an Intervention for Weight Management) trial.

15.3.1.3 POSE Procedure

A new, less invasive surgical option performing gastric plication is the POSE procedure, inspired by the endoscopic technique used to treat pouch dilation after bariatric surgery, named ROSE procedure. Primary Obesity Surgery Endolumenal (POSE) is a new scar-free technique based on the use of the Incisionless Operating Platform® (IOP® – USGI Medical) made of three main components: TransPort Multi-lumen Operating Platform®, a flexible endoscope with four working channels functioning as flexible trocars, with insufflation capability, and allows operators to deploy and use up to three tools simultaneously. The Platform further consists of a g-Prox® tissue grasper, a flexible endoscopic tissue approximation device deployed via one of the four working channels; Expandable Tissue Anchors®, suturing technology designed to overcome the problems of endolumenal suturing in the GI tract by distributing forces over large tissue contact. These anchors also have a semi-compliant nature that accommodates postoperative swelling. Their plasticity allows them to withstand swelling, yet maintain hold on tissue.

To perform POSE, surgeons advance the USGI TransPort® down the oesophagus to the stomach fundus, like a traditional endoscope. The tip of the device is then turned towards the operating site and locked for stabilization. Once the platform is in place, the flexible grasper is delivered to the operative site through a lumen of the TransPort® and is then used to bite a fold of the stomach mucosa on which the anchors are put (Fig. 15.1). Each anchor pair is preloaded into a catheter (g-Cath®), and inserted into the grasper before firing. Several folds are created in this way to reduce gastric fundus and limit its ability to expand. Once the desired capacity is reached, the device is removed through the oesophagus. POSE is reported to be performed successfully in North America, Europe and the Middle East. From 2011 to 2012, a prospective observational study was undertaken by J. C. Espinós et al. involving 45 patients: 75.6 % female; mean age 43.4 ± 9.2 SD (range 21.0–64.0). At baseline: mean absolute weight, 100.8 ± 12.9 (75.5–132.5); BMI 36.7 ± 3.8 (28.1–46.6). All POSE cases were performed with no intraoperative adverse events, no conversions or failed procedures. No mortality was reported; only two minor postoperative adverse events resulted: one case of low-grade

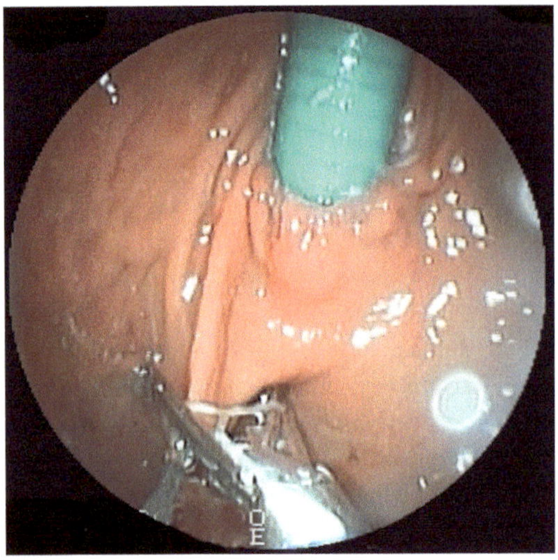

Fig. 15.1 Creation of a gastric fold using IOP® (USGI Medical, Inc.)

fever (resolved with oral antibiotic treatment) and one patient returned to hospital on the second postoperative day with chest pain. Minor postoperative side effects included sore throat, stomach pain, nausea and chest pain. Three cases of vomiting resolved within the first 12 h with no requirement of additional hospital stay. To be noted, all patients were discharged from hospital in less than 24 h. Liquid intake began 12 h post-procedure with full solids by 6 weeks. Follow-up visits were performed in a tight schedule at 1, 2 and 3 weeks, and at 1, 2, 3, 4, 5 and 6 months. The mean 6-month POSE TBWL was 15.5 % and more than 80.0 % of POSE patients had achieved ≥25 %EWL. The overall POSE patient mean EWL was MLT 40.0 % (calculated by metric) and 49.4 % (calculated with BMI 25 as ideal end point). The authors also report that patients in the current POSE cohort who have reached the 9- and 12-month time points have continued their weight-loss trend without complications [25].

15.3.1.4 Overstitch

Similar in concept, the recently redesigned Overstitch, by Apollo Endosurgery, is able to perform transoral endoscopic gastric volume reduction by a series of endoluminally placed, full-thickness, closely spaced interrupted sutures through the gastric wall from the prepyloric antrum to EGJ (Fig. 15.2). Although very fashionable, published data on the procedure is scarce at the time of writing. Among the preliminary experience, Abu Dayyeh in Rochester (Minnesota, USA) performed a transoral endoscopic gastric volume reduction with Overstitch in four subjects. Post-procedural abdominal pain and nausea developed in three patients, while acid reflux symptoms developed in one and resolved with an oral proton pump inhibitor [26]. No data on EWL or TBWL were reported, being only a pilot feasibility study. Long-term safety and efficacy of the procedure are yet to be evaluated.

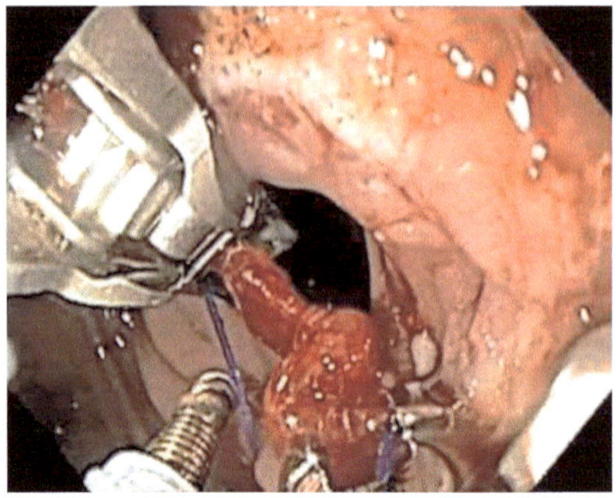

Fig. 15.2 Overstitch® Endoscopic Suturing System (Apollo Endosurgery, Inc.)

15.3.1.5 TERIS

The Trans-oral Endoscopic Restrictive Implant System (TERIS® – Barosense Inc.) uses an endoscopic guidance to trans-orally implant a prosthesis placed at the cardia level to decrease food reservoir size at the upper part of the stomach to induce early and prolonged satiety. Five gastric plications are created about 3 cm below the EGJ using an articulating endoscopic circular stapler. The gastric restrictor is subsequently attached to the gastric wall using silicon anchors inserted through the gastric plications. Primary clinical results, observed in a female patient with a BMI of 46 kg/m^2, showed no major complications during and after the procedure. The EWL was 21 and 26 % at 3 and 6 months, respectively. The observation of a high rate of implant obstruction led to the development of a second-generation implant [27].

Later, Fockens et al. published a study on safety and efficacy using the TERIS implant. This short-term trial included 13 patients with comorbidities (BMI 40–50 kg/m^2 or 35–40 kg/m^2) and a 3-month follow-up. Results reported one patient with intraprocedural gastric perforation related to stapler malfunctioning. Two other patients had a pneumoperitoneum treated conservatively in one case and deflated by a percutaneous hollow needle in the other. Twelve of 13 patients had a successful implant placement. At 3 months of follow-up, a median excess weight loss of 28 % and a median BMI decrease of 4.2 kg/m^2 (from 42.1 to 37.9 kg/m^2) were reported [28].

15.3.2 Derivative Procedures

A device, which applies a concept similar to the biliopancreatic diversion (BPD), is the duodeno-jejunal bypass liner (DJBL), a sterilized, single-use endoscopic device, which is minimally invasive and used under radioscopic control. It is composed of a nitinol anchor with tiny lateral barbs for fixation, and an impermeable plastic conduit made of a fluorine polymer 62 cm in length (Fig. 15.3), which prevents contact of bile–pancreatic secretions with chime prior to the proximal segments of the jejunum [29].

15.3.2.1 Results

The first human experience was registered in 2007 by L. Rodriguez-Grunert et al. with a 12-patient prospective, open-label, single-centre, 12-week study. They reported problems with the fixation of the device and adverse events related to the device itself, including abdominal pain, nausea, vomiting, mainly within 2 weeks of implantation. Implant site inflammation was found in all the patients [30].

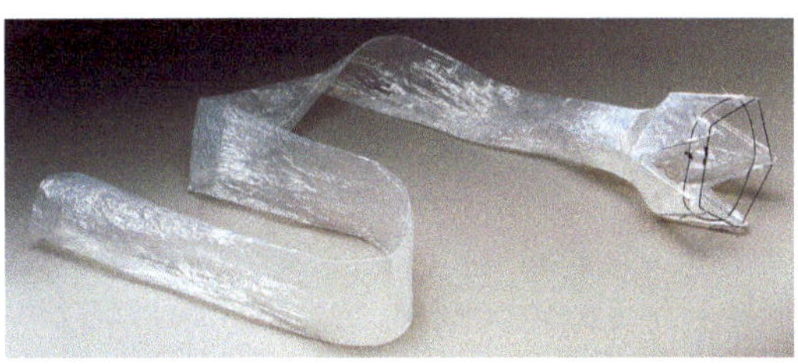

Fig. 15.3 Duodenal-jejunal bypass liner EndoBarrier® (gi-Dynamics, Inc.) from: http://www.gidynamics.com/

Gersin et al. carried out an open-label, sham-controlled trial on obese patients to test weight loss before bariatric surgery due to the implantation of DJBL. The primary end point of the trial was the difference between the two groups, in percentage of excess weight loss (EWL) at week 12. Thirty-seven patients were enrolled in the trial, 13 received the DJBL and 24 patients in the sham group underwent EGD and mock implantation. After 12 weeks, they observed a statistically relevant difference of EWL between the two groups: 62 % of patients in the DJBL achieved 10 % or more EWL compared with 17 % of the subjects in the sham arm. Total weight change in the DJBL arm was -8.2 ± 1.3 kg compared with -2.1 ± 1.1 kg in the sham arm ($P < 0.05$) [31].

In 2009, Gersin et al. published a study on the use of DJBL for type 2 diabetes treatment. They randomized 18 obese diabetic patients in two groups: the first (12 patients) underwent DJBL implantation while the other (6 patients) underwent sham endoscopy. The subjects baseline HbA(1c) was 9.1 ± 1.7 % and body mass index 38.9 ± 6.1 kg/m^2. By week 1, change in fasting glucose in the DJBL arm was -55 ± 21 mg/dL versus $+42 \pm 30$ mg/dL in the sham arm. At week 12, HbA(1c) change was -1.3 ± 0.9 % in the DJBL arm and -0.7 ± 0.4 % in the sham arm, and at 24 weeks, values were -2.4 ± 0.7 % in the DJBL arm and -0.8 ± 0.4 % in the sham arm [32].

Similar results were obtained in the Netherlands by Greve's group [33] that completed a randomized clinical trial including 41 patients: 30 underwent sleeve implantation and the remaining 11 were put on diet as control group. Only 26 devices were implanted and 4 of them had to be explanted prior to study completion due to migration (1), anchor dislocation (1), sleeve obstruction (1), and continuous epigastric pain (1). No procedure related adverse events occurred; however, each patient had at least one adverse event during the first week after implantation, mainly abdominal pain and nausea. Initial mean BMI was 48.9 and 47.4 kg/m^2 for the device and control patients, respectively. Mean EWL after 3 months was 19.0 % for device patients versus 6.9 % for controls. Absolute change in BMI at 3 months was 5.5 and 1.9 kg/m^2, respectively. Type 2 diabetes mellitus was present at baseline in eight patients of the device group and improved in seven patients during the study period (lower glucose levels, HbA1c and medication requirements) [33].

Subsequently, Escalona et al. in 2009 reported a 12-week pilot trial of ten patients treated with EDJBL modified with a 4-mm restrictor orifice distal to the anchor. The baseline BMI was of 40.8 ± 4.0 kg/m^2 (range 35.9–47.8 kg/m^2). After 12 weeks, the EWL range was 22–64 %, corresponding to a total weight loss of 16.7 ± 1.4 kg (range 12.0–26.0) [34].

Notwithstanding the promising results, the authors observed side effects related to the technique as inflammation of the anchoring site, nausea and vomiting.

The group led by Sandlers in California tested a similar concept, but different device, in 2011. A unique gastroduodenojejunal bypass sleeve secured at the EGJ with endoscopic and laparoscopic techniques was designed to create an endoluminal gastroduodenojejunal bypass. Twenty-four patients were enrolled in the trial and 22 underwent endoscopic implant of the bypass sleeve, which was maintained for 12 weeks and then removed endoscopically. Two patients required early explant due to postoperative dysphagia. Observed EWL was 39.7 %, and all patients who presented preoperative diabetes mellitus showed normal blood glucose levels at 12 weeks follow-up [35].

No long-term results are available, considering that DJBL is also a temporary device.

15.4 Translumenal Treatment

Natural Orifice Translumenal Endoscopic Surgery (NOTES) promises to open a new era for surgery. It can be defined as scarless abdominal operations performed with an endoscope passed through a natural orifice, then through an internal incision in the stomach, vagina, bladder or colon (hollow viscous), thus avoiding any external incisions and scars [36].

It requires specific endoscopic instruments introduced into the abdominal cavity. Several experiences of cholecystectomy and appendectomy performed by trans-vaginal or trans-gastric approach in humans have been published [37, 38]. However, "pure" NOTES is still more of a concept than a routine practice. It has also been considered a very promising technique for bariatric surgery, for the particular advantages of a minimally invasive approach to the abdomen of obese patients. Nevertheless, the complexity of bariatric procedures and the lack of appropriate devices remain a main issue, which could be overcome by the future introduction of miniaturized robotic devices.

One major point of criticism to translumenal surgery is the closure of access to the abdominal cavity gained through the viscous, since any complication rate perforating a healthy organ is considered unacceptable, at least conceptually. Several reports mention safe access and closure with new devices as the transmurally placed anchor systems, t-tags or bar-shaped stitches. Moreover, large-scale clips (OTSC; Ovesco), Padlock-G® clip (Aponos Medical) and Jumbo clips® (Endoclips, Olympus Optical Co. Ltd.) have been developed. Technically, the closure of the gastrotomy is obtained either by applying a clip after suction of the surrounding mucosal tissue, or by applying clips first to both ends of the incision and then towards the centre of the same incision [39, 40].

The Queen's NOTES group designed a novel endoscopic method of closing gastrotomies using PolyLoop polyp ligature devices and endoscopic clips [41]. This method for closing the gastric defect after NOTES procedures has been tested in animal trials on five 30-kg pigs. No complication after surgery was reported. Endoscopic examination carried out 1 week after surgery revealed all the closures to be intact and identifiable only by a small ulcer [42].

Linear staplers for flexible endoscopy have also been proposed to close the hole after NOTES procedure. Stapling activation is reported to be simple in endoscopic procedures: application in humans is still under evaluation and the tightness of the closure has been controlled by laparoscopy in the reported experience. However, the visualization and manipulation of tissue and other constrains limit, as of present, the use of this device [43].

Limited literature on clinical procedure hybrid NOTES sleeve gastrectomy has been reported. In 2009, Fischer et al. from the UCSD published a case report of a NOTES laparoscopic-assisted transvaginal sleeve gastrectomy in a 29-year-old woman who already underwent cholecystectomy and umbilical hernia repair. A 12-mm optical trocar was placed transumbilically, to provide insufflation, inspect the abdomen to define the feasibility of the procedure and as an additional instrument during procedure. A 15-cm-long, 15-mm-dilating trocar with a dual lumen cap was placed under direct vision through the posterior cul-de-sac of the vagina into the peritoneal cavity. The operation proceeded using a single channel gastroscope. Operative time was 171 min. The %EWL was 53 % and BMI reduced to 33.2 kg/m^2 after 6 months of follow- up [44].

In 2011, Buesing et al. described a series of 14 cases of sleeve gastrectomies using the trans-vaginal-assisted (hybrid NOTES) technique within a larger group of 200 patients who underwent laparoscopic sleeve gastrectomy. The transvaginal technique decreased the number of required trocars by1–2. In all the 14 cases, the resected stomach was retrieved transvaginally without complications due to the transvaginal access. Results were comparable to sleeve gastrectomy carried out through the routine laparoscopic approach [45]. In a recent paper, Horgan reports 3 cases of trans-vaginal and 18 cases of NOTES sleeve gastrectomy, the latter followed by standard laparoscopic stapler closure of the gastrotomy site. The NOTES specimen extraction in both TG and TV procedures proved to markedly decrease the postoperative pain in patients compared with transabdominal extraction [46].

Nevertheless, these procedures should be considered investigational and not as currently clinical.

Conclusions

As mentioned in the introduction, endolumenal approach to obesity treatment is considered a reliable solution and, maybe, the most suitable in the future, fitting perfectly to the well-established concept of minimal invasiveness. The described devices will probably be replaced by more advanced ones in the near future, but will remain as "pioneers" of a new era of bariatric treatments.

References

1. Cigaina V, Saggioro A, Rigo V, Pinato G, Ischai S. Long-term effects of gastric pacing to reduce feed intake in swine. Obes Surg. 1996;6:250–3.
2. Greenway FL, Zheng J. Electrical stimulation as a treatment for obesity and diabetes. J Diabetes Sci Technol. 2007;1:251–9.
3. Favretti F, De Luca M, Segato G, et al. Treatment of morbid obesity with the transcend implantable gastric stimulator (IGS): a prospective survey. Obes Surg. 2004;14(5):666–70.
4. Shikora SA. "What are the yanks doing?" the U.S. experience with implantable gastric stimulation (IGS) for the treatment of obesity – update on the ongoing clinical trials. Obes Surg. 2004;14:S40–8.
5. Shikora SA, et al. Implantable gastric stimulation for the treatment of clinically severe obesity: results of the SHAPE trial. Surg Obes Relat Dis. 2009;5(1):31–7. Epub 2008 Oct 1.
6. Peles S, Petersen J, Aviv R, Policker S, Abu-Hatoum O, Ben-Haim SA, Gutterman DD, Sengupta JN. Enhancement of antral contractions and vagal afferent signaling with synchronized electrical stimulation. Am J Physiol Gastrointest Liver Physiol. 2003;285(3):G577–85.
7. Sanmiguel CP, Conklin JL, Cunneen SA, et al. Gastric electrical stimulation with the TANTALUS System in obese type 2 diabetes patients: effect on weight and glycemic control. J Diabetes Sci Technol. 2009;3(4):964–70.
8. Bohdjalian A, Prager G, Aviv R, et al. One-year experience with Tantalus: a new surgical approach to treat morbid obesity. Obes Surg. 2006;16(5):627–34.
9. Bohdjalian A, Prager G, Rosak C, Weiner R, Jung R, Schramm M, Aviv R, Schindler K, Haddad W, Rosenthal N, Ludvik B. Improvement in glycemic control in morbidly obese type 2 diabetic subjects by gastric stimulation. Obes Surg. 2009;19(9):1221–7. Epub 2009 Jul 3.
10. Horbach T, Thalheimer A, Meyer G. Meeting abstract: Sicherheit und Effektivität einer "Closed Loop"Magenstimulation bei adipösen Patienten (abiliti®). Deutsche Gesellschaft für Chirurgie. 129. Kongress der Deutschen Gesellschaft für Chirurgie. Berlin, 24.-27.04.2012. Düsseldorf: German Medical Science GMS Publishing House; 2012.

11. Camilleri M, Toouli J, Herrera MF, Kulseng B. Intra-abdominal vagal blocking (VBLOC therapy): clinical results with a new implantable medical device. Surgery. 2008;143:723–31.
12. Tweden KS, Sarr MG, Camilleri M, Kendrick ML, Moody FG, Bierk MD, et al. Vagal blocking for obesity control (VBLOC): studies of pancreatic and gastric function and safety in a porcine model. Surg Obes Relat Dis. 2006;2:301.
13. Kral JG, Gortz L, Hermansson G, Wallin GS. Gastroplasty for obesity: long-term weight loss improved by vagotomy. World J Surg. 1993;17:75–9.
14. Shikora S, Toouli J, Herrera MF, Kulseng B, Zulewski H, Brancatisano R, Kow L, Pantoja JP, Johnsen G, Brancatisano A, Tweden KS, Knudson MB, Billington CJ. Vagal blocking improves glycemic control and elevated blood pressure in obese subjects with type 2 diabetes mellitus. J Obes. 2013;2013:245683. doi:10.1155/2013/245683.
15. Aspire Bariatrics official website: http://aspirebariatrics.com/.
16. Devière J, Ojeda Valdes G, et al. Safety, feasibility and weight loss after transoral gastroplasty: first human multicenter study. Surg Endosc. 2008;22:589–98.
17. Arezzo A, Morino M. Endoscopic closure of gastric access in perspective NOTES: an update on techniques and technologies. Surg Endosc. 2010;24:298–303.
18. Zagol B, Mikami D. Advances in transoral fundoplication for oesophageal reflux. Dig Liver Dis. 2011;43:361–4.
19. Awan AN, Swain CP. Endoscopic vertical band gastroplasty with an en- doscopic sewing machine. Gastrointest Endosc. 2002;55:254–6.
20. Fogel R, De Fogel J, Bonilla Y, et al. Clinical experience of transoral sutur-ing for an endoluminal vertical gastroplasty: 1-year follow-up in 64 patients. Gastrointest Endosc. 2008;68:51–8.
21. Familiari P, Costamagna G, Bléro D, Le Moine O, Perri V, Boskoski I, Coppens E, et al. Transoral gastroplasty for morbid obesity: a multicenter trial with a 1-year outcome. Gastrointest Endosc. 2011;74(6):1248–58. doi:10.1016/j.gie.2011.08.046.
22. Chiellini C, Iaconelli A, Familiari P, Riccioni ME, Castagneto M, Nanni G, Costamagna G, et al. Study of the effects of transoral gastroplasty on insulin sensitivity and secretion in obese subjects. Nutr Metab Cardiovasc Dis. 2010;20(3):202–7. doi:10.1016/j.numecd.2009.03.012.
23. Devière J, Ojeda Valdes G, Cuevas Herrera L, Closset J, Le Moine O, Eisendrath P, Moreno C, et al. Safety, feasibility and weight loss after transoral gastroplasty: first human multicenter study. Surg Endosc. 2008;22(3):589–98. doi:10.1007/s00464-007-9662-5.
24. Brethauer SA, Chand B, Schauer PR, Thompson CC. Transoral gastric volume reduction for weight management: technique and feasibility in 18 patients. Surg Obes Relat Dis. 2010;6:689–94.
25. Espinós J, Turró R, Mata A, Cruz M. Early Experience with the Incisionless Operating Platform™(IOP) for the treatment of obesity. Obes Surg. 2013;510:1375–83. doi:10.1007/s11695-013-0937-8.
26. Abu Dayyeh BK, Rajan E, Gostout CJ. Endoscopic sleeve gastroplasty: a potential endoscopic alternative to surgical sleeve gastrectomy for treatment of obesity. Gastrointest Endosc. 2013;78(3):530–5. doi:10.1016/j.gie.2013.04.197.
27. Biertho L, Hould FS, Lebel S, Biron S. Transoral endoscopic restrictive implant system: a new endoscopic technique for the treatment of obesity. Surg Obes Relat Dis. 2010;6(2):203–5.
28. De Jong K, Mathus-Vliegen EM, Veldhuyzen EA, Eshuis JH, Fockens P. Short-term safety and efficacy of the Trans-oral Endoscopic Restrictive Implant System for the treatment of obesity. Gastrointest Endosc. 2010;72(3):497–504. Epub 2010 Jun 11.
29. de Moura EG, Orso IR, Martins BC, Lopes GS, de Oliveira SL, Galvão-Neto P, Mancini MC, Santo MA, Sakai P, Ramos AC, Garrido-Júnior AB, Halpern A, Cecconello I. Improvement of insulin resistance and reduction of cardiovascular risk among obese patients with type 2 diabetes with the duodenojejunal bypass liner. Obes Surg. 2011;21(7):941–7.
30. Rodriguez-Grunert L, Galvao Neto MP, Alamo M, Ramos AC, Baez PB, Tarnoff M. First human experience with endoscopically delivered and retrieved duodenal-jejunal bypass sleeve. Surg Obes Relat Dis. 2008;4:55–9.
31. Gersin KS, Rothstein RI, Rosenthal RJ, Stefanidis D, Deal SE, Kuwada TS, Laycock W, Adrales G, Vassiliou M, Szomstein S, Heller S, Joyce AM, Heiss F, Nepomnayshy D. Open-label, sham-controlled trial of an endoscopic duodenojejunal bypass liner for preoperative weight loss in bariatric surgery candidates. Gastrointest Endosc. 2010;71(6):976–82. Epub 2010 Mar 20.
32. Rodriguez L, Reyes E, Fagalde P, Oltra MS, Saba J, Aylwin CG, Prieto C, Ramos A, Galvao M, Gersin KS, Sorli C. Pilot clinical study of an endoscopic, removable duodenal-jejunal bypass liner for the treatment of type 2 diabetes. Diabetes Technol Ther. 2009;11(11):725–32.
33. Schouten R, Rijs CS, Bouvy ND, Hameeteman W, Koek GH, Janssen IM, Greve JW. A multicenter, randomized efficacy study of the EndoBarrier Gastrointestinal Liner for presurgical weight loss prior to bariatric surgery. Ann Surg. 2010;251(2):236–43.
34. Escalona A, Yáñez R, Pimentel F, Galvao M, Ramos AC, Turiel D, Boza C, Awruch D, Gersin K, Ibáñez L. Initial human experience with restrictive duodenal-jejunal bypass liner for treatment of morbid obesity. Surg Obes Relat Dis. 2010;6:126–31.
35. Sandler BJ, Rumbaut R, Swain CP, Torres G, Morales L, Gonzales L, Schultz S, Talamini M, Horgan S. Human experience with an endoluminal, endoscopic, gastrojejunal bypass sleeve. Surg Endosc. 2011;25(9):3028–33.
36. D. Rattner, A. Kalloo, and the SAGES/ASGE Working Group on Natural Orifice Translumenal Endoscopic Surgery. White Paper. ASGE/SAGES Working Group

on Natural Orifice Translumenal Endoscopic Surgery October 2005. Surg Endosc. 2006;20:329–33. Gastrointestinal Endoscopy: Volume 63, No.2; 2006.

37. Shin EJ, Jeong GA, Jung JC, Cho GS, Lim CW, Kim HC, et al. Transvaginal endoscopic appendectomy. J Korean Soc Coloproctol. 2010;26(6):429–32.
38. Meining A, Feussner H, Swain P, Yang GZ, Lehmann K, Zorron R, Meisner S, Ponsky J, Martiny H, Reddy N, Armengol-Miro JR, Fockens P, Fingerhut A, Costamagna G. Natural-orifice transluminal endoscopic surgery (NOTES) in Europe: summary of the working group reports of the Euro-NOTES meeting 2010. Endoscopy. 2011;43:140–3.
39. Merrifield BF, Wagh MS, Thompson CC. Peroral trans- gastric organ resection: a feasibility study in pigs. Gastrointest Endosc. 2006;63:693–7.
40. Schurr MO, Baur F, Ho CN, Anhoeck G, Kratt T, Gottwald T. Endoluminal full-thickness resection of GI lesions: a new device and technique. Minim Invasive Ther Allied Technol. 2011;20(3):189–92.
41. Hookey LC, Khokhotva V, Bielawska B, Samis A, Jalink D, Hurlbut D, Mercer D. The Queen's closure: a novel technique for closure of endoscopic gastrotomy for natural-orifice transluminal endoscopic surgery. Endoscopy. 2009;41(2):149–53.
42. Hookey LC, Bielawska B, Samis A, Jalink D, Ellis R, Khokhotva V, Hurlbut D, Mercer D. A reliable and safe gastrotomy closure technique assessed in a porcine survival model pilot study: success of the Queen's closure. Endoscopy. 2009;41(6):493–7. Epub 2009 Jun 16.
43. Ryou M, Fong DG, Pai RD, Rattner DW, Thompson CC. Transluminal closure for NOTES: an ex vivo study comparing leak pressures of various gastrotomy and colotomy closure modalities. Endoscopy. 2008;40:432–6.
44. Fischer LJ, Jacobsen G, Wong B, Thompson K, Bosia J, Talamini M, Horgan S. NOTES laparoscopic-assisted transvaginal sleeve gastrectomy in humans–description of preliminary experience in the United States. Surg Obes Relat Dis. 2009;5(5):633–6. Epub 2009 May 9.
45. Buesing M, Utech M, Halter J, Riege R, Saada G, Knapp A. Sleeve gastrectomy in the treatment of morbid obesity. Study results and first experiences with the transvaginal hybrid NOTES technique. Chirurg. 2011;82(8):675–83.
46. Horgan S, Meireles OR, Jacobsen GR, Sandler BJ, Ferreres A, Ramamoorthy S, Savides T, Katagiri T, Dotai T, Sedrak M, Majid SF, Nijhawan S, Talamini MA. Broad clinical utilization of NOTES: is it safe? Surg Endosc. 2013;27:1872–80. doi:10.1007/s00464-012-2736-z.

16 Adjustable Gastric Banding

Karl A. Miller

16.1 Introduction

Morbid obesity (body mass index ≥40 kg/m^2 or ≥35 kg/m^2 in the presence of comorbidities [1]) is a complex and increasingly prevalent chronic disease that operates at the nexus of genetics, hormones, environment, and behavior [2–4]. There is no known cure for morbid obesity, and life-long treatment in association with lifestyle change is required to minimize its progressive effects. No medical treatment has been successful in maintaining weight loss and reducing the comorbidities of obesity [5–7]; surgical and device technologies, however, have demonstrated their effectiveness [8–10] and safety [11–13] over the intermediate to longer terms (i.e., 5–10 years), providing the impetus for continued innovation in these areas.

Laparoscopic adjustable gastric banding (LAGB) is a proven approach to the treatment of morbid obesity [14, 15] that comprises both an operation and an implantable biomedical device. The efficacy of this purely restrictive bariatric procedure has been tested in the worldwide literature over the past decade in numerous series summarized by systematic review [16–18] and meta-analysis [19, 20]. These report a LAGB percentage excess weight loss of 50–61 % at 2–3 years. Although in the short term, weight loss with the gastric band is exceeded by that of the malabsorptive operations, beyond 2 years, weight loss has been shown to be equivalent [18], with possible metabolic advantages accruing to band patients (e.g., decreased incidence of cholecystitis [21]) due to the gradual nature of weight loss with banding.

Since the introduction of the first gastric band in the early 1980s, the technique used for its implantation has evolved in response to the clinical experience of surgeons, the band's long-term complication profile, and advancements in band and injection-port engineering. This review presents a summary of the development of gastric banding, particularly, the primary operative techniques [22], and a description of a recent innovation in injection-port implantation technology and technique.

16.2 Technical Aspects

In 1978, Wilkinson pioneered the concept of gastric banding in an open procedure by surrounding, and thus constricting, the upper stomach with a 2-cm-wide nonadjustable mesh fabric (Marlex®) [23], an innovation that was ineffective in achieving sufficient weight loss. In 1980, Dacron® graft segmentation of the upper stomach by Molina resulted in unacceptably high rates of

K.A. Miller, MD, FACS
Surgical Department, Hallein Clinic,
Buergermeister Str. 34, Hallein A-5400, Austria
e-mail: karl.miller@kh-hallein.at

M. Lucchese, N. Scopinaro (eds.), *Minimally Invasive Bariatric and Metabolic Surgery: Principles and Technical Aspects*, DOI 10.1007/978-3-319-15356-8_16,

reoperation [24] and was abandoned. Wilkinson and Peloso, in 1981 [25], Kolle, in 1982 [26], and Molina and Oria, in 1983 [27], each introduced a constricting-ring *nonadjustable* gastric band which were, unfortunately, also associated with high rates of reoperation, as the stomach tissue stretched postoperatively and the stoma diameter of the band could not be modulated. In a 1984 meeting presentation and 1989 report, Szinicz and Muller [28] and Szinicz et al. [29] presented the results of their experiments in minipigs implanting a "reversible" gastric band, the forerunner of today's adjustable gastric bands.

In 1985, the Swedish group of Hallberg and Forsell published their first report of an *adjustable* gastric band [30]—the Swedish Adjustable Gastric Band (SAGB)—developed in Huddinge University Hospital, Sweden, and first implanted clinically in an open procedure by Klaiber in Switzerland [31]. The SAGB was designed to accomplish stoma restriction by means of a low-pressure/high-volume mechanism [32–34]. Kuzmak, in 1986 [35–37], described his implantation of a slender (1-cm wide), nonadjustable, silicone band that created an effective 13-mm gastric stoma; in 1986, Kuzmak modified his nonadjustable gastric band to incorporate an inflatable, small-diameter balloon that functioned in a high-pressure/low-volume manner [38] (which later became the Lap-Band®) [39].

In the early 1990s, Catona et al. [40] and Broadbent et al. [41] were the first to *laparoscopically* perform nonadjustable gastric banding. Catona et al. suggested opening the lesser omentum to increase the procedure's speed and simplicity. In 1993, Belachew et al. [42] reported their animal studies of laparoscopic placement of the adjustable band, and in 1994 and 1995, Belachew et al. (Lap-Band) [43, 44], and in 1997, Forsell et al. (SAGB) [33] reported performing the first human implantations of *laparoscopic adjustable* gastric bands (generically, "LAGBs"). Belachew et al. employed a perigastric technique, Forsell et al., the pars flaccida technique, developed specifically for use with the SAGB to reduce the complications associated with nonadjustable banding. Niville et al., in 1998 [45], described creating an extremely small gastric pouch by positioning the posterior aspect of the band at the distal esophagus. In 2000, Weiner et al. [46] presented an amalgam of the advantages of both techniques in their report of a "two-step" (pars flaccida to perigastric) approach.

In 2000, Catona, La Manna, and Forsell [47] reviewed the development of gastric banding, particularly pars flaccida technique, over the previous 13 years, and Fielding and Allen [48] followed by Ren and Fielding [49] reported the improvements that were attainable using the pars flaccida as opposed to the perigastric technique (i.e., reduced incidence of late complications, particularly gastric prolapse, to between 0.6 and 3.5 %). Both bands, in wide use throughout Europe from the mid-1990s, have undergone several design modifications. The Lap-Band was approved for use in the US in 2001 [39]; the SAGB was approved in the US (as the REALIZE™ Band) in 2007 [50].

The most recent innovation in implantation technique is mechanical injection port fixation technology, as opposed to suture fixation of the port. In two prospective, 1-year, randomized studies [51, 52], the Velocity® port (Obtech Medical AG, Baar, Switzerland, distributed by Ethicon Endo-Surgery, Inc., Cincinnati, OH) demonstrated improved stability, speed of fixation, and reduced complications, including diminished port-site pain and use of pain medications; Miller and Pump showed an eightfold improvement in speed-to-implant (i.e., from >8 min to <1 min, $P<0.0001$).

The perigastric approach is summarized, below, followed by a more detailed description of the pars flaccida implantation of the SAGB.

16.2.1 Perigastric Approach

In the perigastric approach, following introduction of the trocars and with the calibration balloon in place in the stomach, an incision of approximately 0.5–1 cm is made at the lesser curvature close to the cardia (Fig. 16.1). A passage is formed along the posterior wall of the stomach from the gastroesophageal (GE) junction above the peritoneal reflection of the bursa omentalis through to

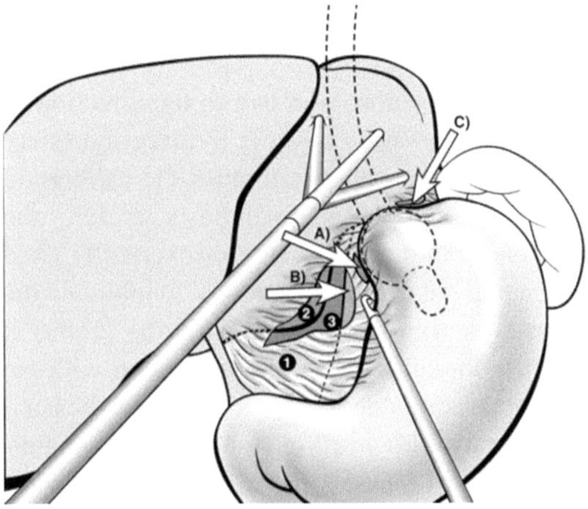

Fig. 16.1 The point of dissection employed in the perigastric (*A*) and pars flaccida (*B*) techniques. (*C*) angle of His; (*1*) lesser omentum (pars flaccida); (*2*) caudate lobe of the liver; (*3*) right crus of the diaphragm

the angle of His. Using the endodissector (Allergan, Irvine, CA), attached to the end of the catheter, the gastric band is placed around the cardia. The calibration balloon is used to gauge final positioning of the band and the creation of the so-called virtual pouch. To prevent band slippage, three or four sutures are placed in the greater curvature. The catheter end of the band is brought outward through the 15- or 18-mm trocar and connected to the port, which is then fixed beneath the anterior rectus sheath using four nonresorbable interrupted sutures [44, 53].

16.2.2 Pars Flaccida Technique

The anatomic landmarks of the LAGB procedure are best identified by bringing the patient into a 30° reverse Trendelenburg position. If necessary, the subcardiac region of the stomach and GE junction should be freed from fat to ensure an optimal view of the field.

16.2.3 Dissection at the Lesser Curvature

To determine the precise location of the GE junction, the anesthetist passes the gastric calibration tube into the stomach and the tube's balloon is slowly filled with 25 mL saline, or air. The balloon is then drawn back up against the GE junction.

The lesser omentum is grasped with forceps to stretch the pars flaccida. An approximately 5-cm incision is made caudal to the GE junction but cranial to the left gastric artery (Fig. 16.1) to avoid opening the omental bursa (lesser sac) and prevent injury to the left gastric artery, the inferior phrenic artery, the branches of the vagal nerve, or an accessory hepatic artery. The right crus of the diaphragm is exposed, and the tissue medial to the right crus, 5 cm distal to the GE junction, is incised approximately 0.5 cm in preparation for eventual retrocardiac tunneling.

At this point, the calibration tube is advanced into the stomach. The fundus is grasped with the forceps and drawn caudally, with the forceps passed to the assistant. The avascular portion of the ligament at the angle of His is incised about 1 cm in width to prepare for eventual placement of the gastric band. This action establishes the direction of the dissection for the retrocardiac tunnel. Finally, the left crus of the diaphragm is exposed approximately 1–1.5 cm.

16.2.4 Introducing the Adjustable Gastric Band (AGB)

The AGB is checked to ensure that it has been properly prepared for insertion and is free of leaks. The band is grasped with forceps at its locking end flap, and positioned so that the balloon side of the band parallels the forceps. The band is introduced into the abdominal cavity through the 15-mm trocar, assisting its introduction, if necessary, through the trocar with the forceps.

16.2.5 Creating the Retrocardiac Tunnel

The Goldfinger instrument (Obtech Medical AG, Baar, Switzerland, distributed by Ethicon Endo-Surgery, Inc.) is introduced in front of the anterior wall of the stomach corresponding to the eventual course of the retrocardiac tunnel. From the incision prepared at the right crus of the diaphragm, the Goldfinger dissector is introduced retrocardially toward the incision at the angle of His until it emerges at that incision. In order to ensure a small pouch size (approximately 15 mL) and to avoid injury to the stomach and esophagus, it is important not to deviate from the plane of dissection during this maneuver. Any suspicion of a perforation should be investigated.

16.2.6 Positioning the Band

The gastric band should be positioned in the retrocardiac tunnel so that the balloon side is oriented toward the stomach wall. Using the forceps, the suture loop of the AGB is brought to the notch of the Goldfinger dissector, which (with the attached band) is pulled, under vision, through the retrocardiac tunnel from the angle of His until the locking end flap is visible at the lesser curvature. The tab end of the AGB on the side of the lesser curvature is grasped with the forceps and the Goldfinger dissector is carefully removed.

16.2.7 Closing the Band, Retrocardiac Technique

The calibration balloon, if used is withdrawn to the point of the GE junction. The possibility of closing the band is checked, with respect to the patient's individual anatomy, by attempting to overlap both ends of the band. If it is not readily possible due to a large amount of perigastric fat, the "two-step" technique (pars flaccida to perigastric) should be employed (see Sect. 16.2.9.1, below).

Closing the band is accomplished by pulling the locking end flap with the forceps until it has passed through the buckle. It is important to ensure that no portion of the stomach or fat has been drawn into the locking mechanism of the band, and that the band is not too tightly fitted around the stomach.

16.2.8 Placing Safety Sutures

The band fastening is drawn in the direction of the lesser curvature in order to place the safety sutures. The anesthetist empties the calibration tube completely and withdraws it into the esophagus to avoid its being inadvertently fixed when placing the safety sutures. To maintain the gastric band in the best position, the fundus is fixed to the left crus of the diaphragm with the first nonabsorbable suture. To surround the band completely with a cuff of stomach wall, the fundus is grasped caudal to the band and pulled in the direction of the crus. The suturing is continued anteriorly with two additional safety sutures between the seromuscular layer of the fundus and the pouch, ensuring that the band fastening is freely accessible. During this process, the assistant should insert a swab above the upper margin of the band to ensure that the band is protected.

16.2.9 Testing for Leaks, Inspecting the Operative Field

The anesthetist advances the calibration tube back into the pouch and fills it with 20 mL of methylene blue solution. If the methylene blue emerges anywhere on the stomach, the source of injury responsible for the leak should be meticulously sought out and repaired. The poorly visible posterior stomach wall, especially, should be examined. The methylene solution should subsequently be suctioned away by the anesthetist and the calibration tube removed.

The operating field is completely inspected for bleeding or injury to organs. The end of the band tubing is grasped with the forceps and pulled out through the trocar in preparation for the extracorporeal attachment of the port system. The 15-mm trocar is carefully removed, avoiding injury to the tubing system, and the fascia at the entry site is closed with fascial suture to avoid hernia formation. All trocars are removed under vision, finally, including the optical trocar.

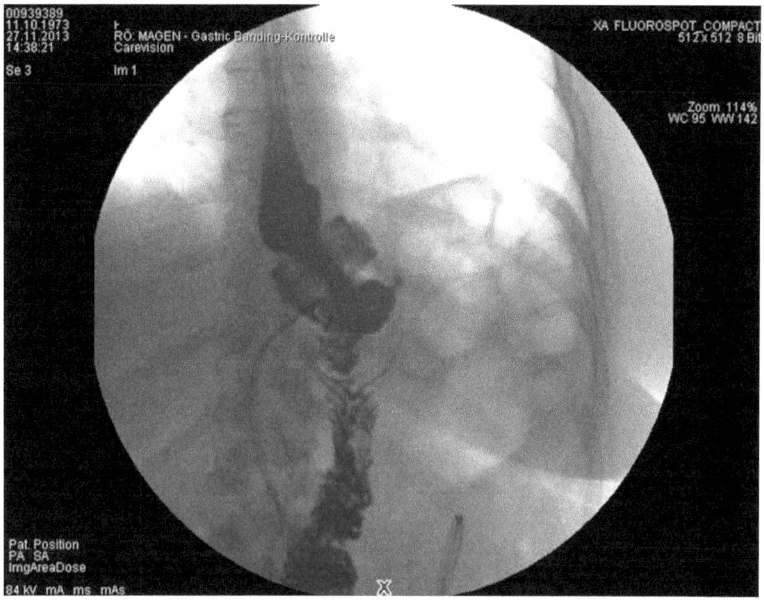

Fig. 16.2 Adjustable banded gastric bypass

16.2.9.1 Two-Step Technique

Another implantation option is the "two-step" maneuver, applicable when perigastric and visceral fat are too extensive to dissect during pars flaccida implantation. The fat at the lesser curvature containing the nerve of Latarjet at the level of the band is separated carefully from the gastric wall in the direction of the right crus until the curvature becomes visible. A blunt articulating dissector is passed through the incision on the lesser curvature side until it is visible at the pars flaccida incision site. The dissector (with attached band) is pulled, under vision and without force, from the incised pars flaccida to the incision at the lesser curvature close to the gastric wall until the locking end flap appears at this site.

16.2.10 Adjustable Banded Gastric Bypass

In case of insufficient weight loss or technical pouch failure after RYGB, we perform an adjustable gastric band to restrict the gastric pouch as a salvage procedure (Fig. 16.2). After exploration of the gastric pouch, an atraumatic grasper is passed through a small opening of the pars flaccida and introduced retrocardially toward the incision at the angle of His on the lesser curve and the gastric pouch 1–2 cm above the horizontal cut edge of the pouch. Following this step, an AGB is introduced via the 15 mm port, drawn around the pouch and locked into place. To prevent slippage, the band is then fixed by suturing the gastric remnant to the gastric pouch both above and below the band with nonabsorbable sutures.

16.2.11 Attaching the Port System

16.2.11.1 Suture Fixation Method

The skin incision is extended to approximately 3.5 cm, and the fat is completely dissected from the fascia of the anterior rectus sheath for safe port placement. The locking connector of the port is placed into the cut end of the tubing and fastened at the port connection. The locking connector is pushed over the tubing toward the port until the tubing is completely fixed at the port.

The port should be positioned on the fascia so as to be readily located and accessible for band adjustments, and placed in a position that will not rotate or migrate. For better visualization of the fascia, the skin is held open using two Langenbeck hooks. Four threads are placed on the fascia; one side of each thread is guided through one of the suture holes of the port and the port is placed in the fascia. The tubing is guided carefully into the abdominal cavity and the threads are knotted to fix the port securely.

16.2.11.2 Mechanical Port Fixation Method

When using the SAGB-compatible Velocity® mechanical port fixation device (or "port applier"), the device description and operating instructions should be carefully read. A skin incision of at least 3 cm must be made to accommodate the mechanical fixation introducer. The fat should be dissected away from the fascia of the anterior rectus sheath. The strain-relief end of the port locking connector is placed onto the cut end of the band tubing until the tubing passes approximately 2 cm beyond the locking connector tab. The band tubing is pushed onto the connection tube extending from the port until the tubing reaches the outer face of the port connection housing. It is important to ensure that locking connector tabs are aligned with the notch in the connection housing before sliding the connector into the housing. The connector is turned clockwise until it stops rotating. Air is aspirated from the port using a Huber needle.

The port is checked to verify that the actuator ring is in the unlocked position, and the fastening hooks of the port are retracted into the port. If hooks are still visible, the actuator ring is rotated again. While the actuator is still in the unlocked position, and the tubing connected, the port is inserted into the applier receptacle with the red safety cap facing opposite the applier and the connection housing fitted into one of the two guide notches. Correctly inserted, the port snaps into place in the applier.

The safety cap is removed from the bottom of the port and the applier's handle is grasped in the palm. The port is placed on the prepared fascia and the applier is inserted at an angle, with the tubing and connector entering the incision first. Light downward pressure is used to situate the port flat on top of the fascia, the safety trigger is released, and the firing lever is compressed with the palm. Maintaining compression on the firing lever, the applier is removed from the field. The port is left attached to the fascia without suture fixation. If proper mechanical fixation is not attainable, the port is secured with sutures using the three holes visible through the actuator ring. In both the suture and mechanical port fixation techniques, a loop of tubing is retained inside the abdomen to facilitate free movement by the patient during exercise without dislodging the band or port system. The band balloon is left uninflated at the conclusion of surgery.

16.3 Clinical Management

The first band adjustment of the LAGB should be performed no sooner than 4–6 weeks postoperatively to avert esophageal dilation and risk of band slippage. The patient should not lose more than 0.5–1 kg of weight per week, there should be no intestinal obstruction, and no abdominal pain should be experienced with eating.

The patient is positioned supine on the X-ray table and the area of skin above the port is disinfected. The table is tilted to a 30–45° reverse Trendelenburg position. A syringe with 3–4 mL of 41 % Jopamidol® injection solution (USP), or sterile 0.9 % NaCl solution is prepared. Port location is identified by palpation, and an atraumatic Huber needle is inserted vertically through the skin into the chamber while holding the port positioned between two fingers. If the port cannot be located in this manner, the puncture should be repeated under fluoroscopic control.

All air is removed from the band system before being filled for the first time.

The water-soluble contrast agent is instilled into the port. The patient swallows a barium-containing contrast agent under fluoroscopic control so that the correct position and filling of the band may be gauged (Fig. 16.3). The angle of the band with respect to the transverse plane should be 40–45°; the contrast agent should move from the pouch into the stomach in a continuous flow of 1–2 peristaltic waves. Some water-soluble contrast agent may be aspirated until optimal

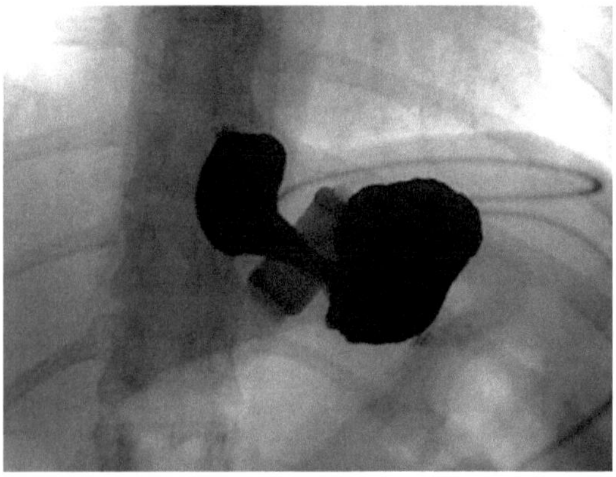

Fig. 16.3 Following barium swallow under fluoroscopic control, the angle of the band with respect to the transverse plane should be 40–45°—the shape of pouch formation and esophageal clearance is of importance

filling can be demonstrated via barium swallow. A maximum volume of 4 mL (depending on band systems) should not be exceeded at the first filling.

16.4 Outcomes

Regardless of the surgical technique employed, long-term success with LAGB is dependent on recognition of the chronic, multifactorial nature of morbid obesity, and thus, the necessity, for the patient, of enduring lifestyle change, and for the surgeon, of long-term follow-up. Although minimally invasive, and performed at an ever-increasing rate in most parts of the world, LAGB is not a simple procedure, and it is associated with distinctive long-term morbidity despite its reputation as the least invasive bariatric operation with the lowest perioperative morbidity and mortality.

Forsell et al., in their early papers on laparoscopic technique and adjustable banding [32–34], stressed four keys to successful technique: correct positioning of the band to avoid gastric injury or perforation, fixation of the band to avoid slippage down along the greater curvature, placement of the port connecting tube so as to avoid kinking, and waiting to inflate the band for 4–6 weeks following surgery. Catona et al. [47] also stressed the importance of high, accurate placement of the band as well as employment of tunneling sutures in fixing the band in place. The early results of mechanical port fixation technology and technique are promising. A potentially more secure port position may be achieved with the velocity port mechanical applier while reducing total operating time by 19 %.

The pars flaccida technique is associated with a decreased rate of gastric prolapse, an asset that may result in improved overall LAGB weight loss and enhanced patient compliance. Gastric band and port implantation technique will continue to evolve in response to the needs of the patient and the goal of increasing safety and efficacy.

O'Brien et al. demonstrate from one center a durable weight loss with 47 % EWL maintained to 15 years. This weight loss occurred regardless of whether any revisional procedures were needed and showed substantial and similar long-term weight losses for LAGB and other bariatric procedures [54]. Nevertheless, numerous reports indicate that LAGB cannot be recommended as a primary procedure to the general morbidly obese population, a careful patient selection is mandatory [55].

Angrisani et al. showed in a long-term follow-up study that LAGB is a safe and effective procedure in patients with a BMI <35 kg/m^2 [56].

The implantation of a LAGB in failed gastric bypass procedures seems to be emerging. The results of all nine studies shown by Vijgen et al. reported a further increase in weight loss after salvage banding for failed RYGB. In case of insufficient weight loss or technical pouch failure after RYGB, all reports suggest that salvage banding is a safe and feasible revisional procedure [57].

The results of the study from Silberhumer et al. demonstrate that LAGB is an effective and safe procedure in adolescents and children with a very carefully selected patient population [58]. In adolescents, the attractiveness of this procedure as first-line surgical treatment in a multidisciplinary setting is due to the reversibility of the procedure without altering the physiological intestinal tract in a very dynamic patient population.

Even adjustable gastric banding is not very popular in many centers around the world; it will be a good alternative procedure in selected patients, adolescents, and low BMI patients and nevertheless a fair salvage procedure for failed gastric bypass procedures.

References

1. Gastrointestinal Surgery for Severe Obesity. NIH Consens Statement 1991;9(1):1–20.
2. Kaila B, Raman M. Obesity: a review of pathogenesis and management strategies. Can J Gastroenterol. 2008; 22(1):61–8.
3. Marti A, Martinez-González MA, Martinez JA. Interaction between genes and lifestyle factors on obesity. Proc Nutr Soc. 2008;67(1):1–8.
4. Mond J, Myers TC, Crosby R, Hay P, Mitchell J. 'Excessive exercise' and eating-disordered behaviour in young adult women: further evidence from a primary care sample. Eur Eat Disord Rev. 2008;16(3):215–21.
5. Goodrick GK, Foreyt JP. Why treatments for obesity don't last. JAMA. 1999;91:1243–7.
6. North American Association for the Study of Obesity (NAASO) and the National Heart, Lung, and Blood Institute (NHLBI). The practical guide: identification, evaluation, and treatment of overweight and obesity in adults. Bethesda; 2000. NIH Publication Number 00–4084.
7. O'Brien PE, Dixon JB, Laurie C, et al. Treatment of mild to moderate obesity with laparoscopic adjustable gastric banding or an intensive medical program: a randomized trial. Ann Intern Med. 2006;144(9): 625–33.
8. O'Connell T. An overview of obesity and weight-loss surgery. Clin Diab. 2004;22:115–20.
9. Vella M, Galloway DJ. Laparoscopic adjustable gastric banding for severe obesity. Obes Surg. 2003;13(4): 642–8. Review.
10. O'Brien PE, Dixon JB, Brown W, et al. The laparoscopic adjustable gastric band (Lap-Band): a prospective study of medium-term effects on weight, health and quality of life. Obes Surg. 2002;12(5):652–60.
11. Sjöström L, Narbro K, Sjöström CD. Effects of bariatric surgery on mortality in Swedish obese subjects. N Engl J Med. 2007;357(8):741–52.
12. Christou NV, Sampalis JS, Liberman M, et al. Surgery decreases long-term mortality, morbidity, and health care use in morbidly obese patients. Ann Surg. 2004;240:416–23.
13. Parikh MS, Laker S, Weiner M, Hajiseyedjavadi O, Ren CJ. Objective comparison of complications resulting from laparoscopic bariatric procedures. J Am Coll Surg. 2006;202(2):252–61.
14. Buchwald H, Consensus Conference Panel. Bariatric surgery for morbid obesity: health implications for patients, health professionals, and third-party payers. J Am Coll Surg. 2005;200(4):593–604.
15. Weiner R, Blanco-Engert R, Weiner S, et al. Outcome after laparoscopic adjustable gastric banding – 8 years experience. Obes Surg. 2003;13:427–34.
16. Fried M, Miller K, Kormanova K. Literature review of comparative studies of complications with Swedish band and Lap-Band. Obes Surg. 2004;14(2):256–60.
17. Chapman AE, Kiroff G, Game P, et al. Laparoscopic adjustable gastric banding in the treatment of obesity: a systematic literature review. Surgery. 2004;135(3): 326–51.
18. O'Brien PE, McPhail T, Chaston TB, Dixon JB. Systematic review of medium-term weight loss after bariatric operations. Obes Surg. 2006;16(8): 1032–4.
19. Buchwald H, Avidor Y, Braunwald E, et al. Bariatric surgery: a systematic review and meta-analysis. JAMA. 2004;292:1724–37.
20. Cunneen SA, Phillips E, Fielding G, et al. Studies of the Swedish adjustable gastric band and Lap-Band: systematic review and meta-analysis. Surg Obes Relat Dis. 2008; 4(2):174–85.
21. Al-Jiffry BO, Shaffer EA, Saccone GT, et al. Changes in gallbladder motility and gallstone formation following laparoscopic gastric banding for morbid obesity. Can J Gastroenterol. 2003;17(3):169–74.
22. Miller K. Operation primer: laparoscopic gastric banding with the Swedish Adjustable Gastric Band (SAGB quick close). Haslemere/Surrey: Euromed Communications, Ltd; 2006.
23. Buchwald H, Buchwald JN. Evolution of operative procedures for the management of morbid obesity 1950–2000. Obes Surg. 2002;12:705–17.
24. Vassallo C, Andreoli M, La Manna A, Turpini C. 60 Reoperations on 890 patients after gastric restrictive surgery. Obes Surg. 2002;11:752–6.
25. Wilkinson LH, Peloso OA. Gastric (reservoir) reduction for morbid obesity. Arch Surg. 1981;116:602–5.
26. Kolle K. Gastric banding. OMGI 7th Congress, Stockholm, 1982;37:145. [Abstract]
27. Molina M, Oria HE. Gastric segmentation: a new, safe, effective, simple, readily revised and fully reversible surgical procedure for the correction of morbid obesity. Sixth Bariatric Surgery Colloquium Iowa City, 2–3 June 1983. [Abstract]
28. Szinicz G, Muller L. A new method in the surgical treatment of pathologic obesity—results of animal experiments. Proceedings of the XI Annual Meeting of the European Society for Artificial Organs; 1984; Alpbach-Innsbruck, Austria. London: W. B. Saunders Company Ltd; 1984. p. 322.
29. Szinicz G, Muller L, Erhart W, et al. "Reversible gastric banding" in surgical treatment of morbid obesity – results of animal experiments. Res Exp Med (Berl). 1989;189:55–60.
30. Hallberg D, Forsell P. Ballongband Vid Behandling av Massiv Overvikt (Balloon band for treatment of massive obesity). Svensk Kirurgi. 1985;43:106.
31. Klaiber C, Metzger A, Forsell P. Laparoscopic gastric banding. Chirurg. 2000;71(2):146–51.

32. Forsell P, Hallberg D, Hellers G. A gastric band with adjustable inner diameter for morbid obesity: preliminary studies. Obes Surg. 1993;3:303–6.
33. Forsell P, Hellers G. The Swedish Adjustable Gastric Banding (SAGB) for morbid obesity: 9-year experience and a 4-year follow up of patients operated with a new adjustable band. Obes Surg. 1997;7:345–51.
34. Forsell P, Hallerback B, Glise H, Hellers G. Complications following Swedish Adjustable Gastric Banding: a long-term follow-up. Obes Surg. 1999;9:11–6.
35. Kuzmak L, Coe F. Gastric banding device. United States Patent No. 4,592,339; 1986.
36. Kuzmak LI. Silicone gastric banding: a simple and effective operation for morbid obesity. Contemp Surg. 1986;28:13–8.
37. Kuzmak LI. A preliminary report on silicone gastric banding for morbid obesity. Clin Nutr. 1986;5:73–7.
38. Kuzmak LI. A review of seven years' experience with silicone gastric banding. Obes Surg. 1991;1:40–8.
39. US Food and Drug Administration: new device approvals. LAP-BAND® Adjustable Gastric Banding (LAGB®) System – P000008: summary of safety and effectiveness data; 5 June 2001.
40. Catona A, Gossenberg M, La Manna A, Mussini G. Laparoscopic adjustable gastric banding: preliminary series. Obes Surg. 1993;3:207–9.
41. Broadbent R, Tracey M, Harrington P. Laparoscopic gastric banding: a preliminary report. Obes Surg. 1993;3(1):63–7.
42. Belachew M, Legrand MJ, Defechereux TH, et al. Laparoscopic adjustable silicone gastric banding in the treatment of morbid obesity: a preliminary report. Surg Endosc. 1994;8:1354–6.
43. Belachew M, Legrand M, Vincent V, et al. Laparoscopic placement of adjustable silicone gastric band in the treatment of morbid obesity: how to do it. Obes Surg. 1995;5:66–70.
44. Belachew M, Legrand M, Vincent V, et al. Laparoscopic adjustable gastric banding. World J Surg. 1998;22:955–63.
45. Niville E, Vankeirsblick J, Dams A, et al. Laparoscopic adjustable gastric banding: a preliminary experience. Obes Surg. 1998;8:39–42.
46. Weiner R, Wagner D, Blanco-Engert R, et al. Eine neue Technik zur laparoskopischen Plazierung des steuerbaren Magenbandes (LAP-Band) zur Vermeidung eines Slippage. Chirurg. 2000;71:1243–50.
47. Catona A, La Manna L, Forsell P. The Swedish Adjustable Gastric Band: laparoscopic technique and preliminary results. Obes Surg. 2000;10:15–21.
48. Fielding GA, Allen JW. A step-by-step guide to placement of the Lap-Band adjustable gastric banding system. Am J Surg. 2002;184:26S–30.
49. Ren CJ, Fielding GA. Laparoscopic adjustable gastric banding: surgical technique. J Laparoendosc Adv Surg Tech A. 2003;13(4):257–63.
50. US Food and Drug Administration: new device approvals. REALIZE™ adjustable gastric band – APPROVAL #P070009. Summary of safety and effectiveness data; 28 Sept 2007.
51. Fried M, Kormanova K, Kasalicky M. Comparison of SAGB QC "classic" titanium port and Velocity™ port: pilot phase prospective randomized study on perioperative and short-term postoperative implantation outcomes. Obes Surg. 2006;16:716–20.
52. Miller K, Pump A. Mechanical vs suture fixation of the port in adjustable gastric banding procedures: a prospective randomized blinded study. Surg Endosc. 2008;22:2478–84.
53. Miller KA. Laparoscopic restrictive procedures: adjustable gastric banding. In: Pitombo C, Jones KB, Higa KD, Pareja JC, editors. Obesity surgery: principles and practice. New York: McGraw-Hill Medical; 2007. p. 169–76.
54. O'Brien PE, MacDonald L, Anderson M, Brennan L, Brown WA. Long-term outcomes after bariatric surgery: fifteen-year follow-up of adjustable gastric banding and a systematic review of the bariatric surgical literature. Ann Surg. 2013;1:87–94.
55. Victorzon M, Tolonen P. Mean fourteen-year, 100 % follow-up of laparoscopic adjustable gastric banding for morbid obesity. Surg Obes Relat Dis. 2013;5:753–7.
56. Angrisani L, Cutolo PP, Formisano G, Nosso G, Santonicola A, Vitolo G. Long-term outcomes of laparoscopic adjustable silicone gastric banding (LAGB) in moderately obese patients with and without comorbidities. Obes Surg. 2013;7:897–902.
57. Vijgen GH, Schouten R, Bouvy ND, Greve JW. Salvage banding for failed Roux-en-Y gastric bypass. SOARD. 2012;8:803–8.
58. Silberhumer GR, Miller K, Pump A, Kriwanek S, Widhalm K, Gyoeri G, Prager G. Long-term results after laparoscopic adjustable gastric banding in adolescent patients: follow-up of the Austrian experience. Surg Endosc. 2011;25:2993–9.

17 Laparoscopic Sleeve Gastrectomy

Giovanni Casella, Emanuele Soricelli, Alfredo Genco, Adriano Redler, and Nicola Basso

17.1 Introduction

Sleeve gastrectomy (SG) is a technically simple surgical procedure with low complications rate and negligible long-term nutritional deficiencies.

SG was proposed and performed in 1988 by Hess and Hess as part of a hybrid malabsorption procedure, the biliopancreatic diversion (BPD) with duodenal switch (DS), because of the high incidence of marginal ulcers at the gastro-ileum anastomosis in the original Scopinaro BPD procedure [1]. In 2000, Ren et al. demonstrated the feasibility of BPD-DS with a laparoscopic approach. Because of the high rate of complications and mortality in their early experience, a two-stage laparoscopic BPD-DS, laparoscopic SG (LSG) first and BPD-DS after an average 11-month interval, was proposed [2, 3].

Results obtained in terms of weight loss and resolution of comorbidities, after SG as first stage of BPD-DS, encouraged and stimulated its spreading with increasing compliance of the patients. At first, the efficacy of SG had been attributed to the reduction of the gastric capacity and the procedure was classified as restrictive. It became soon evident that significant modifications of the gastrointestinal hormones play a preeminent role. Changes in ghrelin (GHR), glucagon-like peptide1 (GLP-1) and protein YY (PYY) induced by the gastric resection are of paramount importance in the weight loss and glucose homeostasis effects of the procedure. In addition, it has been recently shown in the experimental animal that SG induces modifications of the gut microbiota instrumental in the genesis of its metabolic effects [4].

In 2010, the American Society for Metabolic and Bariatric Surgery (ASMBS) issued a position statement recommending LSG as an approved bariatric procedure [5]. In 2011, LSG became the second most performed bariatric operation after gastric bypass (GBP) (27.8 % vs 46.6 %), according to a survey of the International Federation for the Surgery of Obesity and Metabolic Disorders (IFSO), with a fivefold increase when compared to data from a similar questionnaire in 2008, so becoming the bariatric procedure with the highest growth rate [6, 7].

G. Casella • E. Soricelli • A. Redler
Department of Surgical Sciences, "Sapienza" University of Rome, Vle Regina Elena, 324, Rome 00161, Italy
e-mail: Giovanni.casella@uniroma1.it; lelesori@hotmail.com; adriano.redler@uniroma1.it

A. Genco
Department of Surgical Sciences, Sapienza, University of Rome, Viale del Policlinico 155, Rome 00161, Italy
e-mail: Alfredo.genco@uniroma1.it

N. Basso (✉)
Department of Surgical Sciences, "Sapienza" University of Rome, Via Napoli, 51, Rome 00184, Italy
e-mail: nicola.basso@uniroma1.it

M. Lucchese, N. Scopinaro (eds.), *Minimally Invasive Bariatric and Metabolic Surgery: Principles and Technical Aspects*, DOI 10.1007/978-3-319-15356-8_17,

Since 2007, an International SG Summit Conference has been held every 2 years, allowing surgeons performing LSG to share clinical experiences and discuss technical aspects of the procedure. At the 2012 International SG Summit Conference, 130 surgeons reported on 46,133 procedures with a mean follow-up of 5 years [8–12].

17.2 Technical Aspects

The laparoscopic technique has been well standardized by Gagner in 2000 [2]. However, during the following years, several details have been modified. In this chapter, we will emphasize technical points in the light of our own experience of about 900 cases since 2002 [13]. Although LSG is not a technically demanding procedure, important key points should be respected to achieve good long-term results on weight loss and co-morbidities improvement and to minimize the incidence of postoperative complications. Open questions and future perspectives will be discussed.

17.3 Surgical Technique

The patient is positioned in 30° anti-Trendelemburg position with legs abducted. The surgeon stands between the patient's legs, the first assistance, holding the camera, is on the left side of the patient aside the scrub nurse, a second assistant is placed on the right side (Fig. 17.1a). Pneumoperitoneum is generally created using Veress needle placed in the left subcostal margin (Palmer's point). After obtaining a pneumoperitoneum pressure of 15 mmHg, the Veress needle is withdrawn and replaced by a 12-mm optical trocar to allocate the camera. Four additional trocars are placed in the upper abdominal quadrants under direct vision (Fig. 17.1b). The procedure starts with the identification of the pylorus. Using a marked grasper and stretching the gastric wall, a distance of 4–6 cm along the greater gastric curvature is measured and marked. Some authors suggest 2–3 cm as distance from the pylorus where to begin the gastric resection. However, antrum resection may result in a defec-

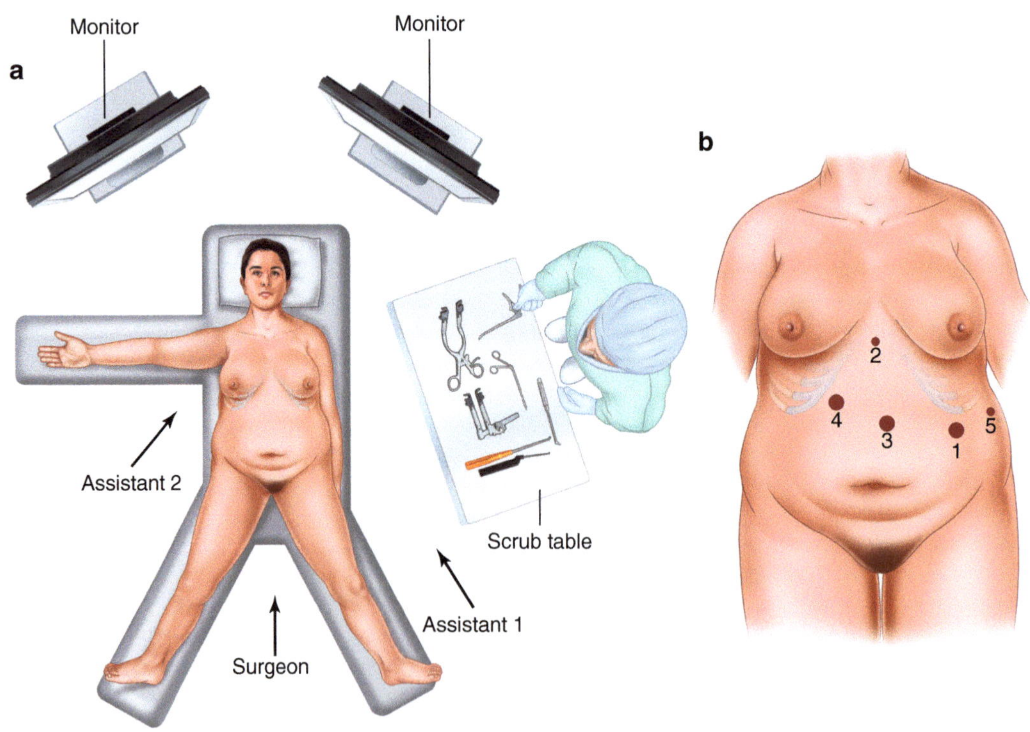

Fig. 17.1 (**a**) Operating room set up. (**b**) Trocar placement scheme. *1* Left subcostal, *2* Subxyphoid, *3* Optical, *4* Right subcostal, *5* Left anterior axillary line

tive pumping mechanism causing nausea to the patient because of delayed gastric emptying. The first maneuver of the procedure is *skeletonization of the greater curvature*. Radiofrequency or ultrasound energy instruments are used. The gastro-colic ligament is dissected close to the gastric wall at the median third of the greater curvature where the ligament is thin. In the antrum area, adhesions between the posterior wall of the stomach and the anterior aspect of the pancreas are often present and may make the access to the omental bursa more difficult. The skeletonization is completed toward the pylorus until the 4–6 cm mark is reached and then it proceeds upward to the angle of His. The *complete mobilization of the fundus* is of primary importance to achieve a correct fundectomy. In this phase, the surgeon uses the left subcostal port for the right hand and the subxiphoid trocar for the left hand. The dissection of the fundus is completed when clear exposure of the left diaphragmatic pillar is obtained (Fig. 17.2A).

Anteriorly redundant Belsey's fat pad may be resected in order to better visualize the gastroesophageal junction and the area where the stapler will be positioned. The posterior gastric wall must be freed by adhesions and occasionally it is necessary to divide posterior gastric vessels, when present, to ensure easy maneuvering of the stomach during resection. At the end of the mobilization the left gastric vessels and the left crus are clearly exposed and the stomach can be easily moved on its axis like "the page of a book" (Fig. 17.2A). Incomplete mobilization of the fundus may cause incomplete fundectomy determining an hourglass aspect of the stomach at the postoperative X-ray images and influencing long-term results.

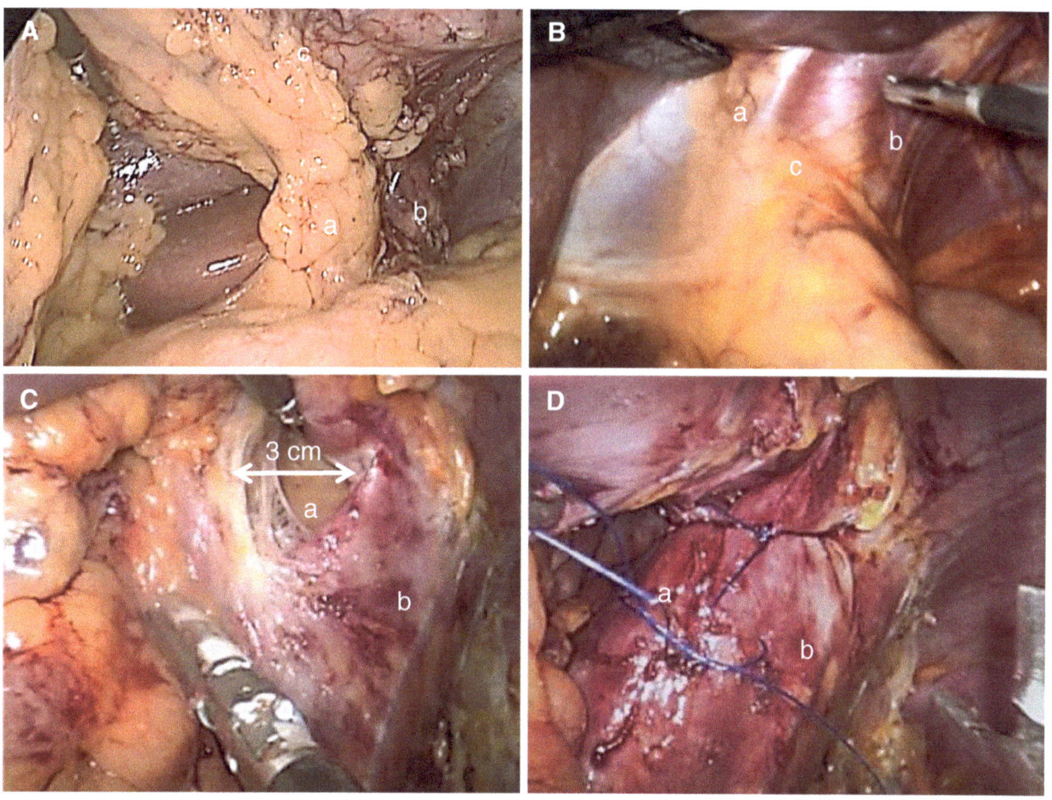

Fig. 17.2 (**A**) – The left gastric vessels (*a*) are visualized together with the left pillar (*b*). The posterior gastric wall (*c*) is completely free. The stomach is moved up like "the page of a book." B – Finger print indentation on the peritoneum covering the hiatus orifice (*c*), right pillar (*a*), and left pillar (*b*). (**C**) Enlarged hiatus (*a*). Left pillar (*b*). (**D**) Hiatoplasty. Right pillar (*a*). Left pillar (*b*)

The ablation of the GHR producing region of the stomach seems to be a crucial factor to ensure a proper functional result when considering EWL and comorbidities resolution: in several studies, it has been demonstrated that GHR concentration in the gastric mucosa increases from the corpus to the fundus. For this reason, the accurate fundectomy is a critical technical point [14, 15]. On the other hand, the accurate gastroesophageal junction mobilization by division of the short gastric vessels, of posterior gastric artery and of phrenic branches when present, in order to perform an ideal fundectomy may hamper the blood supply of this area and facilitate the onset of the gastric leak that occurs quite uniformly at the uppermost part of the suture line. Sound judgment must be used to balance the risks (leak) and the benefits (functional results).

Careful *inspection of the hiatal area* is performed after complete mobilization of the gastric fundus and of the posterior gastric wall. Enlarged hiatus and hiatal hernias must be identified. A 3 cm diameter of hiatal orifice is considered abnormal. As a practical rule in our clinical practice, exploration of the hiatal crura is indicated by a macroscopically evident fingerprint indentation of the diaphragm just above the esophageal emergence from the diaphragm (Fig. 17.2B). In these cases, the dissection of the hiatal crus is indicated and easily performed, because of the mobilized fundus, from the left approach (Fig. 17.2C). When present, the hernia sac and the gastroesophageal fat pad are dissected and reduced within the abdominal cavity. Retrogastric lipomas should be identified and removed to diminish the occurrence of the sliding of the gastric tubule into the mediastinum. A posterior hiatoplasty is performed. The hiatal crus defect is repaired with two or three interrupted nonabsorbable sutures between the right and the left diaphragmatic pillars (Fig. 17.2D) [16].

Once the stomach is completely mobilized, an *oro-gastric tube* is inserted by the anesthesiologist in order to calibrate the resection. A 48-French bougie is pushed down possibly through the pylorus and placed against the lesser curvature. The use of tube sizes from 30- to 60-French bougie is reported in the literature. There is evidence that smaller sizes of bougie (<40 Fr) correlate to a significant increase of gastric leaks [17–19]. On the other hand, it is not clear if the bougie size can significantly affect the capacity of the residual stomach and the postoperative weight loss. In our experience, the capacity of the gastric remnant was dependent not by the bougie size but by other technical points: placement of the stapler well against the bougie, complete gastric fundus dissection, and lateral traction of the gastric walls during the resection.

Gastric resection is performed using a linear stapler. The stapler is applied alongside the calibrating bougie. Because of the decreasing thickness of the gastric wall from the antrum to the corpus and fundus, the cartridges must be chosen accordingly. The staple height used by us is 4.4 or 4.1 mm near the antrum and 3.8 or 3.5 mm on corpus and fundus. In revisional surgery cases, the presence of scar tissue indicates the use of higher staples. The stapler is inserted through the right subcostal trocar for the first and second firing and then through the left subcostal trocar. Occasionally, it can be inserted through the optical trocar and the camera moved to the left subcostal trocar. The stapler branches must be coplanar to the gastric walls to avoid tubule twisting.

Before closing and firing the staplers, the anterior and posterior gastric walls are fully stretched by two graspers precisely positioned on the greater curve and moved along it (Fig. 17.3A).

At the *incisura angularis*, the stretching is somewhat loosened to avoid a functional stricture that may occur at this level (Fig. 17.4C). The last cartridge is fired 1–2 cm away from the angle of His so that the staple line does not fall in the "critical area" (Fig. 17.3B). The staple line is reinforced by buttressing with absorbable polymer membrane (Seamguard, Gore). After moving the stomach specimen away from the left subcostal space, the final end of the membrane is fixed with two nonabsorbable sutures to the left pillar to avoid sliding of the stomach tubule into the mediastinum (Fig. 17.3C). At the end of the procedure, the staple line is meticulously checked and bleeding spots are treated by hemostatic clips or stitches (Fig. 17.3D). A nasogastric tube is positioned in the gastric remnant and a *methylene*

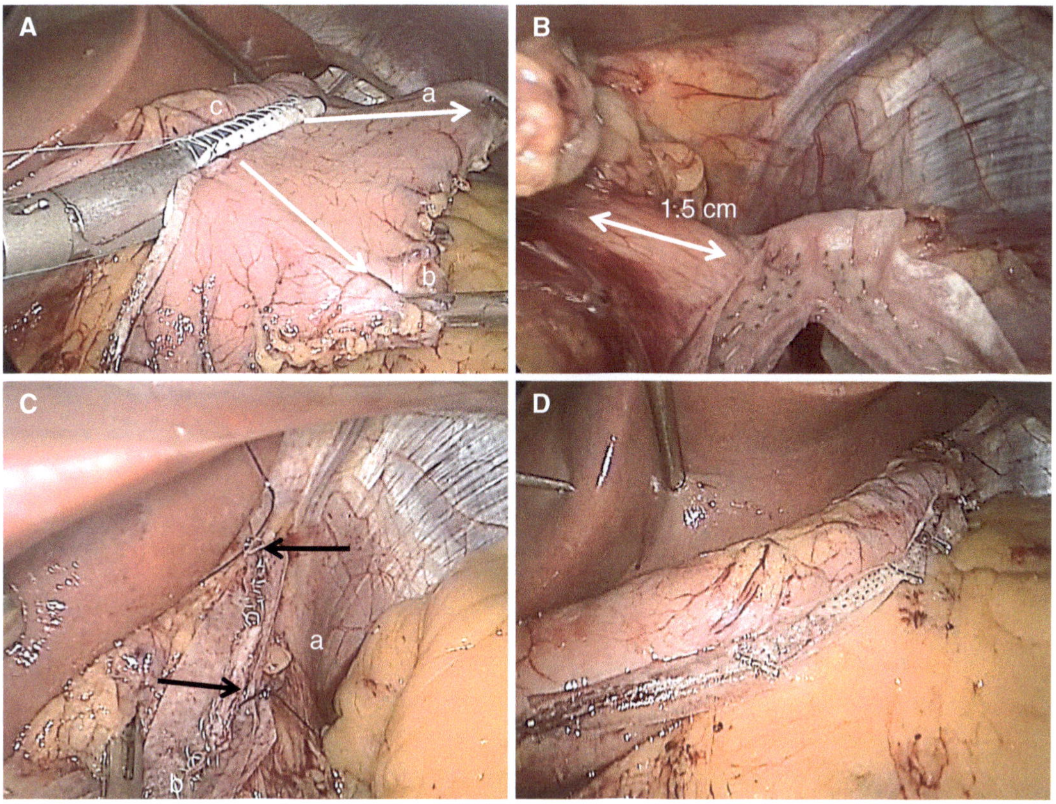

Fig. 17.3 (**A**) Traction on the gastric walls by two graspers (*a*, *b*) on the greater curvature. The suture line (*c*) is alongside the bougie. (**B**) The last stapler is fired 1.5 cm from the angle of His. (**C**) The final end of the buttressing membrane (*b*) is fixed to the left pillar (*a*) by two nylon stitches (*arrows*). (**D**) Final view. Several metal clips complete the hemostasis on the suture line

blue dye test is routinely performed to check the sealing of the staple line and to evaluate the residual gastric capacity, usually 60–80 ml.

The specimen is extracted by grabbing its distal end with a grasper (Fig. 17.4A) and it is easily brought out of the abdominal cavity through the slightly enlarged right subcostal access *without the need of retrieval bags or endo loops* and taking care not to open the specimen during these maneuvers (Fig. 17.4B). A gauze soaked in povidone–iodine solution (betadine) is left for 1–2 min on the retrieval site to avoid infection of the wound [20].

When gallbladder stones are present, cholecystectomy is routinely performed at completion of the SG procedure. The same trocars are used. Occasionally, in complicated cases, an additional 5 mm trocar is added 5 cm laterally to the right subcostal trocar. Drains are not routinely placed and the nasogastric tube is removed at the end of the procedure.

17.4 Postoperative Management

Patients are mobilized on the same day of the operation and maintained with intravenous fluid therapy, proton pump inhibitors, and analgesics. Subcutaneous low-molecular-weight-heparin is administered 6 h after surgery and is continued for 2 weeks. Short-term antibiotic therapy is added. Upper gastrointestinal contrast (Gastrografin) study is performed on the second or third postoperative day. Afterward patients are started on liquid diet and discharged on the fourth postoperative day.

Soft diets with mashed and soft foods are prescribed for 4 weeks after surgery. One month

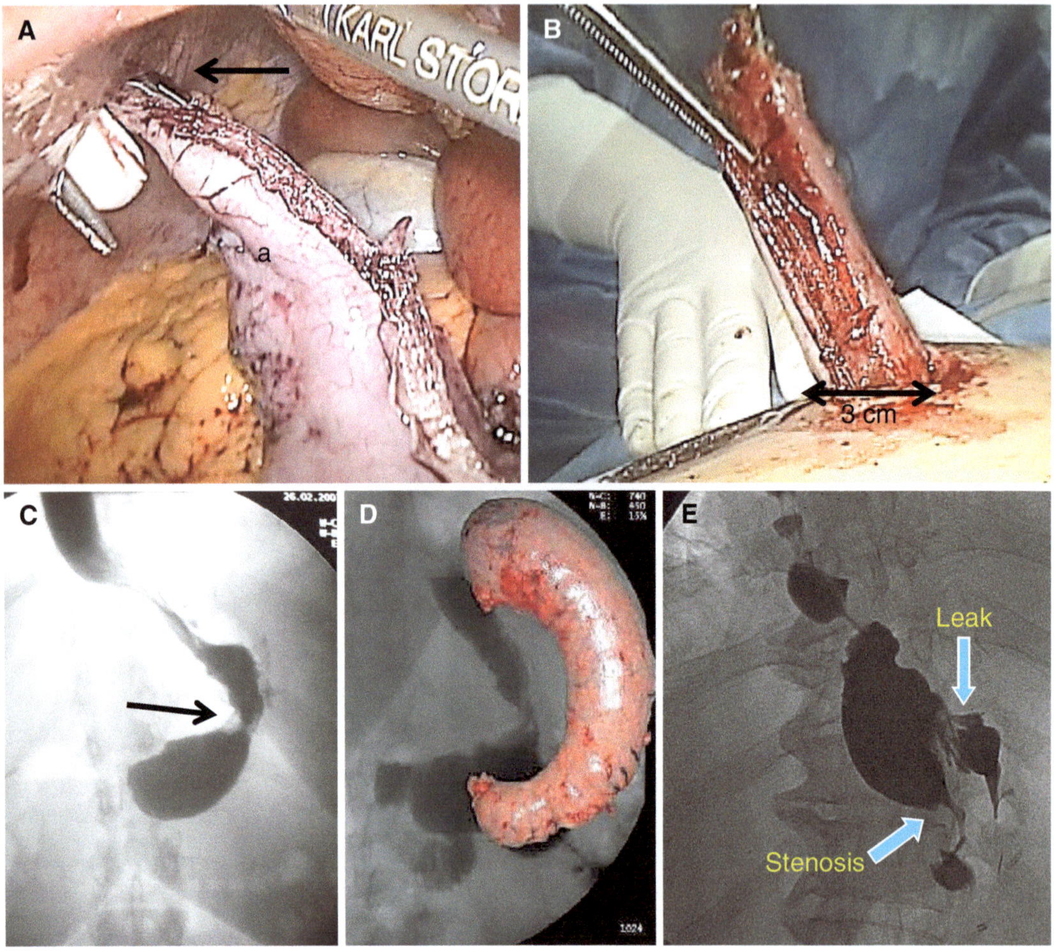

Fig. 17.4 (**A**) Specimen extraction. Grasper (*arrow*) on the antrum end of the gastric specimen (*a*). (**B**) Extraction through a 3 cm enlarged trocar access. (**C**) Functional stenosis at the middle third (*arrow*) of the gastric tubule. The prestenosis segment is not dilated. (**D**) Gastric specimen. In the background: normal post-op X-ray aspect of the gastric tubule. (**E**) Post SG upper GI contrast X-ray: organic stenosis and gastric leak. Dilation of the prestenosis segment

after surgery, patients resume normal diet with the advice of adding one type of food at a time, meat may take longer to be well tolerated. Five small meals are suggested.

Postoperative follow-up is performed at 1, 3, 6, 12, 18, and 24 months after the operation, annually afterward. Controls involve Physical examination, blood tests (including vitamin B12, folate, serum iron, calcium and vitamin D serum levels), upper gastrointestinal contrast (at 1st month and 1st year), liver ultrasound (at sixth month). Endoscopic check is mandatory 2 years after the operation in all patients.

Oral proton pump inhibitors and urso-deoxycholic acid for 6 months and multivitamin tablets for 1 year are prescribed.

17.5 Complications

The postoperative mortality rate varies from 0.1 to 0.5 % and the postoperative morbidity rate ranges from 0.0 to 12 % [5, 10, 12]. Early diagnosis is the most important factor to ensure a positive solution of complications. Treatment is often challenging and should be managed in bariatric centers and by dedicated medical teams. Operative treatment is required only in few selected cases.

Bleeding: Significant hemorrhage occurs in 1.1–8.7 % of cases. Most frequently, bleeding occurs within the first 24–48 h and originates from the staple line [5, 21, 22]. Other sites of bleeding are the gastroepiploic or short gastric vessels divided during the mobilization of the stomach, the trocar accesses, hepatic or splenic injuries. Almost always, the bleeding is into the abdominal cavity, rarely determines hematemesis or melena. Once the hemodynamic parameters are stable, CT-scan is mandatory in order to define the bleeding site and to quantify the hemoperitoneum. In case of hemorrhage from the staple line, the CT images show a hematoma close to the gastric remnant. The treatment is interventional radiology or, in fewer instances, open or laparoscopic surgical exploration. Suture line reinforcement has significantly reduced the occurrence of this complication. Bleeding from the staple line increases the risk of gastric leak.

The two major most debated complications are staple line leak and gastroesophageal reflux disease (GERD). Three main factors should be considered in their pathophysiology: intraluminal pressure, intra-abdominal pressure, and critical vascularization of the gastroesophageal junction.

Leak: Staple line leaks represent the most dangerous and life-threatening complication after LSG, with an incidence between 0 and 7 %. Leaks occur mostly during the first post-op week (early leaks) and, in fewer instances, in the 40 days postoperative period (late leaks) [10, 11]. The most common location of leaks is just below the esophageal gastric junction. Causative factors to be considered in its genesis are: high intragastric pressure, thin wall of the gastric fundus, transitional vascularization (esophageal arteries system above, gastric arteries system below) on the left side of the esophageal-gastric junction ("critical area") causing ischemia [13]. Technical factors include small bougie size and tight sleeves, heat from electrocautery or other energy sources during dissection, or hemostasis which may determine gastric injury.

Some technical details may lessen the incidence of leaks: the final portion of the line of resection should avoid the "critical area" remaining 1–2 cm laterally to the angle of His; the gastric resection should be more loose at the *incisura angularis*, the most frequent site of stenosis.

The treatment of leaks is challenging and different managements have been reported. In our experience, operative treatment is reserved only in patients with hemodynamic instability and signs of acute peritonitis. Peritoneal toilet and proper drainage are recommended. Attempts to repair the fistula are contraindicated: recurrence occurs in most cases. An unsuccessful control of the leak, at occasion, may require total gastrectomy or creation of a Roux limb. In the vast majority of patients, nonoperative management by percutaneous CT-guided drainage, alone or in combination with stent placement and enteral nutrition, is a safe and effective treatment for suture line leaks [23].

In an attempt to reduce the incidence of staple line bleeding and/or leak in recent years several different techniques have been adopted to reinforce the staple line during LSG. The routine use of *reinforcement of staple line* seems to reduce the complications rate. At present, the main options are: oversewing the staple line with a running or inverting absorbable suture, buttressing the staple line with absorbable materials, bovine pericardium strips or porcine small intestine submucosa, applying fibrin glue or hemostatic agents on the staple line [24, 25]. In all published studies, staple line buttressing was reported to reduce significantly the incidence of bleeding; however, the preventive effect on gastric leak was less evident. In a recent review of 88 papers reporting on 8,920 patients, leak rate in LSG was significantly reduced by buttressing the staple line with absorbable polymer membrane compared to over sewing, bovine pericardium strips, or no reinforcement [26].

Stenosis: Stenosis is reported with an incidence ranging from 0.2 to 4 % and usually occurs at the corpus-antrum transition zone (*incisura angularis*) of the gastric tubule. At this site transient functional stenosis (Fig. 17.4C), due to dysmotility because of the muscular layers section, may occur causing high intragastric pressure and so favoring leak occurrence. Mechanical stenosis, causing significant and lasting dysphagia and vomiting, can be determined by an incorrect orientation of the stapler tip during the resection or subsequent to an imbrication of the staple line. Twisted sleeve may cause symptomatic stenosis. An upper gastrointestinal (GI) contrast study is indicated to confirm the gastric outlet obstruction (Fig. 17.4E). Endoscopy has an important role in terms of diagnosis and treatment. Repeated endoscopic dilations are the first therapeutic approach. Placement of endoscopic stents should be considered as alternative solution. In case of persistence of symptoms with nutrition problems, patient's reoperation should be considered [27]. Conversion to Roux-en-Y gastric bypass is a valid therapy. Laparoscopic seromyotomy of the stenotic tract (stricturoplasty) has also been proposed [28].

Hiatal hernia, GERD: In the Fourth International Consensus Summit on SG held in 2012, there was a general agreement that when a hiatal hernia is present it should be repaired at the time of the bariatric procedure. In the same Consensus postoperative GERD was the most frequently reported complication with a mean incidence of 7.9 % [12]. However, the clinical and pathophysiological relationship between SG and GERD is still debated. In some series a postoperative improvement of GERD symptoms has been reported while in other series a worsening has been registered [29–32]. Surgical technique might be of importance for the outcome of GERD after SG, though its effective role has not been defined, yet. In order to explain these conflicting data, the coexistence of different mechanisms, which may respectively promote/worsen or improve GERD symptoms, has been advocated. The former are represented by: impairment of the lower esophageal sphincter's (LES) function due to the section of the sling fibers; sliding of the stomach tubule into the mediastinum determining diminished intraluminal pressure in the cardiac segment; increased intraluminal pressure in the gastric remnant and delayed emptying of the stomach in case of mid-gastric stenosis of the lumen; the latter entail accelerated gastric emptying; reduction of acid secretion; significant weight loss.

In a recent survey of our patients submitted to LSG with a 3–5 years follow-up, a 15 % incidence of peptic esophageal lesions and of non-dysplastic Barrett's esophagus was found with no correlation between the severity of reflux symptoms and the degree of esophageal lesions (unpublished data). For this reason, a careful follow-up schedule is recommended.

17.6 Outcomes

17.6.1 Effect on Excess Weight (EW)

EW is greatly affected by LSG: Several prospective randomized controlled (PRC) studies show that this procedure is more effective than intensive medical and diet regimen or gastric banding and that it is comparable to RYGBP in inducing excess weight loss (EWL) [33]. Because of the relatively recent spreading of LSG in the clinical practice, the majority of studies are related to short- and medium-term results, with a mean EWL ranging from 49 to 81 % [21]. In 2008, Lacy's group reported that SG at 12 months after surgery was as effective as gastric bypass on EW [34]. In 2014, Schauer et al. in a PCR trial found that reductions in body weight, BMI, waist circumference, and waist-to-hip ratio were greater after gastric bypass and after SG than after intensive medical therapy [35]. In 2014, in a PC cohort study by our group BMI diminished from a 41.3 kg/m^2 preoperative value to a 28.3 kg/m^2 value 18 months after SG; intensive medical therapy had no significant effect [36].

Long-term results from large series are lacking. In a recent review a mean EWL of 62.3 % (nine studies enrolling 258 patients) was reported at the 60 months follow-up. At the 72-month follow-up the mean EWL was 53.8 % (three studies with a total of 72 patients) [37]. In the Fourth International Consensus Summit on SG, in an online questionnaire using web-based Survey Monkey® mean EWL at 1, 2, 3, 4, 5, and 6 postoperative years was, respectively, 59.3, 59.0, 54.7, 52.3, 52.4, and 50.6 % [12]. Sarela reports an EWL of 69 % in 13 patients with 8 years follow-up [38].

While the short-term WL effect induced by SG is mostly related to the reduction of the gastric capacity, the durable WL seems to be dependent on additional factors. The mechanisms involve hormonal modifications, in particular dramatic decrease of the circulating GHR (orexigenic hormone) due to the resection of the gastric fundus, main source for this hormone, and the increase of food mediated release of GLP-1 and PYY from the L cells of the small intestine [39]. In experimental studies, Karamanakos et al. showed a significant increase in both fasting and postprandial PYY levels and a marked reduction in fasting GHR levels after SG [40].

17.6.2 Effect on Type 2 Diabetes Mellitus (T2DM) and on Other Comorbidities

Weight-loss surgery has been shown to reduce mortality and comorbidities and most significantly to ameliorate or resolve T2DM in patients with obesity [41, 42]. SG is associated with a high rate of resolution of T2DM and other obesity-associated comorbidities such as hypertension, hyperlipidemia, and sleep apnea. In the ASMBS 2009 position statement, data from ten studies ($n=754$ patients) on the evolution of comorbidities after SG were analyzed. T2DM remission ranged from 14 to 100 %, arterial hypertension from 15 to 93 %, and obstructive sleep apnea (OSA) from 39 to 100 % [5].

In particular the effect on T2DM resulted noteworthy. In 2006, Cottam et al. reported T2DM remission in 81 % of T2DM patients submitted to LSG [43]. In the Moon Han et al. study at 6 months follow–up, the EWL was 71 % and the T2DM remission was 100 % [44]. In the 2007 Vidal et al. study, SG and gastric bypass (GBP) had a similar impact on diabetes (51.4 and 62 %, respectively, $P=.332$) in the short term (4 months) and an identical remission rate (84.6 %, $P=.618$) at 12 months. SG was defined a "metabolic procedure" [34]. In 2012, in two PC studies it has been reported that in diabetic obese patients submitted to SG, results are superior to those after intensive medical treatment both in terms of remission of diabetes and use of medications [35, 36]. The effectiveness of the SG on T2DM remission seems to be related to the β-cell reserve of patients: diabetes duration longer than 10 years, low C-peptide levels, and insulin therapy are negative prognostic factors. In our series, DM remission occurred in 100 % of patients with DM duration <10 years and in 31 % of patients with DM duration >10 years [45].

The beneficial actions of SG on DM occur very early after completion of the procedure. In the study by Peterly, GLP-1 and PYY plasma levels were modified 7 days post-op [46]. In a study by our group, insulin secretion and sensitivity, plasma PYY, and GLP-1 levels improved just 72 h postoperatively independently by food intake. At the same time GHR values were significantly lower than those at pre-op. These data prompted us to formulate a "gastric hypothesis" [47].

The long-term antidiabetic effects of SG are not well documented due to the novelty of the procedure and need more extensive cases and longer follow-up. In a small series of patients, at 5 years follow-up, remission was present in 87.8 % of cases [48]. In our experience in 65 obese and diabetic patients submitted to LSG, remission was present in 57 patients (87 %) and amelioration in 7 patients (10 %) at a mean follow-up of 63 months. Most important, once remission was achieved it was maintained in all cases except two, although weight regain occurred in six patients Soricelli et al. 2015.

SG exerts salutary effects on other comorbidities. In 2006, we reported on the ameliorating outcome of SG on hypertension, OSA, and DM in super-obese patients and subsequently we documented cardiac remodeling with a significant reduction of the Framingham risk score 1.5 years after surgery [49].

When evaluating SG outcome an additional important factor to be considered is patient's satisfaction. Several papers, addressing the topic of QoL after SG, report encouraging results. In the D'Hondt et al. study, the Baros score was "good" to "excellent" in 90 % of patients [50]. In another retrospective study by Alley et al., QoL was superior in SG patients when compared to laparoscopic adjustable gastric banding (LAGB) patients [51].

At present SG is a very popular bariatric procedure both among patients and surgeons. Technically, it is not a very difficult operation although there are crucial technical details that deserve much attention: morbidity and mortality are low; there is no residual "blind stomach"; there are no foreign bodies; malabsorption is minimal; and the treatment of failures is well standardized, second-stage DS, RYGBP, or resleeve. Although long-term results are still lacking, SG is at present an established and reliable procedure that can be confidently maintained in the bariatric armamentarium.

References

1. Hess DS, Hess DW. Biliopancreatic diversion with a duodenal switch. Obes Surg. 1998;8(3):267–82.
2. Ren CJ, Patterson E, Gagner M. Early results of laparoscopic biliopancreatic diversion with duodenal switch: a case series of 40 consecutive patients. Obes Surg. 2000;10(6):514–23.
3. Silecchia G, Boru C, Pecchia A, Rizzello M, Casella G, Leonetti F, Basso N. Effectiveness of laparoscopic sleeve gastrectomy (first stage of biliopancreatic diversion with duodenalswitch) on co-morbidities in super-obese high-risk patients. Obes Surg. 2006;16(9): 1138–44.
4. Ryan KK, Tremaroli V, Clemmensen C, et al. FXR is a molecular target for the effects of vertical sleeve gastrectomy. Nature. 2014;509(7499):183–8.
5. Clinical Issues Committee of the American Society for Metabolic and Bariatric Surgery. Updated position statement on sleeve gastrectomy as a bariatric procedure. Surg Obes Relat Dis. 2010;6(1):1–5.
6. Buchwald H, Oien DM. Metabolic/bariatric surgery Worldwide 2008. Obes Surg. 2009;19(12):1605–11.
7. Buchwald H, Oien DM. Metabolic/bariatric surgery worldwide 2011. Obes Surg. 2013;23(4):427–36.
8. Deitel M, Crosby RD, Gagner M. The First International Consensus Summit for Sleeve Gastrectomy (SG), New York City, October 25–27, 2007. Obes Surg. 2008;18(5):487–96.
9. Gagner M, Deitel M, Kalberer TL, Erickson AL, Crosby RD. The Second International Consensus Summit for Sleeve Gastrectomy, March 19–21, 2009. Surg Obes Relat Dis. 2009;5(4):476–85.
10. Deitel M, Gagner M, Erickson AL, Crosby RD. Third International Summit: current status of sleeve gastrectomy. Surg Obes Relat Dis. 2011;7(6):749–59.
11. Rosenthal RJ; International Sleeve Gastrectomy Expert Panel, Diaz AA, et al. International Sleeve Gastrectomy Expert Panel Consensus Statement: best practice guidelines based on experience of 12,000 cases. Surg Obes Relat Dis. 2012;8(1):8–19.
12. Gagner M, Deitel M, Erickson AL, Crosby RD. Survey on laparoscopic sleeve gastrectomy (LSG) at the Fourth International Consensus Summit on Sleeve Gastrectomy. Obes Surg. 2013;23(12):2013–7.
13. Basso N, Casella G, Rizzello M, et al. Laparoscopic sleeve gastrectomy as first stage or definitive intent in 300 consecutive cases. Surg Endosc. 2011;25(2):444–9.
14. Frezza EE, Chiriva-Internati M, Wachtel MS. Analysis of the results of sleeve gastrectomy for morbid obesity and the role of ghrelin. Surg Today. 2008;38(6):481–3.
15. Chabot F, Caron A, Laplante M, St-Pierre DH. Interrelationships between ghrelin, insulin and glucose homeostasis: Physiological relevance. World J Diabetes. 2014;5(3):328–41.
16. Soricelli E, Iossa A, Casella G, Abbatini F, Calì B, Basso N. Sleeve gastrectomy and crural repair in obese patients with gastroesophageal reflux disease and/or hiatal hernia. Surg Obes Relat Dis. 2013;9(3):356–61.
17. Yuval JB, Mintz Y, Cohen MJ, Rivkind AI, Elazary R. The effects of bougie caliber on leaks and excess weight loss following laparoscopic sleeve gastrectomy. Is there an ideal bougie size? Obes Surg. 2013;23(10):1685–91.
18. Parikh M, Issa R, McCrillis A, Saunders JK, Ude-Welcome A, Gagner M. Surgical strategies that may decrease leak after laparoscopic sleeve gastrectomy: a systematic review and meta-analysis of 9991 cases. Ann Surg. 2013;257(2):231–7.
19. Atkins ER, Preen DB, Jarman C, Cohen LD. Improved obesity reduction and co-morbidity resolution in patients treated with 40-French bougie versus 50-French bougie four years after laparoscopic sleeve gastrectomy. Analysis of 294 patients. Obes Surg. 2012;22(1):97–104.
20. Casella G, Soricelli E, Fantini A, Basso N. A time-saving technique for specimen extraction in sleeve gastrectomy. World J Surg. 2010;34(4):765–7.
21. Trastulli S, Desiderio J, Guarino S, Cirocchi R, Scalercio V, Noya G, Parisi A. Laparoscopic sleeve gastrectomy compared with other bariatric surgical procedures: a systematic review of randomized trials. Surg Obes Relat Dis. 2013;9(5):816–29.
22. Macias CA, Sandler B, Barajas-Gamboa JS, et al. Standardized protocol utilization decreases rate of complications: a study of laparoscopic sleeve gastrectomy in 189 consecutive patients. Surg Endosc. 2013; 27:S489.
23. Casella G, Soricelli E, Rizzello M, et al. Nonsurgical treatment of staple line leaks after laparoscopic sleeve gastrectomy. Obes Surg. 2009;19(7):821–6.
24. D'Ugo S, Gentileschi P, Benavoli D, Cerci M, Gaspari A, Berta RD, Moretto C, Bellini R, Basso N, Casella G, Soricelli E, Cutolo P, Formisano G, Angrisani L, Anselmino M. Comparative use of different techniques for leak and bleeding prevention during laparoscopic sleeve gastrectomy: a multicenter study. Surg Obes Relat Dis. 2014;10(3):450–4.

25. Aurora AR, Khaitan L, Saber AA. Sleeve gastrectomy and the risk of leak: a systematic analysis of 4,888 patients. Surg Endosc. 2012;26(6):1509–15.
26. Gagner M, Buchwald JN. Comparison of laparoscopic sleeve gastrectomy leak rates in four staple-line reinforcement options: a systematic review. Surg Obes Relat Dis. 2014;10(4):713–23.
27. Parikh A, Alley JB, Peterson RM, et al. Management options for symptomatic stenosis after laparoscopic vertical sleeve gastrectomy in the morbidly obese. Surg Endosc. 2012;26(3):738–46.
28. Vilallonga R, Himpens J, van de Vrande S. Laparoscopic management of persistent strictures after laparoscopic sleeve gastrectomy. Obes Surg. 2013;23(10):1655–61.
29. Sheppard CE, Sadowski DC, de Gara CJ, Karmali S, Birch DW. Rates of reflux before and after laparoscopic sleeve gastrectomy for severe obesity. Obes Surg. 2014 [Epub ahead of print].
30. Rebecchi F, Allaix ME, Giaccone C, Ugliono E, Scozzari G, Morino M. Gastroesophageal reflux disease and laparoscopic sleeve gastrectomy: a physiopathologic evaluation. Ann Surg. 2014;260(5): 909–15.
31. Sharma A, Aggarwal S, Ahuja V, Bal C. Evaluation of gastroesophageal reflux before and after sleeve gastrectomy using symptom scoring, scintigraphy, and endoscopy. Surg Obes Relat Dis. 2014;10(4):600–5.
32. Laffin M, Chau J, Gill RS, Birch DW, Karmali S. Sleeve gastrectomy and gastroesophageal reflux disease. J Obes. 2013;2013:741097.
33. Clinical Issues Committee ASMBS. Updated position statement on sleeve gastrectomy as a bariatric procedure. Surg Obes Relat Dis. 2012;8(3):e21–6.
34. Vidal J, Ibarzabal A, Romero F, Delgado S, Momblán D, Flores L, Lacy A. Type 2 diabetes mellitus and the metabolic syndrome following sleeve gastrectomy in severely obese subjects. Obes Surg. 2008;18(9):1077–82.
35. Schauer PR, Bhatt DL, Kirwan JP, Wolski K, Brethauer SA, Navaneethan SD, Aminian A, Pothier CE, Kim ES, Nissen SE, Kashyap SR, STAMPEDE Investigators. Bariatric surgery versus intensive medical therapy for diabetes–3-year outcomes. N Engl J Med. 2014;370(21):2002–13.
36. Leonetti F, Capoccia D, Coccia F, et al. Obesity, type 2 diabetes mellitus, and other comorbidities: a prospective cohort study of laparoscopic sleeve gastrectomy vs medical treatment. Arch Surg. 2012;147(8):694–700.
37. Diamantis T, Apostolou KG, Alexandrou A, Griniatsos J, Felekouras E, Tsigris C. Review of long-term weight loss results after laparoscopic sleeve gastrectomy. Surg Obes Relat Dis. 2014;10(1):177–83.
38. Sarela AI, Dexter SP, O'Kane M, Menon A, McMahon MJ. Long-term follow-up after laparoscopic sleeve gastrectomy: 8-9-year results. Surg Obes Relat Dis. 2012;8(6):679–84.
39. Dimitriadis E, Daskalakis M, Kampa M, Peppe A, Papadakis JA, Melissas J. Alterations in gut hormones after laparoscopic sleeve gastrectomy: a prospective clinical and laboratory investigational study. Ann Surg. 2013;257(4):647–54.
40. Karamanakos SN, Vagenas K, Kalfarentzos F, Alexandrides TK. Weight loss, appetite suppression, and changes in fasting and postprandial ghrelin and peptide-YY levels after Roux-en-Y gastric bypass and sleeve gastrectomy: a prospective, double blind study. Ann Surg. 2008;247(3):401–7.
41. Vest AR, Heneghan HM, Agarwal S, Schauer PR, Young JB. Bariatric surgery and cardiovascular outcomes: a systematic review. Heart. 2012;98:1763–77.
42. Flumm DR, Dellinger EP. Impact of gastric bypass operation on survival: a population-based analysis. J Am Coll Surg. 2004;199:543–51.
43. Cottam D, Qureshi FG, Mattar SG, et al. Laparoscopic sleeve gastrectomy as an initial weight-loss procedure for high-risk patients with morbid obesity. Surg Endosc. 2006;20:859–63.
44. Moon Han S, Kim WW, Oh JH. Results of laparoscopic sleeve gastrectomy (LSG) at 1 year in morbidly obese Korean patients. Obes Surg. 2005;15:1469–75.
45. Casella G, Abbatini F, Calì B, Capoccia D, Leonetti F, Basso N. Ten-year duration of type 2 diabetes as prognostic factor for remission after sleeve gastrectomy. Surg Obes Relat Dis. 2011;7(6):697–702.
46. Peterli R, Wölnerhanssen B, Peters T, et al. Improvement in glucose metabolism after bariatric surgery: comparison of laparoscopic Roux-en-Y gastric bypass and laparoscopic sleeve gastrectomy: a prospective randomized trial. Ann Surg. 2009;250(2):234–41.
47. Basso N, Capoccia D, Rizzello M, et al. First-phase insulin secretion, insulin sensitivity, ghrelin, GLP-1, and PYY changes 72 h after sleeve gastrectomy in obese diabetic patients: the gastric hypothesis. Surg Endosc. 2011;25(11):3540–50.
48. Abbatini F, Capoccia D, Casella G, Soricelli E, Leonetti F, Basso N. Long-term remission of type 2 diabetes in morbidly obese patients after sleeve gastrectomy. Surg Obes Relat Dis. 2013;9(4):498–502.
49. Cavarretta E, Casella G, Calì B, et al. Cardiac remodeling in obese patients after laparoscopic sleeve gastrectomy. World J Surg. 2013;37(3):565–72.
50. D'Hondt M, Vanneste S, Pottel H, Devriendt D, Van Rooy F, Vansteenkiste F. Laparoscopic sleeve gastrectomy as a single-stage procedure for the treatment of morbid obesity and the resulting quality of life, resolution of comorbidities, food tolerance, and 6-year weight loss. Surg Endosc. 2011;25(8):2498–504.
51. Alley JB, Fenton SJ, Harnisch MC, Tapper DN, Pfluke JM, Peterson RM. Quality of life after sleeve gastrectomy and adjustable gastric banding. Surg Obes Relat Dis. 2012;8(1):31–40.

18 Laparoscopic Gastric Plication

Martin Fried

Laparoscopic greater curvature plication (LGCP), referred also as gastric plication (GP), gastric curvature plication (GCP), laparoscopic total gastric vertical plication or vertical sleeve plication, has been introduced to the contemporary bariatric and metabolic field relatively recently. LGCP is not, however, a new procedure.

18.1 History

In 1896, Ewart reports plication of the gastric greater curvature, similar to the current LGCP, as treatment for a diabetic patient with dilatation of the stomach [1].

LGCP as a potential bariatric operation was proposed firstly by Kirk, who reported outcomes of his study experiments on weight loss after LGCP in rats in 1969 [2]. Kirk was followed by Tretbar's and Wilkinson's reports on LGCP in human clinical studies in 1976 and in 1981 [3, 4]. Almost 30 years later, in 2006 and 2007, Fusco and Talebour published reports on LGCP as a procedure resulting in significant weight loss in rats and sheep models [5–7].

M. Fried, PhD
1st Faculty of Medicine, Charles University Prague, Prague, Czech Republic

OB klinika -Center for Treatment of Obesity and Metabolic Disorders , Prague, Czech Republic
e-mail: docfried@volny.cz

Kirk and Fusco focused on safety and efficacy of the procedure in their studies, while comparing different types of gastric plication (the anterior gastric wall plication vs greater curvature plication/LGCP), as well as gastric plication versus sham and simple visceral manipulation. These studies concluded that LGCP results in significant weight loss in comparison with other approaches and modifications. Both of the authors studied as well the possible influence of different suturing materials (braided vs monofilament) and suturing techniques (interrupted vs continuous sutures). Finally, Kirk reported that invagination of the greater curvature of the stomach was a safe and effective method to achieve weight loss in rats.

In 2011, Menchaca and his co-workers published results of a canine study, comparing durability of the gastric plications infoldings achieved with different suturing and fastening mechanisms. Authors demonstrated that in short term, sufficient durability of serosa-to-serosa apposition is achieved with means of interrupted sutures, sutures anchored with t-tags, or staples [8].

18.2 The Procedure

LGCP is mostly referred to as restrictive bariatric procedure which reduces the stomach capacity without a need for gastric resection or placement of an implantable device. The primary goal of

M. Lucchese, N. Scopinaro (eds.), *Minimally Invasive Bariatric and Metabolic Surgery: Principles and Technical Aspects*, DOI 10.1007/978-3-319-15356-8_18,

this procedure is to achieve long-term weight loss while decreasing or even avoiding complications seen with some of the bariatric procedures. However, the most currently published studies reveal that alongside with the restrictive effect of the LGCP, there seems to be a metabolic, weight loss independent component of the operation as well [9, 10].

As with most new procedures, there have been several techniques and personal modifications employed by different surgeons when performing a laparoscopic greater curvature plication. However, with the experience of several thousand LGCP operations performed worldwide in different bariatric centres, the procedure became more uniform, reproducible and standardized from both the indication and contraindication point of view as well as from surgical technique.

18.3 Indication Criteria

For the LGCP apply the same indication criteria as have been recently published in the Interdisciplinary European Guidelines on Metabolic and Bariatric Surgery. These guidelines were created by and endorsed by the European Association for the Study of Obesity (EASO) and the International Federation for the Surgery of Morbid Obesity and Metabolic Disorders – European chapter (IFSO-EC) [11, 12]. According to these guidelines, patients should be in age range from 18 to 60 years, with BMI ≥40 kg/m^2 or with BMI 35–40 kg/m^2 with comorbidity, in which surgically induced weight loss is expected to improve the disorders (such as metabolic disorders, cardiorespiratory disease, severe joint disease, obesity-related severe psychological problems, etc.). The BMI criterion may be the current BMI or previously maximum attained BMI of this severity. Weight loss as a result of intensified treatment before surgery (patients who reach a body weight below the required BMI for surgery) is not a contraindication for the planned bariatric surgery. Bariatric surgery is indicated in patients who exhibited a substantial weight loss in a conservative treatment programme but started to gain weight again, even if the required minimum indication weight for surgery has not yet been attained again. To be considered for surgery, patients should have failed to lose weight or to maintain long-term weight loss, despite appropriate surgical and/or nonsurgical comprehensive medical care. Consideration should be given to reducing the BMI threshold by 2.5 for individuals of Asian genetic background and to the balance between genetic and environmental/dietary factors. Patients should have shown their compliance with scheduled medical appointments.

18.4 Contraindications

General contraindications to bariatric surgery are as well applicable to LGCP patients; however, there are some LGCP specific contraindications.

General contraindications include (but are not limited to):

Absence of a period of identifiable medical management. Patient who is unable to participate in prolonged medical follow-up. Nonstabilized psychotic disorders, severe depression, personality and eating disorders, unless specifically advised by a psychiatrist experienced in obesity. Alcohol abuse and/or drug dependencies. Diseases threatening life in the short term.

Patients who are unable to care for themselves and have no long-term family or social support that will warrant such care [11, 12].

LGCP specific contraindications include several clinical conditions. Among such contraindications may be considered impaired ability to vomit (i.e. status after Nissen fundoplication), as LGCP patients often experience a period of 1–2 days of postoperative vomiting. Impaired ability to vomit may lead to substantial increase of intragastric pressure during attempts to vomit, resulting in tears of gastric wall, or even gastric perforation caused by "cheese wire" effect of plicating sutures and/or staplers. As a contraindication should be considered as well previous complex and complicated upper gastric surgery, or postsurgical complications located in the upper third of the stomach, especially in the fundus region. Among such complications may be considered leaks, peritonitis, reoperations with multiple fibrotic adhesions, prolonged gastric band migrations and others. The rationale is that these complications usually result in compromised blood supply at the region where they occured. Impaired blood supply at the fundus region, coupled with devascularization of the greater curvature which is a routine part of the LGCP, may result in serious devitalization and subsequent necrosis of the plicated stomach wall.

18.5 The LGCP Operation

It is essential and extremely important to underline that although the LGCP at the end of the operation looks anatomically very close to sleeve gastrectomy, and several steps of the LGCP operation may seem almost identical to those applied in sleeve gastrectomy, it is crucial to realize that there are substantial differences in several, critical parts of the operation. If inadequate attention is paid to these differences, there is highly increased risk of major, serious complications after LGCP. Most of the differences in operation technique between LGCP and sleeve gastrectomy will be highlighted in the following sections.

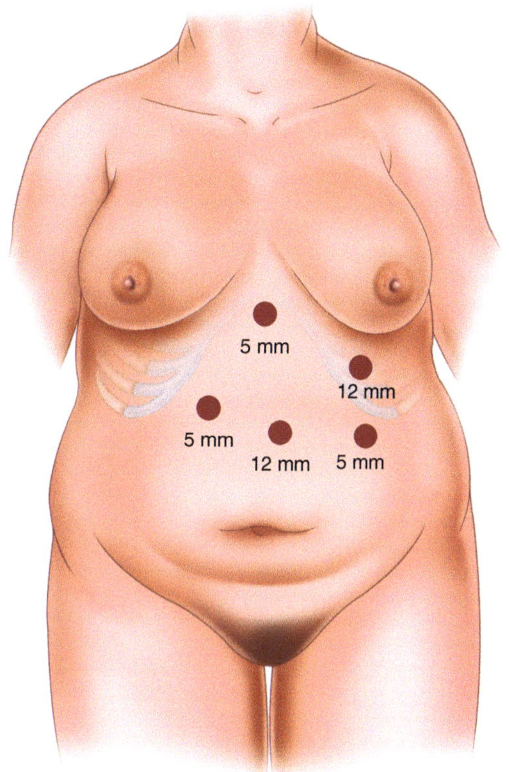

Fig. 18.1 Trocar position and size for LGCP

18.6 Critical Steps of the Operation

18.6.1 Operation Technique

Patient should be placed on the operating table in the supine position with outstretched legs, firmly strapped as steep anti-Trendelenburg position is needed for most of the operation time. The operating surgeon stands in between patient's legs, the assisting surgeon is on patient's left side. Pneumoperitoneum is established with a Veress needle, Hasson's technique or through another institutional standardized approach. The total of five (two 10/12 mm and three 5 mm) trocars are used. Firstly, a 10/12 mm trocar (for laparoscopic optics) is inserted left to the patient's midline, approximately 10 cm below the left costal margin. After that, laparoscopical inspection of the entire abdominal cavity is done. The rest of the trocars were placed in the following positions: 5 mm trocar (for liver retraction) in the uppermost subxiphoid area; another 5 mm trocar (surgeon's left hand working port) in the right upper quadrant, below the first 5 mm trocar, at the mid-clavicular line; 10/12 mm trocar (surgeon's right hand working port) in the left upper quadrant, just below the left costal margin at midclavicular line; and the last 5 mm trocar (for surgical assistance) at the left lower costal margin. Different variations in trocar positioning may be applied according to surgeons'preferences, patient's body size and/or institutional requirements (Fig. 18.1).

18.6.2 Dissection

The operation begins with dissection along the greater curvature of the stomach. The easiest area where to start the dissection is usually at the distal body of the stomach. Dissection should be extended proximally towards the angle of Hiss, however stopping the dissection approximately 1–2 cm distally to the angle of Hiss (preserving the last 2–3 short gastric vessels) is recommended. There are several reasons for leaving the top of the fundus intact, in particular in order to

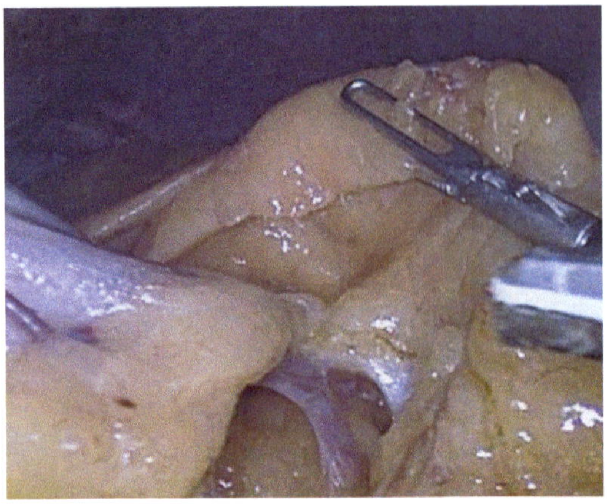

Fig. 18.2 Dissection of the greater curvature performed in distance from the stomach wall

preserve the angle of Hiss anatomical antireflux mechanism, as well as to preserve blood supply of the most proximal fundus area, which is especially susceptible to ischaemia. Stopping the dissection distally from the angle of Hiss helps as well to retain this part of the fundus in place, thus preventing possibility of "valve type," intermittent gastroesophageal obstruction caused by invagination of a floppy fundus if entirely dissected.

In summary, at this stage of the operation two substantial differences from sleeve gastrectomy should be taken into consideration:

(a) Dissection along the greater curvature of the stomach must not be carried out close to the stomach wall. Thus, approximately 1–2 cm "rim/edge" should be preserved between the stomach (greater curvature) tissue and the dissecting instrument. The reason is that in LGCP the stomach (greater curvature) is infolded, and stays in place (is not resected/removed). Therefore, any possible traumatic or thermal injury caused by dissection close to stomach may result into a leak during the early postoperative period. This is a distinct and marked difference from sleeve gastrectomy, in which close to stomach wall dissection plays no role (Fig. 18.2).

(b) Dissection towards the angle of Hiss should stop approximately 1–2 cm distally to the angle of Hiss and the last 2–3 short gastric vessels are to be preserved. This is another obvious difference from sleeve gastrectomy.

Greater curvature dissection stops distally within 4–6 cm from the pylorus.

18.6.3 The First Plication Row (the Inner Layer)

For sizing of the plication, an endoscope or 36 F calibration bougie should be kept in place during the operation. The greater curvature is imbricated, starting 1–2 cm distal to the angle of Hiss up to 4–6 cm of the pylorus. It is recommended to use nonabsorbable running suture, 2-0 or 1-0 size. Stitches should not be more than 1.5–2 cm apart. The stitches may be placed as full thickness, so no action or correction is to be taken in case the stitches are visible on endoscopy. Care must be taken not to cause gastric lumen obstruction, especially from a point of view that the greater curvature is infolded inside the gastric lumen, however not removed. Postoperative gastric wall oedema and venous congestion has to be taken into account as well. Therefore, even though the narrowed stomach may look at the end of the operation wider than after sleeve gastrectomy, the actual volume of the plicated stomach is close to the one after sleeve gastrectomy. Special attention should be paid to the two most common areas of potential obstruction – the GE junction and the incisura angularis. Especially, the distal stomach parts are more susceptible to obstruction. In general, the more distally the plication goes, the more care (more shallow bites) has to be taken to avoid an obstruction (Fig. 18.3).

18.6.4 The Second Plication Row (the Outer Layer)

An additional second plication row (the outer layer) is applied "over" the first imbrication row to achieve appropriate gastric lumen, thus as close as possible to the 36 F calibration. By adding the second plication row, an increased (wider/deeper) gastric fold size is created. Stitches are positioned in the same way as when suturing the

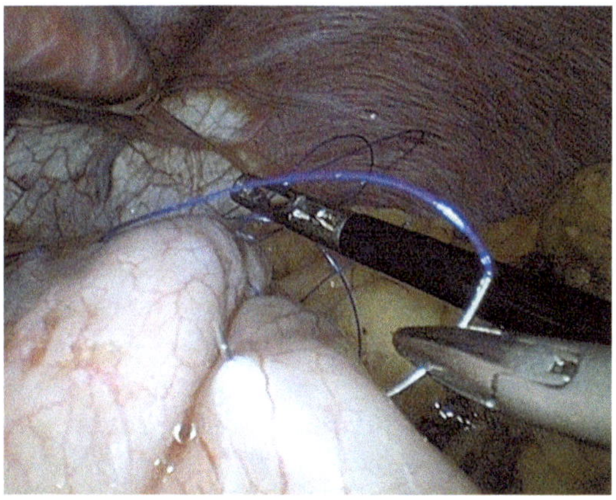

Fig. 18.3 Correct suturing of the greater curvature

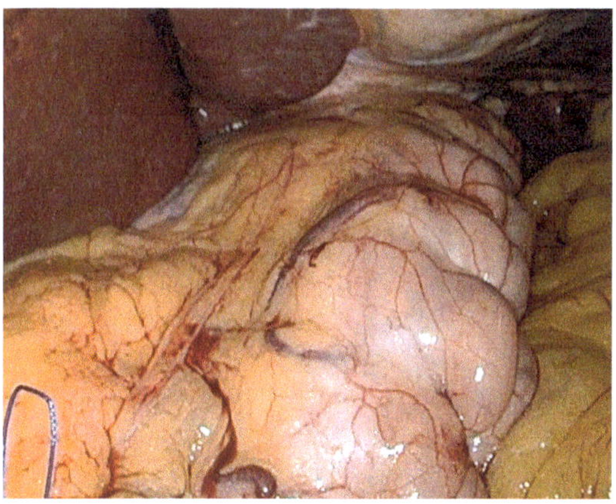

Fig. 18.4 Laparoscopic view of plicated stomach

first row. Care must be taken, not to place the stitches/bites more than 2 cm apart to minimize the risk of underlying gastric wall/tissue herniation through the gaps between the stitches (bites). The procedure ends up with drying up of the operation field, and a leak test, if desired (see the section "Leak Test"). Trocars are removed sequentially under direct visualization at the end of the operation, and the incision sites are closed in institutional standard fashion (Fig. 18.4).

There are reports on using staplers (single stapler/clip firing), instead of the running sutures. The staplers are used in the same way as stitches, thus with a distance of maximum 2 cm between the individual clips. The proximal (1–2 cm below angle of Hiss) and distal (4–6 cm to pylorus) start and end up areas remain unchanged. From author's personal experience with a limited number of patients who underwent stapled LGCP, it seems that a less frequent postoperative nausea and/or vomiting is observed, as well as less noticeable postoperative oedema of the invaginated gastric tissue in short post-period is present. So far reported results of stapled LGCPs are encouraging; however, longer term results are awaited.

18.6.5 Lumen Size Control

As it was described, most of the surgeons use a 36 F calibration bougie for sizing of the plicated stomach while creating the plication folds. However, in the initial phase of starting/learning the LGCP, endoscope kept in place during the procedure, and subsequently used at the end of the procedure for visualization of the lumen of the plicated stomach is a recommended alternative.

18.6.6 Leak Test

Methylene blue, or air insufflation via endoscope, may be used for a leak test at the end of the procedure; however, the leak test is not considered as mandatory. Thus, there is almost negligible risk of causing a leak intraoperatively provided the above-mentioned intraoperative technical precautions are respected. In fact, apart from a massive tissue destruction inflicted during the greater curvature suturing phase, which would be, however, obvious at the time when happened, there 'is no (other) risk of obscured, undetected immediate, intraoperative perforation.

18.7 Intraoperavive and Immediate Postoperative Complications

During the LGCP similar intraoperative complications may occur as with any other gastrointestinal procedure. Immediate postoperative complications include (however are not limited to) nausea, vomiting and sialorrhea. Such complications can be ameliorated with pharmacotherapy, such as ondancetron. In the literature, there are reports on complications following LGCP, including gastric perforation and/or leak, peritonitis, obstruction and infection. Perforation and/or leak may occur due to stomach wall necrosis because of ischaemia induced by dissection of the greater curvature/fundus in the course of the operation, especially in the most susceptible, anterior fundus area. Ischaemia may also occur due to thermic injury to the stomach caused by dissection carried out too close to stomach wall. There are reports on gastric perforation caused by "cheese wire" cutting through effect of the suturing material being a result of compulsive, early postoperative overeating. However, most of these complications are not specific to LGCP, and may be considered among possible complications associated with any upper gastrointestinal restrictive operation.

18.8 Long-Term Complications (Stomach Dilatation/Replication)

Long-term complications include the risk of enlargement of the plicated stomach. Stomach dilatation may result from dietary noncompliance accompanied with repeated, massive overeating or suture line disruption, or a combination of both. Dilatation of plicated stomach appears to be very similar to those reported in a certain number of sleeve gastrectomies. Rarely, psychological intolerance of restriction is reported.

18.9 Clinical Outcomes

In 2012, Fried et al. [9] published results of LGCP in a series of 244 morbidly obese patients in up to 18 months follow-up. Published data showed that in this series, the mean preoperative BMI (±SD) was 41.4±5.5, mean age 46.1±11.0 years and 27.9 % patients had T2DM. Mean operative time was 70.6 min; mean hospitalization, 36 h (24–72). Postoperatively, 27.9 % of the patients experienced nausea and/or vomiting. There was no mortality reported, major complication rate was 1.2 %. The procedure was associated with significant weight loss ($p<0.001$). At 6 months, BMI, %EBMIL and %EWL were 36.1±4.7, 34.8±17.3 and 31.8±15.9, respectively. In patients with preoperative BMI < 40, 18-month %EWL approached 50 % and %EBMIL exceeded 50 %; 96.9 % of patients' T2DM was significantly improved/resolved.

In 2013, Bradnova et al. [12] published results of a study which explored changes in glucose homoeostasis, postprandial triglyceridaemia, and meal-stimulated secretion of selected gut hormones (glucose-dependent insulinotropic polypeptide, GIP; glucagon-like peptide-1, GLP-1; ghrelin and obestatin) in patients with type 2 diabetes mellitus (T2DM) at 1 month and 6 months after LGCP. Results of the study show that LGCP is associated with significant weight loss both at 1 month and 6 months after the LGCP ($p\leq0.002$), mean percent excess weight loss (%EWL) reached 29.7±2.9 % at the 6-month follow-up. Fasting hyperglycaemia and hyperinsulinaemia improved significantly at 1 month and 6 months after the LGCP ($p<0.05$), with parallel improvement in insulin sensitivity and HbA1c levels ($p<0.0001$). Meal-induced glucose plasma levels were also lower at 1 month and 6 months after the LGCP ($p<0.0001$) and postprandial triglyceridaemia was ameliorated at the 6-month follow-up ($p<0.001$). Postprandial GIP plasma levels were significantly increased both at 1 month and 6 months after the LGCP ($p<0.0001$), whereas the overall meal-induced GLP-1 response was not significantly changed after the procedure ($p>0.05$). Postprandial ghrelin plasma levels decreased at 1 and 6 months after the LGCP ($p<0.0001$) with no significant changes in circulating obestatin levels. Overall conclusion is that LGCP induces significant weight loss and improves the metabolic profile of morbidly obese T2DM patients, while also decreases circulating postprandial ghrelin levels and increases the meal-induced GIP response.

Other studies published between 2007 and 2011 have reported that LGCP offers the benefit of gastric restriction while potentially being associated with lower risks of complications in comparison with some other bariatric procedures [7, 13, 14].

Brethauer et al. [15] compared LGCP outcomes after two different gastric plication techniques: anterior gastric plication and the greater curvature gastric plication. In the anterior plication group at 1-year follow-up the %EWL reached 23.3 %, while the % EWL for the greater curvature gastric plication group was 53.4 %. There were no complications in either procedure; however, all of the patients experienced mild to moderate nausea early postoperatively.

Ramos et al. [13] studied 42 morbidly obese patients who underwent laparoscopic greater curvature plication. Eighteen-month data demonstrated an EWL of 62 %. There were no intraoperative complications. Short-term postoperative complications included nausea, vomiting and sialorrhea. A study by Sales [14] reported a 69.6 % EWL at 12 months in 100 patients. Twenty five percent of the patients had a preoperative BMI of <35. No major complications were reported.

Talebpour and Amoli [7] reported results of LGCP performed in 100 patients. The mean %EWL at 6, 12, 24 and 36 months was 54, 61, 60 and 57 %, respectively. Nausea and vomiting were present in all patients. According to Talebpour's report, major complications linked with the LGCP were such as leakage at the suture line, and acute gastric perforation. Reoperation was required in four cases and there were no mortalities.

18.10 Clinical Management

18.10.1 Dietary Recommendations After LGCP

Successful outcomes of LGCP are dependent, among other factors, on patients'compliance with dietary recommendations. Hence, failure to follow up on dietary recommendations either shortly postoperatively, or even in longer term after the LGCP substantially increases the risk of treatment failure.

Generally speaking, suggested dietary changes after LGCP are rather similar to those following sleeve gastrectomy.

Immediately following LGCP, 2 weeks of strictly liquidized diet are recommended, starting on postoperative day two. After that, patient should be kept on a minced/mashed diet for another 2 weeks.

The following are examples of what is recommended in this postoperative period:

Mashed potatoes, minced meat mixed into the mashed potatoes, broth, if vegetable, then liquidized, vegetable soup, with liquidized vegetables (spinach, carrot, etc.), grated apple, mashed banana, children's fruit snacks, steamed and liquidized fruit. It is recommended to avoid food causing flatulence, such as broccoli and cauliflower. All accompanying drinks should be noncaloric, noncarconated and nonalcoholic. The maximum amount of food and/or drinks must not exceed 150 mL at a go. It is recommended to drink either 15 min before starting a meal, or to wait at least 30 min after a meal. The meal should not be mixed with drinks. It should be ensured that, in total, the minimum amount of daily liquid intake is at least 2 L.

18.10.2 Reversibility

So far no clinical study was conducted on reversibility of the LGCP; however, it has been repeatedly clinically confirmed that in case of surgical emergency (e.g. leaks with peritonitis after LGCP), it is possible to fully reverse the gastric plication both short- and long-term postoperatively. The longest period after LGCP which our team has experienced with dismantling the LGCP is 16 months, and the procedure was fully reversible.

18.11 LGCP Emergencies

Most of LGCP related emergencies occur in the early postoperative period. The overall number of serious emergencies (major complications) after LGCP is low (1.2 %) [9]. According to our experience, among the most frequent is gastric leak (0.6 %), followed by gastric obstruction (0.4 %) and ischaemia of anterior fundus wall (0.2 %). Gastric leak may occur in two variations:

(a) "classical" leak caused by clearly visible stomach perforation, for example, due to "cheese wire" effect of the plicating suture, (b) "obscured" leak in which it is impossible to identify a clear stomach perforation, however one or several sites of plicating stitches are oozing.

Management of distinct gastric leaks should include dismantling of both plication layers on the entire length of the plicated stomach, and closure of the leak area in a standard fashion as appropriate in any upper GI surgical complication.

Oozing, obscured leaks at the site of the plicating sutures can be managed in most of the cases just by complete dismantling of both layers of the plication and drainage of the perigastric region. Usually, patients completely recover within a few days after revisional surgery.

Gastric obstruction may be clinically present as total, or intermittent. Obstruction usually occurs in the fundus area, or at the incisura angularis, being a result of too tight suturing invaginating excessively voluminous part of the greater curvature (the invaginated stomach is too bulky and after calibrating bougie is retrieved, the invaginated stomach tissue expands and occupies the entire gastric lumen). Obstruction is rather straight forward to manage, and loosing the suture line at the area of obstruction results in immediate improvement.

In case of ischaemia of the stomach wall, all the plication layers have to be taken down. After the plication layers are taken down, it is recommended to wait for several minutes and see as some parts of what appears as ischaemic gastric wall, may regain vitality. The truly necrotic areas of the stomach wall have to be resected and the defect securely sutured and closed in two layers. After this manoeuvre, the reoperation should be completed as per standard institutional/surgeons custom.

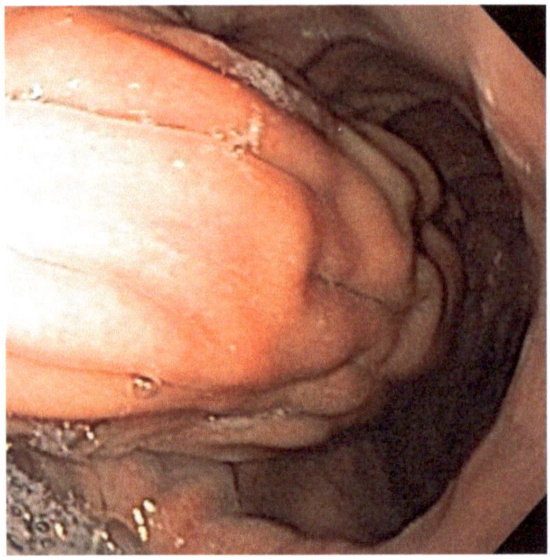

Fig. 18.5 Dilated stomach after LGCP

18.12 LGCP as Re-do Bariatric Procedure

There are several reports on successful indication of the LGCP as a re-do procedure in patients who failed different other bariatric procedures. LGCP was performed as re-do surgery especially after failed gastric bands, and as reoperation in patients who failed LGCP and/or sleeve gastrectomies (in particular due to stomach dilatations). Re-do plication after failed adjustable gastric band is possible if the patient is still willing to undergo another gastric restriction. However, attention must be paid not to perform the LGCP after gastric banding which was associated with peri- or postoperative complications, such as bleeding in the region of the band, band migration or band infection. In such cases, it is highly likely that the blood supply to the fundus/angle of Hiss region is already compromized, so further dissection of the greater curvature would add to substantial risk of impaired blood supply postoperatively, which may result in stomach wall necrosis. Technically, it does not make sense to perform LGCP as re-do operation after failed gastric bypass or biliopancreatic diversion; however, LGCP may be realistically considered as an option in patients who failed previuos LGCP or sleeve gastrectomy. Notably, LGCP may be beneficial in patients who were successful in losing weight or improving their comorbidities after primary sleeve gastrectomy or LGCP, and who were in general satisfied with the primary procedure. In a number of such patients, the primary procedure fails mostly due to stomach dilatation. Thus, re-plication of the dilated LGCP, or re-plication of dilated sleeve gastrectomy is one of the preferred and rather straightforward alternatives (Fig. 18.5).

18.13 Summary

Even though experience with the LGCP is still limited, and more long-term data is needed, it may be concluded that 3-year follow-up of several thousands of gastric plication patients show that LGCP results in acceptable weight loss, significant amelioration of type 2 diabetes mellitus, which appears to be weight loss independent, and reduction of several other, obesity-related comorbidities. LGCP exhibits very low complication rates both in short- and mid-term follow-up postoperatively.

References

1. Ewart W, et al. A case of dilatation of the stomach treated by an operation believed to be new. Lancet. 1896;148(3801):8–10.
2. Kirk RM. An experimental trial of gastric plication as a means of weight reduction in the rat. Br J Surg. 1969;56(12):930–2. Tretbar LL, Taylor TL, Sifers EC. Weight reduction: gastric plication for morbid obesity.J Kans Med Soc. 1976;77:488–90.
3. Tretbar LL, Taylor TL, Sifers EC. Weight reduction:gastric plication for morbid obesity. J Kans Med Soc. 1976;77:488–90.
4. Wilkinson LH, Peloso OA. Gastric (reservoir) reduction for morbid obesity. Arch Surg. 1981;116: 602–5.
5. Fusco PEB, et al. Comparison of anterior gastric wall and greater gastric curvature invaginations for weight loss in rats. Obes Surg. 2007;17:1340–5.
6. Fusco PEB, et al. Evaluation of gastric greater curvature invagination for weight loss in rats. Obes Surg. 2006;16:172–7.
7. Talebpour M, Amoli BS. Technical report- laparoscopic total gastric vertical plication in morbid obesity. J Laparoendosc Adv Surg Tech. 2007;17(3):793–8.
8. Menchaca HJ, et al. Gastric plication: a preclinical study of the durability of serosa-to-serosa apposition. Surg Obes Relat Dis. 2011;7(1):8–14.
9. Fried M, Dolezalova K, Buchwald JN, et al. Laparoscopic greater curvature plication (LGCP) for treatment of morbid obesity in a series of 244 patients. Obes Surg. 2012;22:1298–307.
10. Fried M, Yumuk V, Oppert JM, et al. Interdisciplinary European guidelines on metabolic and bariatric surgery. Obes Facts. 2013;6:449–68.
11. Fried M, Yumuk V, Oppert JM, et al. Interdisciplinary European guidelines on metabolic and bariatric surgery. Obes Surg. 2014;24:42–55.
12. Bradnova O, Kyrou I, Hainer V, et al. Laparoscopic greater curvature plication in morbidly obese women with type 2 diabetes: effects on glucose homeostasis, postprandial triglyceridemia and selected gut hormones. Obes Surg. 2014;24:718–26.
13. Ramos A, et al. Laparoscopic greater curvature plication: initial results of an alternative restrictive bariatric procedure. Obes Surg. 2010;20(7):913–8.
14. Sales Puccini CE. Surset gástrico de Sales: una alternative para cirugía bariátrica restrictive. Revista Colombiana De Cirugía. 2008;23(3):131–5.
15. Brethauer SA, et al. Laparoscopic gastric plication for the treatment of severe obesity. Surg Obes Relat Dis. 2011;7:15–22.

Laparoscopic Roux-en-Y Gastric Bypass: Technical Aspects, Clinical Management, and Outcomes

19

Kelvin D. Higa

19.1 Introduction

The laparoscopic Roux-en-Y gastric bypass was first performed by Wittgrove et al. in 1993 and was an act of genius [1]. This procedure helped to bring treatment options to millions of individuals with the disease of morbid obesity and became the tipping point for the discipline of minimally invasive surgery as a whole. For the first time, a complex, reconstructive operation was more than a novelty; it became the standard of care. Although difficult, with a long learning curve, the tremendous patient adoption and lower complication rates over open, traditional procedures helped to fuel an industry and define our specialty. Over 20 years later, although there have been modifications by others, this original technique is still being practiced today—a testimony to the sagacity of its inventors.

Despite its criticisms, the Roux-en-Y gastric bypass has established itself as the standard to which all other procedures are compared. Although not the most powerful metabolic procedure, long-term outcomes studies and quality of life factors make it the best option for most patients. It is not only modifiable but also reversible (unlike the vertical sleeve gastrectomy). Fortunately, most, if not all, complications of the gastric bypass have minimally invasive solutions. Unfortunately, the most frustrating problem—weight recidivism or lack of control of metabolic disease—is a complex problem. Conversion to duodenal switch or biliopancreactic diversion is a daunting task after gastric bypass.

Little was known of physiology of the gastric bypass conceived by Mason and Ito in the 1960s [2]. This operation and further modifications were erroneously based on concepts of mechanical "restriction" or "malabsorption." Early evolution of the procedure was focused on lowering complications and side effects of the Billroth II based procedure. Conversion of the short-loop gastro-enterostomy to a Roux-en-Y configuration eliminated bile reflux. Transitioning from a horizontal to a vertically oriented gastric pouch improved alimentation while creating a more stable, less distensible reservoir. With the advent of laparoscopy and the ability to create much smaller pouches, this did not correlate with improved weight loss. This clinical observation serves to underscore current concepts of the role of incretins, bile acids [3], and gut microbiota [4] on satiety and food acquisition. Overall size of the gastric pouch or stability of the gastro-jejunostomy is thought to be no longer relevant to

K.D. Higa, MD, FACS, FASMBS, UCSF
Minimally Invasive and Bariatric Surgery,
Fresno Heart and Surgical Hospital,
Advanced Laparoscopic Surgery Associates,
205 E. River Park Circle, Suite 460,
Fresno, CA 93720, USA
e-mail: higanoid@yahoo.com

M. Lucchese, N. Scopinaro (eds.), *Minimally Invasive Bariatric and Metabolic Surgery: Principles and Technical Aspects*, DOI 10.1007/978-3-319-15356-8_19,

performance, although may be critical in complications such as marginal ulceration or reactive hypoglycemia.

If modification of the gastric pouch and/or the gastro-jejunostomy has no effect on weight loss, then the primary trigger must be in the bypass. Whether configured as a Roux-en-Y or an omega loop [5], there is little difference in weight loss. Modifications of altering limb lengths, then, should have pronounced effects on performance. However, the current literature does not support this [6]. Our current studies on distalizing the bypass (shortening the alimentary tract by increasing the biliopancreatic limb length) are encouraging, but inconclusive at this time.

Therefore, given the lack of standardization regarding gastric pouch size, anastomotic stability, and limb lengths in conjunction with the consistent weight loss and metabolic effects among varying researchers, one can only conclude that the mechanism of action of the gastric bypass is not attributable to a single cause; it is a symphony of effects as a result of the anatomic construct, and as of yet, unknown.

19.2 Surgical Construct

The evolution of the gastric bypass has been to make smaller pouches, with exclusion of the distensible fundus. This has had little effect on long-term weight loss when one compares open and laparoscopic series (assuming that smaller pouches are achieved laparoscopically), but we would hope this would lead to fewer complications such as marginal ulceration or GERD [7–9]. Proponents of the banded gastric bypass argue that pouch stability is an important component for both initial and sustained weight loss as indicated in Obrien's systematic review of medium-term weight loss [10] and Schauer's short- term comparative trial [11], but Herrera's randomized controlled study of banded versus non-banded gastric bypass failed to support this hypothesis [12].

There are three primary methods of gastro-jejunostomy: the hand-sewn, the linear stapler, and the circular stapler [13]. Leaks at the gastro-jejunostomy are feared as one of the most devastating complications of this procedure. Surgeons are understandably concerned with patient safety, but they are also concerned with operative time and cost. The circular stapler technique as proposed by Wittgrove and Clark [14] using an endoscopically retrieved guidewire to pull the anvil of the stapler transorally into the pouch was later modified by Jacob and Gagner [15] using only a modified anvil and NGT without the need for an endoscope. Another modification was by Scott and de la Torre [16] who used a transgastric placement of the anvil. All of these techniques are successful, reproducible, and safe. The major drawbacks are the need to use an entry port larger than 12 mm to accommodate the stapler, the cost of the stapler, and an increase in wound infections if the entry site was unprotected when withdrawing the contaminated tip [17].

The linear stapled anastomosis popularized by Williams and Champion [18], Schauer et al. [19] and others avoided the issues with the circular-stapled anastomosis, but required manual suturing to close the enterotomy. In addition, it was more difficult to calibrate the size of the anastomosis. The completely hand-sewn technique avoided many of the issues of the stapled anastomosis, but admittedly was the most difficult to master [20].

Clearly, no single best technique has emerged as all are in use today, with excellent results [21]. However, when one considers the increasing number of revisional surgical procedures, it is in these, the most complex situations, that manual suturing skills are necessary for superior outcomes and damage control.

Small bowel obstruction after gastric bypass is a particularly troublesome issue because of the vulnerability of the isolated gastric remnant prone to distension and possible ischemic necrosis. As opposed to bowel infarction due to adhesions that is often limited, the entire small bowel and right colon can be at risk with an internal hernia. This phenomenon has been described for the open gastric bypass, but is observed much less often than in the laparoscopic procedures due to a greater degree of post-surgical adhesions in the former. Delay in treatment and diagnosis has led to disastrous consequences emphasizing

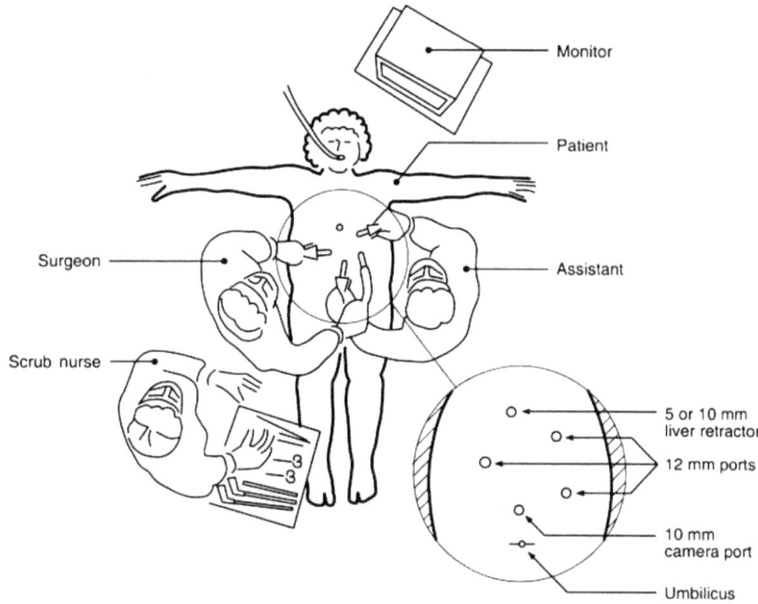

Fig. 19.1 Position and port placement

the need for formal education of general surgeons called upon to treat post-gastric bypass patients.

Our initial experience was based on our open gastric bypass, closing potential internal hernia spaces (except for Petersen's) with absorbable sutures. We quickly found this to be inadequate and decreased the incidence of this problem to less than 1 % using continuous permanent sutures [22]. Others eliminated the meso-colic defect of the traditional retro-colic bypass by routing the Roux limb ante-colic, but this did not eliminate the need to close the jejunal and Petersen's defects [23]. Most authorities agree that closure of mesenteric defects with nonabsorbable suture material is highly advisable, but will not conclusively prevent internal hernias.

Optimal port placement allows for dissection of the small bowel without compromising the exposure of the proximal stomach. Extremes of size can be challenging: adequate space to allow the formation of the Roux limb in smaller patients can be as problematic as the inadequate length of instrumentation and difficulties associated with visualization of the proximal stomach in larger patients. It is of interest that authors maintain how critical proper port placement is to the success of the operation; yet there is no consistency as to a dominant port configuration amongst these experts. We use five ports as per the illustration (Fig. 19.1), but it is obvious that port placement is at the discretion of each individual surgeon. Our current arrangement also allows for concomitant cholecystectomy if necessary at the time of the operation or later as indicated.

Rather than use external landmarks such as the umbilicus or xyphoid to determine port placement, we feel it better to place the trocars based on internal anatomy and visceral relationships. In this way, triangulation and visualization will be preserved, accommodating for variations in the size of the liver, or length of the patient's torso.

Attention must not only be given to individual trocar placement, but also the angle in which the trocar enters the skin. Some individuals' thick, muscular abdominal walls do not allow for the range of motion necessary to achieve the objective, forcing redirection of the trocar internally, through the same skin incision, but different fascial opening, or by placement of another trocar. In general, the optimal placement is to orient all trocars toward the midline, pointing to the base of the mesocolon.

Extra long trocars may be necessary and although some surgeons prefer to limit the number of 12 mm trocars (necessary to accommodate stapling devices), this may limit proper stapler orientation and compromise the anatomic construct. The hernia risk is minimized by either closing the trocar defects, or preferably, using non-bladed trocars without fascial closure to minimize postoperative pain.

Our port placement scheme is as follows; it illustrates the rationale necessary for consistency of this technique and represents an evolutionary process that has taken over 12 years to develop (Fig. 19.1).

Initial trocar (*12 mm*) – Left, upper quadrant, subcostal, mid-clavicular line. This is often an optical entry without prior insufflation. The rationale is that many patients have had previous procedures, pelvic or otherwise—this area is rarely affected with intra-abdominal adhesions from common open procedures. This allows dissection of midline adhesions, inspection of the size of the liver, and determination of the best level for the primary optical port. This will also be the primary port for vertical stapling of the gastric pouch. Once adhesions are mobilized, then the optical port can be thoughtfully placed as to see the ligament of Treitz as well as hiatus without having to "turn around." Also, by keeping the initial entry away from the midline, the vena cava and aorta are not as vulnerable to injury.

Primary optical trocar (*12 mm*) – Placement has been described above. Optimal placement allows for forward visualization of the proximal small bowel and the hiatus. Once this trocar is placed, the camera is moved to this port for subsequent trocar placement. I have not found the current 5-mm scopes to provide enough light delivery and therefore resolution for optimal visualization in most patients.

Right-sided trocar (*12 mm*) – This trocar must be placed thoughtfully just as all others. Exterior landmarks are irrelevant. It must come in below the liver edge, just to the right of the midline so as to be able to triangulate on the hiatus as well as the ligament of Treitz; therefore, it should be angled toward the root of the mesocolon, rather than perpendicular to the abdominal wall. It must be 12 mm to accommodate the stapler that will define the inferior gastric pouch.

Left-inferior trocar (*12 mm*) – This is often at the same level as the primary optical trocar and in the same line as the initial trocar. This will be the primary stapler entry site for the jejuno-jejunostomy and along with the right-upper quadrant trocar will triangulate very well for a comfortable manual gastro-jejunostomy.

Liver retractor – The most optimal placement appears to be subxyphoid. A 5-mm port can be used here, depending on the liver retractor of choice. We have found that a simple 5-mm instrument or similar device will provide excellent exposure and therefore is often placed without a trocar, through direct puncture, as it will not be removed until the end of the case.

The omentum is displaced cephalad to expose the ligament of Treitz. In patients whose omentum is adherent to pelvic structures or involved in an incarcerated ventral hernia, we prefer to incise the gastrocolic omentum and open the transverse mesocolon from above, thus exposing the ligament of Treitz directly. Ventral hernias are repaired at a later date when optimal weight loss and nutrition ensure a greater degree of primary success and the use of prosthetic mesh is not compromised by contamination of enteric contents.

The proximal jejunum is transected with a 2.5- to 3.8-mm linear stapler, depending on the thickness of the bowel, and the mesentery is divided with another firing of the stapler or with an ultrasonic scalpel. The Roux limb is measured and a side-to-side linear anastomosis is performed (Fig. 19.2). Typically, the length of the Roux limb can be up to 150 cm without an associated increased incidence of malabsorptive complications [24]. The enterotomy is closed with a single layer of absorbable suture. The mesenteric defect must be closed with a continuous, nonabsorbable suture to limit the possibility of internal herniation (Fig. 19.3).

The Roux limb is passed through a retrocolic tunnel and fixed to the transverse mesocolon with nonabsorbable sutures, which also includes closing the Petersen's space (Figs. 19.4 and 19.5), again, to help prevent possible internal herniation. Alternatively, some surgeons prefer an

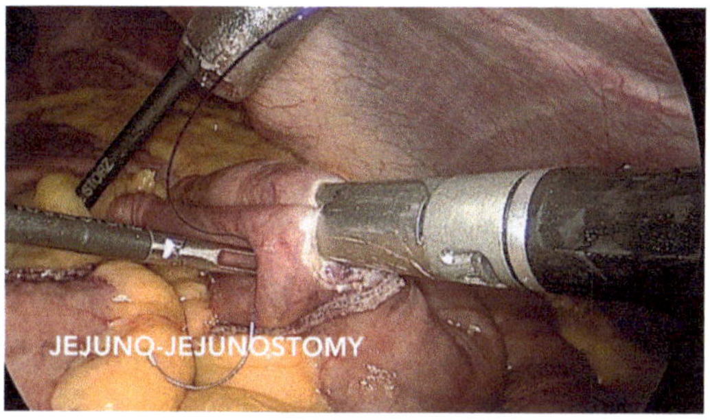

Fig. 19.2 Jejuno-jejunostomy

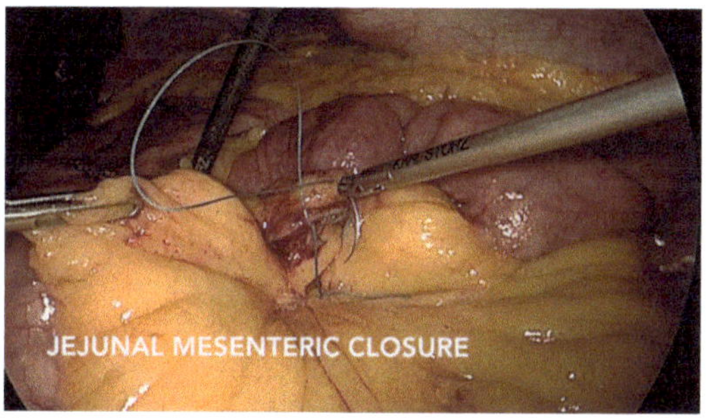

Fig. 19.3 Jejunal mesenteric closure

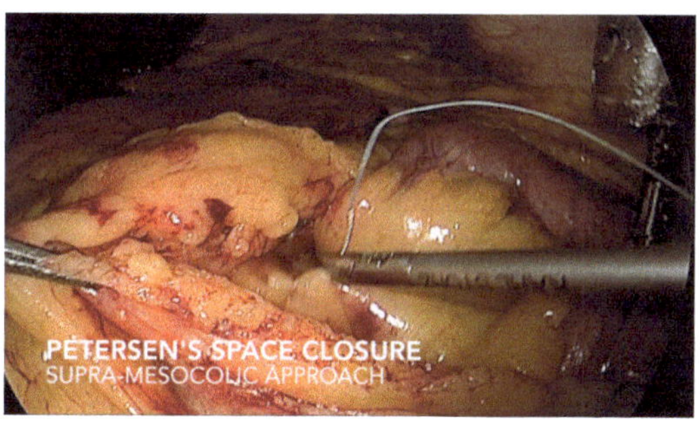

Fig. 19.4 Petersen's space closure

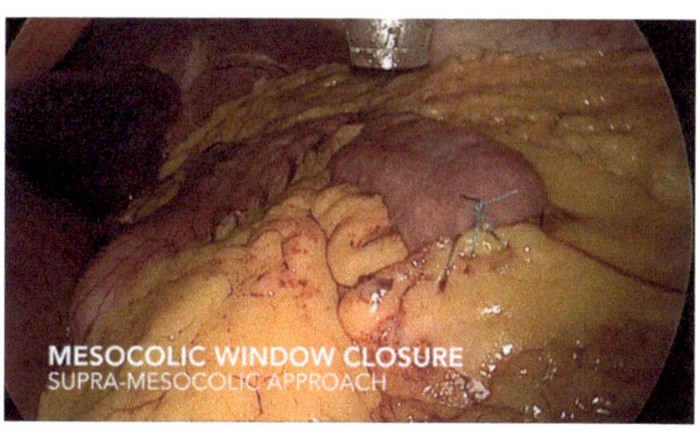

Fig. 19.5 Mesocolic window closure

antecolic route for the Roux limb, claiming a lower incidence of postoperative bowel obstructions [25].

There are times when the mesocolon is uncomfortably short and will not allow for the safe passage of a retrocolic Roux limb. In these rare instances, the decision to route the Roux limb antecolic must be made before the transection of the jejunum. This site must be more distal from the ligament of Treitz, typically 50–100 cm, to limit the tension on the gastro-jejunal anastomosis. By lengthening the biliopancreatic limb, iron and calcium absorption may be less efficient, and the incidence of these deficiencies may be theoretically increased or more difficult to manage with oral supplementation alone.

Controversy exists as to whether the large resultant Petersen's space associated with an antecolic Roux limb requires closure. Clearly, these patients are still at risk for intestinal volvulous [26]. Therefore, our philosophy is to eliminate the risk of postoperative bowel obstruction rather than simply settling for a reduction in the incidence. However, the long-term stability of suture closure of these defects is still to be determined.

The liver retractor is now placed to allow dissection of the proximal stomach. Occasionally, a very large liver will not allow for sufficient visualization—an indication for open conversion. However, displacement of the liver to the right, rather than anterior, will allow sufficient exposure in the largest of patients. Alternatively, the surgeon may decide to abort the procedure, evaluate the cause of hepatic enlargement (usually steatosis), and institute therapy (medical weight reduction) in anticipation of performing the procedure at a later time under more ideal circumstances. In this way, surgical restraint and proper judgment may reduce the morbidity associated with these operations.

The pouch is formed by sequential firing of a laparoscopic linear cutter, stapling device around a 34 Fr. orogastrically placed bougie. The first firing is horizontal, introducing the stapler from the RUQ port (Fig. 19.6), beginning no more than 5 cm distal to the esophagogastric junction, using 3.8- to 4.1-mm cartridges, depending on stomach

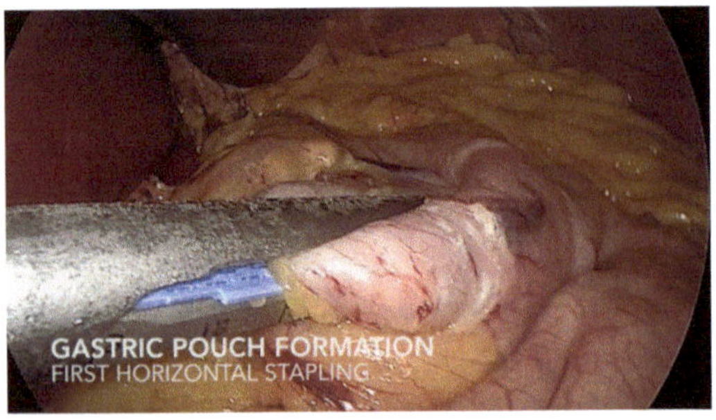

Fig. 19.6 Gastric pouch formation

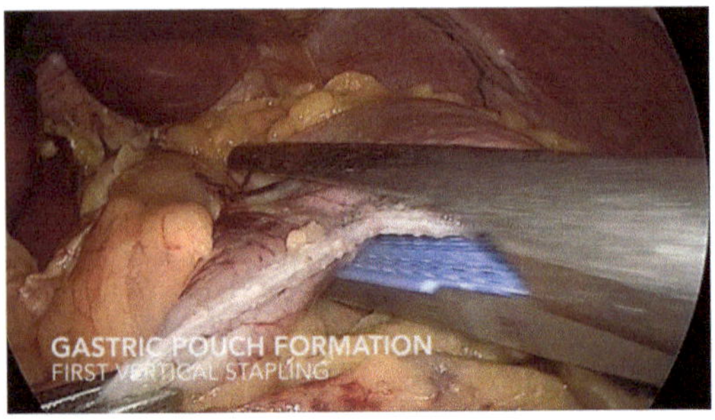

Fig. 19.7 Gastric pouch formation

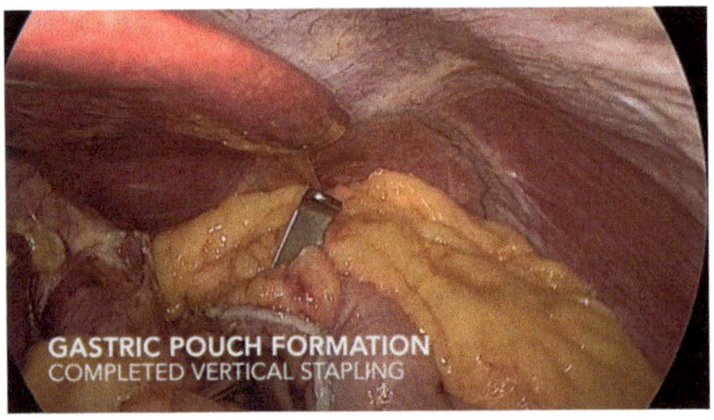

Fig. 19.8 Gastric pouch formation

thickness. It is important to orient the stapler slightly cephalad to angulate the stapler line. Subsequent firings are vertically oriented to the angle of His, introducing the stapler from the LUQ port (Figs. 19.7 and 19.8). By using this port configuration, extra-long staplers are unnecessary for the majority of patients.

One of the critical steps in creation of the gastric pouch is posterior visualization at the level of the hiatus. Many surgeons will "bluntly" dissect behind the stomach, but given the variable level of adhesions to the pancreas and the splenic

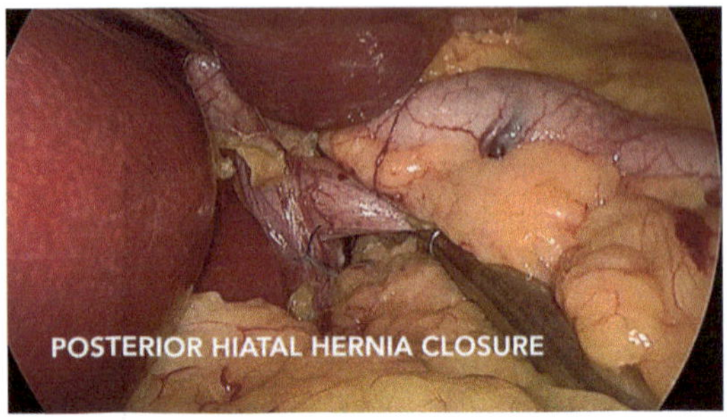

Fig. 19.9 Posterior hiatal hernia closure

vessels, this is unwise. Optimally, it is better to enter the lesser sack through the gastrocolic omentum and free the posterior gastric adhesions up to the esophageal hiatus. This protects the pancreas and the occasional tortuous splenic artery from inadvertent injury. After this, the lesser curve, perigastric dissection can be performed with more confidence and placement of the stapler more precisely as not to "twist" the stomach pouch. This occurs when posterior gastric adhesions prevent the initial horizontal stapler from capturing equal amounts of anterior and posterior gastric wall. The resultant twist is not as critical as in the gastric sleeve but is not esthetically pleasing.

Controversy exists as to whether or not to dissect the hiatus and repair a hiatal hernia when present. Autopsy studies show that a hiatal hernia is present in up to 70 % of individuals, similar to our observations. However, dissection of the hiatus can add additional time and potential complications to an already complicated procedure. Our studies have not shown that preoperative endoscopy accurately predicts the absence of a hiatal hernia; the only way to determine its presence is circumferential dissection of the esophagus. The absence of the "anterior" dimple is not reliable as the hernia space is often taken up by a large para-esophageal lipoma that can be easily reduced into the abdomen once identified. Once identified, the hiatal hernia is best repaired posteriorly (Fig. 19.9).

The question remains: "Is it important to repair every hiatal hernia at the time of gastric bypass?" The answer is not clear. If one assumes that precise dissection and formation of the gastric pouch is important to limit postoperative complications, then it would be appropriate to absolutely identify the location of the gastro-esophageal junction, often hidden in a "sea of fat," to better perform more consistent reconstruction. It has been our observation that almost 100 % of patients we have reoperated after gastric bypass have a significant hiatal hernia at the time of reoperation – something not appreciated at the time of the first intervention.

Dissection of the hiatus and repair of the hiatal hernia along with removing the fat pad overlying the angle of His may allow for more precise and consistent pouch formation and subsequent better long-term performance and lower complications, but this has not been proven. Although this may add up to 5–10 min of operative time, which is significant, the added exposure may make for a safer operation. Each surgeon will need to evaluate this perception in the context of his or her individual experience and skill level. Suffice it to say, to perform a good laparoscopic gastric bypass, the surgeon must be expert at hiatal dissection.

Routing of the Roux limb is best determined by the patient's internal anatomy. As stated previously, the risk of internal herniation is the same, whether routed antecolic or retrocolic as long as potential internal hernia spaces are closed with nonabsorbable sutures. It is important that there is as little tension on the anastomosis as possible. In most cases, an antegastric orientation makes gastro-jejunal anastomosis more visible and easier for subsequent revision if necessary. However, the retrogastric orientation is a more direct route and offers unobstructed access to the anterior stomach.

The method of gastro-jejunal anastomosis is not critical. Whether stapled, or hand-sewn, primary or reinforcing, sutures should be absorbable to prevent suture migration or ulcer formation. Choice of suture material, braided or monofilament, single- or two-layer, is left to the discretion and results of each individual surgeon (Figs. 19.10, 19.11, 19.12, 19.13, 19.14, and 19.15).

The anastomosis and proximal staple lines can be tested with blue dye, air insufflation via the orogastric tube, or operative endoscopy. Routine drainage is unnecessary. The port sites are

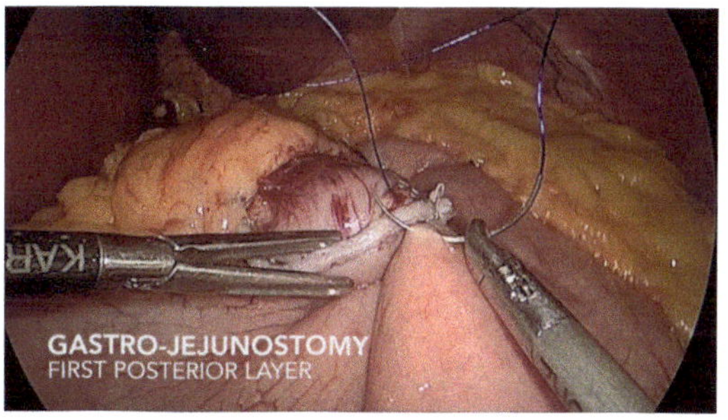

Fig. 19.10 Gastro-jejunostomy

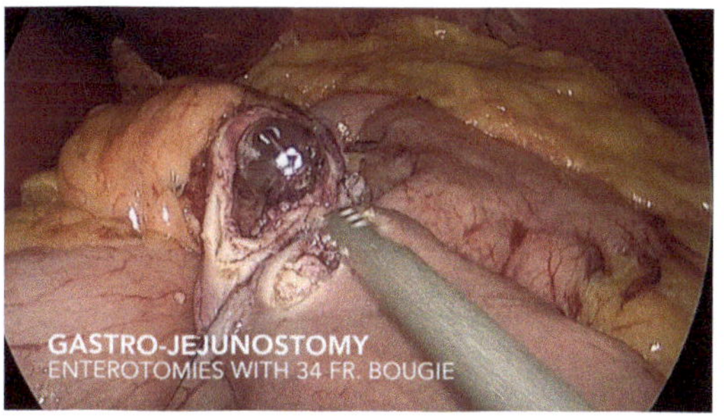

Fig. 19.11 Gastro-jejunostomy

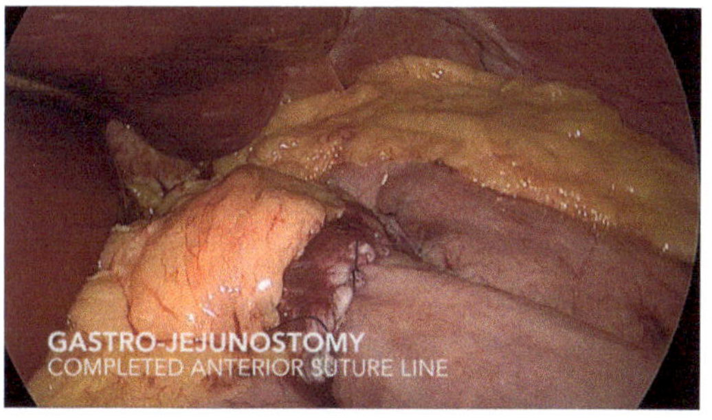

Fig. 19.12 Gastro-jejunostomy

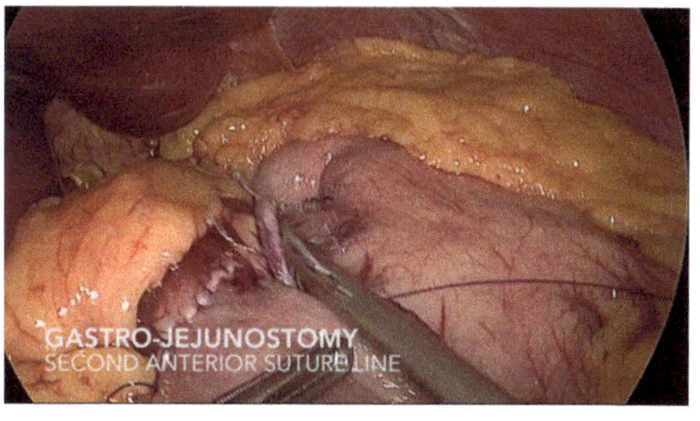

Fig. 19.13 Gastro-jejunostomy

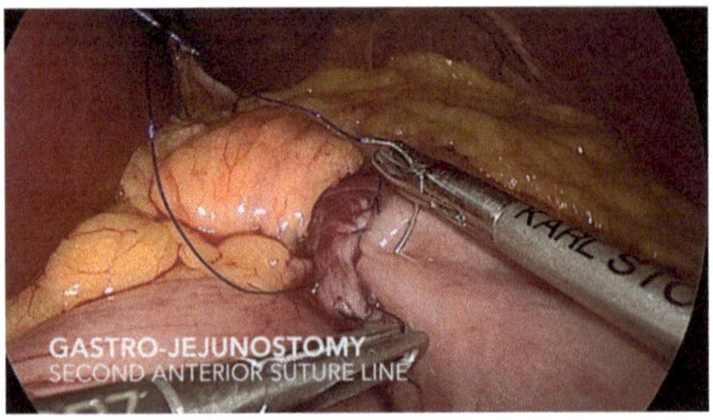

Fig. 19.14 Gastro-jejunostomy

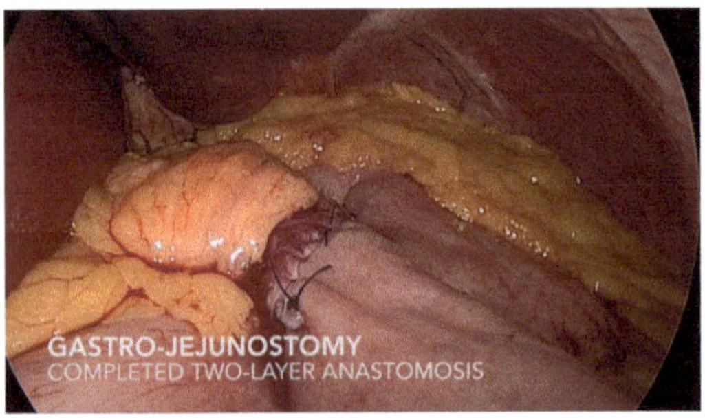

Fig. 19.15 Gastro-jejunostomy

inspected for bleeding on withdrawal of the trocars and the skin is closed with simple absorbable monofilament sutures.

19.3 Postoperative Management

Perioperative antibiotic is continued for 24 h, while thromboembolism prophylaxis continues until the patient is discharged. Analgesia is in the form of patient controlled narcotic delivery systems and intravenous ketorolac or acetaminophen. Oral narcotics are offered when clear liquids are tolerated. Metoclopramide is administered routinely and a variety of antiemetic pharmacologic agents are available for nurses to use at their discretion.

Routine postoperative contrast studies add little to the management of these patients and serve only to delay discharge secondary to nausea [27]. A normal postoperative upper gastrointestinal (UGI) study should not preclude the surgeon's intervening based on clinical suspicion of a leak [28].

Patients are started on clear liquids the day of surgery and are required to ambulate with assistance. Preoperative oral medications can be resumed as soon as the patient can tolerate clear liquids. Most patients are discharged by the second postoperative day, the majority on the first postoperative day.

Patients are continued on a clear liquid diet for 1 week and slowly advanced to solids over a 3- to 4-week period. Patients are instructed to take either an H2-blocker or proton pump inhibitor for 30 days. Routine follow-up visits are at 1, 3 weeks, and quarterly for the first year, and then on a yearly basis. Ongoing nutritional, emotional, exercise counseling, and support groups are provided. Complete nutritional assessment occurs on a yearly basis or when symptoms or clinical suspicion dictates.

19.4 Results

Long-term data regarding the laparoscopic Roux-en-Y gastric bypass have been lacking due the difficulty with patient follow-up. Despite tremendous effort, we were only able to obtain a 27 % sample regarding our 10-year results [8]. However, we found no difference in results in comparing patients who consistently followed up in our office and those who did not, so it is not unreasonable to extrapolate our results and they are similar to Himpens' 9-year data [29] as well as from the open era.

As important as is weight maintenance, resolution of medical comorbidities and metabolic syndrome is well illustrated with our data and this emulates other reports [30] (Tables 19.1 and 19.2).

19.5 Complications

Although our perioperative mortality remains low (0.2 % overall), potential complications must be looked at in the context of the chronicity

Table 19.1 Reported long-term weight loss

Investigator	Patients (*n*)	Follow-up (years)	Patients eligible for follow-up (*n*)	Patients at follow-up, *n* (%)	%EWL	Postoperative BMI (kg/m²)
Jones [31]	352	10	71	36(51)	62	30
Pories et al. [32]	608	10	NR	158 (NR)	55	35
Sugerman et al. [33]	1,025	10–12	361	135 (37)	52	36
Christou et al. [34]	272	12	272	161 (59)	68	38
Higa et al. [8]	242	10	242	65 (27)	57	33
Himpens et al. [29]	126	9	126	77 (61)	63	30

NR not-reported

Table 19.2 Outcomes of 242 patients: 10-year follow-up

Comorbid condition	Patients (*N*)	% of 242	Resolved or improved (%)
Osteoarthritis	110	45	84
Diabetes	45	19	83
Dyslipidemia	6	2	67
Hypertension	108	45	87
Infertility	5	2	50
Obstructive sleep apnea	45	19	76
Asthma	23	10	100
Gastroesophageal reflux disease	121	50	89
Urinary stress incontinence	35	14	69
Varicose veins	21	9	100

of the disease and the permanent derangement of the anatomic construct. A marginal ulceration or internal hernia that occurs 15 years after a laparoscopic Roux-en-y gastric bypass is still a complication of the procedure, regardless. An overall 10-year complication rate of 45 % seems high, but it accurately reflects our experience and is indicative of underreporting common to the literature. As an example, our initial internal hernia rate was not captured in our first report [22]; internal hernias are a lifelong risk and can present years after the procedure, so a 16 % rate without proper closure of the defects is to be expected. (Our current internal hernia rate is approximately 1 %.) Biliary tract disease and substance abuse may not be directly related to the gastric bypass, but there is an association. Marginal ulcers and vitamin

Table 19.3 Early morbidity (242 patients)

	N	%
Incomplete stomach division	4	1.7
Staple-line failure	2	0.8
Leak due to thermal injury	1	0.4
Marginal ulcer perforation	1	0.4
Bleeding (observation only)	1	0.4
Stenosis: gastro-jejunostomy	12	5.0
Stenosis: mesocolon	1	0.4
Fever and readmission	6	2.5
Hypoglycemia	1	0.4
Central pontine myelinolysis	1	0.4
Total	31	12.8

Table 19.4 Late morbidity (242 patients)

	N	%
Internal hernia	39	16.1
Marginal ulcer	11	4.5
Gastrogastric fistula	1	0.4
Gallstones	17	7.0
Alcohol dependency	6	2.5
Other substance abuse	1	0.4
Hernia, trocar	3	1.2
Total	78	32.2

deficiencies may be entirely due to patient choices (tobacco, NSAIDs), but it is still relevant that they occurred after the procedure. What is also relevant is the overwhelming evidence that the gastric bypass, as well as other operations can improve longevity as well as control of metabolic syndrome compared with nonoperative alternatives [35–38] (Tables 19.3, 19.4, and 19.5).

Table 19.5 Cumulative 10-year nutritional deficiencies (136 patients)

	N	%
Vitamin B_{12}	81	60
Hemoglobin	71	52
Albumin	46	34
Intact parathyroid hormone	36	26
Vitamin B_6	23	17
Calcium	18	13
Folate	2	1.0

References

1. Wittgrove AC, Clark GW, Tremblay LJ. Laparoscopic gastric bypass, Roux-en-Y: preliminary report of five cases. Obes Surg. 1994;4:353–7.
2. Mason EE, Ito C. Gastric bypass in obesity. Surg Clin North Am. 1967;47:1345–51.
3. Pournaras DJ, Glicksman C, Vincent RP, et al. The role of bile after Roux-en-Y gastric bypass in promoting weight loss and improving glycemic control. Endocrinology. 2012;153(8):3613–9.
4. Kong LC, Tap J, Aron-Wisnewsky J, Pelloux V, Basdevant A, Bouillot JL, Zucker JD, Doré J, Clément K. Gut microbiota after gastric bypass in human obesity: increased richness and associations of bacterial genera with adipose tissue genes. Am J Clin Nutr. 2013;98(1):16–24.
5. Lee WJ, Yu PJ, Wang W, Chen TC, Wei PL, Huang MT. Laparoscopic Roux-en-Y versus mini-gastric bypass for the treatment of mor- bid obesity: a prospective randomized controlled clinical trial. Ann Surg. 2005;242: 20–8.
6. Orci L, Chilcott M, Huber O. Short versus long Roux-limb length in Roux-en-Y gastric bypass surgery for the treatment of morbid and super obesity: a systematic review of the literature. Obes Surg. 2011;21(6): 797–804.
7. Coblijn UK, Goucham AB, Lagarde SM, Kuiken SD, van Wagensveld BA. Development of ulcer disease after Roux-en-Y gastric bypass, incidence, risk factors, and patient presentation: a systematic review. Obes Surg. 2014;24(2):299–309.
8. Higa K, Ho T, Tercero F, Yunus T, Boone K. Laparoscopic Roux-en-Y gastric bypass: 10-year follow-up. Surg Obes Relat Dis. 2011;7:516–25.
9. Gilmore MM, Kallies KJ, Mathiason MA, Kothari SN. Varying marginal ulcer rates in patients undergoing laparoscopic Roux-en-Y gastric bypass for morbid obesity versus gastroesophageal reflux disease: is the acid pocket to blame? Surg Obes Relat Dis. 2013; 9(6):862–6.
10. O'Brien PE, McPhail T, Chaston TB, Dixon JB. Systematic review of medium-term weight loss after bariatric operations. Obes Surg. 2006;16(8):1032–40.
11. Heneghan H, Annaberdyev S, Eldar S, Rogula T, Brethauer S, Schauer P. Banded Roux-en-Y gastric bypass for the treatment of morbid obesity. Surg Obes Relat Dis. 2014;10(2):210–6.
12. Zarate X, Arceo-Olaiz R, Montalvo Hernandez J, García-García E, Pablo Pantoja J, Herrera MF. Long-term results of a randomized trial comparing banded versus standard laparoscopic Roux-en-Y gastric bypass. Surg Obes Relat Dis. 2013;9(3):395–7.
13. Madan AK, Harper JL, Tichansky DS. Techniques of laparoscopic gastric bypass: on-line survey of American society for bariatric surgery practicing surgeons. Surg Obes Relat Dis. 2008;4(2):166–72.
14. Wittgrove AC, Clark GW. Combined laparoscopic/endoscopic anvil placement for the performance of the gastroenterostomy. Obes Surg. 2001;11(5):565–9.
15. Jacob BP, Gagner M. New developments in gastric bypass procedures and physiological mechanisms. Surg Technol Int. 2003;11:119–26.
16. de la Torre RA, Scott JS. Laparoscopic Roux-en-Y gastric bypass: a totally intra-abdominal approach–technique and preliminary report. Obes Surg. 1999;9(5):492–8.
17. Alasfar F, Sabnis A, Liu R, Chand B. Reduction of circular stapler-related wound infection in patients undergoing laparoscopic Roux-en-Y gastric bypass, Cleveland clinic technique. Obes Surg. 2010;20(2):168–72.
18. Williams MD, Champion JK. Linear technique of laparoscopic Roux-en-Y gastric bypass. Surg Technol Int. 2004;13:101–5.
19. Schauer PR, Ikramuddin S, Hamad G, Eid GM, Mattar S, Cottam D, Ramanathan R, Gourash W. Laparoscopic gastric bypass surgery: current technique. J Laparoendosc Adv Surg Tech A. 2003;13(4):229–39.
20. Higa KD, Boone KB, Ho T, Davies OG. Laparoscopic Roux-en-Y gastric bypass for morbid obesity: technique and preliminary results of our first 400 patients. Arch Surg. 2000;135(9):1029–33.
21. Bendewald FP, Choi JN, Blythe LS, Selzer DJ, Ditslear JH, Mattar SG. Comparison of hand-sewn, linear-stapled, and circular-stapled gastrojejunostomy in laparoscopic Roux-en-Y gastric bypass. Obes Surg. 2011;21(11):1671–5.
22. Higa KD, Ho T, Boone KB. Internal hernias after laparoscopic Roux-en-Y gastric bypass: incidence, treatment and prevention. Obes Surg. 2003;13(3):350–4.
23. Obeid A, McNeal S, Breland M, Stahl R, Clements RH, Grams J. Internal hernia after laparoscopic Roux-en-Y gastric bypass. J Gastrointest Surg. 2014;18(2):250–5.
24. Brolin RE, Kenler HA, Gorman JH, Cody RP. Long-limb gastric bypass in the super obese: a prospective randomized trial. Ann Surg. 1991;215:387–95.
25. Champion JK. Small bowl obstruction after laparoscopic Roux-en-Y gastric bypass. Obes Surg. 2002;12: 197–8.
26. Khanna A, Newman B, Reyes J, Fung JJ, Todo S, Starzl TL. Internal hernia and volvulus of the small bowel following liver transplantation. Transpl Int. 1997;10(2):133.
27. Sims TL, Mullican MA, Hamilton EC, et al. Routine upper gastrointestinal Gastrografin swallow after

laparoscopic Roux-en-Y gastric bypass. Obes Surg. 2003;13:66–72.
28. Singh R, Fisher B. Sensitivity and specificity of post-operative upper GI series following gastric bypass. Obes Surg. 2003;13:73–5.
29. Himpens J, Verbrugghe A, Cadière G, Everaerts W, Greve J. Long-term results of laparoscopic Roux-en-Y gastric bypass: evaluation after 9 years. Obes Surg. 2012;22:1586–93.
30. Buchwald H, Avidor Y, Braunwald E, et al. Bariatric surgery: a systematic review and meta-analysis. JAMA. 2004;292:1724–37.
31. Jones K. Experience with the Roux-en-Y gastric bypass, and commentary on current trends. Obes Surg. 2000;10:183–5.
32. Pories W, Swanson M, MacDonald K. Who would have thought it? An operation proves to be the most effective therapy for adult-onset diabetes mellitus. Ann Surg. 1995;222:339–50.
33. Sugerman HJ, Wolfe LG, Sica DA, Clore JN. Diabetes and hypertension in severe obesity and effects of gastric bypass-induced weight loss. Ann Surg. 2003;237:751–8.
34. Christou NV, Look D, Maclean LD. Weight gain after short- and long-limb gastric bypass in patients followed for longer than 10 years. Ann Surg. 2006;244:734–40.
35. Sjöström L, Peltonen M, Jacobson P, et al. Bariatric surgery and long-term cardiovascular events. JAMA. 2012;307:56–65.
36. Schauer PR, Kashyap SR, Wolski K, et al. Bariatric surgery versus intensive medical therapy in obese patients with diabetes. N Engl J Med. 2012;366:1567–76.
37. Adams TD, Gress RE, Smith SC, Halverson RC, Simper SC, Rosamond WD, Lamonte MJ, Stroup AM, Hunt SC. Long-term mortality after gastric bypass surgery. N Engl J Med. 2007;357(8):753–61.
38. Christou NV, MacLean LD. Effect of bariatric surgery on long-term mortality. Adv Surg. 2005;39:165–79.

20 Laparoscopic Biliopancreatic Diversion

Nicola Scopinaro

20.1 Introduction

This chapter is a very good occasion to clarify a concept which still today seems not to have been understood by a large part of the bariatric surgeons: biliopancreatic diversion (BPD) is not a particular operation, it is a mechanism of action, essentially consisting of delaying the meeting between food and biliopancreatic juices with the aim of reducing digestion, and thus intestinal absorption of the high-caloric nutrients which need to be digested for being absorbed. The mechanism itself does not necessarily provoke the obtainment of the goal, unless the time of contact between food and biliopancreatic secretions is insufficient to cause a complete digestion-absorption.

The creation of a BPD necessarily requires an alteration of the normal GI continuity. The basic components of the mechanism, no matter how it is constructed, are as follows: (1) an intestinal segment, immediately following the duodenum, where the meeting between food and digestive juices is prevented, called biliopancreatic limb (BPL) as it only leads the biliodigestive juices to the point of meeting with food; (2) an intestinal segment leading food from the stomach to the point where aliments meet the biliopancreatic secretions, called alimentary limb (AL); (3) an intestinal segment, between the point of meeting and the ileocecal valve (ICV), where biliopancreatic digestion starts and the products of it can be absorbed (common limb or CL).

The BPD mechanism, as described above, should not disturb the intestinal absorption of the microaliments, except for the possible bypass of intestinal segments with specific active absorption (e.g., duodenum for active absorption of Ca and Fe), provided that the AL be long enough for their complete absorption, whilst it should be effective on reduction of fat absorption, provided that the CL be short enough not to allow its completion. A big question mark would obviously remain for protein absorption. However, for a better comprehension of what can happen in differently constructed BPD mechanisms, let us consider the behavior of the three intestinal limbs in the standard BPD, which is far the most studied model.

Standard BPD [1] (Fig. 20.1) consists of a distal gastrectomy, including the entire antrum, with a long Roux-en-Y reconstruction where the enteroenterostomy (EEA) is placed 50 or 75 (exceptionally 100) cm proximal to the ileocecal valve, thus identifying the length of the CL, while, in the current model, the GEA is 250 cm far from the EEA (AL), and the remaining small bowel, from the duodenum to the EEA, belongs to the BPL. As our about 3,000 measurements (all done with the small bowel fully stretched)

N. Scopinaro, FACS (Hon)
Department of Surgery, University of Genoa
Medical School, Genova 16132, Italy
e-mail: nicola.scopinaro@gmail.com

M. Lucchese, N. Scopinaro (eds.), *Minimally Invasive Bariatric and Metabolic Surgery: Principles and Technical Aspects*, DOI 10.1007/978-3-319-15356-8_20,

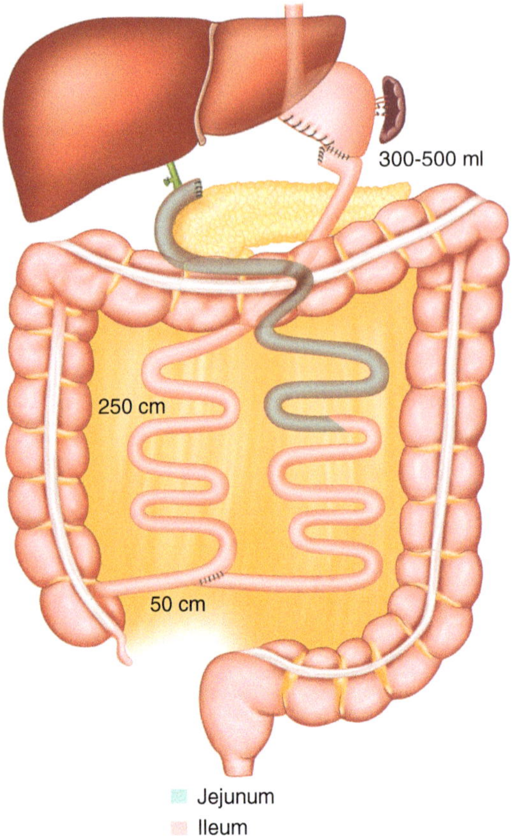

Fig. 20.1 Scopinaro's biliopancreatic diversion, 1979

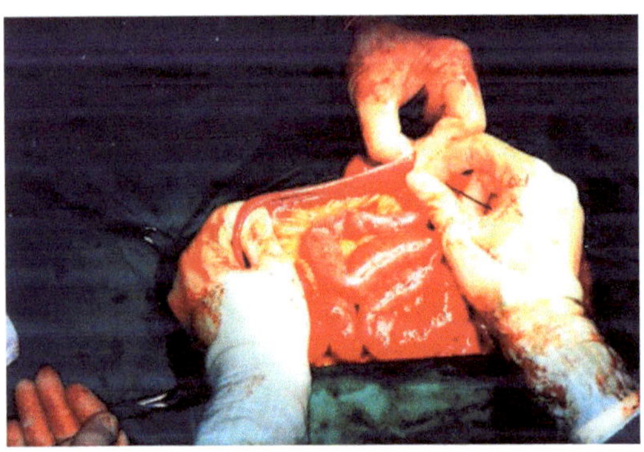

Fig. 20.2 Intestinal measurement in open surgery

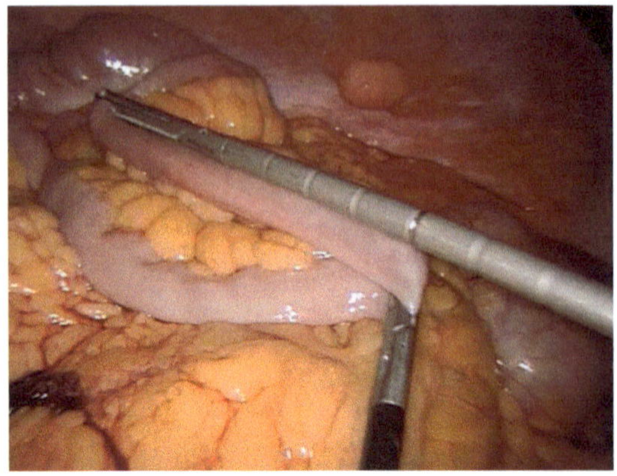

Fig. 20.3 Intestinal measurement in laparoscopic surgery

(Figs. 20.2 and 20.3) demonstrated a mean small bowel length of about 800 cm, and the jejunum is considered to correspond to the first 2/5 of the small bowel, almost invariably the EEA is a gastro-ileal anastomosis, and the BPL is the longest of the three intestinal limbs. Pancreatic enzymes are slowly digested and absorbed in the long BPL, and our studies demonstrated that little if any of them actually reach the CL, so that no pancreatic digestion occurs in it. Protein and starches are uniformly digested and absorbed in the entire intestinal segment from the GEA to the ICV (as well as simple sugars and short-chain fatty acids) thanks to the action of the enterocyte brush-border enzymes, while, due to the necessity of bile salts, only fat absorption is limited to the CL [2]. Therefore, the longer the AL the greater is the protein absorption, but, due to digestion-absorption of complex carbohydrates, the energy absorption is also greater and thus higher is the weight of stabilization. Moreover, colon plays an important role in protein-energy absorption, through the digestive enzymes of its bacterial flora. In fact, colon has a great protein digestive-absorptive capacity [3], which is fully exploited in standard BPD, otherwise there would not be protein malabsorption, which, contrary to what happens for fat, is a percent of the intake corresponding to only about 30 % [4]. This is why, despite the about fivefold increased loss of endogenous nitrogen (up to 5 g/day, mainly consisting of desquamated cells and dead bacterial bodies) protein-energy malnutrition (PEM), potentially the most severe nutritional complication of BPD, is a rare event with the intestinal lengths currently in use. Finally, an unfavorable event is to be considered, that is, the capacity of colonic enzymes to cause fermentation of fiber to fatty acid and lactate, which are then absorbed in this caloric form, thus increasing calorie absorption. It was calculated that up to 500 kcal/day can be absorbed with this mechanism [5].

In summary, except for the unavoidable reduction of calcium and iron, due to the duodenal-jejunal bypass, and of liposoluble vitamins, consequent to the reduced fat absorption, assuming that simple sugars are fully absorbed by the small bowel in the alimentary stream, the absorption of all the other high-caloric nutrients in the standard BPD essentially depends on the volume of the gastric remnant (which, if too small, can cause a rapid gastric emptying and intestinal transit, thus reducing absorption capacity) and on the length of the intestinal limbs. The BPL should be long enough to allow complete digestion-absorption of pancreatic enzymes; the AL plus the CL should be long enough to guarantee, together with the colon, a protein absorption sufficient to counteract the endogenous nitrogen loss, as well as a sufficient water, electrolyte, and water-soluble vitamin absorption, still not allowing an excessive polysaccharide digestion-absorption; CL should be short enough to reduce as much as possible fat absorption, still allowing a bile salt absorption sufficient not to cause bile acid diarrhea. Incidentally, the loss of bile salt into the colon, together with the lack of gallbladder contraction, causes the constant presence of a lithogenic bile, which in turn would cause gallstone formation in the almost totality of operated patients, if a prophylactic cholecystectomy were not added to the operation in all cases.

It is very important to remember that the characteristics of very long term individual and interindividual weight maintenance, together with accurate studies of energy, fat, and protein intestinal absorption [4], and of postoperative changes of resting energy expenditure [2], lead to the hypothesis, subsequently verified by an overfeeding study [2], that a maximum daily intestinal absorption capacity exists for each standard BPD individual for fat and starch, while simple sugars are entirely absorbed, and protein absorption is a percent of the intake, corresponding to about 70 % [4]. In other words, the original intestinal lengths and gastric volume being equal, the interindividual variability of the weight of stabilization in BPD subjects is accounted for by interindividual differences of: (1) the original energy absorption capacity per unit of intestinal surface; (2) the entity of postoperative intestinal adaptation phenomena; (3) the intestinal transit time (which, in addition to gastric volume, can be influenced by the intake of fluids); (4) the simple sugar and protein intake; (5) the number of meals per day and the meal duration; (6) the body weight itself and the energy expenditure per unit of body mass. However, in each BPD individual the weight of stabilization cannot be modified by any increase or decrease of fat and starch intake, provided that the intake is greater than the maximum daily absorption capacity (also defined as "maximum transport threshold").

Apart from the many overt modifications of the standard BPD, like preservation of the distal stomach [6] or of the entire stomach [7], or modifications of the intestinal limb lengths [8] (Figww. 20.4), and, more recently, the so-called duodenal switch [9, 10] (Fig. 20.5), which will be the object of another chapter of this book, once the BPD as a mechanism of action has been clearly described it is easy to recognize it in bariatric operations which have apparently nothing to do with BPD. The most obvious

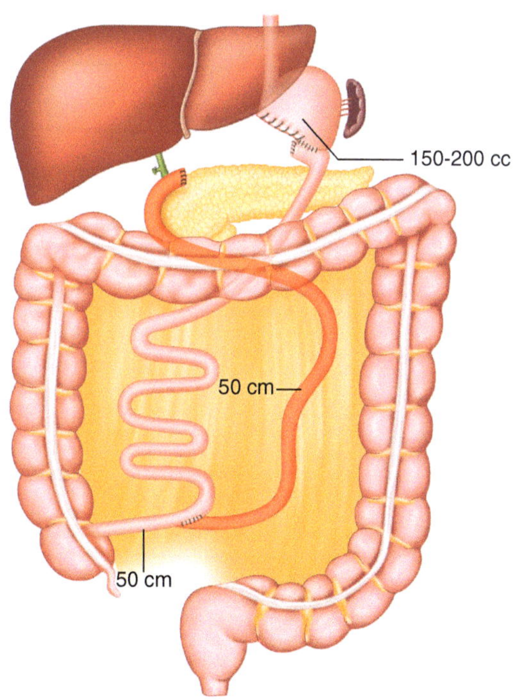

Fig. 20.4 Larrad's biliopancreatic diversion

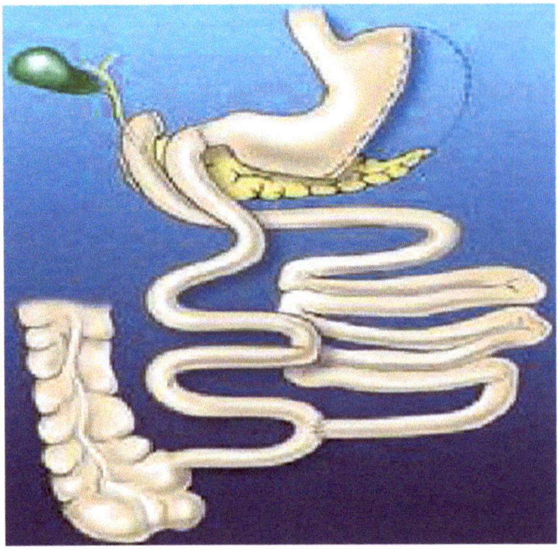

Fig. 20.5 BPD with sleeve gastrectomy and duodenal switch (BPD/DS) [9]

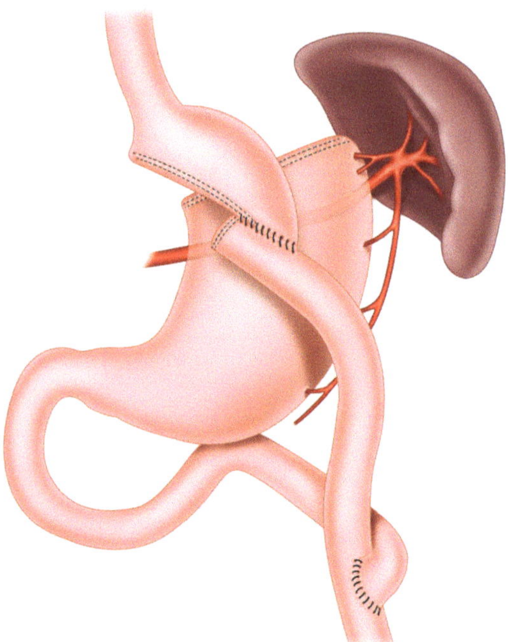

Fig. 20.6 Miller's divided gastric bypass, 1979

example is Roux-Y gastric bypass, where, even in its classic version with short BPL and AL [11–13] (Fig. 20.6), the meeting between food and biliopancreatic juices is delayed. In this operation it is generally assumed that the mechanism for calorie absorption reduction is ineffective, because the length of the CL is such that a complete calorie-rich aliment occurs. This is only partially true, as in many subjects with standard RYGB we have found a mild to moderate steatorrhea, in most cases confined to the first postoperative year. Anyway, it seems that the BPD mechanism is active, the threshold for intestinal fat absorption being exceeded, even if only minimally and temporarily, and that the initial weight reduction after RYGB is initially at least partially due to calorie malabsorption. The close similarity of RYGB to BPD is witnessed by the many surgeons who, with the very questionable aim of adding energy malabsorption to gastric restriction, use longer AL, or BPL, or both, thus originating operations called "distal GB" [14], or "long-limb GB" [15, 16], or even "very very long-limb GB" [17]. These operations, prompted by poor knowledge of the BPD mechanism, are very dangerous, because it was repeatedly demonstrated that to add malabsorption to gastric restriction is either just useless or even harmful for protein nutrition [14, 18].

Another evident case of misunderstanding is the so-called mini-gastric bypass or MGB, which should be more correctly and meaningfully named "single anastomosis GB" or "loop GB." Pioneered by Rutledge [19], MGB consists of a GB where the pouch is created much longer than usual (to prevent esophageal reflux), and the Roux-Y anastomosis is replaced by a loop one, placed in all cases 200 cm distal to the ligament of Treitz, with the aim of sparing one enteroenterostomy. The operation was severely criticized in the USA, but it is being increasingly performed in many non-American countries, where the authors generally report the same good weight loss result as in the standard RYGB, but with less complications and shorter hospital stay. Interestingly, with the exception of Sanchez-Pernaute [20], who replaced the classic gastric pouch with a sleeve gastrectomy in order to avoid also gastric bile reflux (Fig. 20.7), none of the surgeons who perform MGB (including the originator) seems to have realized that the operation is a BPD, already published as such by Scopinaro in 1980 [21] as one of the possible versions of the standard BPD (Fig. 20.8), where no AL exists, as the gastric remnant directly empties into the common

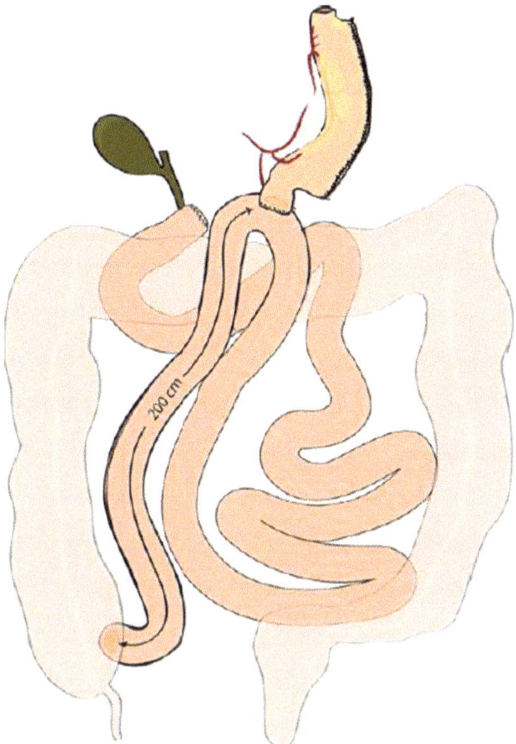

Fig. 20.7 Single anastomosis duodeno-ileal bypass with sleeve gastrectomy (SADI-S, 2010)

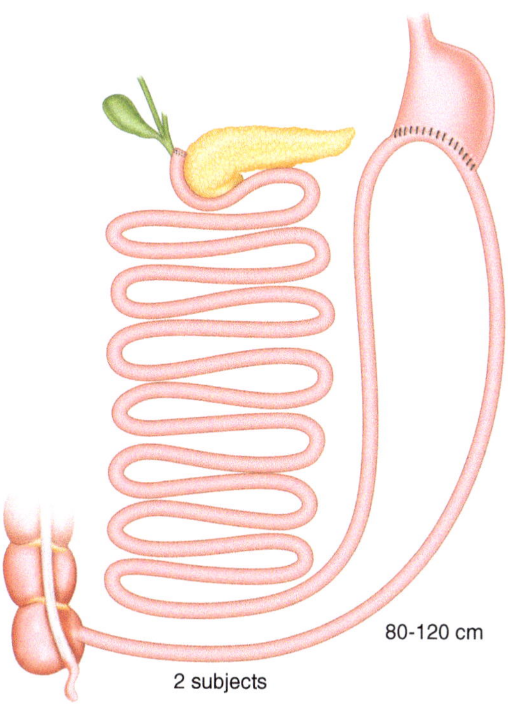

Fig. 20.8 Scopinaro's 1980 standard biliopancreatic diversion (bypass) with loop gastroenterostomy

limb, which, also exerting the functions of the AL, determines the existence, the quality, and the entity of malabsorption, and consequently is the one that should be measured. As almost no surgeon measures the small bowel in condition of full reproducibility, that is fully stretched, in case of short small bowel (e.g., around 400 cm, which is not a very infrequent case), the 200 cm that Rutledge and the vast majority of the other authors measure distal to the ligament of Treitz, thus totally ignoring what is left distal to the GEA, could very well leave them with a common limb, whose length is not known to the surgeon, short enough to cause severe energy and protein malnutrition.

An interesting example of unacknowledged BPD is the so-called endobarrier gastrointestinal liner [22], a short intraluminal sleeve anchored to the pylorus that delays the meeting of food with biliopancreatic juices, thus causing a certain degree of energy malabsorption and consequent weight loss. The device, 60–100 cm long, can be left in place only temporarily (generally 6 months), and it is used today to obtain a pre-surgical weight loss prior to bariatric surgery.

Evidently, the number of different types of BPD (laparoscopic or not) currently in use today is so huge that a description of each of them would be as impossible as useless. Therefore, we will only describe the technical aspects, the clinical management, and the outcome of the laparoscopic standard BPD (LSBPD) in our experience of little less than 300, and as reported by the few bariatric surgeons who used the same model of operation (laparoscopic or not).

20.2 Technical Aspects

The surgical technique [23] entails the use of five trocars, placed in the positions illustrated in Fig. 20.9. The patient is placed in a moderate anti-Trendelenburg position (20–25°). As a rule, we prefer to do first the cholecystectomy, which can be annoying due to the non standard trocar positions. The gastrocolic ligament is incised at about its midpoint and

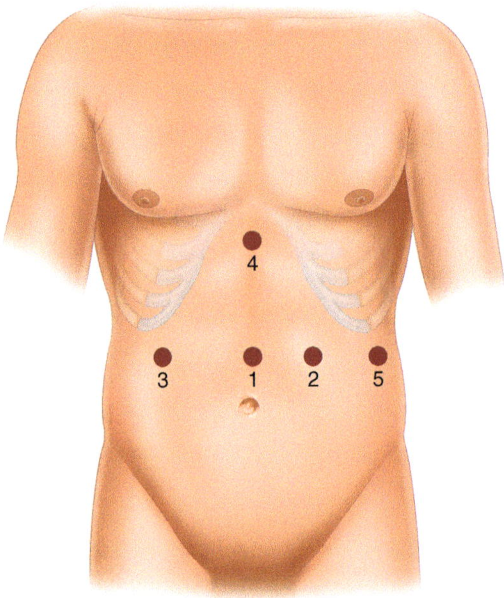

Fig. 20.9 Trocar position in laparoscopic standard BPD. *1*: supraumbilical (10–12 mm), on the midline, 3–4 cm above the superior margin of the umbilicus; *2*: left hypondriac (10–12 mm), along the left midclavicular line, about 6 cm below the costal margin; *3*: right hypondriac (10–12 mm), along the right midclavicular line, about 6 cm below the costal margin; *4*: xiphoid (10–12 mm), on the midline, 3 cm below the xiphoid; *5*: left subcostal (5 mm), on the left costal margin, along the left middle axillary line

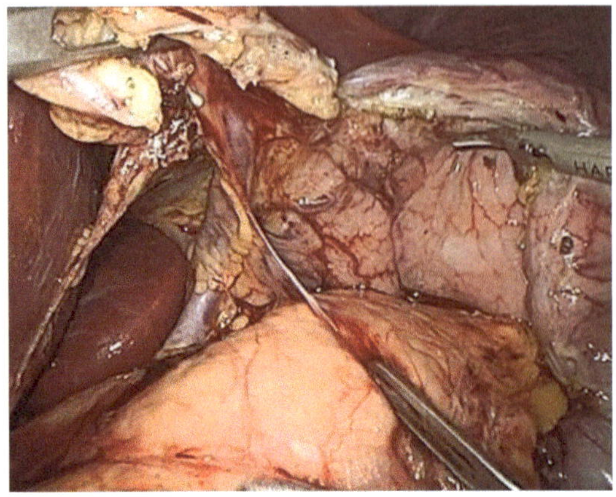

Fig. 20.10 Left gastric vessels

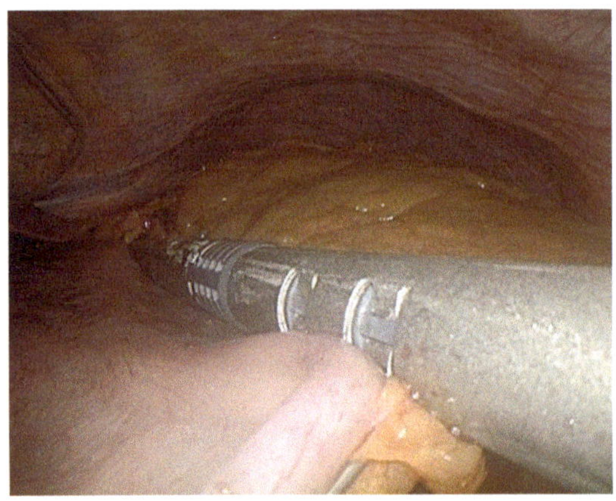

Fig. 20.11 Gastric measurement along the greater curve

the dissection, which is carried out with a harmonic scalpel, is performed until the traction of the large curve allows for the mobilization of the gastric fundus, which implies that the avascular area is always sectioned. The first short vessel is rarely sectioned, exceptionally the second. The dissection of the lower greater curve and the sectioning of the right gastroepiploic and the right gastric vessels complete the isolation of the duodenum, which is divided with single application of endoGIA 60. The small curve is then isolated cranially with the ultrasound scissors, stopping 1 or 2 cm before the trunk of the left gastric artery (Fig. 20.10), and the gastric resection is carried out by repeated firing of endoGIA 60. To measure the gastric stump is very easy by filling with water (35 cm H_2O) a condom which has been tied at the end of a nasogastric tube. Gastric volume should be measured until the surgeon becomes able to evaluate it by sight. Roughly, a gastric sectioning from the greater curve, moderately stretched, at approximately 15 cm from the cardias (Fig. 20.11) to the lesser curve at 5 cm from the cardias corresponds to a gastric volume of about 300 mL (Fig. 20.12). A distance of 20 cm along the greater curve corresponds to a volume of about 400 mL. This applies both to the laparoscopic and the open technique, as it was demonstrated by a check done in all cases of conversion (which, being due to problems with the GEA construction, was generally done after division of the stomach) at the beginning of our experience with the laparoscopic technique, when we started measuring again the gastric volume in order to reacquire the ability the gastric stump [23].

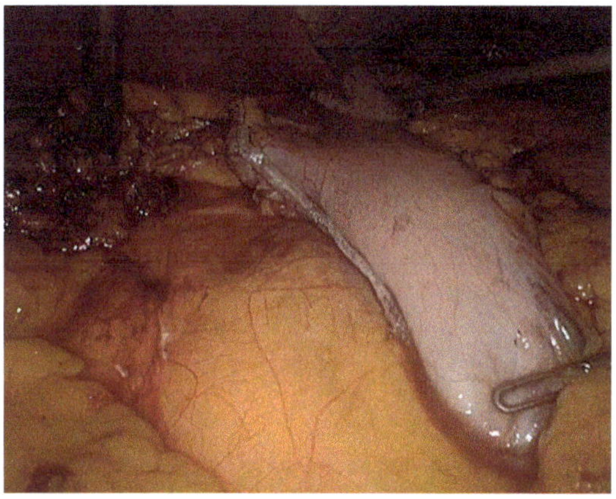

Fig. 20.12 Gastric stump of approximately 300 mL

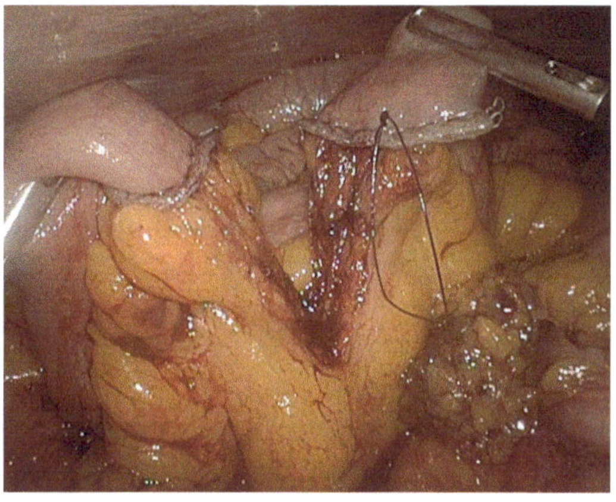

Fig. 20.13 Ileal division

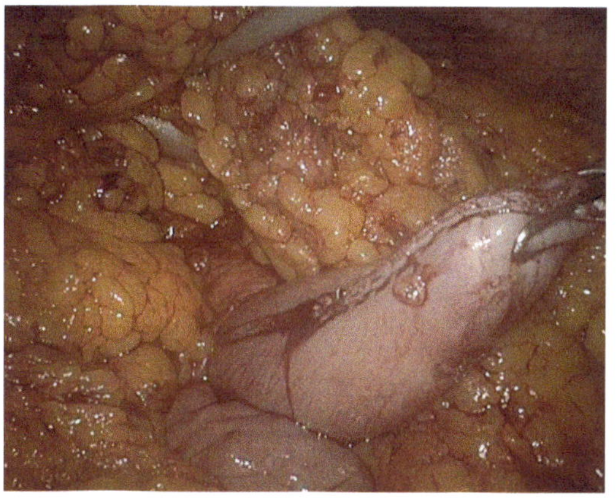

Fig. 20.14 Gastric stump attraction through the mesocolic rent

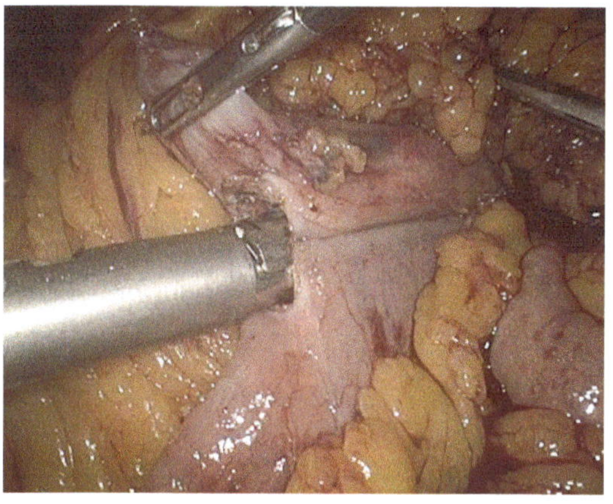

Fig. 20.15 Gastroenteroanastomosis

The patient is then placed in a slightly Trendelenburg position (about 10°). The small bowel is measured backward from the cecum, fully stretched (Fig. 20.3), using two forceps marked at 10 cm in alternating movements. A mark is left at 50 cm, the ileum is divided at 300 cm by using an endoGIA 45, and the mesentery is sectioned in depth with the ultrasonic scissors, taking care to proceed perpendicularly to its root (Fig. 20.13). The EEA is fashioned with a latero-lateral technique, with an endoGIA 45 through two small enterotomies made by the harmonic scalpel. The conjoined defect is closed with a manual running seromuscular suture.

The left angle of the gastric stump is then identified, grasped, and pulled into the submesocolic space through an incision performed in the transverse mesocolon over the ligament of Treitz (Fig. 20.14). The distal intestinal stump is identified, checked for possible torsion, and perforated with the ultrasonic scissors at a distance from the suture line equal to the operative length of the endoGIA 45. The latter is used to perform a latero-lateral isoperistaltic GEA on the posterior wall of the stomach, as close as possible to the distal angle and at midway between the suture line and the greater curve (Fig. 20.15), with manual closure of the conjoined defect. After the leak test with methylene blue introduced through the nasogastric tube, the GEA is anchored by two stitches to the mesocolic rent, in order to avoid intestinal kinkings and internal hernias (Fig. 20.16). We always close the distal mesenteric defect and never the proximal one (Patterson).

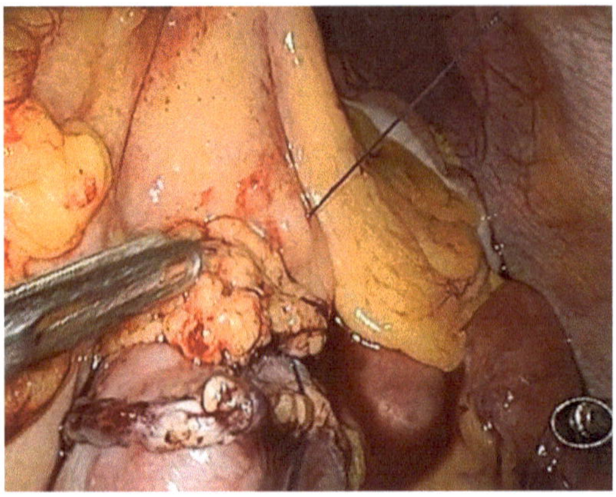

Fig. 20.16 Fixation of the GEA to the mesocolic rent

A liver wedge biopsy is always obtained. The last maneuver, as in open surgery, is the final intestinal check, starting from the ileocecal valve, with the surgeon following the AL and the first aid the BPL. It takes time, but it is the only way to make sure that no 360° intestinal torsion exists. As an alternative, the two mesenteric edges are carefully inspected from the anastomoses to the start of the mesenteric division.

The distal stomach, as well as the gallbladder, is extracted through the supraumbilical opening, which sometimes needs to be widened. Two drains are left in the Douglas pouch and under the liver. The trocars are removed under visual control. The fascial defect is sutured in the supraumbilical hole. The others are left as they are, with simple skin suturing.

As to the possible modifications of gastric volume and intestinal lengths, being similar all the other conditions, a larger gastric remnant generally, but not necessarily, results in a higher weight of stabilization, and certainly in a lower risk of protein malnutrition. It can be used precautionally in patients with lower compliance, never forgetting that low compliance should be considered in principle a contraindication to BPD, or in case of low BMI type 2 diabetic or hypercholesterolemic patients, when the aim of the operation is the exploitation of the specific actions for those conditions, with little or no weight loss (see below). On the contrary, a smaller gastric volume results in a more rapid weight loss with lower stabilization weight. The lower acceptable limit for gastric volume is about 300 mL (Fig. 20.12), as a smaller stomach has proven, in our [2, 18, 24] and in other authors' experience [14], to entail a great risk of energy-protein malnutrition (PEM).

It is very important to remember that the small bowel is to be measured fully stretched, midway between the mesenteric and the antimesenteric border (Figs. 20.2 and 20.3), in order to make the measurements reproducible both in the sane and in different hands. At the beginning of our experience with laparoscopic BPD, when the conversions to open surgery were more frequent, a check of intestinal lengths measured after conversion never showed a difference greater than 10 % between the two measurements [23], so, at least in our experience, we can refer to the intestinal lengths independently of the conditions (open or laparoscopic) in which the measurements were done. The length of 250 cm for the AL is the results of decades of experience, and should not be changed, unless a longer AL is requested to reduce to the minimum the weight loss, as in the above mentioned particular indications. An AL shorter than 250 cm entails a progressively increasing risk of PEM.

The CL length of 50 cm has been our gold standard since the completion of the early experimental phase, and it has remained the same during more than 30 years, always giving excellent and indefinitely maintained weight results. However, it demonstrated to be incompatible with a gastric volume smaller than 300 mL, the so-called very little stomach BPD causing, besides a 90 % loss of the excess weight, an incidence of 30 % PEM, with more than 10 % recurrent form requiring surgical revision [2, 18, 24]. This was confirmed by Sugerman et al. [14] who had overwhelming PEM problems when, leaving the very small gastric pouch, they converted standard RYGB into BPD with 200 cm AL and 50 cm CL (so-called distal gastric bypass). In our experience with BPD evolution, the progressive enlargement of the gastric remnant brought the PEM down to around 3 % with 1 % recurrence rate, and the additional lengthening of the AL from 200 to 250 cm made this important nutritional complication to essentially disappear, still leaving the permanent loss of the excess weight around 70 % [24]. With similar more than 300 mL gastric remnant, Clare [25] reported good results with 50 cm CL and equal AL and BPL (as our "half-half" BPD [26]), with little less weight loss than the standard model and only 2 % of hypoproteinemia. The same good results were obtained by Marceau [27] with the 50 cm CL standard BPD. Still, the problems remained of side effects, mainly represented by diarrhea, present in 13 % of operated patients.

More recently, Garcia et al. [28] compared standard BPD (50 CL – 200 AL cm) with a modified version (75–225 cm), showing an astonishing fall of malnutrition from 16 to 2 %, with slight lower weight loss. These findings go into the same direction of the preliminary ones of a prospective randomized trial we are carrying out on our patients, where a 75 cm CL results in modest reduction of weight loss accompanied by a significant reduction of side effects, mainly diarrhea but also gas problems and foul smelling stools.

For the rest, different intestinal lengths were used in modified RYGB in order to achieve a greater weight loss, especially in the super-obese patients. To understand what the authors actually did is made difficult due to the apparently different semantics they use when defining the intestinal limbs. First, Brolin et al. in 1992 proposed the "long-limb" RYGB [15], consisting of a "defunctionalized jejunum" (and then a BPL) of 150 cm compared with a BPL of 75 cm. The first operation caused a greater weight loss when compared to the second one only in the super-obese patients, when weight loss did not change in the morbidly obese ones. These results were confirmed by MacLean et al. in 2001 [16] and subsequently by Brolin himself in 2005 [29]. The confusion arises when the "very very long limb" RYGB is considered. This operation, described first by Murr et al. in 1999 [17] and then by Nelson et al. in 2006 [30], both belonging to the same group of the Mayo Clinic, Rochester, Minnesota, apparently consists of a gastric bypass with a short (60 cm) "pancreatobiliary limb," which evidently corresponds to what we call BPL, a 100-cm "common channel," and thus our CL, while all the rest of the small bowel, from the GEA to the EEA, ranging in length between 400 and 500 cm, which is evidently our AL, is named "Roux-limb." The authors refer to the Sugerman "distal gastric bypass" [14], who uses the same terminology, that is, "Roux-limb" = AL. Therefore, the Brolin and MacLean "long-limb" is apparently named "Roux-limb" and corresponds to the biliopancreatic limb (BPL), while the definition "Roux-limb" in the Sugerman distal gastric bypass and in the Rochester group "very very long limb" is evidently referred to the alimentary limb (AL). This gross semantic confusion, that I have repeatedly indicated as one of the greatest problems in bariatric surgery (I even wrote a chapter in the Deitel's book entitled "Semantics in obesity surgery" [31]), certainly does not help the reader to understand how these operations are structured, and, even less, how they work.

At the beginning of the introduction, when describing the BPD as a basic mechanism of action, we underlined that the mechanism is effective in causing a reduction, or, to say better, a limitation of calorie absorption only if the time of contact between food and biliopancreatic secretions is reduced enough to cause incomplete digestion and absorption of calorie rich aliment. At this point, in order to fully understand the importance of the intestinal limb lengths, it is important to remember that not necessarily the BPD operation causes weight loss. BPD simply leads the body weight to the value corresponding to the amount of daily calorie absorption which is allowed by its mechanism of action. As we said, there is for each BPD individual a maximum energy absorption capacity which, in that specific subject, if all the other conditions mentioned above remain constant, also remains constant and corresponds to a determined weight of stabilization. If the starting body weight of the BPD subject corresponds to a daily energy consumption higher than the operation energy absorption threshold, a negative calorie balance takes place causing the reduction of body weight which will stop only when the body energy expenditure will equal the energy absorption threshold. Assuming, for example, that the threshold is 1,600 kcal/day, corresponding to the body energy expenditure of 85 kg, the latter will be the weight of stabilization of that subject for that operation. Any starting body weight higher than this will be forced by the negative calorie balance to reduce to 85 kg, when the energy balance is reached between daily intestinal energy absorption and daily body energy expenditure. The result will be a weight loss equal to the starting body weight minus 85 kg. However, if the starting body weight is already stable at 85 kg, this means that the BPD individual is eating and consuming as much as the operation allows to absorb. Consequently, the operation causes no negative energy balance, neither weight change. The same obviously applies to the case of starting body weight lower than 85 kg. The BPD subject eats and consumes less energy than what the BPD allows to absorb, then again nothing would change in calorie balance and no weight change would occur.

BPD possesses some metabolic specific actions which are totally independent of the weight loss, the best known being the serum cholesterol lowering and the beneficial effect on glycemic control. Consequently, the morbidly obese patient, in case of hypercholesterolemia or type 2 diabetes mellitus, besides weight loss will also benefit of these two weight-independent actions. They depend on the structure of the operation, the first being due to the loss of bile salts in the colon, caused by the short segment of bile salt absorbing terminal ileum in continuity, which causes increased bile acid neosynthesis in the liver which happens at the expenses of the cholesterol pool. The beneficial action on type 2 diabetes, first reported by us in 1984 [26], is caused by hormonal changes due to the bypass of the duodenum and by the presence of aliments in the ileum. If these anatomic conditions are preserved, the two beneficial specific actions remain active also in case of no weight loss. Therefore, the operation is precious, because it can be used for the treatment of hypercholesterolemia and of type 2 diabetes mellitus also in lean individuals, with no risk of undue weight loss. In those cases, as we do not know which the exact value of energy absorption threshold will be, in order not to take the risk of undue weight loss, we deliberately increase its level by elongating by 50 cm both the CL and the AL, which become 100 and 300 cm, respectively, thus obtaining the preservation of the above specific actions with minimal or no weight loss at all [24, 32]. Obviously, in these conditions, an increase of energy intake would cause weight gain, but this only exceptionally happens, and the same applies to the hypothetical weight gain resulting from the better glycemic homeostasis.

In conclusion, the good knowledge and the wise use of the intestinal limbs absorption characteristics makes BPD an extremely ductile operation, as it can operate in such a wide range of action that it can cause from the greatest weight loss obtainable with any bariatric operation down to even no weight loss at all, still maintaining its specific actions, like the two mentioned above.

20.3 Clinical Management

20.3.1 Postoperative Management

One single antibiotic shot is given preoperatively, when thromboembolic prophylaxis is started, that is continued for the entire first postoperative month. The patient is ambulating the day of operation. Analgesia consists of morphine and ketorolac by means of a continuous delivery system for 3 days, with paracetamol on demand. Metoclopramide is administered routinely together with intravenous fluids, that is, 3 days.

NG tube is removed on the first postoperative morning. GEA transit is checked on the 2nd day by X-ray oral contrast (leak diagnosis is based on clinical signs). Clear liquids are allowed on the 3rd day, when i.v. fluids are discontinued. Solid food is given within the first week, according to the gastric emptying as shown by X-ray check. Patients are discharged on 4th or 5th day (the vast majority of them live far from Genoa).

Patients are called for routine follow-up visits (with all the laboratory exams done) at 1, 4, 12, 24, and 36 months. Subsequently, they are not called anymore, but strongly recommended to continue coming yearly, or at least sending their complete lab exams by fax or e-mail.

PPI are prescribed for 1 year, oral Fe, Ca (2 g/day), and multivitamins for life. The minimum daily protein intake recommended is 90 g/day.

Patients are encouraged to call us for any unpleasant clinical symptoms, even if judged not important. Our availability by phone is 24 h for life.

In the patients with type 2 diabetes as the main or the only indication to surgery the postoperative management is essentially the same, with the addition of oral glucose tolerance test (OGTT) or acute insulin response to intravenous glucose load (AIR), or both, plus frequent controls of serum glucose level.

20.4 Outcomes

BPD has many aspects that makes it the opposite of what could be considered the ideal operation for a bariatric surgeon. It requires a very accurate patient selection, especially as far as compliance is concerned; it is relatively difficult to perform, even if the laparoscopic approach, at least up to a BMI of about 50, facilitates some of its technical steps; it gives origin to a huge number of micronutrient and vitamin potential deficiencies, requiring lifelong supplementation; finally, it is the possible cause of the most dangerous nutritional complications in bariatric surgery, that is the hypoalbuminemic form of protein-energy malnutrition (PEM), a problem that can be prevented up to near disappearance only at the price of an accurate lifetime surveillance which represents a heavy engagement both for the patient and the person in charge for follow-up, generally the surgeon.

On the other side, BPD is the bariatric operation which yields far the best weight loss results, being able to obtain a satisfactory weight reduction in the vast majority of the super-obese patients (BMI >50 kg/m) [2], as well as to guarantee an indefinite weight maintenance. Furthermore, it is the operation with the best metabolic effects, and the best procedure for conversional surgery, especially when multiple other operations have failed.

Consequently, the bariatric surgeon is not eager to perform BPD, but he is obliged to use it in case of super, and especially super-superobesity (BMI >60), in case of severe metabolic complications, especially type 2 diabetes, in case of single or multiple failure of previous bariatric operations, and in case of very young patients. This last indication is controversial; however, we have no doubts that the solution of such a major problem for the entire life is well worth all the possible risks (generally limited to the first postoperative years) entailed by the only operation able to yield an excellent weight loss result maintained for 50 years or more. On the contrary, a 60-year-old patient will be very happy with an operation which can give him a satisfactory 5–6 year long weight reduction, with good quality of life, resolution of comorbidities, and no risk of late complications or rehospitalization, even if this will be followed by a slow weight regain, which can be anyway reasonably controlled.

The result is that the majority of bariatric surgeons have BPD in their armamentarium, but they do very few cases, generally obtaining good weight loss results, which are unavoidable if the right technique is used, but never reaching the experience that is necessary to avoid complications. The series are small, the follow-up is short, and the overall results not such as to justify a clinical publication. We were able to find less than 30 published articles on standard BPD, most regarding initial experience [33–36], specific studies in small series, such as diabetes surgery [37–39], hormonal research studies [40–44], reports of exceptional complications [45–49], or comparisons between standard versus differently modified intestinal limb lengths [50, 51]. Moreover, the majority of these publications refer to the operation done in open surgery, so that, in order to have a minimum of published material to refer to for comparison with our experience, all the material found was reported in this chapter independently of the open or laparoscopic adopted technique.

Therefore, the only way to describe standard LBPD outcome is to report results and complications of our large series of patients, occasionally reporting other authors' data (laparoscopic or not) when it is of some clinical interest.

20.4.1 Follow-up Rate

Follow-up rate reflects the outcome of your patients' population only if a direct contact is established with the near totality of your patients and biochemistry values are obtained for each of them. Therefore, even tracking all operated patients every year can result in a poor, and thus meaningless follow-up rate, due to the patients' mobility, which, in countries like the USA, can prevent all attempts to have a reliable image of your operated patients' population. One of the many other possible biases is the geographic distance and the diffusion of the bariatric surgery, which can push the patient to find a closer surgeon to take care of him in case of necessity. Patient's expectation can also affect the meaning of the follow-up rate. If the patient is aware of the high probability of failure to lose weight or of weight regain, in case this happens there is no reason to complain with the surgeon, while if good weight loss results were expected the patient goes to the surgeon to ask the why of the failure. In this perspective a patient with gastric banding lost to follow-up is probably a failure, while the opposite may be true for a BPD patient.

We call our operation patients up to the third year, assuming then that if they do not show up this probably means that they are happy with the results. Therefore, our poor 20 years follow-up includes both patients with late postoperative problems, generally caused by long-term deficiencies, and those who, as the vast majority of them live very far from us (generally in the southern Italy), occasionally pass near to Genoa and take the occasion to come and visit us, to say hello, thank you, and to show how good are their results. They tell us about their operated friends, and this, compared with the small number of patients who contact us for any complaint, can be considered as an indirect demonstration that the vast majority of our operated patients do not have significant long-term problems.

An exception is represented by our patients operated on because of type 2 diabetes, where we have another substantial indirect proof that the near totality of our many operated patients at very long term are well and have satisfactory weight loss results. The 100 % follow-up rate in this group is simply due to the fact they are not so many and we are very interested in their results, so we call all of them at least once a year, we find them, and they are happy to come to Genoa to get reassured that everything is going well with their "special" operation.

Something similar explains the why of the excellent 67 % follow-up rate we have with our laparoscopically operated patients. Especially those who were operated a relatively long time ago, when the laparoscopic approach was not so common for major surgery, feel their surgical event as something "special," so they tend to come to us much more often than the others, with a 67 % follow-up rate at 10 years very similar to the 61 % at 20 years we had when we called all of our very old BPD morbidly obese type 2 diabetic patients. The patients where T2DM was the main or the only indication to LBPD were all included in prospective controlled or randomized controlled studies and they have a maximum 6-year follow-up with 100 % follow-up rate.

20.4.2 Case Material and Weight Loss Results

Our 290 LBPD patients (70 M, mean age 39 ± 16 years), operated on from April 2000 to June 2014 for morbid obesity, had a mean preoperative weight of 125.9 ± 13.7, with a mean BMI of 45.7 ± 4.4. Mean BMI and % loss of the IEW at 1, 3, and 10 years were, respectively, 30.9 ± 3.6 with 66.0 ± 16,6 % (mean follow-up rate 100 %), 29.8 ± 3.6 with 68.2 ± 15.1 % (93.3 %), and 29.6 ± 4.0 with 68.4 ± 17.4 % (67.3 %).

The mean reduction of the IEW is slightly smaller when compared with that obtained in open surgery (~70 %). This is most probably due to the great care taken in order not to provoke any intestinal damage when stretching it for measurements, resulting in slightly longer alimentary and common limb.

Interestingly, the initial BMI of the 655 (264 M) patients operated on in open surgery after starting the use of laparoscopic approach, was 52.5±7.3, which is much higher than the 47±9.2 unselected patients operated on before, that is in turn higher than the 45.7±4.4 in the laparoscopic series.

The improvement of our laparoscopic technical skill is indicated by the fact that the mean BMI of our first 50 laparoscopic patients was 42.8, versus the mean BMI of 49.6 of the last 50 operated patients.

In another 52 patients, operated on from May 2007, the indication was mild obesity (BMI 30–34.9) and type 2 diabetes, with mean BMI 33.1±2.0. Finally, 47 T2DM nonobese patients (BMI 25–29.9) underwent LBPD from July 2007, with a mean BMI of 27.7±1.9. Those groups, in a maximum 6-year follow-up stabilized around BMI 27 and 26, respectively.

20.4.3 Perioperative Complications

Conversion to open surgery was less than 5 %, the more frequent causes being hepatomegalia and anesthetic problems. Early complications were GEA edema (only exceptionally frank ulcer) 8 %, always resolved with intravenous PPI administration, rhabdomyolysis (CPK >1,000 mg/dL) 20 %, treated by massive hydratation, without any renal problems, intraperitoneal bleeding 1 %, two cases of GEA leak, and one case of nonfatal pulmonary embolism. Overall operative mortality was 0.3 %.

20.4.4 Beneficial and Unpleasant Side Effects

The other benefits of BPD in our population at 1, 3, and 10 years, together with the preoperative incidence of the condition, are listed in Table 20.1, while unpleasant side effects are reported together with late complications in Table 20.2.

Sleep apnea syndrome, Pickwickian syndrome, and somnolence are quickly resolved after standard LBPD, as already observed with the open operation. Similarly, hypercholesterolemia early disappears and hypertriglyceridemia, though much reduced, is still present only in a small minority of cases. Differently, arterial hypertension gradually reduces but, though greatly reduced in all cases, still exists in a sizeable percent of cases at 10 years, and, as expected due to the chronic damages in many cases, leg stasis shows an immediate disappearance in less than half of cases, and then improves with time but is only modestly reduced or even unchanged in some patients at long term. On the contrary, as it is the rule in the morbidly obese patients, type 2 diabetes quickly disappears at short time in the near totality of patients. The use of LBPD for the treatment of T2DM in nonobese

Table 20.1 Other beneficial effects of BPD

	Pre-op.	1 year	3 years	10 years
Follow-up rate (%)		100	93	67
Sleep apnea syndrome (%)	25	0	0	0
Pickwickian syndrome[a] (%)	2	0	0	0
Somnolence[b] (%)	8	0	0	0
Hypertension[c] (%)	62	13	9	10
Leg stasis[d] (%)	43	23	17	18
Hypercholesterolemia[e] (%)	58	1	0.5	1
Hypertiglyceridemia[f] (%)	31	4	3	3
Type 2 diabetes[g] (%)	22	0.3	0.3	1

[a]Somnolence with cyanosis, polycythemia, and hypercapnia
[b]In absence of one or more features of the Pickwickian syndrome
[c]Systolic pressure ≥140 mmHg, diastolic pressure ≥90 mmHg
[d]Moderate or severe
[e]More than 200 mg/dL
[f]More than 150 mg/dL
[g]ADA definition

Table 20.2 Unpleasant side effects and late complications of BPD

	Pre-op.	1 year	3 years	10 years
Follow-up rate (%)		100	93	67
Anemia[a] (%)	0	7	8	14
Stomal ulcer (%)	0	6	1	1
Intestinal obstruction (%)	0	1	1	1
Diarrhea (%)	0	1	1	1
Meteorism (%)	0	17	4	1
Foul smelling stools (%)	0	6	1	1

[a]Hb ≤10 mg/dlc

patients will be described below. As to the negative effects of BPD, diarrhea is almost absent already by the first year, while a nice surprise is offered by the changes in meteorism and foul smelling stools, which, though being unavoidable consequences of malabsorption, are strongly reduced at 3 years and reported as a problem only in few cases at long term, generally due to adaptation of the eating habits. On the contrary, again as expectable, all problems of iron, calcium, and vitamin deficiencies inexorably increase in incidence with time.

Preoperative comorbidity is lower, and postoperative comorbidity resolution is better, as it happens with postoperative unpleasant side-effect severity and long-term reduction, when the laparoscopic series is compared with the population of patients operated on in open surgery. This is easily explained by the fact that the super-obese patients are generally excluded from laparoscopic approach. The lower mean BMI in the laparoscopic group, since the maximum absorption capacity and the consequent weight of stabilization are more or less the same, causes a lower degree of malabsorption with all the malabsorption consequences being obviously reduced. Needless to say, this especially applies to the cases where type 2 diabetes is the main or the only indication to LBPD.

20.4.5 Metabolic Effects

The two main specific actions of BPD, that on serum cholesterol and that on type 2 diabetes, were synthetically mentioned above. In reality, all bariatric procedures have a beneficial effect on T2DM, simply because they reduce body fat, which is mainly responsible for insulin resistance. As BPD is the procedure with the greatest weight reduction effect, this would be already sufficient to make it the most effective among the bariatric operations on glycemic control [52]. However, insulin resistance alone would not be able to cause diabetes in presence of a healthy beta-cell, which can increase indefinitely its insulin production, thus counteracting the resistance caused by any amount of body fat and maintaining normoglycemia. This is why only about 20 % of the morbidly obese patients are diabetic. The real problem of type 2 diabetes is a beta-cell more or less genetically damaged, with a limited capacity to increase insulin secretion. When beta-cell becomes unable to effectively counteract the insulin resistance caused to the increasing amount of body fat, diabetes occur, which can be defeated only by increasing the insulin production capacity of the endocrine pancreas. Unfortunately, medical therapy has in metformin a powerful weapon against insulin resistance, but there are not drugs active on beta-cell function. On the contrary, both gastric bypass and biliopancreatic diversion have proven to possess a beneficial action on beta-cell, which is mainly based on food stimulation of the ileum to produce GLP-1, a powerful incretin (gut hormone able to stimulate insulin secretion by the beta-cell) which demonstrated to possess the capacity not only to increase insulin production [53] even by the genetically damaged beta-cell, but even to increase the beta-cell mass, by stimulating regeneration [54] and reducing apoptosis [55], all this independently of weight loss. Therefore, while the antidiabetic effect of all bariatric operation gradually reduces with reduction of body weight, RYGB and BPD exert their weight-independent action also in nonobese diabetic patients. It must be said that, comprehensibly, the lower the initial body weight the greater the beta-cell damage, with the ones of the nonobese diabetic patient being so weak that they cannot effectively counteract the very small insulin resistance produced by the corresponding minimal amount of fat. Since RYGB on one side possesses a smaller capacity of GLP-1 food stimulation, thus being essentially ineffective on the very damaged beta-cell of the nonobese patient, on the other side it could not be employed in these patients due to the risk of causing severe underweight. On the contrary, GLP-1 food stimulation is maximal in BPD, where the stomach directly empties in the ileum, and, as we saw, BPD can be transformed, by lengthening the CL and the AL, into an operation which does not cause weight loss, still maintaining its specific effect on glycemic control. In conclusion BPD, far the most effective antidiabetes bariatric operation [56] is today the only weapon we possess to beneficially act on nonobese diabetic patients. Its effect is smaller than that in the morbidly obese patients, where, in a large series of 443 preoperatively diabetic patients, due to the very good response of an only slightly damaged beta-cell, 97 % were normoglycemic at 1 and 10 years, and 91 % at 20 years, with a very good 61 % follow-up rate [57]; the BPD effect is less good in the nonobese patients not because its action is reduced, but because the beta-cell response is much weaker. Nonetheless, BPD proven able to obtain at 5 years diabetes remission (HbA1c ≤6 %) or control (HbA1c ≤7 %) in 60 % of an unselected (mean BMI 28.0, HbA1c 9.4 %, diabetes duration 14 years, preoperative insulin therapy 60 %) population of 15 diabetic nonobese patients, all the other operated patients having anyway considerably improved. If we only consider the seven patients in this group with diabetes duration lower than 10 years, the percent of remission plus control goes up to 100 %. Interestingly, all but one of those seven patients were not on insulin before operation. Similarly, if we consider the eight patients in the same group on preoperative oral therapy, success was obtained in seven of them or 88 %. It is then possible to obtain excellent results with BPD also in the nonobese patients, but only at the price of selecting the lower risk subjects.

20.4.6 Late Complications

Stomal ulcer was observed in up to 6 % of cases. Its incidence is essentially concentrated in the first postoperative years but it can occur also at long term, especially in the smokers. The prevalence of marginal ulcer after BPD is certainly largely underestimated, due to the prompt use of PPI by the family doctors without endoscopic diagnosis confirmation.

Supraumbilical incisional hernia is probably also underestimated, having been observed in 10 % of cases. Internal hernia was never observed in our series, most likely due to the mesocolic rent well closed by the fixation to the GEA, and to the deep mesenteric incision which prevents the occurrence of tension in the Petterson space, which is never closed at operation.

An interesting complication were two cases of portal vein thrombosis which caused severe small bowel necrosis starting from the ligament of Treitz and ending before the enteroenterostomy, thus allowing the complete salvage of the operation by resecting the whole biliopancreatic limb and creating a temporary short jejunostomy, with subsequent reconnection of the BPL to the AL. A third similar case was immediately and successfully treated with massive heparin therapy and did not require operation.

20.4.7 Deficiencies

Laparoscopic BPD was started when the alimentary limb had already been lengthened to 250 cm, which, together with our more than 30 year experience, caused the almost disappearance of the most dangerous complication. In fact only two cases of PEM (one recurrent requiring elongation) were observed in our series of LBPD.

On the contrary, as already reported above, all problems of iron, calcium, and vitamin deficiencies progressively increase with time.

For detailed information of all possible LBPD macro- and micronutrient deficiencies, compared with other operations, as well as of protein malnutrition and its physiology, see Chap. 27 in this book.

20.4.8 Reoperations

No conversions to other type of surgery were done so far in our laparoscopic BPD series, nor any restoration was necessary. The only reoperation was an elongation of the common limb which was necessary in a case of recurrent hypoalbuminemic form of protein-energy malnutrition.

Conclusions

Biliopancreatic diversion is unanimously considered the surgical procedure that yields the best weight loss and metabolic results in bariatric surgery. Differently from all other bariatric procedures, the actions of BPD are lifelong, and consequently its beneficial effects are also for a lifetime. However, for the same reason, the negative effects of BPD are also for life, and this must be very clear both to the surgeon and the patient.

BPD gives origin to a long list of potential micro- and macronutrient deficiencies which, if not prevented, may cause severe nutritional complications. Moreover, some of its unpleasant side effects are strictly connected with the functioning of the operation. Therefore, they can greatly reduce with time, but never totally disappear.

On one hand, patients undergoing BPD must be carefully informed that they will need micronutrient supplementation for the entire life, and guarantee a lifelong minimum protein and calcium intake. The noncompliance with these rules may result in even lethal complications, and this is the price to be paid for the indefinite beneficial effect of the operation.

On the other hand, the surgeon who wants to use BPD must first of all learn all the details of its mechanisms of actions and of its possible negative consequences. Then, he takes the responsibility of selecting highly compliant patients, of carefully informing them of their future requirements and responsibilities, and of being prepared to an indefinite follow-up, which may need to be an active one in case of risky situations. Finally, the surgeon must make sure that, in case of his inability to take care of his patients, somebody else will do it, without forgetting that the interdisciplinary team may be of enormous help to the surgeon, but it cannot replace him.

Great compliance on one side, and full availability on the other, will make a lean, healthy, happy, and safe operated subject.

References

1. Scopinaro N, Gianetta E, Civalleri D, Bonalumi U, Bachi V. Biliopancreatic bypass for obesity: II. Initial experience in man. Br J Surg. 1979;66:618–9.
2. Scopinaro N, Adami GF, Marinari GM, Gianetta E, Traverso E, Friedman D, Camerini G, Baschieri G, Simonelli A. Biliopancresatic diversion. World J Surg. 1998;22:936–46.
3. Bonalumi U, Cafiero F, Caponnetto A, Gianetta E, Reboa G, Civalleri D, Piccardo A, Berti Riboli E, Scopinaro N. Protein absorption studies in biliopancreatic bypass patients. Int J Obesity. 1981;5:543 (abstract).
4. Scopinaro N, Marinari GM, Camerini G, Pretolesi F, Papadia F, Murelli F, Marini P, Adami GF. Energy and nitrogen absorption after biliopancreatic diversion. Obes Surg. 2000;10:436–41.
5. Mortensen PB, Hove H, Clausen MR, Holtug K. Fermentation to short-chain fatty acids and lactate in human faecal batch cultures. Intra- and inter-individual variations versus variations caused by changes in fermented saccharides. Scand J Gastroenterol. 1991;26:1285–94.
6. Polyzogopoulou EV, Kalfarentzos F, Vagenakis AG, Alexandrides TK. Restoration of euglycemia and normal acute insulin response to glucose in obese subjects with type 2 diabetes following bariatric surgery. Diabetes. 2003;52:1098–103.
7. Vassallo C, Negri L, Della Valle A, Salvaneschi M, Vegezzi G, Griziotti A, Dono C, Mussi P, Bausardo MG, Pietrobono P. Biliopancreatic diversion with transitory gastroplasty preserving duodenal bulb: 3 years experience. Obes Surg. 1997;7:30–3.
8. Larrad-Jiménez A, Díaz-Guerra CS, de Cuadros Borrajo P, Lesmes IB, Esteban BM. Short-, mid- and long-term results of Larrad biliopancreatic diversion. Obes Surg. 2007;17(2):202–10.
9. Hess DS, Hess DW. Biliopancreatic diversion with a duodenal switch. Obes Surg. 1998;8:267–82.
10. Marceau P, Biron S, Bourque RA, Potvin M, Hould FS, Simard S. Biliopancreatic diversion with a new type of gastrectomy. Obes Surg. 1993;3:29–35.
11. Mason EE, Ito C. Gastric bypass in obesity. Surg Clin North Am. 1967;47:1345–51.
12. Griffen Jr WO. Gastric bypass for morbid obesity. Surg Clin North Am. 1979;59:1103–12.
13. Wittgrove AC, Clark GW. Laparoscopic gastric bypass, Roux-en-Y: preliminary report of five cases. Obes Surg. 1994;4:353–7.
14. Sugerman HJ, Kellum JM, DeMaria EJ. Conversion of proximal to distal gastric bypass for failed gastric bypass for superobesity. J Gastrointest Surg. 1997;6:517–24.

15. Brolin RE, Kenier HA, Gorman JH, Cody RP. Long-limb gastric bypass in the superobese. A prospective randomized study. Ann Surg. 1992;215:387–95.
16. MacLean LD, Rhode BM, Nohr CW. Long- or short-limb gastric bypass? J Gastrointest Surg. 2001;5:525–30.
17. Murr MM, Balsiger BM, Kennedy FP, Mail JL, Sarr MG. Malabsorptive procedures for severe obesity: comparison of pancreatobiliary bypass and very very long limb Roux-en-Y gastric bypass. J Gastrointest Surg. 1999;3:607–12.
18. Scopinaro N, Marinari G, Camerini G, Papadia F. Biliopancreatic diversion for obesity: state of the art (2004 ASBS Consensus Conference). Surg Obes Relat Dis. 2005;1:317–28.
19. Rutledge R. The mini-gastric bypass: experience with the first 1,274 cases. Obes Surg. 2001;11:276–80.
20. Sánchez-Pernaute A, Herrera MA, Pérez-Aguirre ME, Talavera P, Cabrerizo L, Matía P, Díez-Valladares L, Barabash A, Martín-Antona E, García-Botella A, Garcia-Almenta EM, Torres A. Single anastomosis duodeno-ileal bypass with sleeve gastrectomy (SADI-S). One to three year follow-up. Obes Surg. 2010;20:1720–6.
21. Scopinaro N, Gianetta E, Civalleri D, Bonalumi U, Bachi V. Two years of clinical experience with biliopancreatic bypass for obesity. Am J Clin Nutr. 1980;33:506–14.
22. Schouten R, Rijs CS, Bouvy ND, Hameeteman W, Koek GH, Janssen IM, Greve JW. A multicenter randomized efficacy study of the EndoBarrier Gastrointestinal Liner for presurgical weight loss prior to bariatric surgery. Ann Surg. 2010;216:236–43.
23. Scopinaro N, Marinari GM, Camerini G. Laparoscopic standard biliopancreatic diversion: technique and preliminary results. Obes Surg. 2002;12:241–4.
24. Scopinaro N. Thirty-five years of biliopancreatic diversion: notes on gastrointestinal physiology to complete the published information useful for a better understanding and clinical use of the operation. Obes Surg. 2012;22:427–32.
25. Clare MW. Equal biliopancreatic and alimentary limbs: an analysis of 106 cases over 5 years. Obes Surg. 1993;3:289–95.
26. Scopinaro N, Gianetta E, Friedman D, Adami GF, Traverso E, Bachi V. Evolution of biliopancreatic bypass. Clin Nutr. 1986;5:137–46. First international symposium on obesity surgery, Genoa, Italy, October 1984.
27. Marceau S, Biron S, Lagacé M, Hould FS, Potvin M, Bourque RA, Marceau P. Biliopancreatic diversion, with distal gastrectomy, 250 cm and 50 cm limbs: long-term results. Obes Surg. 1995;5:302–7.
28. Garcia JA, Martinez M, Aguilella V, Elia M, Royo P. Postoperative morbidity of biliopancreatic diversion depending on common limb length. Obes Surg. 2007;17:1306–11.
29. Brolin RE. Long limb Roux en Y gastric bypass revisited. Surg Clin North Am. 2005;5:807–17.
30. Nelson WK, Fatima J, Houghton SG, Thompson GB, Kendrick ML, Mai JL, Kennel KA, Sarr MG. The malabsorptive very, very long limb Roux-en-Y gastric bypass for super obesity: results in 257 patients. Surgery. 2006;140:517–22; discussion 522–3.
31. Scopinaro N. Physiology and semantics in obesity surgery. In: Deitel M, Cowan JR, editors. Update: surgery for the morbidly obese patients. Toronto: FD Communication Inc; 2000. p. 69–72.
32. Scopinaro N, Adami GF, Papadia FS, Camerini G, Carlini F, Briatore L, D'Alessandro G, Parodi C, Weiss A, Andraghetti G, Catalano M, Cordera R. The effects of biliopancreatic diversion on type 2 diabetes mellitus in patients with mild obesity (BMI 30–35 kg/m2) and simple overweight (BMI 25–30 kg/m2): a prospective controlled study. Obes Surg. 2011;21:880–8.
33. Paiva D, Bernardes L, Suretti L. Laparoscopic biliopancreatic diversion: technique and initial results. Obes Surg. 2002;12(3):358–61.
34. Resa JJ, Solano J, Fatás JA, Blas JL, Monzón A, García A, Lagos J, Escartin J. Laparoscopic biliopancreatic diversion: technical aspects and results of our protocol. Obes Surg. 2004;14:329–33.
35. de Luis DA, Pacheco D, Izaola O, Romero A, Marcos JL, Pelaz J, Barrera A, Cabezas G, Terroba MC, Cuellar L, Anta A. Early clinical and surgical results of biliopancreatic diversion. Obes Surg. 2005;15:799–802.
36. de Luis DA, Pacheco D, Izaola O, Terroba MC, Cuellar L, Martin T. Clinical results and nutritional consequences of biliopancreatic diversion: three years of follow-up. Ann Nutr Metab. 2008;53:234–9.
37. Vila M, Ruíz O, Belmonte M, Riesco M, Barceló A, Perez G, Moreiro J, Salinas R. Changes in lipid profile and insulin resistance in obese patients after Scopinaro biliopancreatic diversion. Obes Surg. 2009;19:299–306.
38. Murri M, García-Fuentes E, García-Almeida JM, Garrido-Sánchez L, Mayas MD, Bernal R, Tinahones FJ. Changes in oxidative stress and insulin resistance in morbidly obese patients after bariatric surgery. Obes Surg. 2010;20:363–8.
39. Garrido-Sanchez L, Murri M, Rivas-Becerra J, Ocaña-Wilhelmi L, Cohen RV, Garcia-Fuentes E, Tinahones FJ. Bypass of the duodenum improves insulin resistance much more rapidly than sleeve gastrectomy. Surg Obes Relat Dis. 2012;2:145–50.
40. García-Unzueta MT, Fernández-Santiago R, Domínguez-Díez A, Vazquez-Salví L, Fernández-Escalante JC, Amado JA. Fasting plasma ghrelin levels increase progressively after biliopancreatic diversion: one-year follow-up. Obes Surg. 2005;15:187–90.
41. Alagna S, Cossu ML, Gallo P, Tilocca PL, Pileri P, Alagna G, Maninchedda P, Sini AL, Pilo L, Rovasio PP, Noya G, Masala A. Biliopancreatic diversion: long-term effects on gonadal function in severely obese men. Surg Obes Relat Dis. 2006;2:82–6.
42. Moreiro J, Ruiz O, Perez G, Salinas R, Urgeles JR, Riesco M, García-Sanz M. Parathyroid hormone and bone marker levels in patients with morbid obesity before and after biliopancreatic diversion. Obes Surg. 2007;17:348–54.

43. Garcia-Fuentes E, Garrido-Sanchez L, Garcia-Almeida JM, Garcia-Arnes J, Gallego-Perales JL, Rivas-Marin J, Morcillo S, Cardona I, Soriguer F. Different effect of laparoscopic Roux-en-Y gastric bypass and open biliopancreatic diversion of Scopinaro on serum PYY and ghrelin levels. Obes Surg. 2008;18:1424–9.
44. Hernández Hernández JR, López-Tomassetti Fernández E, Caballero Díaz Y, Molina Cabrillana J, Morales García D, Núñez Jorge V. Remission of female sexual dysfunction in morbidly obese female patients with the Scopinaro procedure. Surg Obes Relat Dis. 2013;9:987–90.
45. Quaranta L, Nascimbeni G, Semeraro F, Quaranta CA. Severe corneoconjunctival xerosis after biliopancreatic bypass for obesity (Scopinaro's operation). Am J Ophthalmol. 1994;118:817–8.
46. Cossu ML, Fais E, Meloni GB, Profili S, Masala A, Alagna S, Rovasio PP, Spartà C, Pilo L, Tilocca PL, Noya G. Impact of age on long-term complications after biliopancreatic diversion. Obes Surg. 2004;14:1182–6.
47. Boldery R, Fielding G, Rafter T, Pascoe AL, Scalia GM. Nutritional deficiency of selenium secondary to weight loss (bariatric) surgery associated with life-threatening cardiomyopathy. Heart Lung Circ. 2007;16:123–6.
48. Ferrer Márquez M, Carvia Pousaillè C, Velasco Albendea J, Rico Morales Mdel M, Casado Martín M, Belda Lozano R, Ferrer Ayza M. Influence of bariatric surgery on the non-alcoholic liver steatosis. A histological evaluation. Cir Esp. 2009;86:94–100.
49. Geerts A, Darius T, Chapelle T, Roeyen G, Francque S, Libbrecht L, Nevens F, Pirenne J, Troisi R. The multicenter Belgian survey on liver transplantation for hepatocellular failure after bariatric surgery. Transplant Proc. 2010;42:4395–8.
50. Gracia-Solanas JA, Elia M, Aguilella V, Ramirez JM, Martínez J, Bielsa MA, Martínez M. Metabolic syndrome after bariatric surgery. Results depending on the technique performed. Obes Surg. 2011;21:179–85.
51. Frenken M, Cho EY. Metabolic intestinal bypass surgery for type 2 diabetes in patients with a BMI <35 kg/m2: comparative analysis of 16 patients undergoing either BPD, BPD-DS, or RYGB. Obes Facts. 2011;4 Suppl 1:13–7.
52. Buchwald H, Avidor Y, Braunwald E, Jensen MD, Pories W, Fahrbach K, Schoelles K. Bariatric surgery: a systematic review and meta-analysis. JAMA. 2004;292:1724–37.
53. Doyle ME, Egan JM. Mechanisms of action of glucagone-like peptide 1 in the pancreas. Pharmacol Ther. 2007;113:546–93.
54. Xu G, Stoffers DA, Habener JF, Bonner-Weir S. Exendin-4 stimulates both beta-cell replication and neogenesis, resulting in increased beta-cell mass. Diabetes. 1999;48:2270–6.
55. Farilla L, Bulotta A, Hirshberg B, Li Calzi S, Khoury N, Noushmehr H, Bertolotto C, Di Mario U, Harlan DM, Perfetti R. Glucagon-like peptide 1 inhibits cell apoptosis and improve glucose responsiveness of freshly isolated human islets. Endocrinology. 2003;144:5149–58.
56. Buchwald H, Estok R, Fahrbach K, Banel D, Jensen MD, Pories WJ, Bantle JP, Sledge I. Weight and type 2 diabetes after bariatric surgery: systematic review and meta-analysis. Am J Med. 2009;122:248–56.
57. Scopinaro N, Papadia F, Camerini G, Marinari G, Civalleri D. A comparison of a personal series of biliopanreatic diversion and literature data on gastric bypass help to explain the mechanisms of resolution of type 2 diabetes by the two operations. Obes Surg. 2008;18:1035–8.

21 Laparoscopic Duodenal Switch

Antonio Iannelli and Francesco Martini

21.1 Introduction

Duodenal switch (DS)—the modified version of biliopancreatic diversion (BPD) originally described by Scopinaro in 1979 [1]—was first reported in the United States and Canada by Hess and Hess [2] and by Marceau et al. [3], followed by Baltasar et al. in Spain [4]. Gagner then introduced the laparoscopic approach in 1999 [5].

This complex bariatric procedure consists of a vertical gastrectomy with duodenal preservation (sleeve gastrectomy [SG]), division of the first portion of the duodenum, and reconnection to the distal 250 cm of ileum. The bypassed duodenum, jejunum, and proximal ileum (biliopancreatic limb) are then reconnected to create a Roux-en-Y anatomy with a common channel of 100 cm and an alimentary channel of 150 cm (Fig. 21.1).

The DS is mainly used in super-obese patients (BMI >50 kg/m^2) as it results in an excess weight loss (EWL) which is far better than what is reported for other bariatric procedures such as gastric banding (AGB) or gastric bypass (RYGB) [6–9].

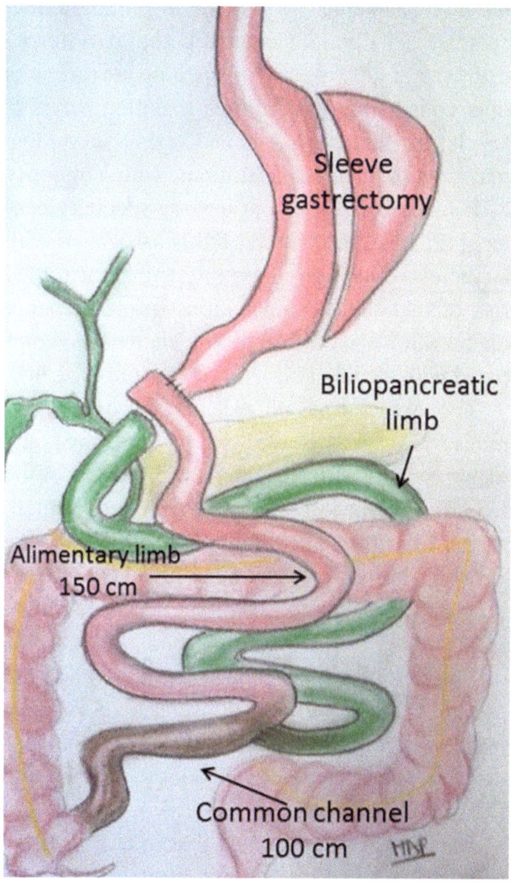

Fig. 21.1 Illustration of the duodenal switch procedure: the operation consists of a sleeve gastrectomy, creation of an alimentary limb approximately of 150 cm and a common channel length of 100 cm

A. Iannelli (✉) • F. Martini
Service de Chirurgie Digestive et ttransplantation hépatique – Hôpital Archet 2, Centre Hospitalo-Universitaire Université de Nice Sophia Antipolis, 151 route ST Antoine de Ginestière, Nice 06202, France
e-mail: Iannelli.a@chu-nice.fr

M. Lucchese, N. Scopinaro (eds.), *Minimally Invasive Bariatric and Metabolic Surgery: Principles and Technical Aspects*, DOI 10.1007/978-3-319-15356-8_21,

A recent paper by Buchwald and Oien, which surveyed the International Federation for the Surgery of Obesity and Metabolic Disorders member nations with an 84 % response rate, revealed that the proportion of DS procedures in relation to all bariatric surgeries declined from 6.1 % in 2003 to 2.1 % in 2011 [10]. A study by Lazzati et al. [11], analyzing bariatric surgery trends in France from 2005 to 2011, showed a reduction in the proportion of this procedure from 1 to 0.7 %.

The reasons why the procedure with the greatest weight loss, evidence of lasting effect, and reversal of obesity-related comorbidities [7, 8] is the least performed worldwide are multiple and complex. Firstly, its technical complexity (especially using laparoscopy) plays a major role: it is time consuming and requires a skilled surgeon. Likely, the learning curve and operative volume may be important considerations, with a majority of DS being performed at tertiary specialty centers [12, 13]. Furthermore, DS is associated with an increased operative mortality and an increased risk of metabolic complications (protein energy malnutrition and other nutrient deficiencies) compared with the other bariatric procedures [14, 15].

The application of the laparoscopic technique to DS soon showed that laparoscopy is the ideal procedure for SG, the restrictive part of the DS. Thus, laparoscopic SG has been used to obtain substantial weight loss in high-risk patients, before proceeding with either DS or RYGB [16]. Given the excellent results obtained in the short term, it was argued that the SG might work as a stand-alone procedure [17]. SG rapidly gained enormous consensus among bariatric surgeons, because of its several advantages compared with laparoscopic RYGB and DS [18–21].

It has been demonstrated that in the hands of experienced surgeons and in high-volume bariatric centers, DS can be performed safely as a single-step procedure [2, 8, 22]. The theoretical advantages of performing DS with the staged approach (SG followed by DS) include the opportunity to detect patients who might achieve good results with SG alone, thus avoiding the morbidity linked to the malabsorption; the selection of patients for the second step who are compliant and attend the follow-up visits; simplification of the surgical technique and a reduction of postoperative morbidity [23].

21.2 Surgical Technique

21.2.1 The First Step: The Sleeve Gastrectomy

The patient is placed in the supine position with both arms appropriately padded and tucked to the sides. The SG is performed first with a six-port approach (Fig. 21.2). The greater curvature of the stomach is dissected free with the harmonic scalpel starting 6 cm proximal to the pylorus up to the *angle of His*. Care is taken to dissect the whole gastric fundus posteriorly, where the left pillar is carefully identified and dissected free over its anterior aspect. In all cases, the vertical gastrectomy is done over a 40 Fr intraluminal boogie with green or gold staple cartridges. The gastric antrum is systematically spared, and the last stapling is fired 1 cm lateral to the esophagogastric junction. Seamguard (Gore-Tex, Flagstaff, AZ) to buttress the staple lines is selectively used.

21.2.2 The Second Step: The Duodenal Switch

Patient's position and port placements are the same as those of the SG (Fig. 21.2). The duodenum is divided using a linear stapler with a blue cartridge 4 cm distal to the pylorus at the level of the gastroduodenal artery (Fig. 21.3). The small bowel is measured with a 50-cm-long tape along the unstretched antimesenteric border. It is then divided with the linear stapler 250 cm from the ileocecal valve, and the distal end is anastomosed to the proximal duodenum with an intracorporeal hand-sewn continuous absorbable suture (Fig. 21.4). The proximal end of the divided bowel is anastomosed to the ileum 100 cm from the ileocecal valve to create a 100-cm common channel and a 150-cm alimentary limb. The mesenteric and Petersen spaces are closed with nonabsorbable running sutures. A leak test (air bubbles and blue dye) is performed at the end of the procedure.

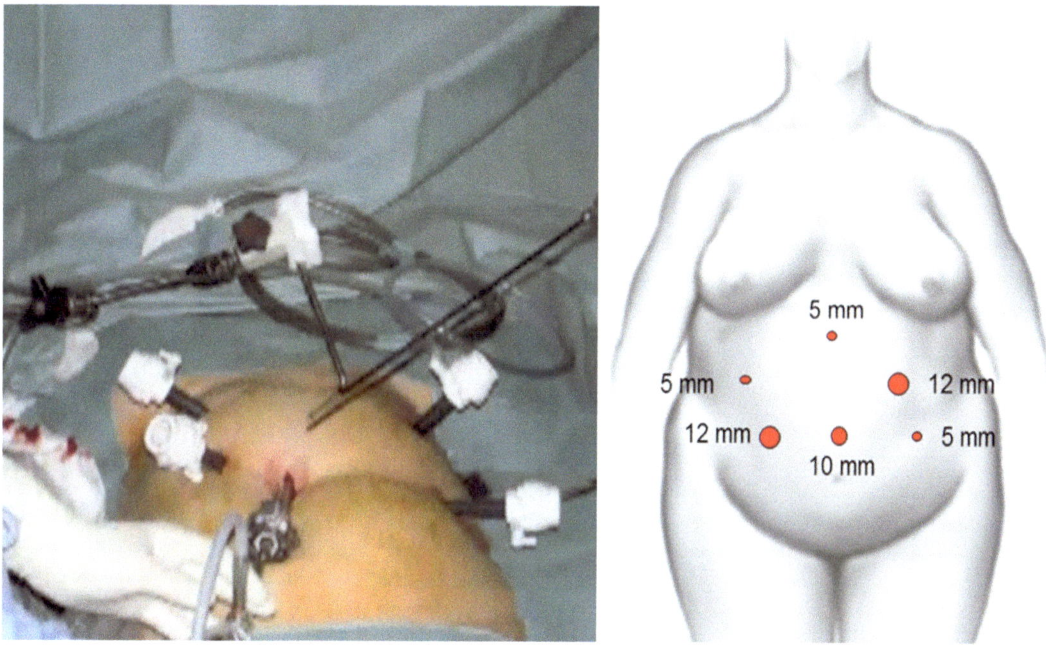

Fig. 21.2 Positioning of the six ports

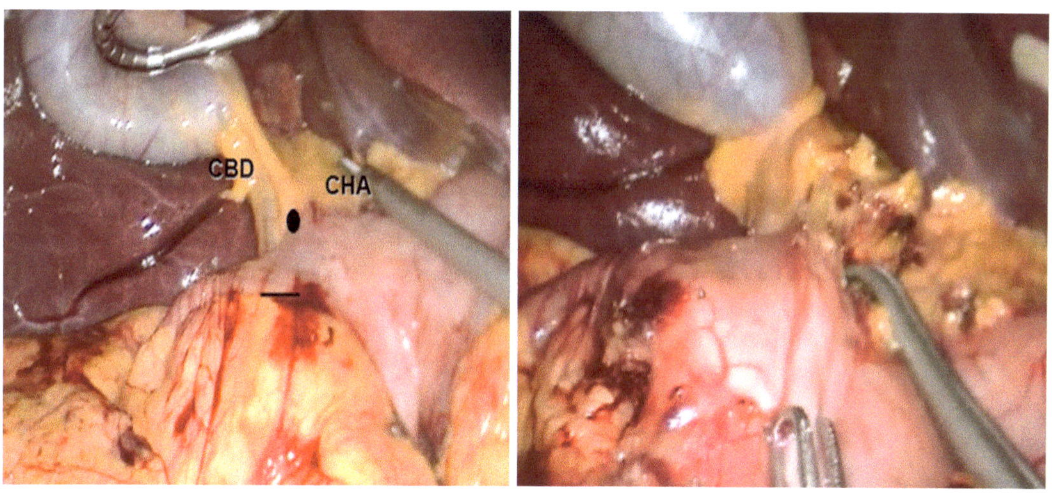

Fig. 21.3 A dissector is passed behind the duodenal bulb from top (*black circle*) to bottom (*black line*) at the level of the gastroduodenal artery, about 4 cm distal to the pylorus. A tape is then passed at this level to lift up the duodenum and guide the introduction of the linear stapler which is then used to divide the duodenum. *CBD* common bile duct, *CHA* common hepatic artery

21.3 Results

21.3.1 Weight Loss

DS has proven to be successful in achieving and maintaining significant weight loss in the super-obese population. Table 21.1 shows the long-term results of the main series of DS published to date concerning EWL and diabetes resolution [7, 23–28]. In all these series, except for the one of Biertho et al. [25] the mean BMI is >50 and the EWL ranges between 66 and 76 %.

The systematic review and meta-analysis by Buchwald et al. [7] included 621 studies for a

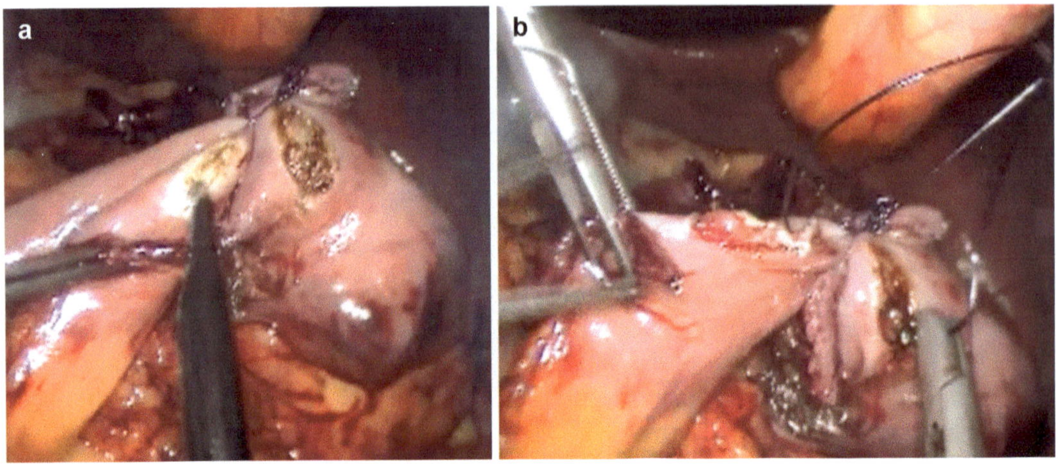

Fig. 21.4 (**a**) A duodenotomy is created on the posterior aspect of the duodenal bulb parallel and close to the staple line with monopolar electrocautery hook, then an enterotomy is created on the antimesenteric border of the jejunal loop. (**b**) The duodeno-jejunostomy is fashioned with an intracorporeal hand-sewn continuous absorbable suture

Table 21.1 Main series of duodenal switch: long-term results concerning weight loss and diabetes resolution

Author, year	No. of pts	Access	BMI[a]	Leaks (%)	Mortality <30 days (%)	Follow-up	EWL[a] (%)	Diabetes resolution (%)
Anthone et al. (2003) [24]	701	O	52.8	1	1.4	50 pts at 5 years	66	NR
Hess (2005) [26]	1,150	O	50.9	0.7	0.6	148 pts at 10 years	74	98
Marceau et al. (2007) [27]	1,356	O	51.5	0.9	1.1	284 pts at 10 years	69	92
Buchwald et al. (2009) [7]	7,761	7,147 O 604 L	50.5	NR	NR	1,520 pts at 2 years	74	96
Prachand et al. (2010) [28]	198	L	58.8	NR	0.5	38 pts at 3 years	69	100
Biertho et al. (2010) [25]	810	O	44.2	2.1	0.6	8.6 years[a]	76	93
Iannelli et al. (2013) [23]	140	L	55.1	3.6	0	3 years[a]	73	86

pts patients, *BMI* body mass index, *EWL* excess weight loss, *O* laparotomy, *L* laparoscopy
[a]Mean

total of 135,246 patients and compared bariatric surgical procedures for weight loss and type 2 diabetes mellitus (T2DM) resolution. This review indicates that BPD/DS is the most effective operation with a EWL of 73 % at 2 years follow-up, followed by RYGB (63 %), vertical banded gastroplasty (56 %), and AGB (49 %).

The only randomized trial comparing DS and RYGB, considered by most as the gold standard for bariatric procedure, was conducted by Sovik et al. [14], who randomized 60 super-obese patients (BMI 50–60 kg/m^2). One year after surgery percentage of excess BMI loss (EBL) was found to be 54.4 % following RYGB compared to 74.8 % following DS. Similarly, Prachand et al. [29] retrospectively analyzed 350 super-obese patients who underwent either DS or RYGB. Preoperative BMI was significantly greater in the DS group compared to the RYGB group (58.8 kg/m^2 versus 56.4 kg/m^2, $P=0.0014$). Percentage of EWL at 36 months was significantly greater in the DS group compared to RYGB: 68.9 % versus 54.9 %. The systematic review and meta-analysis by Hedberg et al. [9] including 16 studies and 874 DS patients and 1,149

RYGB patients, showed the superiority of DS in terms of weight loss.

Biertho et al. [25] in a series of 810 morbidly obese patients with mean BMI of 44.2 ± 3.6 kg/m^2 showed an EWL of 76 % that was maintained at 8.6 years follow-up concluded that DS was appropriate for non–super-obese patients. Concordantly, Anthone et al. [24] in a series including 701 DS patients with preoperative BMI ranging from 34 to 95 kg/m^2 found a EWL of 66 % after 5 or more years of follow-up.

21.3.2 Evolution of Obesity-Related Comorbidities

DS has a marked effect on obesity-related metabolic comorbidities, specifically T2DM (Table 21.1). In the main surgical series of DS, the reported rates of T2DM resolution vary between 86 and 100 % [5, 17–22].

The systematic review and meta-analysis by Buchwald et al. [7] showed that, at 2 years follow-up, diabetes remission was by far the greatest for patients undergoing BPD/DS (96 %), followed by RYGB (71 %), and least for pure restrictive procedures.

Recently Mingrone et al. [30] conducted a randomized controlled trial on 60 morbidly obese patients with a history of at least 5 years of T2D and a glycated hemoglobin level of 7.0 % or more. Patients were randomly assigned to receive conventional medical therapy (lifestyle modifications and hypoglycemic agents) or undergo either RYGB or BPD. At 2 years, T2D remission occurred in 75 % of patients undergoing the RYGB versus 95 % of those undergoing the BPD group ($P<0.001$ for both comparisons). None of the patients in the medical-therapy group showed remission of T2D.

The same group [31] conducted a case-controlled trial with 10-year follow-up including 50 patients (28 medical therapy, 22 BPD), which showed resolution of T2DM in all BPD patients 12 months after surgery. The remission was definitive because none of the patients experienced diabetes again in the course of the study. Similarly, Tsoli et al.'s nonrandomized trial [32] including 24 patients (12 BPD, 12 SG) showed resolution of T2DM in all BPD patients 12 months after surgery.

In the systematic review and meta-analysis by Hedberg et al. [9], T2DM remission rate after DS was 88 %, compared with 76 % in RYGB patients ($P=0.18$). The difference was not statistically significant because of the low number of patients (112 DS, 105 RYGB). Glycated hemoglobin levels were significantly lower after DS compared with RYGB.

Concordantly with T2DM results, hypertension showed marked improvement following BPD/DS (54–95 % resolution rate), as well as dyslipidemia (72–100 % resolution rate) [25, 31–40]. Obstructive sleep apnea was resolved in 90–100 % of patients [25, 27, 33, 36, 39].

21.4 Complications

21.4.1 Perioperative Morbidity and Mortality

Buchwald et al. [15], in his meta-analysis of 361 studies including 85,048 patients reported an overall mortality of 0.28 % within 30 days of bariatric surgery. BPD/DS had the highest early mortality with a rate of 0.29–1.23 % for open and 0–2.7 % for laparoscopic procedures.

The operative mortality for large DS series by laparotomy is approximately 1 % with a range of 0.6–1.4 % (Table 21.1) [24–27]. Laparoscopic approach seems to be associated with a lower mortality, ranging from 0 to 0.5 %, although laparoscopic series report a smaller number of patients. Postoperative mortality is most commonly associated with pulmonary embolus, respiratory failure, and anastomotic leaks. In the aforementioned series [23–28] the leak rate varied between 1 and 3.6 %.

Biertho et al. [41] analyzed a series of 1,000 BPD/DS patients, comparing the laparoscopic (228 cases) and open (772 cases) groups. In this series they reported only 1 postoperative death (0.1 %) due to pulmonary embolus in the laparoscopy group. Major complications occurred in 7 % of the patients, with no significant differences between the two groups (7 % vs 7.4 %, $P=0.1$). No differences were found in the overall leak or intra-abdominal abscess rate (3.5 % vs 4 %, $P=0.1$).

An important consideration is that BPD/DS is the procedure of choice for super-obese patients and it can be argued that surgical risk in this group is higher at baseline.

Flum et al. [42] in the Longitudinal Assessment of Bariatric Surgery, a prospective multicenter observational study, including 4,776 patients, analyzed 30-day outcomes after bariatric surgery and showed that extreme values of BMI were significantly associated with increased risk of major adverse outcomes (death; venous thromboembolism; percutaneous, endoscopic, or operative reintervention; and length of stay greater than 30 days). Similar conclusion were found by Kim et al. [43], who carried out a retrospective study of 54 super-super-obese patients (BMI >60) operated on for DS with a laparoscopic approach in 26 cases and open in 28 cases. Major morbidity occurred in 23 % of patients in the laparoscopic group and in 17 % of patients in the open group ($P=0.63$). There were two deaths in the laparoscopic group (7.6 % mortality) and one death (3.5 % mortality) in the open group ($P=0.51$).

However, other investigators showed that the DS can be safely performed in patients with a BMI > 50 kg/m^2 as a single-stage procedure without significantly increasing the mortality [8]. Topart et al. showed that BMI becomes less predictive of complications once the learning curve for laparoscopic DS is overcome [22].

Iannelli et al. [23] conducted a case-control study in order to compare single-stage DS (110 patients) with a staged strategy (110 patients) consisting in a laparoscopic sleeve SG followed by laparoscopic DS in selected patients. The authors found a trend toward fewer postoperative complications in the staged strategy group that did not reach statistical significance on univariate analysis. However, single-stage DS was the only variable significantly associated with the risk of postoperative complications on multivariate analysis. Furthermore, six patients (5.5 %) in the single-stage DS group required conversion to open surgery and none did so in the staged group ($P<.05$) indicating that the staged approach simplifies the surgical procedure. The main advantage of the staged approach resides in the selection of patients who do not need the malabsorptive component of the complete DS procedure. In this series, 72.7 % of super-obese patients achieved 50.8 % EWL after SG at a mean follow-up of 3 years. These results are in accordance with those reported by Himpens et al. who recorded a 27 % rate of second-stage DS in a series of 41 morbidly obese patients undergoing SG at a follow-up of >6 years.

21.4.2 Close Loop Obstruction

Diversion of the biliopancreatic secretions from the alimentary stream has a potential for closed loop obstruction, which may not be diagnosed by common symptoms and signs of bowel obstruction—vomiting may not occur, and air-fluid level on a plain abdominal radiogram may not be present. Abdominal computed tomography (CT) scan in this situation is a study of choice and reveals a dilated, fluid-filled biliopancreatic limb and the distended distal isolated stomach, which can progress to gastric necrosis, perforation, or pancreatitis [44, 45]. This type of obstruction will not be decompressed by insertion of the nasogastric tube and requires urgent laparotomy [45].

21.4.3 Metabolic Related Complications

DS has proven to be more malabsorptive compared to other bariatric surgeries and is therefore associated with the highest rate of perioperative malnutrition/metabolic related complications. Iron-deficiency anemia, protein calorie malnutrition, hypocalcemia, and deficiency of fat soluble vitamins, vitamin B1, vitamin B12, and folate are common [46]. Aasheim et al. [47] randomized 60 super-obese patients to receive either RYGB or DS comparing 25-hydroxy vitamin D, vitamin A, and vitamin B1 up to 1 year postoperatively. DS patients had lower mean 25-hydroxy vitamin D and vitamin A concentrations, as well as a steeper decline in vitamin B1 compared to RYGB. All patients must begin supplementation postoperatively and a close follow-up is mandatory. However, there is no standardized approach to replacement and data on patients' compliance are lacking [48, 49].

Here, we discuss two specific complications that are usually underemphasized and sometimes life threatening: the protein deficiency syndrome and the intestinal bacterial overgrowth syndrome.

21.4.3.1 Protein Deficiency Syndrome

After DS, protein metabolism is compromised both by decreased absorption and by increased endogenous loss. The capacity to absorb protein is limited by three mechanisms: the contribution of the stomach to protein hydrolysis is decreased, the intestinal absorptive surface is reduced, and the pancreatic enzymatic activity is delayed. Anatomical changes can cause protein loss by exposing intestinal mucosa to peptic action without the buffer protection of bile, by increasing fermentation in the colon and by disrupting intestinal flora.

Scopinaro et al. [44] measured protein absorption and loss after BPD, finding that protein absorption was decreased by 30 %, and endogenous fecal loss was increased from a normal 6 g/day in controls to 30 g/day. This means that daily dietary protein requirements are doubled after a Scopinaro-type BPD, from 40 g/day normally to 90 g/day. This protein intake can be easily met when a patient eats normally, for example, the normal American style diet contains about 100 g/day. However, patients can be susceptible to protein deficiency when dietary intake is decreased (dieting), when additional protein loss occurs (bacterial overgrowth), or when protein requirements increase (infection).

In the experience of Marceau et al. [27, 50], the prevalence of albumin deficiency, that is, level between 32 and 36 g/L, was about 10 % and severe deficiency (below 32 g/L) was 2 %. They observed a temporary decrease in serum protein 6 months after surgery when about 20 % of patients were found to have a level <36 g/L. There was then a gradual improvement, and 2 years after the operation, protein levels were <36 g/L in only 6 % of patients.

Mild hypoalbuminemia is usually asymptomatic and must be sought by routine measurements. It mandates dietary review and suggestions, protein supplements, and monthly follow-up. An albumin level between 25 and 30 g/L is often accompanied by pitting edema at the ankles and represents a serious clinical condition. It requires immediate medical treatment with intravenous human albumin, dietary supplements, and diuretics. Severe hypoalbuminemia <25 g/L is life threatening and requires hospitalization [51–53].

When hypoalbuminemia is resistant or recurrent, surgical revision is the option of choice [54, 55]. Revision for protein deficiency was necessary in 6 of 1,100 patients (0.5 %) in the series of Marceau et al. [27, 50] and consisted of reintroducing a segment of the biliary channel into the alimentary channel, resulting in a lengthening of both the alimentary and the common channel. The length chosen varied from 50 to 225 cm based on the surgeon's appreciation. Revision was successful in four, and in one other patient, a second revision was necessary.

When revision is not followed by normalization of albumin levels, protein loss is most likely the basic causal mechanism rather than insufficient absorption. Excessive protein loss caused by bacterial overgrowth is then the most probable cause responsible for hypoalbuminemia.

21.4.3.2 Bacterial Overgrowth Syndrome

Bacterial overgrowth remains the most serious concern after any type of BPD/DS. There are several factors that may induce changes in intestinal flora and alter microbial equilibrium in the intestinal lumen, resulting in bacterial overgrowth: the absence of bile in a segment of intestine [56, 57], the shortness of the gut [58], the decreased gastric acidity, the dysmotility [59], the protein deficiency [59–61], and the presence of undigested food reaching the colon. There is no study of bacterial count after DS compared to normal bowel. However, beneficial effects of antimicrobial agents serve as indirect evidence that bacterial overgrowth has an impact after DS.

In about 80 % of patients, the only symptoms are increased malodorous gas and discomfort, which are well tolerated. Fifteen percent of patients can present also episodes of bloating and diarrhea, which are self-limited and reduced while fasting or avoiding certain foods. A trial of metronidazole and/or a probiotic agent for 3–5 days alleviates these symptoms [62, 63]. If so, they can be given periodically, usually monthly.

In about 2–3 % of patients, clinical manifestations may include proctitis, nocturnal diarrhea, and painful abdominal distension with pseudoobstruction sometimes accompanied by mental confusion [64, 65]. This can occur many years after BPD and requires oral antibiotics. Usually metronidazole is sufficient, but nonabsorbable antibiotics like neomycin, vancomycin, or aminoglycoside by mouth may occasionally be necessary.

In rare cases Crohn's disease-like a syndrome can be observed, presenting as an acute abdomen or incomplete intestinal obstruction [66]. Symptoms include cramps and persistent abdominal pain with nausea and vomiting, chills and fever, arthralgias, and prostration. CT may reveal thickened dilated intestines. At laparotomy a thickened intestinal segment is found, with inflamed and adherent serosa that bleeds easily. Marceau et al. [27, 50] reported 6 such cases while following 1,500 post-BPD/DS patients. In this series, total reversal was performed in 11 patients (0.8 %) at mean of 66 (range 20–126) months after BPD/DS: 8 after Scopinaro-type BPD and 3 after DS, with an incidence of 3.5 % and 0.3 %, respectively. All reversals were performed for complaints related to bacterial overgrowth.

References

1. Scopinaro N, Gianetta E, Civalleri D, et al. Biliopancreatic bypass for obesity: II. Initial experience in man. Br J Surg. 1979;66(9):618–20.
2. Hess DS, Hess DW. Biliopancreatic diversion with a duodenal switch. Obes Surg. 1998;8(3):267–82.
3. Marceau P, Biron S, Bourque RA, et al. Biliopancreatic diversion with a new type of gastrectomy. Obes Surg. 1993;3(1):29–35.
4. Baltasar A, del Rio J, Escriva C, et al. Preliminary results of the duodenal switch. Obes Surg. 1997;7(6):500–4.
5. Ren CJ, Patterson E, Gagner M. Early results of laparoscopic biliopancreatic diversion with duodenal switch: a case series of 40 consecutive patients. Obes Surg. 2000;10(6):514–23; discussion 524.
6. Buchwald H, Avidor Y, Braunwald E, et al. Bariatric surgery: a systematic review and meta-analysis. JAMA. 2004;292(14):1724–37.
7. Buchwald H, Estok R, Fahrbach K, et al. Weight and type 2 diabetes after bariatric surgery: systematic review and meta-analysis. Am J Med. 2009;122(3):248–56.e5.
8. Buchwald H, Kellogg TA, Leslie DB, et al. Duodenal switch operative mortality and morbidity are not impacted by body mass index. Ann Surg. 2008;248(4):541–8.
9. Hedberg J, Sundstrom J, Sundbom M. Duodenal switch versus Roux-en-Y gastric bypass for morbid obesity: systematic review and meta-analysis of weight results, diabetes resolution and early complications in single-centre comparisons. Obes Rev. 2014;15:555–63.
10. Buchwald H, Oien DM. Metabolic/bariatric surgery worldwide 2011. Obes Surg. 2013;23(4):427–36.
11. Lazzati A, Guy-Lachuer R, Delaunay V, et al. Bariatric surgery trends in France: 2005–2011. Surg Obes Relat Dis. 2014;10(2):328–34.
12. Nguyen NT, Paya M, Stevens CM, et al. The relationship between hospital volume and outcome in bariatric surgery at academic medical centers. Ann Surg. 2004;240(4):586–93; discussion 593–4.
13. Ballantyne GH, Belsley S, Stephens D, et al. Bariatric surgery: low mortality at a high-volume center. Obes Surg. 2008;18(6):660–7.
14. Sovik TT, Taha O, Aasheim ET, et al. Randomized clinical trial of laparoscopic gastric bypass versus laparoscopic duodenal switch for superobesity. Br J Surg. 2010;97(2):160–6.
15. Buchwald H, Estok R, Fahrbach K, et al. Trends in mortality in bariatric surgery: a systematic review and meta-analysis. Surgery. 2007;142(4):621–32; discussion 632–5.
16. Regan JP, Inabnet WB, Gagner M, et al. Early experience with two-stage laparoscopic Roux-en-Y gastric bypass as an alternative in the super-super obese patient. Obes Surg. 2003;13(6):861–4.
17. Hamoui N, Anthone GJ, Kaufman HS, et al. Sleeve gastrectomy in the high-risk patient. Obes Surg. 2006;16(11):1445–9.
18. Gagner M, Deitel M, Kalberer TL, et al. The second international consensus summit for sleeve gastrectomy, March 19–21, 2009. Surg Obes Relat Dis. 2009;5(4):476–85.
19. Himpens J, Dobbeleir J, Peeters G. Long-term results of laparoscopic sleeve gastrectomy for obesity. Ann Surg. 2010;252(2):319–24.
20. Iannelli A, Dainese R, Piche T, et al. Laparoscopic sleeve gastrectomy for morbid obesity. World J Gastroenterol. 2008;14(6):821–7.
21. Peterli R, Wolnerhanssen B, Peters T, et al. Improvement in glucose metabolism after bariatric surgery: comparison of laparoscopic Roux-en-Y gastric bypass and laparoscopic sleeve gastrectomy: a prospective randomized trial. Ann Surg. 2009;250(2):234–41.
22. Topart P, Becouarn G, Ritz P. Should biliopancreatic diversion with duodenal switch be done as single-

stage procedure in patients with BMI>or=50 kg/m2? Surg Obes Relat Dis. 2010;6(1):59–63.
23. Iannelli A, Schneck AS, Topart P, et al. Laparoscopic sleeve gastrectomy followed by duodenal switch in selected patients versus single-stage duodenal switch for superobesity: case–control study. Surg Obes Relat Dis. 2013;9(4):531–8.
24. Anthone GJ, Lord RV, DeMeester TR, et al. The duodenal switch operation for the treatment of morbid obesity. Ann Surg. 2003;238(4):618–27; discussion 627–8.
25. Biertho L, Biron S, Hould FS, et al. Is biliopancreatic diversion with duodenal switch indicated for patients with body mass index <50 kg/m2? Surg Obes Relat Dis. 2010;6(5):508–14.
26. Hess DS. Biliopancreatic diversion with duodenal switch. Surg Obes Relat Dis. 2005;1(3):329–33.
27. Marceau P, Biron S, Hould FS, et al. Duodenal switch: long-term results. Obes Surg. 2007;17(11):1421–30.
28. Prachand VN, Ward M, Alverdy JC. Duodenal switch provides superior resolution of metabolic comorbidities independent of weight loss in the super-obese (BMI>or=50 kg/m2) compared with gastric bypass. J Gastrointest Surg. 2010;14(2):211–20.
29. Prachand VN, Davee RT, Alverdy JC. Duodenal switch provides superior weight loss in the super-obese (BMI>or =50 kg/m2) compared with gastric bypass. Ann Surg. 2006;244(4):611–9.
30. Mingrone G, Panunzi S, De Gaetano A, et al. Bariatric surgery versus conventional medical therapy for type 2 diabetes. N Engl J Med. 2012;366(17):1577–85.
31. Iaconelli A, Panunzi S, De Gaetano A, et al. Effects of bilio-pancreatic diversion on diabetic complications: a 10-year follow-up. Diabetes Care. 2011;34(3):561–7.
32. Tsoli M, Chronaiou A, Kehagias I, et al. Hormone changes and diabetes resolution after biliopancreatic diversion and laparoscopic sleeve gastrectomy: a comparative prospective study. Surg Obes Relat Dis. 2013;9(5):667–77.
33. Crea N, Pata G, Di Betta E, et al. Long-term results of biliopancreatic diversion with or without gastric preservation for morbid obesity. Obes Surg. 2011;21(2): 139–45.
34. Papadia FS, Adami GF, Marinari GM, et al. Bariatric surgery in adolescents: a long-term follow-up study. Surg Obes Relat Dis. 2007;3(4):465–8.
35. Nelson D, Beekley A, Carter P, et al. Early results after introduction of biliopancreatic diversion/duodenal switch at a military bariatric center. Am J Surg. 2011;201(5):678–84.
36. Baltasar A, Bou R, Bengochea M, et al. Duodenal switch: an effective therapy for morbid obesity–intermediate results. Obes Surg. 2001;11(1):54–8.
37. Vage V, Nilsen RM, Berstad A, et al. Predictors for remission of major components of the metabolic syndrome after biliopancreatic diversion with duodenal switch (BPDDS). Obes Surg. 2013;23(1):80–6.
38. Dorman RB, Rasmus NF, al-Haddad BJ, et al. Benefits and complications of the duodenal switch/biliopancreatic diversion compared to the Roux-en-Y gastric bypass. Surgery. 2012;152(4):758–65; discussion 765–7.
39. Pata G, Crea N, Di Betta E, et al. Biliopancreatic diversion with transient gastroplasty and duodenal switch: long-term results of a multicentric study. Surgery. 2013;153(3):413–22.
40. Benetti A, Del Puppo M, Crosignani A, et al. Cholesterol metabolism after bariatric surgery in grade 3 obesity: differences between malabsorptive and restrictive procedures. Diabetes Care. 2013;36(6): 1443–7.
41. Biertho L, Lebel S, Marceau S, et al. Perioperative complications in a consecutive series of 1000 duodenal switches. Surg Obes Relat Dis. 2013;9(1):63–8.
42. Flum DR, Belle SH, King WC, et al. Perioperative safety in the longitudinal assessment of bariatric surgery. N Engl J Med. 2009;361(5):445–54.
43. Kim WW, Gagner M, Kini S, et al. Laparoscopic vs. open biliopancreatic diversion with duodenal switch: a comparative study. J Gastrointest Surg. 2003;7(4): 552–7.
44. Scopinaro N, Adami GF, Marinari GM, et al. Biliopancreatic diversion. World J Surg. 1998;22(9): 936–46.
45. Macgregor AM. Small bowel obstruction following gastric bypass. Obes Surg. 1992;2(4):333–9.
46. Aills L, Blankenship J, Buffington C, et al. ASMBS Allied Health nutritional guidelines for the surgical weight loss patient. Surg Obes Relat Dis. 2008;4(5 Suppl):S73–108.
47. Aasheim ET, Bjorkman S, Sovik TT, et al. Vitamin status after bariatric surgery: a randomized study of gastric bypass and duodenal switch. Am J Clin Nutr. 2009;90(1):15–22.
48. Faintuch J, Matsuda M, Cruz ME, et al. Severe protein-calorie malnutrition after bariatric procedures. Obes Surg. 2004;14(2):175–81.
49. Marceau P, Biron S, Lebel S, et al. Does bone change after biliopancreatic diversion? J Gastrointest Surg. 2002;6(5):690–8.
50. Marceau P, Hould FS, Lebel S, et al. Complications specific to biliopancreatic diversion. Curr Surg. 2003; 60(3):274–9.
51. Hardin TC, Page CP, Schwesinger WH. Rapid replacement of serum albumin in patients receiving total parenteral nutrition. Surg Gynecol Obstet. 1986;163(4):359–62.
52. Moss G. The role of albumin in nutritional support. J Am Coll Nutr. 1988;7(6):441–2.
53. Moss G. Malabsorption associated with extreme malnutrition: importance of replacing plasma albumin. J Am Coll Nutr. 1982;1(1):89–92.
54. Scopinaro N, Gianetta E, Friedman D, et al. Surgical revision of biliopancreatic diversion. Gastroenterol Clin North Am. 1987;16(3):529–31.
55. Clare WM. An analysis of 37 reversals on 504 biliopancreatic surgeries over 12 years. Obes Surg. 1993;3(2):169–73.

56. Deitch EA, Sittig K, Li M, et al. Obstructive jaundice promotes bacterial translocation from the gut. Am J Surg. 1990;159(1):79–84.
57. Slocum MM, Sittig KM, Specian RD, et al. Absence of intestinal bile promotes bacterial translocation. Am Surg. 1992;58(5):305–10.
58. Wilmore DW, Robinson MK. Short bowel syndrome. World J Surg. 2000;24(12):1486–92.
59. Deitch EA, Winterton J, Berg R. Effect of starvation, malnutrition, and trauma on the gastrointestinal tract flora and bacterial translocation. Arch Surg. 1987; 122(9):1019–24.
60. Li M, Specian RD, Berg RD, et al. Effects of protein malnutrition and endotoxin on the intestinal mucosal barrier to the translocation of indigenous flora in mice. JPEN J Parenter Enteral Nutr. 1989;13(6): 572–8.
61. Reynolds JV, O'Farrelly C, Feighery C, et al. Impaired gut barrier function in malnourished patients. Br J Surg. 1996;83(9):1288–91.
62. Fuller R. Probiotics in human medicine. Gut. 1991; 32(4):439–42.
63. Vanderhoof JA, Young RJ, Murray N, et al. Treatment strategies for small bowel bacterial overgrowth in short bowel syndrome. J Pediatr Gastroenterol Nutr. 1998;27(2):155–60.
64. Stolberg L, Rolfe R, Gitlin N, et al. d-Lactic acidosis due to abnormal gut flora: diagnosis and treatment of two cases. N Engl J Med. 1982;306(22):1344–8.
65. Mason PD. Metabolic acidosis due to D-lactate. Br Med J (Clin Res Ed). 1986;292(6528):1105–6.
66. Passaro Jr E, Drenick E, Wilson SE. Bypass enteritis. A new complication of jejunoileal bypass for obesity. Am J Surg. 1976;131(2):169–74.

Revisional Surgery: Gastric Banding Failure

22

Jacques M. Himpens

22.1 Introduction

Up until recently, laparoscopic adjustable gastric banding (LAGB) was the most popular bariatric procedure in the world [1]. Hence, nowadays, thousands of patients carry an adjustable band. Considering the fact that a great number of individuals do not experience satisfactory outcomes after LAGB, a large pool of patients is seeking for a solution to address this issue. Quite often, this solution will consist of an alternate surgical procedure.

22.2 Common Causes of Band Failure and Possible Surgical Solutions

In a great number of individuals who underwent LAGB for weight loss, the band is of a high-pressure type and was placed by the perigastric technique. There is substantial evidence that the combination of this "old type" of band and the by now obsolete insertion technique is characterized by a high incidence of complications [2, 3]. Typical complications include pouch dilatation/band slippage and band erosion, conditions that invariably require a reoperation. Despite the fact that some authors recommend a rebanding procedure to address these severe complications [4, 5], there is a general consensus that band ablation and conversion to another procedure is preferable [6]. Another frequent, perhaps less obvious cause of failure for the band procedure is intractable gastro-esophageal reflux disease (GERD) that may cause respiratory symptoms [7] or may be accompanied by severe esophageal dysmotility [8]. Finally, some patients experience failure of LAGB because of extreme food intolerance [9]. Band deflation is the first treatment of GERD, esophageal dysmotility, and food intolerance, but in a number of patients, band deflation will not suffice to cure the disease, or the condition will return as soon as the band is reinflated. Actually, according to most surgeons, the indications for band salvage procedures are limited to technical material mishaps, such as band-tubing disconnection or local access port problems, including membrane leak or displacement hampering percutaneous adjustment. Considering the above, quite logically, a high incidence of band loss was experienced by most authors [6, 10]. Conversely, O'Brien's team quite uniquely reported a very low incidence of band loss [11]. In our experience, however, close to 50 % of patients suffered band ablation within 10 years after LAGB [12]. When removal of the band is deemed necessary for whatever reason, weight regain will invariably occur [12, 13].

J.M. Himpens, MD, PhD
The European School of Laparoscopy,
St Pierre University Hospital, Brussels, Belgium
e-mail: Jacques_himpens@hotmail.com

M. Lucchese, N. Scopinaro (eds.), *Minimally Invasive Bariatric and Metabolic Surgery: Principles and Technical Aspects*, DOI 10.1007/978-3-319-15356-8_22,

In everyday practice, the most frequent indication for corrective surgery after LAGB remains poor weight loss or weight regain. A bariatric procedure is considered satisfactory in terms of weight loss when excess weight loss surpasses 50 % of the initial excess weight and/or when the residual body mass index (BMI) is under 35 kg/m^2 [14], results that the LAGB does not achieve in the experience of most bariatric surgeons. It is likely that the very weight loss mechanism of LAGB is to blame for the rather poor outcomes in terms of weight loss. Despite rare reports questioning the strictly restrictive nature of LAGB [15], for most investigators, LAGB primarily is a caloric intake limiting procedure. As such, intestinal hormonal implications such as Ghrelin secretion inhibition consecutive to the surgical procedure are limited [16, 17]. The lack of interference with orexogenic peptides might be the most significant cause of the inferior weight loss of LAGB compared to other bariatric procedures [18, 19].

Hence when LAGB does not result in satisfactory weight loss, it appears sensible to search for alternate procedures that imply different weight loss mechanisms. Thus, several alternate bariatric procedures may be considered to replace the LAGB. These procedures include (but are not limited to) the laproscopic sleeve gastrectomy (LSG), the Roux-en-Y gastric bypass (RYGB), the omega-loop gastric bypass (OLGB, also called the mini-gastric bypass), and the malabsorptive procedures such as biliopancreatic diversion (BPD) and duodenal switch (DS). In this chapter, we will not mention more experimental procedures such as the gastric plication, the sleeve gastrectomy with ileal interposition, or the bipartitioning procedure advocated by Santoro.

Logically, patients who experienced insufficient weight loss after LAGB despite an adequate follow-up, likely will benefit the most from a procedure with different mechanism of action (Fig. 22.1). Hence, most surgeons will elect a procedure that is less restrictive in nature. The most commonly chosen procedures are the RYGB, the OLGB, and the typical malabsorptive procedures DS and BPD. Some surgeons will adjust the procedure to obtain additional malabsorption, by lengthening the afferent limb in OLGB [20], or by distalizing the RYGB construction [21]. Recently, Greve and co-workers described a technique for performing a RYGB while leaving the band in place [22]. We usually prefer not to select this procedure, mainly because of its alleged restrictive character, as well as some specific factors that are inherent to the technique, such as anatomical situation of the stomach and the presence of GERD.

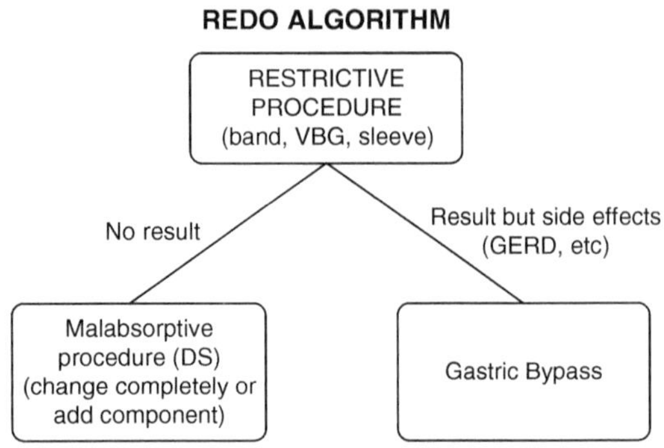

Fig. 22.1 General algorithm for revisional bariatric surgery for other reasons than surgical complications. *VBG* means vertical banded gastroplasty, *SG* means sleeve gastrectomy, *GERD* means gastro-esophageal reflux disease, *DS* duodenal switch

Anatomical situation of the stomach: We mentioned above the two typical complications after LAGB, i.e., the band erosion and the band slippage. The anatomical changes induced by these complications may preclude safe accomplishment of some procedures. Thus, many surgeons will be reluctant to perform LSG after band erosion because of the significant danger for leaks in an area that is already at stake because of poor vascular supply [23].

Presence of GERD: Patients who experienced significant GERD after LAGB should probably not be converted to LSG because of documented concerns that LSG aggravates GERD on midterm follow-up [24].

22.3 Technical Aspects of Conversion Procedures After LAGB Failure

Band erosion (also known as intragastric migration of the band) constitutes a specific and peculiar situation. Symptoms of this condition may include frank septic symptoms, but more subtle signs may be present, such as vague abdominal discomfort and loss of restriction experienced by the patient [25]. Once the condition has been diagnosed, band retrieval by endoscopic approach is to be preferred [26]. Alternatively, laparoscopic gastrotomy performed at a distance from the band may be carried out, allowing for band removal through the opening in the stomach [27]. This approach avoids the phlegmonous area surrounding the erosion site and deals with the risk of persisting gastric fistula.

Except for the specific case of band erosion that precludes immediate conversion, once the decision has been made to proceed with band ablation for other indications, the question remains if the band removal should be complemented by another bariatric procedure at the same stage, versus after a lag time. Staged conversion to RYGB reportedly is characterized by a reduced incidence of anastomotic stricture [28]. Other sources, however, favor the completion of the corrective procedure concomitantly with the band removal [29]. In our department, we prefer to perform band ablation and conversion to a new bariatric construction in one stage. We believe that the band constitutes a highly visible landmark as well as a handy retraction tool. In fact, we usually leave the band in place until full dissection of the upper pole of the stomach has been performed. Conversely, when one decides to proceed with the delayed approach, it is important to anticipate on possible problems during the revisional procedure. Hence, the gastrogastric stitches overlying the band should be severed; to avoid the risk of stapling across a double layer of tissues should one decide to perform a gastric bypass or LSG as revisional procedure. It is probably preferable as well to incise or even to remove the pseudo-capsule under the band, because this may reduce the risk of stenosis after the final procedure, as described some 20 years ago [30].

22.3.1 Dissection of the Adjustable Band

In this paragraph, we will try to highlight the essential steps of band removal and conversion to another procedure, as we usually perform it, i.e., in one stage.

Unlike some, we believe that the conversion procedure should imply a complete dissection of the upper pole of the stomach and of the hiatus. Dissection of the hiatus will possibly unveil a sliding or para-esophageal hernia that must be cured. It may also reveal a diastasis of the crurae, a condition that may favor the development of an intramediastinal migration of the remnant, as experienced by two of our patients who underwent band ablation and conversion to RYGB (unpublished data). One should, however, be aware of the possible hazards involved with the dissection around the hiatus, especially in the presence of substantial deformations caused by scar tissue around the band. One of the most dangerous steps of the dissection pertains to the freeing of the right crus. The vena cava is located in this very area and may be obscured by the scar tissue. The essential landmark in the area is the caudate lobe of the liver. After severance of the anterior adhesions of the liver to the upper part of the stomach, the bare surface of the stomach, obscuring the band to a certain degree, as well as the phreno-esophageal ligament become visible. Lateral traction of the band tubing allows for dissection of the lateral edge of the caudate lobe (Fig. 22.2).

The thick peritoneal layer overlying the edge of the lobe should be incised sharply, hereby opening the angle between the liver and the right crus. This angle should not be dissected any further to avoid lacerating the vena cava. Rather, the right crus should be adequately located and, again aided by forceful retraction of the band tubing in a lateral direction, the peritoneal layer overlying the crus should be incised. This latter maneuver readily reveals the distal esophagus (Fig. 22.3), which, in turn, will allow safe dissection of the adhesions overlying the buckle of the band and the right side of the band. Care must be taken not to damage the left gastric pedicle in this vicinity, and in case of doubt, this step should be delayed until later. Dissection should now be directed towards the apex of the hiatus and the left crus should be dissected from anterior going dorsally, but staying short of the angle of His (Fig. 22.4). Once the right side of the band has been freed, the lateral aspect of the band should be dissected.

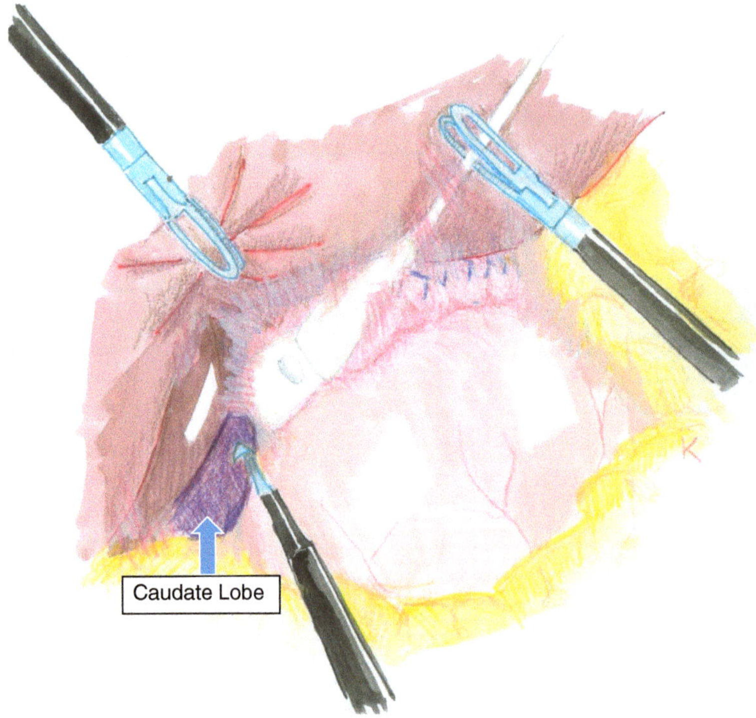

Fig. 22.2 The upper pole of the stomach is usually plastered with the liver. After freeing the anterior adhesions, dissection should be oriented towards the edge of the caudate lobe. Opening the space at the edge of the caudate lobe opens the way to the right crus

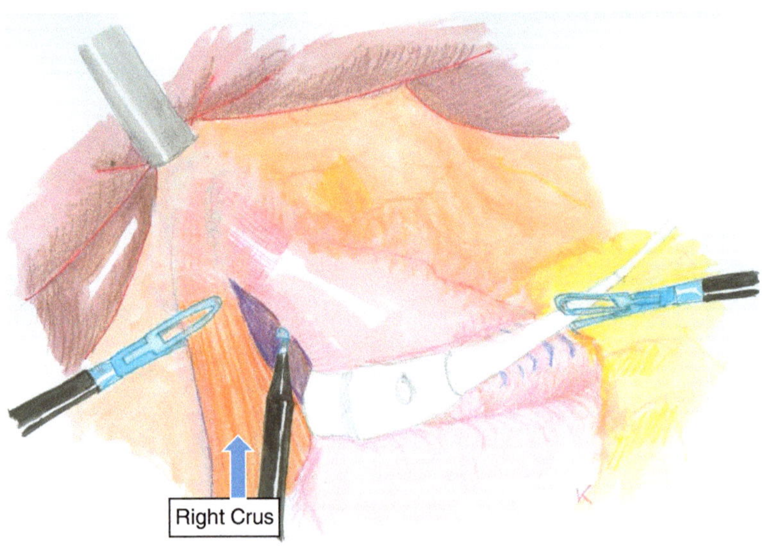

Fig. 22.3 The peritoneum overlying the right crus is incised which allows for exposing the esophagus. The presence of the band is advantageous for forceful retraction of the upper pole of the stomach

Starting at the previously dissected area of the band and going to the left, the gastro-gastric bridge overlying the band can now be dealt with, usually by following the several stitches that had been placed to fix the band (Fig. 22.5). Whenever the plane between the proximal and the distal part of the gastro-gastric bridge is not readily visible, one should rather err towards the distal side, because distal accidental opening of the gastric lumen is less of an issue than a proximal perforation. Severance of the gastro-gastric stitches must be complete, but sometimes the most lateral portion is difficult to reach from the right side and this step should be deferred until later. Dissection

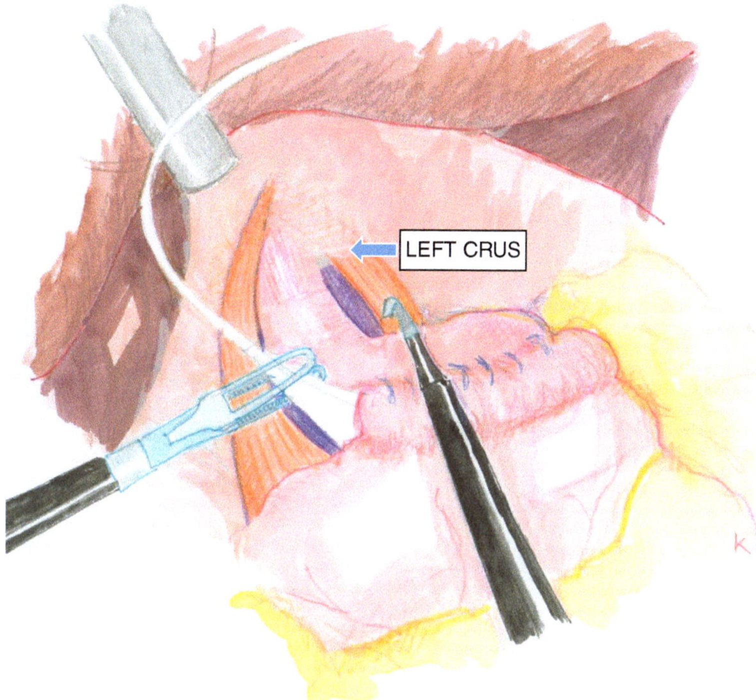

Fig. 22.4 Forceful retraction of the band to the right side of the patient helps with dissecting the left crus, while the esophagus is well visible and out of harm's way

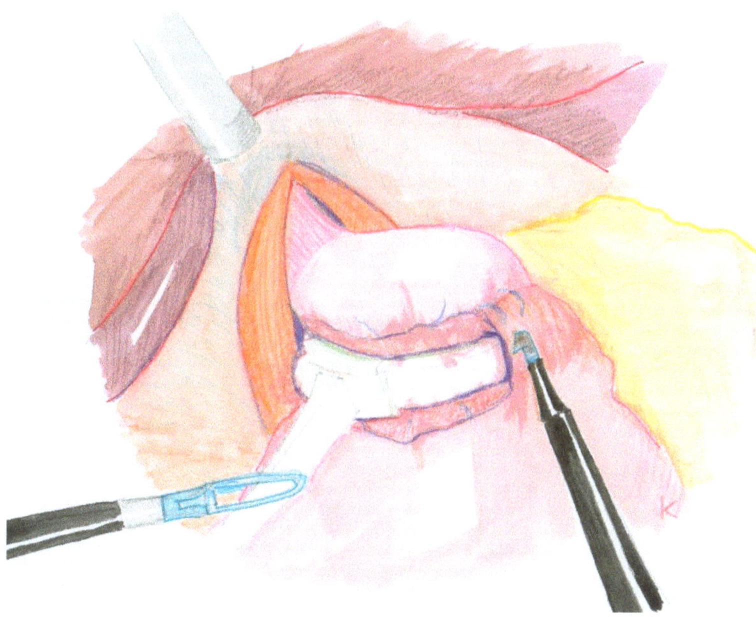

Fig. 22.5 Before attempting to dissect the angle of His, the stomach bridge overlying the band should be incised to reveal the ventral face of the band, lateral to the buckle. The stitches unting the gastrogastric bridge constitute an excellent landmark

thus closes in on the angle of His, which quite often is the most difficult step. One should be aware that in an effort to provide additional stability when inserting the band, some surgeons place a stitch from the stomach distal to the band to the root of the left crus, which obviously obscures the field during a revision. We believe it is advantageous at this stage to halt the dissection in the vicinity of the His angle and to resume dissection at the interface between spleen and upper fundus.

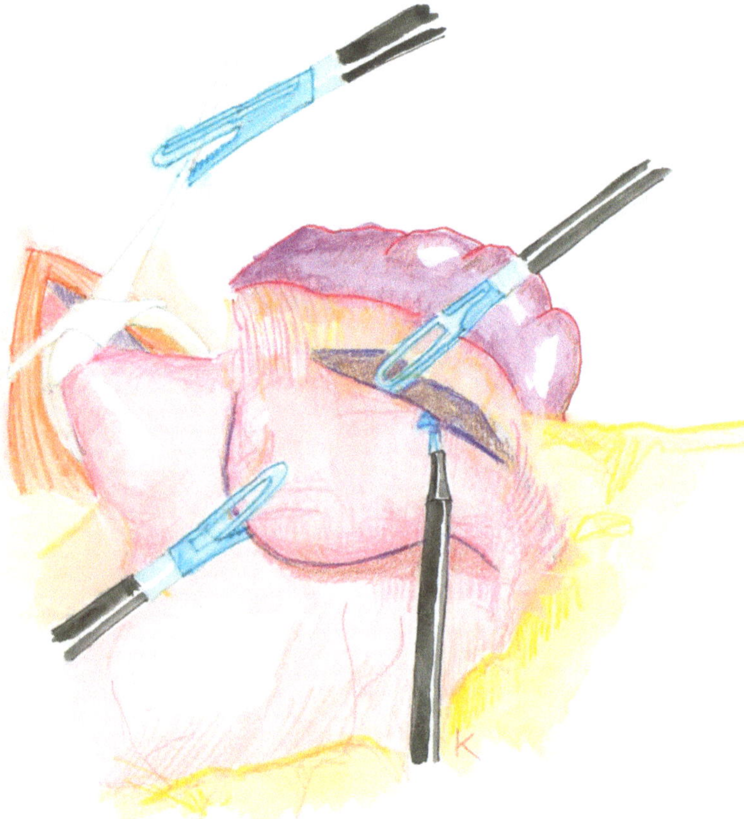

Fig. 22.6 A good strategy in preparing the dissection of the His angle is to open the space between the fundus of the stomach and the spleen, which is achieved by severance of the uppermost short gastric vessels. This maneuver widely opens the lesser sac. Subsequent ventral retraction of the fundus reveals the adhesions between band and angle of His, that can now safely be dealt with

The first few short vessels may now be ligated, which will create a distance between the lateral edge of the fundus and the spleen and give access to the lesser sac (Fig. 22.6). By retracting the freed edge of the fundus anteriorly and from left to right, the usually untouched posterior aspect of the stomach becomes readily visible. The thus created space posterior to the stomach has the shape of a pyramid, with the edge of the fundus anteriorly as base, the pancreas posteriorly and the and spleen edge laterally, while the apex is constituted by the adhesions overlying the posterior aspect of the band, with, to the right of this area, the left gastric pedicle (Fig. 22.7). The posterior adhesions overlying the band, including the ones at the extreme left side may now be safely transected. The final dissection of the angle of His, substantially facilitated by the complete freeing of the tissues all around the area, concludes the preparation for the removal of the band. The fully dissected hiatus should be thoroughly inspected and the surgeon should not hesitate to perform adequate closure of the crurae. The band should still be present at this stage because it significantly helps in a safe and correct hiatoplasty. We usually perform a posterior closure and use one or more figure of 8 stitches of polypropylene material, buttressed by cellulose pledgets (Surgicel, Johnson & Johnson) to avoid cutting through the tissues when the sutures are tied (Fig. 22.8). After completion of the hiatoplasty, the repair should fit snugly around a 34-French orogastric tube. With the band completely free, and the hiatal repair performed, transection or opening of the band can now be carried out. The pseudo-capsule caused by the impression of the band should be incised at this time (Fig. 22.9).

After removal of the band, the surgeon should inspect the freshly dissected upper portion of the stomach and evaluate the possibilities. Significant damage to the tissues may thus preclude safe stapling or suturing and may lead the surgeon to perform a gastric bypass with eso-enteral anastomosis. Conversely, if local conditions did not

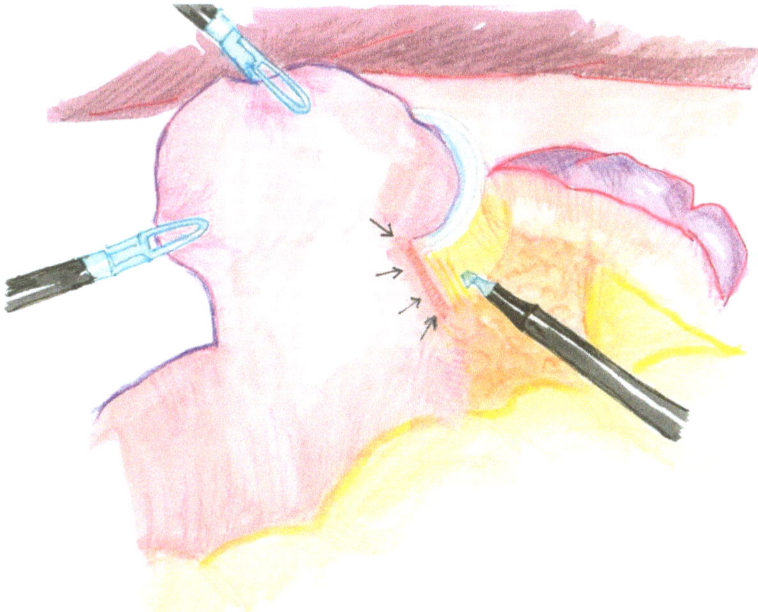

Fig. 22.7 The dissection of the upper pole of the stomach, including the hiatal crurae, is now complete. Now is the right time to perform the hiatal closure, which is carried out by at least one posterior figure of 8 stitches, buttressed by resorbable pledgets

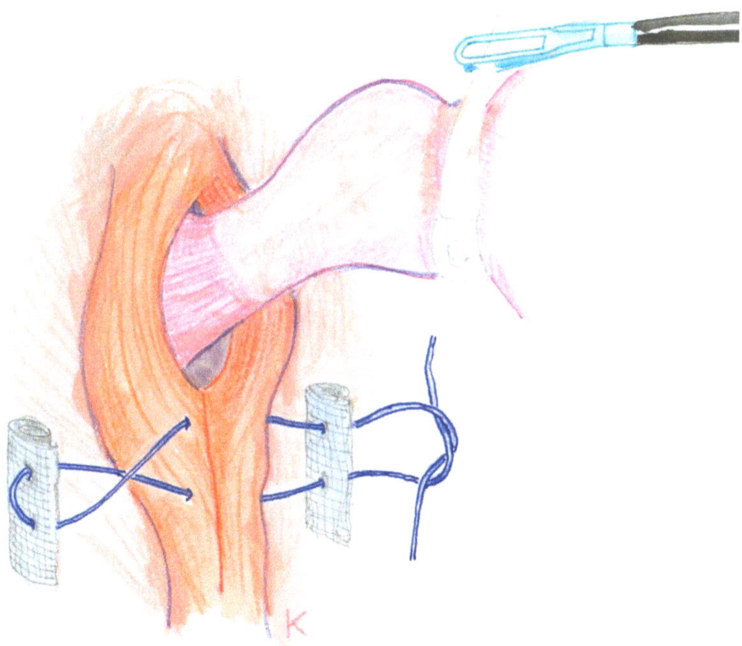

Fig. 22.8 By lifting the fundus from left to right, the posterior aspect of the band is well visible and can be freed from its last attachments. The main trunk of the left gastric artery (*arrows*) can be spotted at the superior edge of the pancreas, more often than not in very close vicinity of the band

allow thorough dissection of the band before removing it, it may be wise to abandon the efforts to obtain a small pouch and to prefer the option of performing a BPD. Usually, however, integrity of the tissues is satisfactory and will permit the planned procedure, i.e., either a gastric bypass or (seldom) an LSG. For either technique, we are concerned about possible damage to the main trunk of the left gastric artery. This is why during the preparation of a gastric bypass or a LSG, we limit the dissection at the lesser curvature to a strict minimum and will focus on the greater curvature.

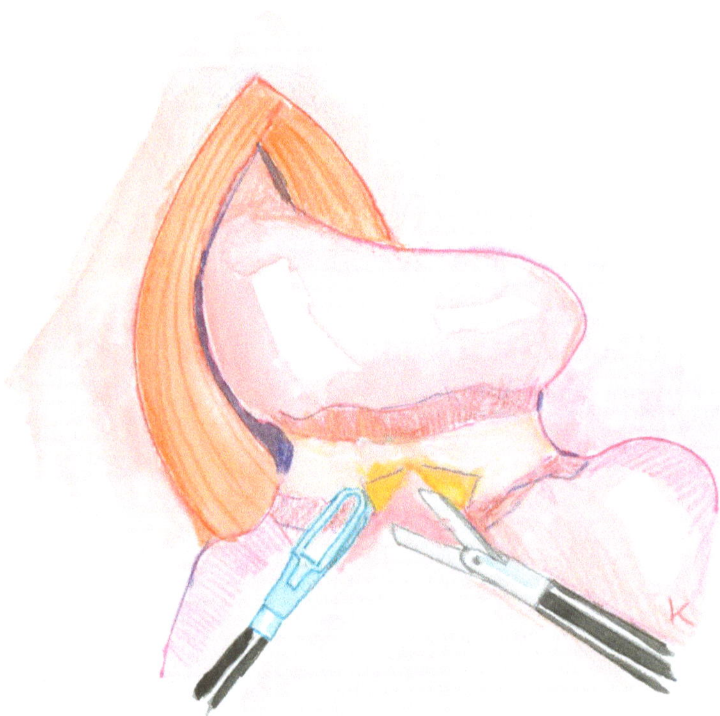

Fig. 22.9 The band has been removed. The underlying pseudo-capsule should be resected or transected (as shown here) to avoid subsequent stenosis

22.3.2 Transection of the Stomach

Over the years, we have gathered experience with over 500 band removals and conversions to RYGB (or, seldom, OLGB and LSG). We have tried to standardize the technique and to develop a strategy that would be similar for whatever construction. The strategy implies the resection of the upper part of the fundus, even in case of gastric bypass. This maneuver has the advantage of diminishing the risk of gastro-gastric fistula formation in revisional procedures [31] and to interfere with the production of Ghrelin, which in turn may improve weight loss [32].

We previously described that the uppermost short gastric vessels are routinely sacrificed during the freeing of the band. With this technique, the lesser sac is widely opened, which gives free access to the posterior surface of the stomach.

- When the foreseen procedure is a gastric bypass, the lesser curvature can now be approached posteriorly. The level of dissection will depend on the type of bypass, i.e., RYGB versus OLGB, and be performed rather close to the band impression for the former and more distally for the latter. In all cases, however, the dissection of the lesser curvature is initiated posteriorly, distally to the previous band placement, where tissues are supple and tissue distortion minimal. By lifting the stomach anteriorly, the tissues at the lesser curvature are placed under traction and the space between the vessels and the stomach itself can safely be dissected by the coagulating hook or by the harmonic scissors, until the tip of the dissecting tool emerges on the ventral aspect of the edge of the lesser curvature. The thus created opening in the peritoneal sheet constitutes the aim for the linear stapler when it transversally transects the stomach. Transection is performed from left to right, approximately at a right angle with the long axis of the stomach (Fig. 22.10). Thanks to the dissection performed at the lesser curvature, lesion to the main arterial trunk should be avoided and bleeding kept minimal.

After complete transverse transection of the stomach, the entire lateral proximal part of the stomach (i.e., the fundus) is forcefully pulled laterally and a 34-French orogastric tube is advanced

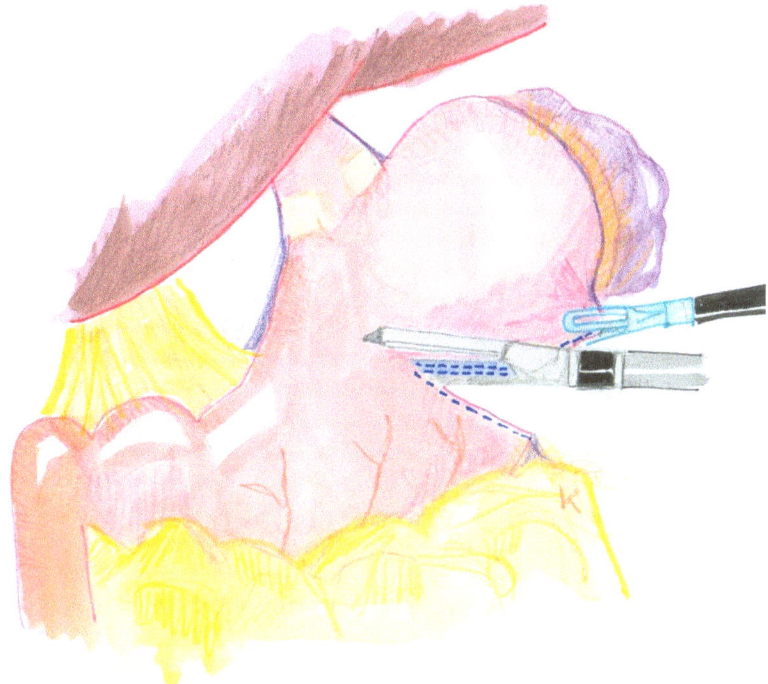

Fig. 22.10 The stomach is now transected from left to right, hereby avoiding dissection of the lesser curvature, that may be distorted by adhesions. The vessels at the lesser curvature are dissected from posterior, in the lesser sac that usually has remained untouched

by the anesthesiologist and is maneuvered close to the lesser curvature until it hits the transverse staple line. This maneuver is essential to obtain a narrow gastric tube, and may prove difficult, especially in the presence of a dilated pouch. However, because of the thoroughness of dissection prior to removal of the band, it should be possible to place a grasper from the left upper quadrant trocar posterior to the stomach, and, keeping it close to the lesser curvature, advance it to the root of the left crus, which will facilitate the correct placement of the large bore tube. With the 34-French tube in place, vertical stapling can be carried out, again while exerting adequate outward traction on the fundus to avoid making the gastric pouch too wide (Fig. 22.11). After complete transection of the stomach, as described, the fundic part has been entirely isolated and should now be removed, care being taken to sever all possible remaining attachments. After extraction of the isolated fundus, the proximal gastric pouch should be inspected. If it is deemed too long (as for RYGB) it can now safely be trimmed to an appropriate size before performing a gastro-enterostomy.

- When the corrective procedure is an LSG, the window at the greater curvature is widened in a caudal direction, until the antral area is reached. Here as well a transverse transection, perpendicular on the long axis of the stomach is performed by application of a linear stapler, but transection obviously remains incomplete to maintain a lumen that easily accommodates a 34-French intraluminal orogastric tube. Correct positioning of the large bore tube can be obtained as explained above for the bypass. Vertical stapling is performed as usual, care being taken not to make the tube too wide and avoiding a corkscrew deformity, which can be prevented by maintaining consistent outward traction on the greater curvature side of the stomach.

22.4 Outcomes of Conversion Procedures After Band Ablation

There is a general consensus that revisional surgery after adjustable band is sentenced by a higher incidence of complications. It appears, however, that revisional surgery after LAGB, is characterized by fewer complications than after other bariatric operations [33]. Nevertheless, in a population-based analysis covering 3,132 patients treated by band removal and conversion to RYGB,

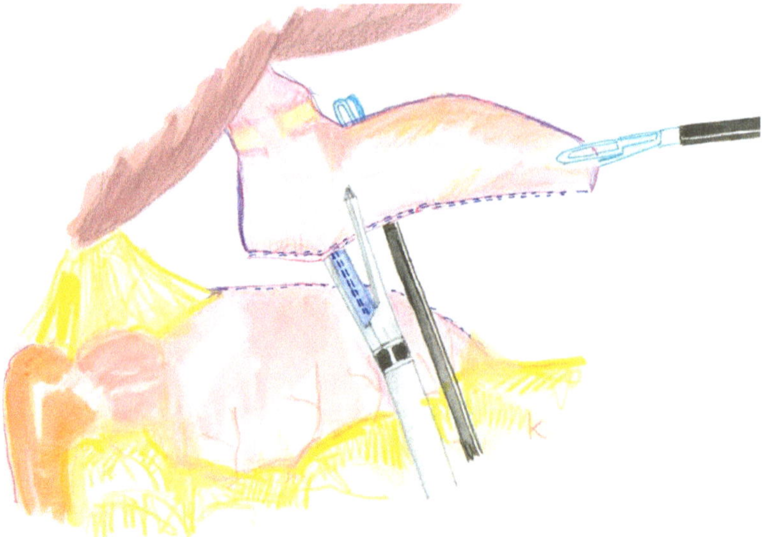

Fig. 22.11 After complete transverse transection of the stomach, at a distance from the band impression, a large bore orogastric tube is advanced by the anesthesiologist, while the fundus is being retracted by posterior and outward retraction with the assistant's grasper. This is an important step that may be time consuming especially when the fundus is very large, as in case of pouch dilation

Womi et al. [34] found a significantly higher incidence of preoperative and postoperative complications compared to primary gastric bypass (63,171 patients). In a retrospective study pertaining to 108 patients treated by RYGB for band failure [35], our group recorded a significantly higher (22.2 %) incidence of early complications, versus 10.2 % in a group of 362 patients treated by primary RYGB in the same time period. In addition, late complications occurred in 30.6 % of the patients in the revisional gastric bypass group, which was significantly higher than in the primary bypass group (12.7 %). Interestingly, we found no difference in terms of weight loss between the primary and the revisional gastric bypass [35]. Similarly, Hii et al. [36] found a good weight loss after conversion of LAGB into LRYGB, but their study confirmed a high incidence of severe complications linked with the procedure (13.4 % of major complications).

Concerning the conversion of LAGB to LSG, according to some, revisional LSG is characterized by a higher incidence of major complications (including mortality) than revisional RYGB [29]. In a review article, Coblijn et al. [37] found a significantly higher leak rate for LSG compared to primary LSG (5.6 % versus 0.35–2.40 %), which was substantially higher than the leak incidence in LRYGB (0.9 %). In addition, in this study, weight-loss figures were better after RYGB than after LSG. In our experience [38, 39], conversion of LAGB to LSG appeared to be safe, but additional weight loss was modest, which unfavorably compares with RYGB. Consequently, in our department conversion of LAGB to LSG is merely considered a first step to the completion of a DS [40].

Considering that LAGB is a purely restrictive procedure, in case of poor weight loss, conversion to a malabsorptive procedure seems logical, at least theoretically. Initially it was thought that "The BPD/DS, as opposed to the Roux-en-Y gastric bypass (RYGB), is well suited for LASGB revision, as its proximal anastomosis is at the duodenum, away from the gastric band scar tissue" [41].

The technique of conversion of LAGB to LDS was fine-tuned by its pioneer, Michel Gagner [42]. The initial indication for conversion to BPD/BPDDS was recurrent band slippage [43]. Lack of success was described in over 10 % of the cases [44], but some authors claim better results for conversion of LAGB to BPD than to RYGB [45]

22.5 Patient Education

An important element for success of a corrective procedure after LAGB is to influence eating behavior and overall life hygiene of the patient.

Especially in cases where the band procedure has failed despite adequate follow-up and despite the absence of surgical complications, poor weight loss is quite often due to the development of poor eating habits on the patient's side, usually sweet eating. It is obviously utopical to think that the simple fact of changing the anatomical situation should automatically condition the patient's eating behavior differently. There is evidence that the RYGB construction implies new and different alimentary preferences in patients [46]. According to our experience, however, this change for the better is rather short lived. Moreover, the dumping syndrome, that allegedly deters the patients from sweets eating after a RYGB [47], is quite infrequent and disappears with time. Conversely, some authors believe that sweet eating encourages more sweet eating, polyphagia (grazing), and weight regain [48] in patients who were treated by RYGB. In addition, sweet eating may on the long-term trigger the development of postprandial hypoglycemia [49], which can evolve to nesidioblastosis.

Similar concerns around dietary habits exist for LSG. We have shown that the long-term outcomes for this procedure typically show a tendency towards weight regain, and that dietary issues appear to be the culprit of this unwanted evolution [50]. Weight regain after LSG can be linked to overeating (hyperphagia) and often parallels the development of GERD. After the procedure, this latter condition becomes prevalent as time goes by. As mentioned before, concerns about GERD logically may deter surgeons from converting the LAGB procedure into LSG.

Finally, the "philosophically" most logical choice for treating LAGB failures, i.e., the malabsorptive procedures (Fig. 22.1), while the least sensitive to dietary flaws, do not allow for unbridled sweet eating, as abuse of fast carbohydrates will be sentenced by diarrhea and flatulence. Hence, dietary counseling remains imperative in these procedures as well.

Conclusion

LAGB is fraught with a substantial number of failures in most bariatric centers. Conversion to other weight loss constructions is technically feasible, but there is a general consensus that the conversion procedure is characterized by a rather high complication rate. In terms of weight loss, however, most corrective procedures prove more effective than the LAGB.

References

1. Buchwald H, Oien DM. Metabolic/bariatric surgery worldwide 2011. Obes Surg. 2013;23(4):427–36.
2. Di Lorenzo N, Furbetta F, Favretti F, et al. Laparoscopic adjustable gastric banding via pars flaccida versus perigastric positioning: technique, complications, and results in 2,549 patients. Surg Endosc. 2010;24(7):1519–23.
3. Singhal R, Bryant C, Kitchen M, et al. Band slippage and erosion after laparoscopic gastric banding: a meta-analysis. Surg Endosc. 2010;24(12):2980–6.
4. Foletto M, Bernante P, Busetto L, et al. Laparoscopic gastric rebanding for slippage with pouch dilation: results on 29 consecutive patients. Obes Surg. 2008; 18(9):1099–103.
5. Niville E, Dams A, Van Der Speeten K, et al. Results of lap rebanding procedures after Lap-Band removal for band erosion – a mid-term evaluation. Obes Surg. 2005;15(5):630–3.
6. Suter M, Calmes JM, Paroz A, et al. A 10-year experience with laparoscopic gastric banding for morbid obesity: high long-term complication and failure rates. Obes Surg. 2006;16(7):829–35.
7. Avriel A, Warner E, Avinoach E, et al. Major respiratory adverse events after laparascopic gastric banding surgery for morbid obesity. Respir Med. 2012;106(8): 1192–9.
8. Naef M, Mouton WG, Naef U, et al. Esophageal dysmotility disorders after laparoscopic gastric banding–an underestimated complication. Ann Surg. 2011;253(2): 285–90.
9. Dargent J. Isolated food intolerance after adjustable gastric banding: a major cause of long-term band removal. Obes Surg. 2008;18(7):829–32.
10. Brown JJ, Boyle M, Mahawar K, et al. Laparoscopic adjustable gastric band survival in a high-volume bariatric unit. Br J Surg. 2013;100(12):1614–8.
11. O'Brien PE, MacDonald L, Anderson M, et al. Long-term outcomes after bariatric surgery: fifteen-year follow-up of adjustable gastric banding and a systematic review of the bariatric surgical literature. Ann Surg. 2013;257(1):87–94.
12. Himpens J, Cadière GB, Bazi M, et al. Long-term outcomes of laparoscopic adjustable gastric banding. Arch Surg. 2011;146(7):802–7.
13. Aarts EO, Dogan K, Koehestanie P, et al. What happens after gastric band removal without additional bariatric surgery? Surg Obes Relat Dis. 2014;10(6):1092–6.

14. Reinhold RB. Critical analysis of long term weight loss following gastric bypass. Surg Gynecol Obstet. 1982;155(3):385–94.
15. Kampe J, Stefanidis A, Lockie SH, et al. Neural and humoral changes associated with the adjustable gastric band: insights from a rodent model. Int J Obes (Lond). 2012;36(11):1403–11.
16. Gelisgen R, Zengin K, Kocael A, et al. Effects of laparoscopic gastric band applications on plasma and fundic acylated ghrelin levels in morbidly obese patients. Obes Surg. 2012;22(2):299–305.
17. Wang Y, Liu J. Plasma ghrelin modulation in gastric band operation and sleeve gastrectomy. Obes Surg. 2009;19(3):357–62.
18. Caiazzo R, Pattou F. Adjustable gastric banding, sleeve gastrectomy or gastric bypass. Can evidence-based medicine help us to choose? J Visc Surg. 2013; 150(2):85–95.
19. Ionut V, Burch M, Youdim A, et al. Gastrointestinal hormones and bariatric surgery-induced weight loss. Obesity (Silver Spring). 2013;21(6):1093–103. doi:10.1002/oby.20364.
20. Lee WJ, Wang W, Lee YC, et al. Laparoscopic mini-gastric bypass: experience with tailored bypass limb according to body weight. Obes Surg. 2008;18(3): 294–9.
21. Srikanth MS, Oh KH, Fox SR. Revision to malabsorptive Roux-en-Y gastric bypass (MRNYGBP) provides long-term (10 years) durable weight loss in patients with failed anatomically intact gastric restrictive operations: long-term effectiveness of a malabsorptive Roux-en-Y gastric bypass in salvaging patients with poor weight loss or complications following gastroplasty and adjustable gastric bands. Obes Surg. 2011;21(7):825–31.
22. Meesters B, Latten G, Timmermans L, et al. Roux-en-Y gastric bypass as revisional procedure after gastric banding: leaving the band in place. Surg Obes Relat Dis. 2012;8(6):717–22.
23. Perez M, Brunaud L, Kedaifa S, et al. Does anatomy explain the origin of a leak after sleeve gastrectomy? Obes Surg. 2014;24(10):1717–23.
24. Laffin M, Chau J, Gill RS, et al. Sleeve gastrectomy and gastroesophageal reflux disease. J Obes. 2013; 2013:741097.
25. Brown WA, Egberts KJ, Franke-Richard D, et al. Erosions after laparoscopic adjustable gastric banding: diagnosis and management. Ann Surg. 2013; 257(6):1047–52.
26. El-Hayek K, Timratana P, Brethauer SA, et al. Complete endoscopic/transgastric retrieval of eroded gastric band: description of a novel technique and review of the literature. Surg Endosc. 2013;27(8):2974–9.
27. Spitali C, De Vogelaere K, Delvaux G. Removal of eroded gastric bands using a transgastric SILS device. Case Rep Surg. 2013;2013:852747.
28. Van Nieuwenhove Y, Ceelen W, Van Renterghem K, et al. Conversion from band to bypass in two steps reduces the risk for anastomotic strictures. Obes Surg. 2011;21(4):501–5.
29. Fernando Santos B, Wallaert JB, Trus TL. Band removal and conversion to sleeve or bypass: are they equally safe? Surg Endosc. 2014;28(11):3086–91.
30. Broadbent R. Endoscopically assisted gastric stomal dilation for reflux and vomiting after gastric banding. Obes Surg. 1994;4(1):47–50.
31. Patel S, Szomstein S, Rosenthal RJ. Reasons and outcomes of reoperative bariatric surgery for failed and complicated procedures (excluding adjustable gastric banding). Obes Surg. 2011;21(8):1209–19.
32. Chronaiou A, Tsoli M, Kehagias I, et al. Lower ghrelin levels and exaggerated postprandial peptide-YY, glucagon-like peptide-1, and insulin responses, after gastric fundus resection, in patients undergoing Roux-en-Y gastric bypass: a randomized clinical trial. Obes Surg. 2012;22(11):1761–70.
33. Stefanidis D, Malireddy K, Kuwada T, et al. Revisional bariatric surgery: perioperative morbidity is determined by type of procedure. Surg Endosc. 2013;27(12):4504–10.
34. Worni M, østbye T, Shah A, et al. High risks for adverse outcomes after gastric bypass surgery following failed gastric banding: a population-based trend analysis of the United States. Ann Surg. 2013;257(2):279–86.
35. Cadière GB, Himpens J, Bazi M, et al. Are laparoscopic gastric bypass after gastroplasty and primary laparoscopic gastric bypass similar in terms of results? Obes Surg. 2011;21:692–8.
36. Hii MVV, Lake AC, Kenfield C, et al. Laparoscopic conversion of failed gastric banding to Roux-en-Y gastric bypass: short-term follow-up and technical considerations. Obes Surg. 2012;22(7):1022–8.
37. Coblijn UK, Verveld CJ, van Wagensveld BA, et al. Laparoscopic Roux-en-Y gastric bypass or laparoscopic sleeve gastrectomy as revisional procedure after adjustable gastric band – a systematic review. Obes Surg. 2013;23(11):1899–914.
38. Himpens J, De Schepper M, Dapri G. Laparoscopic conversion of adjustable gastric banding to sleeve gastrectomy: a feasibility study. Surg Laparosc Endosc Percutan Tech. 2010;20(3):162–5.
39. Dapri G, Cadière GB, Himpens J. Feasibility and technique of laparoscopic conversion of adjustable gastric banding to sleeve gastrectomy. Surg Obes Relat Dis. 2009;5(1):72–6.
40. Dapri G, Cadière GB, Himpens J. Laparoscopic conversion of adjustable gastric banding and vertical banded gastroplasty to duodenal switch. Surg Obes Relat Dis. 2009;5(6):678–83.
41. de Csepel J, Quinn T, Pomp A, et al. Conversion to a laparoscopic biliopancreatic diversion with a duodenal switch for failed laparoscopic adjustable silicone gastric banding. J Laparoendosc Adv Surg Tech A. 2002;12(4):237–40.
42. Gagner M, Steffen R, Biertho L, et al. Laparoscopic adjustable gastric banding with duodenal switch for morbid obesity: technique and preliminary results. Obes Surg. 2003;13(3):444–9.
43. Dolan K, Fielding G. Bilio pancreatic diversion following failure of laparoscopic adjustable gastric banding. Surg Endosc. 2004;18(1):60–3.

44. Slater G, Duncombe J, Fielding GA. Poor weight loss despite biliopancreatic diversion and subsequent revision to a 30-cm common channel after initial laparoscopic adjustable gastric banding: an analysis of 8 cases. Surg Obes Relat Dis. 2005;1(6):573–9. Epub 2005 Oct 27.
45. Topart P, Becouarn G, Ritz P. Biliopancreatic diversion with duodenal switch or gastric bypass for failed gastric banding: retrospective study from two institutions with preliminary results. Surg Obes Relat Dis. 2007;3(5):521–5.
46. Scholtz S, Miras AD, Chhina N, et al. Obes patients after gastric bypass surgery have lower brain-hedonic responses to food than after gastric banding. Gut. 2014;63(6):891–902.
47. Sugerman HJ, Starkey JV, Birkenhauer R. A randomized prospective trial of gastric bypass versus vertical banded gastroplasty for morbid obesity and their effects on sweets versus non-sweets eaters. Ann Surg. 1987;205(6):613–24.
48. Roslin MS, Oren JH, Polan BN, et al. Abnormal glucose tolerance testing after gastric bypass. Surg Obes Relat Dis. 2013;9(1):26–31.
49. McLaughlin T, Peck M, Holst J, et al. Reversible hyperinsulinemic hypoglycemia after gastric bypass: a consequence of altered nutrient delivery. J Clin Endocrinol Metab. 2010;95(4):1851–5.
50. Himpens J, Dobbeleir J, Peeters G. Long-term results of laparoscopic sleeve gastrectomy for obesity. Ann Surg. 2010;252(2):319–24.

23 Revisional or Conversion Procedures for Roux-en-Y Gastric Bypass Failure

Luigi Angrisani, Antonella Santonicola, Giampaolo Formisano, Ariola Hasani, and Michele Lorenzo

Surgery for morbid obesity has been carried out since 1950s, but only after the introduction of biliopancreatic diversion by Scopinaro the surgical approach gain worldwide consensus and diffusion [1, 2]. During the years, gastric restrictive, malabsorptive or combined procedures were introduced in the bariatric surgical praxis [3, 4]. Several experiences reported risk and benefit of each procedure, and the even increasing number of operated patients run parallel with a similar increase of re-do operations [5, 6]. Re-do bariatric surgical procedures are mainly indicated for two reasons. The first reason is the presence of an acute or chronic complication or a side effect of the primary bariatric procedure or metabolic and nutritional sequel. The second is the absence of postoperative weight loss or the weight regain after a successful period, untreatable with conservative approach [7–11]. Re-do bariatric procedures can be divided into conversions and revisions. Conversion surgery is defined as the exchange of a bariatric procedure to another one. Revision surgery is defined as the modification of the primary bariatric procedure without changes of its anatomical scheme.

Inadequate weight loss, according to Reynhold criteria, is considered if %EWL remains <25 % [12]. According to body mass index Maclean defines failures or poor results of those patients with BMI <30 kg/m [2, 13]. Success can be also defined as a resolution of comorbidities and/or improvement of quality of life.

Roux-en-Y gastric bypass was considered by many authors not only as the primary bariatric procedure of choice, but also as the re-do procedure to prefer after unsuccessful restrictive procedure [14–16]. Unfortunately, the bypass can also result in an acute or chronic failure needing a re-do procedure (Table 23.1). As regarding the weight loss, Fobi after 10 years of follow up reported 20 % of weight loss failure [17]. Power reported 30 % of failure in super-obese patients [18]. These data were also confirmed by other experiences with a weight loss failure between 10 and 20 % after 2–3 years of follow up [19, 20]. The Roux-en-Y gastric bypass produces its effects with both restriction and malabsorption. To understand the weight loss failure or

Table 23.1 Causes of chronic failure of Roux-en-Y gastric bypass

Gastro-jejunal stricture
Marginal ulcer
Excessive weight loss (severe malnutrition)
Absence of weight loss or weight regain

L. Angrisani, MD (✉) • A. Santonicola, MD
G. Formisano, MD • A. Hasani, MD
M. Lorenzo, MD, PhD
UOC Chirurgia Generale, Laparoscopica e d'Urgenza, Ospedale "S.Giovanni Bosco" ASL Napoli 1 centro, Naples, Italy
e-mail: luigiangrisani@chirurgiaobesita.it; michele.lorenzo@gmail.com

M. Lucchese, N. Scopinaro (eds.), *Minimally Invasive Bariatric and Metabolic Surgery: Principles and Technical Aspects*, DOI 10.1007/978-3-319-15356-8_23,

Table 23.2 Roux-en-Y gastric bypass weight loss failure: therapeutic options

Restrictive procedures
Endoscopy
Gastro-entero anastomosis suture
Sealants injection
Internal plication (mucosal or full thickness)
Laparoscopy
Nonadjustable ring positioning
Adjustable band positioning
Pouch resection/Fundectomy
External plication
Malabsorptive procedures
BPD -DS
Length limb modification

recidivism, it has been postulated that the loss of the restriction is in relationship with the enlargement of the gastric pouch, or the gastro-jejunostomy, or both [21, 22]. Honeghan et al. in a multivariate analysis identified stomal dilation as independently associated with weight recidivism. The stoma dilation can be functionally linked to a greater quantity of food being needed to distend the gastric pouch, causing the sensation of satiety. It has been reported to occur as early as 6 months from gastric bypass. Obviously, the primary pouch dilation has the same effects on satiety. Moreover, Yimcharoen et al. demonstrated that an enlarged gastric pouch was observed in almost one-third of RYGB operated patients with weight regain.

Another reason of weight regain in gastric bypass is the presence of a gastro-gastric fistula. This is an abnormal communication between the excluded stomach and the gastric pouch. It is a rare complication (1.5–6 %) [23]. The gastro-gastric fistula is responsible of weight regain for the loss of both of restrictive and malabsorptive pathway [23, 24]. In fact by the fistula the food not passing through the stoma and bypassed intestine, causing weight regain. One of most important reasons to weight loss failure is intestinal adaptation. Scopinaro, while describing the malabsorptive properties of the biliopancreatic diversion, say that the massive intestinal adaptation phenomenon causes an increased absorptive surface. Between the gastro-entero anastomosis and the jejuno-jejunal anastomosis the intestinal tract increases in thickness with a corresponding increase in the length of gastrointestinal *villae*.

Re-do surgery for Roux-en-Y gastric bypass was considered a challenge in the field of bariatric surgery, with high risk of complication rate and patients discomfort. Recently, many authors have reported several endoscopic or laparoscopic bariatric options, above all for the problem of weight regain or absence of weight loss (Table 23.2).

23.1 Restrictive Procedures

23.1.1 Endoscopic Procedures

Endoscopic option for weight recidivism linked to dilated gastro-jejunal anastomosis has been suggested in several experiences to be safe with minimal morbidity. Catalano et al. showed that the injection of sclerotic agents to reduce the size of gastro-jejunal anastomosis result in weight loss after weight regain [25]. Thompson et al. showed that endoscopic suturing was also safe and feasible to reduce the gastrointestinal anastomosis to an average of 10 mm, leading to weight loss in 75 % of RYGBP patients and resulting in loss of 23.4 % of EBWL [23]. Recently, a viable endoscopic alternative to reduce the pouch volume was proposed, with mucosal or total wall plication, reshaping the pouch with dedicated instruments [1, 23]. Eid et al. have reported a randomized clinical trial comparing multiple full-thickness plications to sham endoscopy procedure after weight loss failure of RYGB [26]. They suspended the trial prematurely because preliminary results indicated the failure to achieve the primary efficacy end point at last in 50 % of patients treated with plication.

23.1.2 Laparoscopic Procedure

Parikh et al. suggest resecting the pouch and alimentary loop in a longitudinal fashion. But this procedure was not considered safe and effective enough [27]. Hamdi et al. also suggest resizing the gastric pouch by resection and recreating the gastrojejunostomy. Perioperaitive complication rate was 8 % [28]. After 24 months of follow up they observed 44 % of %EWL. They conclude that this re-do procedure can be performed with significant weight loss, but additional studies are requested [28]. Gumbs et al., in case of tissue suffering from previous scars or fistulas or postoperative leak, suggest an external plication mimicking the longitudinal resection suggested by Parikh, and inspired by the gastric plication technique [1]. This plication was performed with nonabsorbable stitches across a 34 French orogastric tube. This revisional option was safe and attractive in terms of safety, but long-term results of these techniques are not reported.

Another laparoscopic option to treat the pouch enlargement is the positioning of an external ring. Essentially two options have been described. Fobi showed that the addition of ring proximally to the gastrointestinal anastomosis is enough to reduce the food ingestion [29]. More recently were described some patients with an adjustable gastric banding positioned around the upper part of the gastric pouch. Chin et al. described their experience with ten patients who underwent revisional surgery positioning an adjustable gastric banding around the RYGB pouch [30]. After 2 years of follow up the %EWL was 48.7 % (range 21.8–98.1 %) without life threatening complications. Bessler et al. reported their experience with 27 patients who underwent RYGB revision with adjustable gastric band [31]. At 60 months of follow up they observed 47 % of %EWL; also, in this report life threatening complications were absent and two port-related complications and one band slippage were recorded. They conclude that the addiction of the adjustable silicone gastric banding causes significant weight loss in patients with weight recidivism or poor weight loss after RYGB. The absence of anastomosis or changes in limbs length makes this revisional option safe and attractive. Recently, Vijgen reported a review of the studies on the effects of salvage pouch banding after failed RYGB [32]. In their review were included patients with both adjustable and non-adjustable gastric banding operated via laparotomy or laparoscopy. In the seven studies considered, all the authors support the opinion that the adjustable gastric banding around the pouch is a safe and feasible revisional procedure after failed RYGB [32]. Moreover, despite these studies, long-term results on a large patient population who underwent pouch banding are scarce, waiting for an evidence-based confirmation.

23.2 Malabsorptive Procedures

Parikh et al. have suggested a conversion procedure to duodenal switch in cases of weight loss failure after Roux-en-Y gastric bypass [33]. This procedure was initially reported on 13 patients and was performed in two steps. The first step is the conversion of gastric bypass to sleeve gastrectomy after gastro-jejunal anastomosis removal and the reconnection of the gastric pouch to the stomach remnant. The second step was to complete the duodenal switch several months after the sleeve. In this series, mortality, leaks, and malabsorptive problems were not observed. Four patients developed a stenosis of gastro-gastric stricture resolved by endoscopy in three cases. Authors conclude on the bases of their early results that the conversion of failed RYGB in DS in expert hands is a valid therapeutic option with 63 % of %EWL and BMI loss of 11 kg/m^2. The complication rate was acceptable, but the number of operated patients was too small and the follow-up too short. Himpens suggested a slight modification of this approach to make the procedure more safer, with a first stage involving reversal to normal anatomy, followed after 3 months by a sleeve gastrectomy, and then a duodenal switch after 9 months from the first stage [34].

An alternative considered is to switch the RYGB in a distal RYGB, with a higher malabsorptive power. This option was considered uneventful by some authors, dangerous by other.

23.3 Causes of Gastric Bypass Revision or Conversion Not Related to Weight Loss

The most common indication for conversion or revision of Roux-en-Y gastric bypass is gatrointestinal anastomosis stricture and marginal ulcers [35–37]. The rate of incidence of gastro-jejunal stricture has been reported with a wide range: 4–36 %. In these cases the endoscopic dilation was safe and effective in 80–90 % of cases with low complication rate (perforation). In negative therapeutic results, a more invasive approach was indicated as in marginal ulcers. The incidence of marginal ulcer after RYGP is 1–16 %. This complication was linked to several factors such as eroded suture, drugs (NSAID), smoking, *Helicobacter pylori* infection, and acid exposure (gastro-gastric fistula). The treatment of these complications is medical by removal of all risk factors with administration of proton pump inhibitors and/or other drugs. In patients refractory to medical therapy or preventive measures or endoscopic attempts, a re-do was suggested to avoid serious complication such as perforation or bleeding. In these cases, the resection of primary gastro-jejunal anastomosis re-doing a new communication was suggested with safe results.

Conclusion

The Roux-en-Y gastric bypass is considered one of the bariatric approach of choice both in primary and in secondary surgical procedures. Moreover, also in this procedure a wide range of unsuccessful weight loss was recorded. In the past, the conversion or the revision of gastric bypass was considered a surgical challenge. The introduction of laparoscopic or endoscopic procedure has recently lowered the minor and major complications to an acceptable rate. Both restrictive and malabsorptive re-do procedures were reported with different success rates in terms of weight loss. Comparative studies among these techniques are scarce, and cost/benefit analysis are lacking. More experiences with lager number of patients are needed.

References

1. Gumbs AA, Pomp A, Gagner M. Revisional Bariatric Surgery for inadequate weight loss. Obes Surg. 2007;17:1137–45.
2. Scopinaro N. Biliopancreatic mechanism of action and long term results. Obes Surg. 2006;16:683–9.
3. Mognol P, Chosidow D, Marmuse JP. Laparoscopic sleeve gastrectomy (LSG): review of a new bariatric procedure and initial results. Surg Technol Int. 2006;15:47–52.
4. Angrisani L, Furbetta F, Doldi SB, et al. Lap Band® – Adjustable Gastric Banding System. The Italian experience with 1863 patients operated on 6 years. Surg Endosc. 2003;17:409–12.
5. Lim CS, Liew V, Talbot ML, et al. Revisional bariatric surgery. Obes Surg. 2009;19:827–32.
6. Karmali S, Brar B, Shi X, Sharma AM, de Gara C, Birch DW. Weight recidivism post-bariatric surgery: a systematic review. Obes Surg. 2013;23:1922–33.
7. Elnahas A, Graybiel K, Farboukhyar F, Gmora S, Anvari M, et al. Revisional surgery after failed laparoscopic adjustable gastric banding: a systematic review. Surg Endosc. 2013;27:740–5.
8. Robert M, Poncet G, Boulez J, Mion F, Espalieu P. Laparoscopic gastric bypass for failure of adjustable gastric banding: a review of 85 cases. Obes Surg. 2011;21:1513–9.
9. Victorzon M. Revisional bariatric surgery by conversion to gastric bypass or sleeve. Good short term outcomes at high risks. Obes Surg. 2012;22:29–33.
10. Coblijn UK, Verveld CJ, van Nagensveld BA, Lagarde SM. Laparoscopic Roux-en-Y Gastric Bypass or Laparoscopic Sleeve gastrectomy as revisional procedure after adjustable Gastric band. A systematic review. Obes Surg. 2013;23:1899–914.
11. Angrisani L, Borrelli V, Lorenzo M, et al. Conversion of LapBand to Gastric bypass for dilated gastric pouch. Obes Surg. 2001;11:232–4.
12. Reinhold RB. Critical analysis of long term weight loss following gastric bypass. Surg Gynecol Obstet. 1982;155:385–94.
13. MacLean LD, Rhodes BM, Nohr CW. Late outcome of isolated gastric bypass. Ann Surg. 2000;231:524–8.
14. Schouten R, Japink F, Meesters B, et al. Systematic literature review of reoperations after gastric banding: is a stepwise approach justified? Surg Obes Relat Dis. 2011;7:99–109.
15. Angrisani L, Lorenzo M, Santoro T, Nicodemi O, Persico G, Tesauro B. Videolaparoscopic treatment of gastric banding complications. Obes Surg. 1999;9:58–62.
16. Ardestani A, Lautz DB, Tavakkolizadeh A. Band revision versus Roux-en-Y gastric bypass conversion as salvage operation after laparoscopic adjustable gastric banding. Surg Obes Relat Dis. 2011;7:33–7.
17. Fobi MA. Surgical treatment of obesity: a review. J Natl Med Assoc. 2004;96:61–75.
18. Powers PS, Rosemurgy A, Boyd F, Peres A. Outcome of gastric restriction, procedure, weight, psychiatric diagnoses and satisfaction. Obes Surg. 1997;7:471–7.
19. Christou N, Look D, MacLean L. Weight gain after short and long limb gastric bypass in patients followed for longer than years. Ann Surg. 2006;244:734–40.
20. Spivak H, Abdelmalek MF, Beltram OR, Ng AW, Kitabama S. Long term outcomes of laparoscopic adjustable gastric banding and laparoscopic

Roux-en-Y gastric bypass in the United States. Surg Endosc. 2012;26:1909–19.
21. Honeghan HM, Yimcaroen P, Brethauer SA, et al. Influence of pouch and stoma size on weight loss after gastric bypass. Surg Obes Relat Dis. 2012;8:408–15.
22. Yimcaroen P, Honeghan HM, Singh M, et al. Endoscopic findings and outcomes of revisional procedures for patients with weight recidivism after gastric bypass. Surg Endosc. 2011;25:3345–52.
23. Thompson CC, Slattery J, Bundga ME, et al. Peroral endoscopic reduction of dilated gastrojejunal anastomosis after Roux-en-Y gastric bypass: a possible new option for patients with weight regain. Surg Endosc. 2006;20:1744–8.
24. Filho AJ, William K, Nassif LS, et al. Gastrogastric fistula, a possible complication of Roux-en-Y gastric Baypass. JSLS. 2006;10:326–31.
25. Catalano MF, Rudic G, Anderson AJ, et al. Weight gain after bariatric surgery as a result of a large gastric stoma: endotherapy with sodium morrhuate may prevent the need for surgical revision. Gastrointest Endosc. 2007;66:240–5.
26. Eid GM, McCloskey CA, Eapleton JK, Lee LB, Conscaulas AP. Stomaphix Vs sham procedure for revisional surgery to reduce regained weight to Roux-en-Y gastric bypass patients. A randomized clinical trial. JAMA Surg. 2014;141:372–9.
27. Parich M, Heacock L, Gagner M. Laparoscopic 'gastrojejunal reduction' as a revision procedure for weight loss failure after Roux-en-Y gastric bypass. Obes Surg. 2011;21:517–23.
28. Hamdi A, Julien C, Brown P, et al. Midterm outcomes of revisional surgery for a gastric pouch and gastrojejunal anastomosis enlargement in patients with weight regain after gastric bypass for morbid obesity. Obes Surg. 2014;24(8):1386–90. Epub March 16.
29. Fobi MA. Placement of the GaBP ring system in the banded gastric bypass operation. Obes Surg. 2005;15:1196–201.
30. Chin PL, Ali M, Francis K, LePort PC. Adjustable gastric band placed around gastric bypass pouch as revision operation for failed gastric bypass. Surg Obes Relat Dis. 2009;5:38–42.
31. Bessler M, Daud A, DiGiorgi MF, et al. Adjustable gastric banding as revisional bariatric procedure after failed gastric bypass – intermediate results. Surg Obes Relat Dis. 2010;6:31–5.
32. Vijgen GHEJ, Shouten R, Bouvy ND, Greve JWM. Salvage banding for failed Roux-en-Y gastric bypass. Surg Obes Relat Dis. 2012;8:803–8.
33. Parikh M, Pomp A, Gagner M. Laparoscopic conversion of failed gastric bypass to duodenal switch: technical considerations and preliminary outcomes. Surg Obes Relat Dis. 2007;3:611–8.
34. Himpens J, Dapri G. Redo Bariatic procedures. In: Frezza EE, Gagner M, Li MKW, editors. International principles of laparoscopic surgery. Cine-Med: Woodbury; 2010. p. 393–404.
35. Mathew A, Veliuoma MA, DePalma FJ, et al. Gastrointestinal stricture after gastric bypass and efficacy of endoscopic intervention. Dig Dis Sci. 2009;54:1971–8.
36. Radtka III JF, Puleo FJ, Wang L, Cooney RN. Revisional bariatric surgery: who, what, where and when? Surg Obes Relat Dis. 2010;6:635–42.
37. El-Hayek K, Timratana P, Shimizu H, Chand B. Marginal ulcer after Roux-en-Y gastric bypass: what have we really learned? Surg Endosc. 2012;26:2789–96.

24 Revisional Surgery: Biliopancreatic Diversion Failure

Valerio Ceriani, Ferdinando Pinna, Tiziana Lodi, and Paolo Gaffuri

24.1 Characteristics and Results of Classic Biliopancreatic Diversion as Proposed by Scopinaro

Biliopancreatic diversion (BPD), as proposed by Scopinaro, is a malabsorptive procedure for the treatment of morbid obesity, which has shown excellent results in terms of percentage excess weight loss (EWL) and improvement of co-morbidities.

In the Scopinaro's series, BPD yielded the following EWL: 74 %, 75 % and 78 % at 2 years, 4 and 12 years, respectively [1]. In addition, complete disappearance of type 2 (T2) diabetes and hyper-cholesterolemia was observed in 100 % of the patients [1].

Similar results have been confirmed by other authors. Guedea reported 70 % EWL at 5 years, with similar results in the morbid obese and super-obese and satisfying quality of life (QoL) [2]. In a recent meta-analysis, Buchwald reported the disappearance of T2 diabetes in 98.9 % of patients and of hyper-lipidaemia in 99.1 % of patients, following BPD. However, some studies included in the meta-analysis used the so-called duodenal switch variant, instead of the classic BPD [3].

The procedure initially described by Scopinaro consists of two third of distal gastrectomy with a 200–500 ml gastric stump draining into a long-limb Roux–en-Y ileal conduit, 250 cm long. The biliopancreatic limb is anastomosed to the alimentary limb, 50 cm proximally to the ileo-cecal valve, leaving a short common channel and excluding both duodenum and jejunum from the alimentary transit (Fig. 24.1) [4].

After BPD, the first phase of rapid weight loss occurs, lasting between several months to 1 year, mainly due to the reduced alimentary intake caused by the distal gastrectomy, and the post-feeding syndrome, owing to the interaction of the ingested material with the distal ileum. The long-term weight loss is then maintained by the malabsorptive effect of the Roux-en-Y limb.

24.2 Type and Incidence of Post-operative Complications

BPD is a safe operation, with low post-operative morbidity and mortality [5]. Nevertheless, chronic malabsorption which is crucial for the

V. Ceriani • T. Lodi • P. Gaffuri
Department of General Surgery, IRCCS Multimedica, Via Milanese 300, Sesto San Giovanni, Milan 20099, Italy
e-mail: valerio.ceriani@multimedica.it; tiziana.lodi@multimedica.it

F. Pinna (✉)
Second General Surgery, Ospedale San Giuseppe, Via San Vittore 12, Milano 20123, Italy
e-mail: ferdinando.pinna@tiscali.it

M. Lucchese, N. Scopinaro (eds.), *Minimally Invasive Bariatric and Metabolic Surgery: Principles and Technical Aspects*, DOI 10.1007/978-3-319-15356-8_24,

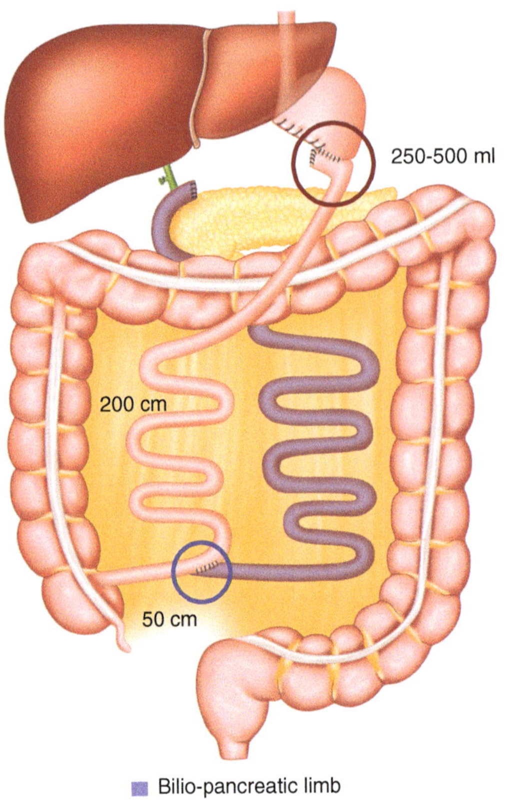

Fig. 24.1 Biliopancreatic diversion as described by Nicola Scopinaro

therapeutic effects can be responsible for some negative side effects.

24.2.1 Protein Malnutrition

This condition represents the most severe side effect of BPD. Its patophysiology is linked to several aspects of the intevention: the gastric volume affects the amount of food, and then proteins that can be assumed, while the length of the alimentary limb conditions the amount of small bowel suitable for proteic absorbption. Moreover, after BPD, there is an increased loss of endogenous nitrogen [1, 6], requiring a higher intake of dietary proteins. Severe hypo-proteinemia may result, owing to an improper nutritional regime.

The incidence of protein malnutrition is higher in the first two years after the intervention, and reduces thereafter.

Guedea reported protein malnutrition in 10 % of 74 patients, who underwent BPD and who had a 5-year-follow-up [2]. In a recent series of 287 patients with classical BPD, severe hypoproteinemia was observed in 1.7% of patients at year 1 [7].

According to Scopinaro, protein malnutrition can be reduced to 1 %, with a recurrence rate of 0.5 %, by correctly balancing the volume of the gastric pouch and the length of the alimentary limb in accordance with the patients' alimentary habits and the desired EWL% [8].

24.2.2 Chronic Anaemia

Distal gastrectomy and the exclusion of the duodenum and proximal jejunum impair absorption of iron and folates, facilitating chronic anaemia. Whereas macrocytic anaemia, due to vitamin B12 deficiency, is rarely seen, if adequate supplementation is provided, iron-deficiency–related microcytic anaemia can be observed more frequently, namely in the presence of chronic bleeding. In particular, fertile women are at high risk of developing iron-deficiency anaemia after BPD. Guedea et al., in a 5-year follow-up study, showed post-operative anaemia in 59.5 % of fertile women; despite oral nutritional integrations [2]. The incidence of iron-deficiency anaemia after BPD can be reduced to 5 % using adequate iron and folate integration [1].

24.2.3 Secondary Hyperparathyroidism

An association between morbid obesity and secondary hyperparathyroidism is well documented, as elevated levels of parathyroid hormone (PTH) and 1,25-OH vitamin D, together with reduced levels of 25-OH Vitamin D, have been observed in up to 50 % of patients before the operation [9]. Hamoui observed a correlation between PTH levels and BMI in obese patients [10]. After BPD, altered absorption of calcium can be responsible for hypo-calcemia and further elevation of PTH levels, even after appropriate supplementation of vitamin D [11]. As a consequence, increased bone reabsorption, bone demineralization, osteoporosis and osteomalacia may occur [12]. Scopinaro showed histopathological bone demineralization in one third of patients after BPD, mainly during the first 4 years post-operatively [8].

High post-operative levels of markers of bone turnover, and decreased bone-density were observed 1 year after BPD (a peculiar variant), irrespective of high doses of calcium integration, and in the absence of secondary hyperparathyroidism.

Decreased bone mass was considered an adaptive phenomenon of the skeleton, secondary to decreased mechanical load after bariatric surgery [13].

After BPD with duodenal switch, in a 10-year-follow-up study, Marceau observed bone fractures in 17 % of patients with classic BPD [14]. However, recent studies seem to exclude an increased risk of bone demineralization, osteoporosis and bone fracture after bariatric surgery, in comparison with a healthy population [15, 16], thus leaving some uncertainty concerning the clinical significance of secondary hyperparathyroidism and calcium metabolism after BPD.

24.2.4 Proctologic Sequelae

Altered composition of faeces (lower pH in comparison to healthy people), together with increased frequency of bowel movements per day after BPD, account for the occurrence in some patients of proctologic disorders, such as anal fissure, prolapsing haemorrhoids, perianal abscesses and fistulas.

After the implementation of adaptive mechanisms, the incidences of these conditions tend to decrease over time. Nevertheless, their persistence may severely impair the QoL and, together with the "foul smell" of stools, which is characteristic of subjects with BPD, may significantly affect the patient's social life.

24.3 Indications to Surgical Revision

A variable rate of surgical revisions has been required in the long term after BPD. Surgical revision may include remodelling of the length of the bowel limb, bowel continuity restoration or surgical revisions of the gastro-enteric-anastomosis (GEA). In addition to GEA revision, due to stenosis or marginal peptic ulcers, bowel remodelling is sometimes required to treat side effects of chronic malabsorption, insufficient weight loss or weight regain, whereas restoration of the small bowel continuity can be the final option for severe relapsing protein malnutrition. In the experience of Scopinaro, 6.3 % of patients required surgical revision after a 19-year-follow-up [8], whereas in a series comparing BPD with duodenal switch, Marceau reported that 18.5 % of 248 BPD patients had surgical revision during a 10-year-follow-up study [14]. However, the need to restore the continuity of the small bowel was comparable in the two series (2 % and 2.7 %, respectively).

Relapsing protein malnutrition is the most frequent reason for surgical revision. The first step of the treatment must aim at restoring an adequate nutritional status before surgery, usually using parenteral nutrition.

For a proper planning of surgery, a thorough clinical and nutritional evaluation must be used to detect whether chronic malabsorption is attributable to insufficient intestinal absorption of proteins or to insufficient nutritional intake. On a clinical basis, the presence of diarrhoea and the overall food intake must be evaluated.

Diarrhoea usually means a reduced tolerance towards the malabsorptive component of the BPD.

In this case, in the presence of adequate daily food intake, elongation of the common channel at the expense of the biliary limb could be the treatment of choice.

In the absence of diarrhoea, elongation of the alimentary channel, moving the common channel proximally along the biliary limb, can provide a longer ileal tract improving protein absorption, without affecting the fat-related malabsorption. In the absence of adequate oral nutrition, the restoration of the small bowel continuity should be considered.

Among the other side effects of chronic malabsorption, proctologic sequelae and chronic diarrhoea, in addition to "foul-smelling" stools, these can be improved by an elongation of the common channel, moving proximally the biliary limb along the alimentary one. In this case, possible weight regain must be anticipated.

Other conditions, such as iron-deficiency anaemia and hyperparathyroidism, as well as micronutrient imbalances, should be evaluated from a wider perspective, together with protein asset, desired %EWL and diarrhoea, in order to personalize surgical re-intervention as a "tailor's suite".

Insufficient weight loss: BPD is an extremely effective procedure, affording an excellent EWL% in the vast majority of patients. Nevertheless, suboptimal compliance to dietary recommendations and lifestyle modifications may significantly reduce the effectiveness of the procedure, thus preventing satisfactory results.

Moreover, in spite of an overall EWL% higher than 50 %, some patients may display a BMI which is still in the obesity range (i.e. >30). These results should be evaluated on an individual basis, considering on the one hand the overall QoL, the presence of significant side effects of chronic malabsorption and the way the patients are able to cope with them, and, on the other, the patient's compliance to post-operative integration and nutritional advices.

Weight regain: Excessive adaptive phenomena after BPD may account for a significant long-term weight regain, but this is still open to question. Conversely, an increased dietary intake of alcohol and carbohydrates, such as mono and disaccharides – which can still be absorbed along the alimentary limb – determines an increase of both energy intake and overall weight. If this is the case, the proper management should be nutritional advice, as no surgical revision could conveniently cope with a wrong alimentary regime.

If weight regain occurs, but no wrong alimentary habit can be documented, and no significant side effect of chronic malabsorption is clinically evident, the shortening of the common channel to increase malabsorption could be the correct solution. Conversely, the possibility of reducing the gastric pouch, in order to increase the restrictive component, requires a word of caution, because of the risk of insufficient protein intake.

24.4 Physiopathological Basis of Limb Remodelling in BPD

Proteins and starch can be reabsorbed along the whole length of the alimentary limb, from the gastro-enteric-anastomosis to the ileo-cecal valve. Moreover, the cecum and ascending colon, because of intestinal adaptive phenomena, become an additional site of protein absorption. Simple sugars and alcohol can be reabsorbed along the whole alimentary limb as well. The short common channel remains the only site for effective reabsorption of fatty acids and bile salts, thus significantly reducing the total amount of energy absorbed from food.

These aspects must be thoroughly considered to explain the clinical results of BPD, and its adverse effects. However, they are of crucial importance in cases of surgical revision.

Varying the length of the common channel at the expense of the alimentary limb affects fat and energy absorption, without directly affecting starch and proteins.

Shortening the common channel below 50 cm or elongating it along the alimentary limb determines a consensual variation in the threshold of fat and energy absorption. Accordingly, relative effects on steatorrhea, diarrhoea and "foul-smelling" stools can be expected.

Elongating the common channel at the expense of the biliopancreatic limb determines increased absorption of macronutrients and energy, as a result of the elongation of the entire alimentary circuit.

Elongating the alimentary limb at the expense of the biliopancreatic limb improves the absorption of protein and starch, without modifying the amount of fat.

Before modifying the relative length of bowel limbs after BPD, the surgeon must take into account the effectiveness of the adaptive mechanisms that occur after the first operation. Moreover, the overall capacity to eat, that is greatly dependent on the total capacity of the gastric pouch, must be evaluated, concomitantly and in addition to the absorptive function of the alimentary circuit.

In other words, a proper strategy before redo surgery can be formulated only after an 18- to 24-month interval following BPD, when proper adaptive mechanisms have already occurred, and the eating capability has been restored completely.

24.5 Problems and Specific Aspects of Redo Bariatric Surgery

Approach: Although the laparoscopic approach can be chosen for a redo procedure even in case of previous open bariatric surgery [17], we prefer to perform a re-laparotomy when initial BPD had been performed using open surgery. In our opinion, further indications to open approach include the presence of a large incisional ventral hernia and the requirement for additional surgery other than cholecystectomy.

When the laparoscopic approach is chosen, we routinely induce pneumoperitoneum using the Veress needle in the left subcostal region.

Removal of previous adhesions: Extensive post-operative adhesions are unusual after uncomplicated laparoscopic BPD (Fig. 24.3). The most severe adhesions are usually restricted to the region of the lesser curvature of the stomach and gastro-ileal anastomosis. On the contrary, there are usually no significant adhesions in close proximity to both the entero-enteric anastomosis and common limb.

Adhesion removal can be safely performed either with a monopolar hook or a harmonic scalpel. The liver border represents an excellent anatomical landmark. Following the liver edge, the exposure of the lesser curvature is greatly facilitated.

Staplers: The presence of scars and the thickness of tissues requiring transection must be accurately evaluated, in order to choose the most appropriate staple cartridges. A vascular cartridge is usually preferred to transect the small bowel far from scar tissue and for the ileo-ileal anastomosis. A blue or violet cartridge is preferred for the stomach and to perform a gastro-ileal anastomosis. The same cartridge is chosen to transect the small bowel in the presence of significant scar and to take down a previous anastomosis.

The staple lines must be carefully inspected for bleeding and leaks, but we do not routinely perfom a methilene blue test in the operative room when the gastric pouch is resized, or a new gastric anastomosis is constructed.

Drains: Redo surgery has an increased risk of anastomotic leakage and fistulas, bleeding and infections. Therefore, surgical drains are frequently used. If the gastric pouch is revised or a new gastric anastomosis is performed, a Jackson-Pratt drain is usually fitted, passing through the Morrison cavity and draining the peri-anastomotic space. A drain is not routinely placed close to the jejuno-ileal anastomosis.

24.6 Technical Notes

24.6.1 Common Limb Elongation

Common limb elongation along the biliopancreatic limb can be required to cure relapsing protein malnutrition with diarrhoea and normal food intake.

The aim is to provide a longer alimentary tract for effective protein absorption, together with a longer common channel for absorption of fat and energy. Scopinaro proposes elongating the common channel from 50 to 150 cm along the biliopancreatic limb, thus reaching a total length of 400 cm for the alimentary circuit. As a result of the enhanced energy absorption, weight regain can be expected, thus making the procedure suitable for patients with an excess weight loss [8].

Elongation of the common channel, leaving the total length of the alimentary circuit unchanged, should be reserved to treat proctologic sequelae, persistent diarrhoea and intolerance to "foul-smelling" stools. In this case, the biliopancreatic limb should be moved proximally along the alimentary limb, so creating a common channel of 150 cm, which has been shown to be effective for this specific aim [8].

24.6.2 Surgical Restoration

Complete (or near complete) restoration of the small bowel length should be reserved for patients with severe relapsing protein malnutrition and normal food intake. In fact, this condition is characterized by an insufficient absorptive capacity of the alimentary canal.

Various technical solutions have been proposed. Perhaps the simplest solution is moving the alimentary limb proximally, along the biliopancreatic limb, just distally to the ligament of Treitz [8]. In this way, the duodenum is still excluded from the transit, thus preserving some favourable effects relating to glucose metabolism and T2 diabetes. If the transit through the duodenum is maintained, in order to improve iron and calcium absorption, the alimentary limb can be sectioned from the common channel and anastomosed to the duodenal stump. The only residual negative effect would be a moderate reduction of food intake derived from gastric resection.

24.6.3 Structural Remodelling of BPD for Unfavourable Results of the Procedure

While initially addressing the problem of proctologic sequelae in a group of patients who underwent Scopinaro's classic BPD, we succeeded in achieving two aims: (1) control of symptoms from chronic diarrhoea and (2) avoidance of weight regain.

To reduce the malabsorptive effects of surgery, we elongated the common limb from 50 to 200 cm at the expense of the alimentary limb, and simultaneously, with the aim of avoiding weight

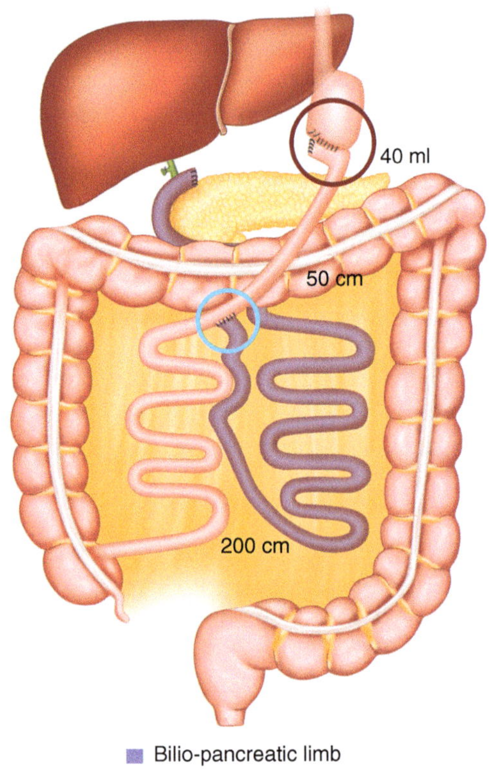

Fig. 24.2 Structural remodelling of biliopancreatic diversion

gain, we reduced the gastric pouch from 500 to 40 ml. The new procedure may resemble a long-limb distal gastric bypass, but, owing to its direct derivation from Scopinaro's BPD, we refer to it as the "structural remodelling of classic BPD" (Fig. 24.2).

After increased experience with the new procedure, favourable effects on calcium metabolism and PTH levels were also observed, together with a tendency for further weight loss. Thus we also extended the indications to the "structural remodelling after BPD" to patients with severe secondary hyperparathyroidism and to those with unsatisfactory weight loss after classic BPD.

As the technique has not been previously described, we will describe it in detail. We will refer to this technique being performed using the laparoscopic approach, since the open procedure can be performed following the same principles

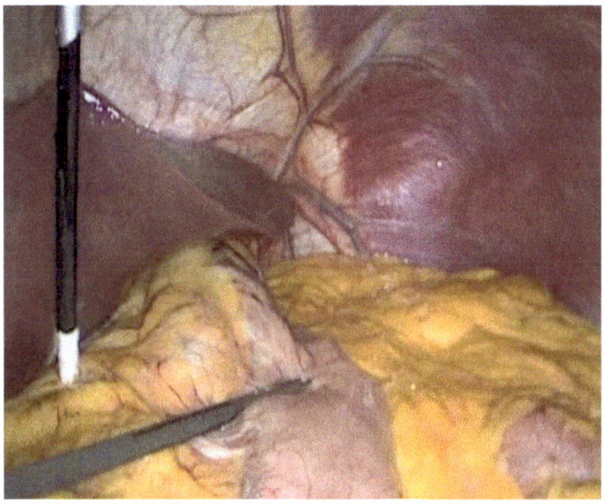

Fig. 24.3 The surgical field is free from significant adesions

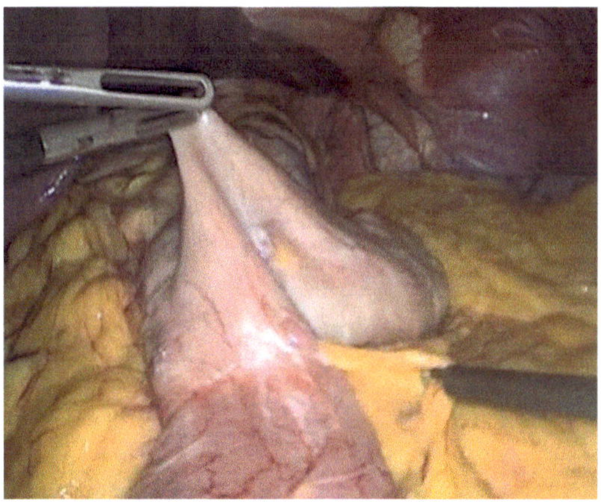

Fig. 24.4 The gastric pouch is inspected and the gastro-ileostomy identified, and dissected free from adhesions, using a monopolar hook

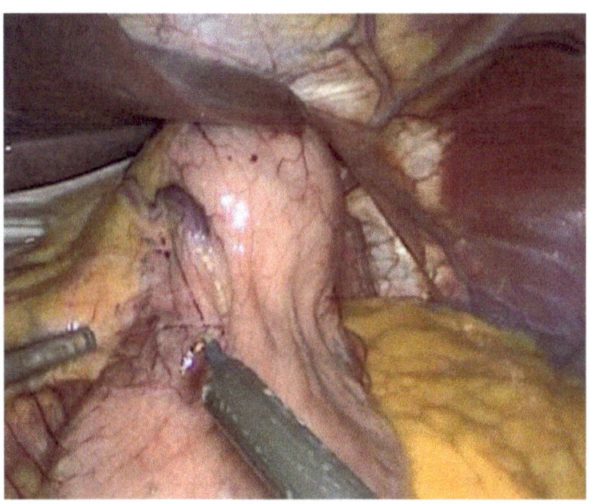

Fig. 24.5 An oro-gastric calibration balloon is inserted, inflated to 40 ml and finally retracted against the cardias

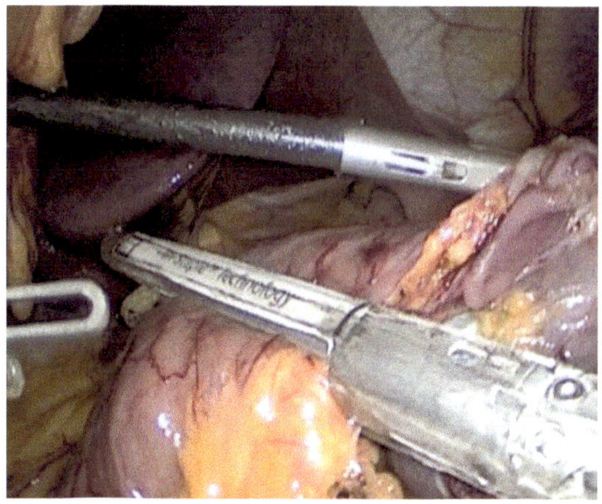

Fig. 24.6 The alimentary limb is transected immediately beside the gastro-ileostomy with a 60-mm tan cartridge

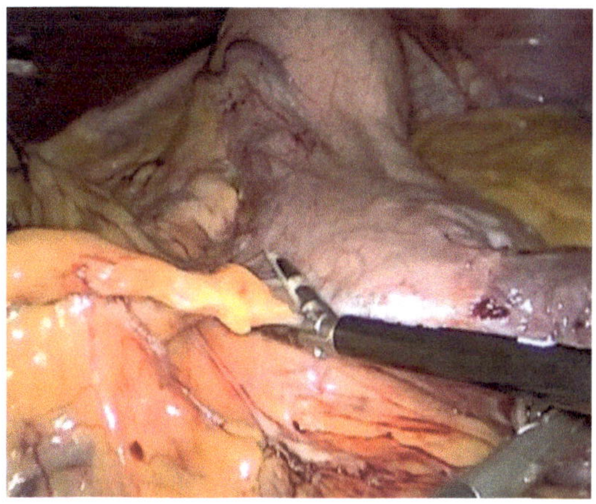

Fig. 24.7 The lesser curvature is freed proceeding upward to the level of the intragastric balloon

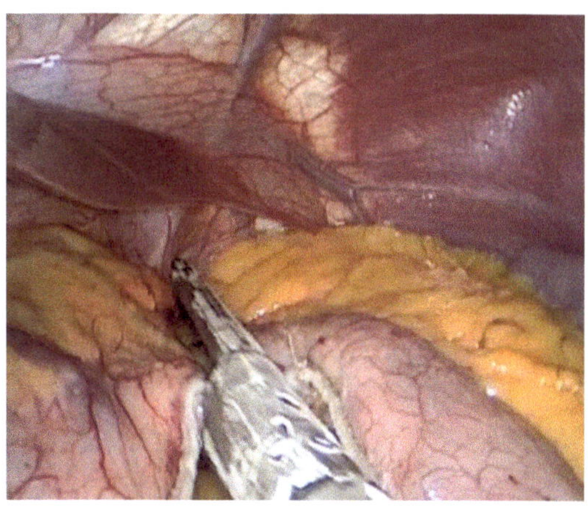

Fig. 24.8 The gastric pouch is trimmed on the gastric balloon with blue or violet cartridge

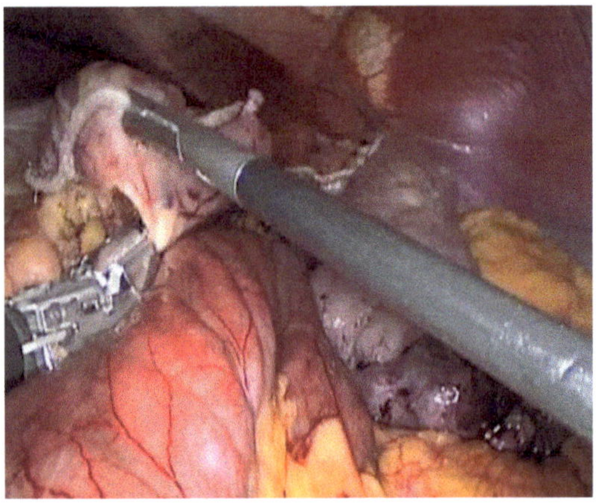

Fig. 24.9 A new gastro-ileostomy is performed, between the alimentary limb and the posterior aspect of the new gastric pouch

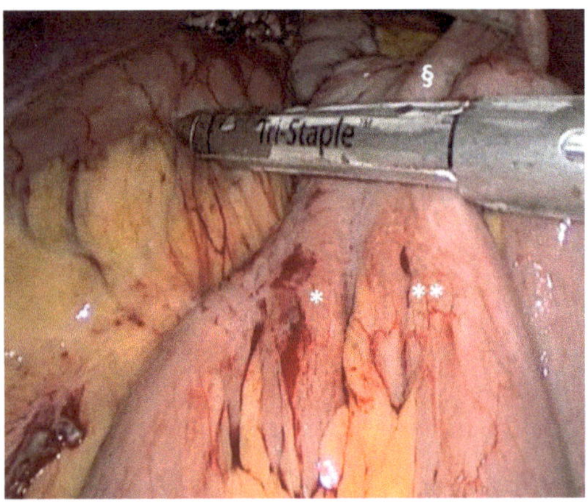

Fig. 24.10 The biliopancreatic limb is identified at the anastomotic level and taken down *Alimentary limb, **common channel, § biliopancreatic limb

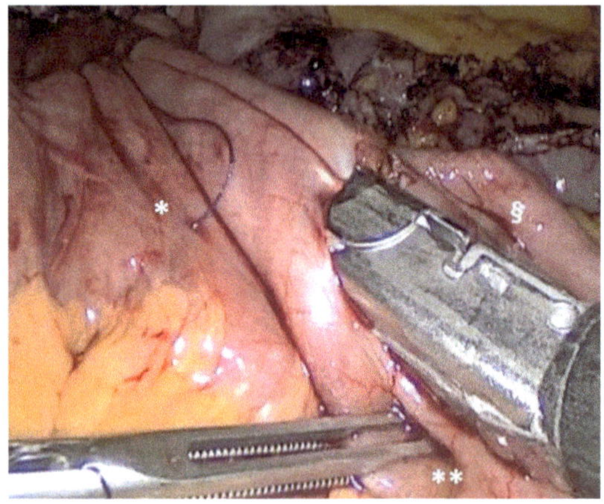

Fig. 24.11 A new common channel, 200 cm long is then created, anastomosing the biliopancreatic limb to the alimentary limb, at 50 cm from the gastric pouch *Alimentary limb, **common channel, §biliopancreatic limb

and surgical steps (Figs. 24.3, 24.4, 24.5, 24.6, 24.7, 24.8, 24.9, 24.10 and 24.11).

The patient is placed in a moderate reverse Trendelenburg position. Pneumoperitoneum is induced and maintained at 14–16 mmHg using the Veress needle, which has been placed in the left subcostal region. One 10–12-mm port is placed in the midline, 20 cm caudally from the xiphoid process. Two 12-mm ports are placed in the right and left flank, at the level of the umbilicus, forming an equilateral triangle. One additional 5-mm port is placed in the subxiphoid region, on the left side of the falciform ligament and another 5-mm port is placed very laterally in the right hypochondrium, below the hepatic edge.

When required, cholecystectomy is performed as the first step.

The gastric pouch is inspected and the gastro-ileostomy is identified, and dissected free from adhesions, using a monopolar hook or a radio frequency device. The alimentary limb is transected immediately beside the gastro-ileostomy with a 60-mm white or tan cartridge.

The dissection proceeds on the lesser curvature of the gastric pouch, freeing it from adhesions with the liver surface up to the cardias, sparing the gastric vessels on this side. After exposure of the cardias and of the right diaphragmatic crus, dissection starts on the greater curvature, which is progressively freed from the omentum up to the left crus. After dissection of the posterior surface of the stomach from the pancreas, an oro-gastric calibration balloon is inserted, inflated to 40 ml and finally retracted against the cardias. The lesser curvature is freed proceeding upward to the level of the intragastric balloon. The gastric pouch is trimmed on the gastric balloon with a blue or violet cartridge, analogously to the similar step in the Roux-en-Y gastric bypass. The surgical specimen is then placed in a plastic bag, to be retrieved at the end of the procedure.

A new gastro-ileostomy is performed (termino-lateral, isoperistaltic), between the alimentary limb and the posterior aspect of the

Table 24.1 Results of structural remodelling of BPD in our experience, on 27 patients with a post-operative follow-up of 2 years

	Preop	Month 1	Month 3	Year 1	Year 2	*p*
BMI	33.6	31.3	32.5	26.9	28.7	.001
Proteinemia	6.8	6.9	7.0	6.8	6.9	ns
Sideremia	48.8	70.9	79.7	82.7	74.8	.01
PTH (ng/l)	134.1	69.8	75.3	71.7	79.3	ns
Calcemia (mmol/l)	2.14	2.21	2.22	2.3	2.31	ns
Bowel movements/day (median)	4 (1–7)	3 (1–4)	2 (1–3)	2(1–4)	2 (1–4)	.003

new gastric pouch, using a 45-mm violet linear cartridge. Several interrupted full thickness stitches are used to complete the anastomosis.

The alimentary limb is followed distally and its surface is marked at 50 cm from the gastro-ileostomy. Following the alimentary limb, the biliopancreatic limb is identified at the anastomotic level and taken down and anastomosed, using a 60-mm blue or violet cartridge, on the biliopancreatic side, avoiding stricture of the common limb.

A new common channel, 200 cm long is then created, anastomosing the biliopancreatic limb to the alimentary limb, at 50 cm from the gastric pouch. A latero-lateral, antiperistaltic anastomosis is performed, using a 45-mm white cartridge, and several full-thickness interrupted stitches are placed to close the remaining defect. Mesenteric defects are left open.

A Jackson-Pratt drainage is left close to the gastric anastomosis and the surgical specimen(s) is (are) is finally retrieved in the plastic bag. Subcuticular sutures are used to close the skin.

Table 24.1 resumes our results with the procedure on 27 consecutive patients, operated from 2008 to 2012, with a post-operative follow-up of 2 years. The structural remodelling of BPD afforded a significant reduction of bowel movements per day and of PTH levels were observed, not only preventing weight regain, but definitely increasing the excess weight loss.

References

1. Scopinaro N, Adami GF, Marinari GM, Giannetta E, Traverso E, Friedman D, Camerini G, Bascheri G, Simonelli A. Biliopanceratic diversion. World J Surg. 1998;22:936.
2. Guedea ME, Arribas del Amo D, Solanas JA, Marco CA, Bernadó AJ, Rodrigo MA, Diago VA, Díez MM. Results of biliopancreatic diversion after five years. Obes Surg. 2004;14(6):766–72.
3. Buchwald H, Estok R, Fahrbach K, Banel D, Jensen MD, Pories WJ, Bantle JP, Sledge I. Weight and type 2 diabetes after bariatric surgery: systematic review and meta-analysis. Am J Med. 2009;122(3):248–256.e5.
4. Scopinaro N, Gianetta E, Adami GF, Friedman D, Traverso E, Marinari GM, Cuneo S, Vitale B, Ballari F, Colombini M, Baschieri G, Bachi V. Biliopancreatic diversion for obesity at eighteen years. Surgery. 1996; 119(3):261–8.
5. Buchwald H, Avidor Y, Braunwald E, Jensen MD, Pories W, Fahrbach K, Schoelles K. Bariatric surgery: a systematic review and meta-analysis. JAMA. 2004; 292(14):1724–37.
6. Scopinaro N. Thirty-five years of biliopancreatic diversion: notes on gastrointestinal physiology to complete the published information useful for a better understanding and clinical use of the operation. Obes Surg. 2012;22(3):427–32.
7. Crea N, Pata G, Di Betta E, Greco F, Casella C, Vilardi A, Mittempergher F. Long-term results of Biliopancreatic diversion with and without gastric preservation for morbid obesity. Obes Surg. 2011;21:139–145.
8. Scopinaro N, Marinari G, Camerini G, Papadia F. Biliopancreatic Diversion: physiological and metabolic aspects. In Bariatric Surgery. Multidisciplinary approach and Surgical techniques. 2nd edn. Aosta: Società valdostana di chirurgia; Quart: Musumeci: 2007.
9. Lozano O, García-Díaz JD, Cancer E, Arribas I, Rubio JL, González-García I, Galván M, Alvarez J, Martín-Duce A. Phosphocalcic metabolism after biliopancreatic diversion. Obes Surg. 2007;17(5): 642–8.
10. Hamoui N, Anthone G, Crookes PF. Calcium metabolism in the morbidly obese. Obes Surg. 2004;14(1): 9–12.
11. Balsa JA, Botella-Carretero JI, Peromingo R, Zamarrón I, Arrieta F, Muñoz-Malo T, Vázquez C. Role of calcium malabsorption in the development of secondary hyperparathyroidism after biliopancreatic diversion. J Endocrinol Invest. 2008;31(10):845–50.
12. Balsa JA, Botella-Carretero JI, Peromingo R, Caballero C, Muñoz-Malo T, Villafruela JJ, Arrieta F,

Zamarrón I, Vázquez C. Chronic increase of bone turnover markers after biliopanceratic diversion is related to secondary hyperparathyroidism and weight loss relation with bone mineral density. Obes Surg. 2010;20:468–73.

13. Tsiftsis DDA, Mylonas P, Mead N, Kalfarentzos F, Alexandrides TK. Bone mass decreases in morbidly obese women after long limb-biliopancreatic diversion and marked weight loss without secondary hyperparathyroidism. A physiological adaptation to weight loss? Obes Surg. 2009;19(11):1497–503.
14. Marceau P, Biron S, Hould FS, Lebel S, Marceau S, Lescelleur O, Biertho L, Simard S. Duodenal Switch improves standard biliopancreatic diversion: a restrospective study. Surg Obes Relat Dis. 2009;5:43–7.
15. Scibora LM, Ikramuddin S, Buchwald H, Petit MA. Examining the link between bariatric surgery, bone loss, and osteoporosis: a review of bone density studies. Obes Surg. 2012;22:654–67.
16. Lalmohamed A, de Vries F, Bazelier MT, Cooper A, van Staa TP, Cooper C, Harvey NC. Risk of fracture after bariatric surgery in the United Kingdom: population based, retrospective cohort study. BMJ. 2012;345:e5085.
17. Kellogg TA. Revisional bariatric surgery. Surg Clin N Am. 2011;91:1353–71.

Internal Hernia After Bariatric Procedures

25

Enrico Facchiano, Giovanni Quartararo, Alessandro Sturiale, and Marcello Lucchese

25.1 Introduction

Internal hernia (IH) represents the most common cause of small bowel obstruction after laparoscopic RYGBP, accounting for up to 61 % of cases of small bowel obstruction [1, 2]. The anatomic changes following bariatric surgery, the use of laparoscopy, the postoperative weight loss account for the high incidence of IH after bariatric procedures [1].

There are three anatomical spaces resulting from the Roux-en-Y reconstruction where IH may occur [1]:

1. Through the transverse mesocolon defect, in case of trans-mesocolic Roux-en-Y limb
2. The entero-enterostomy space, resulting from the union of mesentery at the jejuno-jejunal anastomosis
3. The Petersen's space between the mesentery of the Roux limb and the transverse mesocolon (Fig. 25.1).

However, even if the occurrence of IH has been described above all after RYGBP, this complication can potentially occur after all the bariatric procedures in which a Roux-en-Y limb is fashioned because of the creation of mesenteric defects [3]. A mean rate of 2.51 cases of IH after Roux-en-Y gastric bypass has been reported [1]. The rate of IH should raise up to 8.4 % in case of non-closure of mesenteric defects [2].

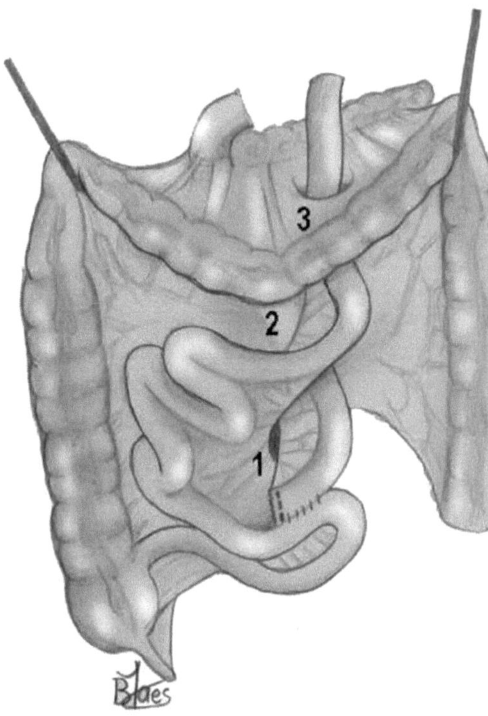

Fig. 25.1 Potential hernia sites in laparoscopic RYGBP. (*1*) entero-enterostomy mesenteric defect; (*2*) space between mesentery of Roux and transverse mesocolon (Petersen's space); (*3*) transverse mesocolon defect. All the procedures fashioning a Roux-en-Y limb result in mesenteric defects that may potentially cause IH (From Iannelli et al. [1])

E. Facchiano, MD (✉) • G. Quartararo, MD
A. Sturiale, MD • M. Lucchese, MD
Department of Surgery, Bariatric and Metabolic Surgery Unit, Azienda Sanitaria Firenze, Santa Maria Nuova Hospital, Piazza Santa Maria Nuova, 1, Florence 50122, Italy
e-mail: enricofacchiano@yahoo.it

M. Lucchese, N. Scopinaro (eds.), *Minimally Invasive Bariatric and Metabolic Surgery: Principles and Technical Aspects*, DOI 10.1007/978-3-319-15356-8_25,

As a matter of fact, the ever increasing use of laparoscopic approach results in an increased incidence of IH when compared to open procedures, maybe because of the reduced formation of postoperative adhesions [4].

Finally, even the weight loss plays an important role in the high incidence of IH as a consequence of the reduction of intra-abdominal adiposity that may lead to the expansion of pre-existent mesenterical defect [1, 5].

IH often remains a misdiagnosed disease or an incidental finding because symptoms may be very vague and other clinical hypothesis are advocated. On the other side, it can present with an acute and dramatic clinical picture that can oblige the general surgeon to face an unusual disease.

An appropriate knowledge of bariatric techniques may help the general surgeon to recognize this potentially lethal complication in order to refer suspect cases of IH to bariatric surgeons and to assure the best care to patient presenting with most urgent symptoms.

25.2 Clinical Presentation and Management

The occurrence of IH after laparoscopic bariatric surgery has largely been reported in the literature and it is well known by bariatric surgeons. However, it still represents a challenge for general surgeons who do not have a specific knowledge of the bariatric techniques. Moreover, a certain diagnosis is often difficult because of the clinical presentation that can be vague and not so easy to recognize.

IH may present as either an acute or chronic clinical picture. In the first case, symptoms are usually evident and the surgeon has to face a dramatic acute abdomen secondary to intestinal ischemia or small bowel necrosis or perforation. When an acute clinical presentation is present, the indication to emergency surgery is evident and a surgical operation is always required. In these cases, an IH must always be researched by examining the whole small bowel. The laparoscopic exploration is a valid option if the surgeon is skilled in laparoscopy and if he knows the technical details of the reconstructions of bariatric surgery.

The diagnosis of IH may be more difficult if the patient presents with less evident clinical picture. In case of chronic IH, symptoms are little evident and not easy to recognize, laboratory and traditional radiological work-up are often unhelpful [6]. CT scan could help for the diagnosis of IH but a clear diagnosis remains difficult because often only indirect signs of intestinal obstruction can be found [7].

CT scan should be systematically examined by skilled radiologist and surgeons for these findings: direct or indirect signs of small bowel obstruction, mesenteric swirl, a thicken shape of the mesentery, mesenteric vessel engorgement, small bowel behind the superior mesenteric artery, displacement of the mesenteric trunk and jejuno-jejunostomy standing on the right side [2, 8].

A chronic IH hernia often presents with vague, colicky pain, which may change or disappear in the lateral decubitus. Nausea and postprandial vomiting may be present. The pain can mainly be localized in the left upper quadrant, even if other localizations are possible, and often resolves spontaneously [1, 9].

The presence of recurrent abdominal pain in a patient with a past history of RYGBP, even in absence of pathological laboratory or radiological findings, should raise the suspicion of a misdiagnosed IH. In these cases, a surgical exploration should be advocated and should be performed by laparoscopy by a surgeon with a good knowledge of bariatric techniques.

At the surgical exploration, the bowel can have an inflammatory aspect with signs of intestinal obstruction. In some cases, a chylous ascites can be found, associated or not with a white coat on the mesentery, maybe because of a lymphatic stagnation secondary to the intermittent torsion of the mesenteric vessels (Fig. 25.2).

At the surgical exploration, the whole small bowel must be examined and all the potential mesenteric defects must be researched. The aspect of the herniated bowel must be observed in each case in order to evaluate if a resection is needed. All mesenteric defects identified, above all if they gave origin to a symptomatic IH, should be closed.

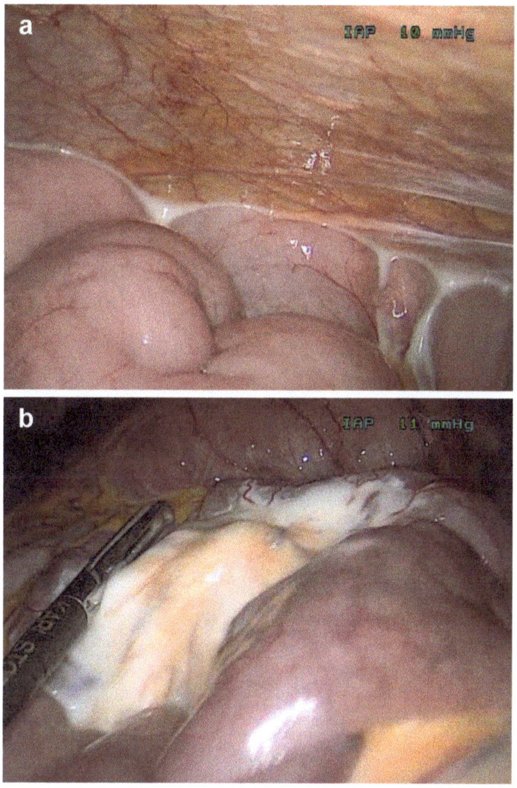

Fig. 25.2 Chylous asitis (**a**) and white mesenteric coat (**b**) in a case of internal hernia. This phenomenon may be due to lymphatic stagnation secondary to the intermittent torsion of the mesenteric vessels

We herein describe the technique that we usually use to perform laparoscopic exploration in patients with clinical or radiological suspicion of IH.

The patient is placed in the supine position with both legs in the straight position and secured to the operating table to allow for subsequent tilting. The surgeon stands on the patient's right side with the assistant on his right side and the monitor is placed at the right side of the operating bed. The first 10-mm trocar is placed at the umbilicus, using an open technique and two 5-mm trocars are placed in the right flank. The 10-mm port will be used to introduce a 30° camera. The operating bed is tilted to the right side.

The procedure should start with the identification of the gastro-enterostomy. If the anastomosis is not evident because of some adhesions between the gastric pouch and the liver, it is probably better not to dissect but just to identify the alimentary limb.

In case of trans-mesocolic placement of the alimentary limb, an IH at the transverse mesocolon defect must be researched. An IH hernia at this site is often easy to recognize.

After the examination of the transverse mesocolon defect or in case of antecolic placement, the alimentary limb should be followed up to the jejuno-jejunal anastomosis. This operation may be difficult in case of IH because the herniated bowel may be blocked in the mesenteric defect and it can be difficult to reduce it in the physiological position by simple traction. In case of IH at the Petersen's defect, the rotation of the mesentery always occurs counterclockwise. We believe that the passage of the jejuno-jejunal anastomosis through a mesenteric defect represents the real point of no return in the pathophysiology of the IH since in all the cases it represent the most difficult part of the herniation to reduce at the surgical exploration. If the jejuno-jejunal anastomosis cannot be reached by following the alimentary limb, it can be because of an IH at the Petersen's defect that cannot be reduced by simple traction. In this case, we suggest moving the limb to the left part of the abdomen in order to have the edge of its mesentery on the right. Once the right part of transverse colon and mesocolon has been identified, the Petersen's space can be now easily recognized between the mesentery of the Roux limb and the transverse mesocolon. If an IH is present, some herniated intestinal loops are evident at this level (Fig. 25.3). The IH must be obviously reduced before closing the Petersen's defect. The herniated bowel must be gently pushed *clockwise* through the mesenteric defect till the entire herniated bowel and the jejuno-jejunal anastomosis are passed through the mesenteric defect. In case of difficulties to identify the sense of the rotation, the ileocecal valve can be identified and the bowel can be run from distal to proximal. When the entire herniated bowel has been passed, the mesenteric defect can finally be closed starting caudally, at the convergence between the transverse mesocolon and the mesentery of the alimentary loop using a running suture and proceeding cephalad. The use of knotless barbed suture may be helpful.

Once the Petersen's defect has been closed, the whole bowel must be explored, starting at the

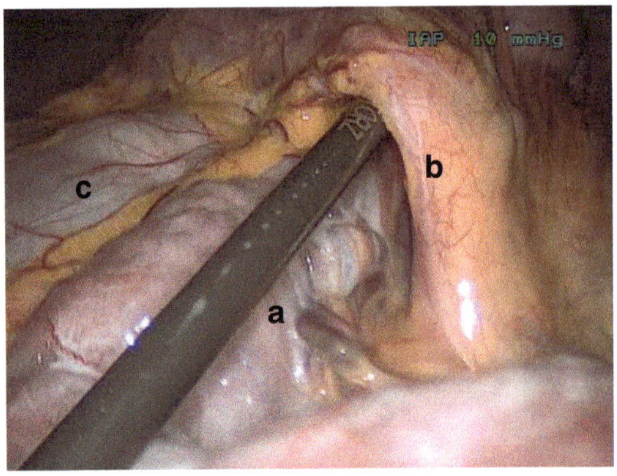

Fig. 25.3 Internal hernia at the Petersen's defect. The upper part of the image is oriented towards the head of the patients. The herniated intestinal loop (**a**) come from a counterclockwise rotation of the mesentery through the defect delimited by the mesentery of the alimentary limb (**b**) and transverse mesocolon (**c**). To be reduced, the herniated bowel must be gently pushed in the sense of the *arrow* till all the herniated bowel and the jejuno-jejunal anastomosis is passed

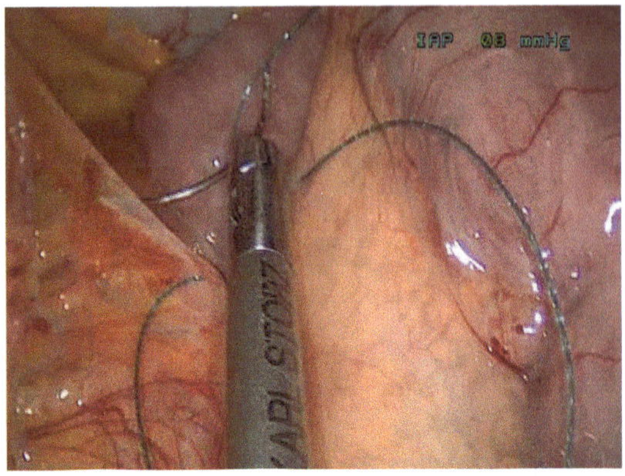

Fig. 25.4 Closure of the Petersen's defect starting at the convergence between the transverse mesocolon and the mesentery of the alimentary loop using a running suture

beginning of the alimentary loop and proceeding up to the jejuno-jejunal anastomosis. At this site, the other mesenteric defect must be researched. In case of evident strangulation or torsion, the diagnosis of IH is often easy. However, above all if the abdominal exploration is done by laparoscopy, it can be difficult to identify the sense of the torsion. In these cases, the ileocecal valve can be identified first and the bowel can be run from distal to proximal. This maneuver can be easier since the distal portion of the bowel is decompressed and easier to manipulate and the hernia may reduce as the small bowel is run [2] (Fig. 25.4).

As the IH can be a potentially fatal complication, in case of difficulties the conversion to open surgery is mandatory.

25.3 To Close or Not to Close Mesenteric Defects?

Several studies report that the closure of mesenteric defects when performing bariatric surgery cannot eliminate the risk of internal hernia, but can consistently reduce its incidence [1, 2, 9].

On the other side, some authors still report that the closure of mesenteric defects are not necessary and do not recommend their systematic closure [10, 11]. The arguments reported for non-routine closure of mesenteric defects include anatomical considerations, the intention to reduce complications linked to mesenteric closure (i.e., hematomas, injury to mesenteric vessels) and the idea that mesenteric closure may result in added costs in terms of operating time and suture materials [10, 11].

We think that no anatomical or surgical details (i.e., a long jejuno-jejunostomy configuration of the Roux limb [10]), other than mesenteric closure, can prevent the formation of IH. Even if some technical features can reduce the size of mesenteric defects at the time of surgery, this does not imply that the anatomy may change after a significant loss of weight [1, 9, 12]. Consideration about cost and complications appear not appropriate because the closure of mesenteric defects usually takes only few minutes to a skilled surgeon and mesenteric hematomas are usually rare and easy to manage [9, 10].

We currently recommend to close all the mesenteric defects at the time of bariatric surgery using, if possible, an ante-colic Roux limb positioning, thus reducing the number of potential mesenteric defects. Absorbable or non-absorbable sutures are both useful in the lack of controlled studies. Barbed knotless sutures may help in case of technical difficulties, above all in patients with visceral fat distribution.

Other technical features such as the division of the omentum and a minimal division of the mesentery cannot be considered effective in the reduction of IH rate since the reduction of the abdominal fat secondary to weight loss can modify the thickness of the omentum and the mesentery producing an expansion of the defects.

Conclusion

In conclusion, when a patient who has previously undergone a gastric bypass or other bariatric procedures with a Roux limb presents with a clinical picture of intestinal obstruction should raise the suspicion of IH. In these cases, a CT scan should be performed and examined for specific findings of IH such as mesenteric swirl, right sided jejuno-jejunostomy, and abnormal position or aspect of the mesenteric trunk. However, as radiological findings are often not easy to recognize, a negative CT scan should not be used to exclude the diagnosis of IH.

In case of clinical suspicion of IH, even in case of normal laboratory and radiological findings, a surgical exploration is indicated and, when the general conditions of the patients make it feasible, it should be attempted laparoscopically. Conversion to open procedure must be considered in case of technical difficulties in the manipulation of the bowel or in the identification of the sense of the rotation of the herniated bowel.

If possible, patients with symptoms consistent with a chronic IH should be referred to a specialized bariatric center or to a surgeon with a specific knowledge of bariatric surgery for a laparoscopic surgical exploration. Acute presentation of IH remains a surgical emergency and a surgical operation should not be delayed.

Even in the absence of randomized studies, it is recommended to close all the mesenteric defects performing procedures that imply the creation of a Roux limb. The routine closure of all the mesenteric defects do not completely avoid IH formation; however, it results in reduced incidence of this complication as reported in several studies.

As bariatric surgery is gaining raising popularity with a great number of procedures performed yearly worldwide, it is probable that general surgeons will be called to face complications of bariatric surgery with an increasing frequency. A specific knowledge of bariatric technique should be required to general surgeons to recognize and treat in emergency specific complications such as IH.

References

1. Iannelli A, Facchiano E, Gugenheim J. Internal hernia after laparoscopic Roux-en-Y gastric bypass for morbid obesity. Obes Surg. 2006;16(10):1265–71.
2. Obeid A, McNeal S, Breland M, et al. Internal hernia after laparoscopic Roux-en-Y gastric bypass. J Gastrointest Surg. 2014;18(2):250–5; discussion 255–6.
3. Khwaja HA, Stewart DJ, Magee CJ, et al. Petersen hernia complicating laparoscopic duodenal switch. Surg Obes Relat Dis. 2012;8(2):236–8.
4. Garrard CL, Clements RH, Nanney L, et al. Adhesion formation is reduced after laparoscopic surgery. Surg Endosc. 1999;13(1):10–3.
5. Quebbemann BB, Dallal RM. The orientation of the antecolic Roux limb markedly affects the incidence of internal hernias after laparoscopic gastric bypass. Obes Surg. 2005;15(6):766–70; discussion 770.
6. Champion JK, Williams M. Small bowel obstruction and internal hernias after laparoscopic Roux-en-Y gastric bypass. Obes Surg. 2003;13(4):596–600.
7. Onopchenko A. Radiological diagnosis of internal hernia after Roux-en-Y gastric bypass. Obes Surg. 2005;15(5):606–11.
8. Comeau E, Gagner M, Inabnet WB, et al. Symptomatic internal hernias after laparoscopic bariatric surgery. Surg Endosc. 2005;19(1):34–9.
9. Facchiano E, Iannelli A, Gugenheim J, Msika S. Internal hernias and nonclosure of mesenteric defects during laparoscopic Roux-en-Y gastric bypass. Obes Surg. 2010;20(5):676–8.
10. Madan AK, Lo Menzo E, Dhawan N, Tichansky DS. Internal hernias and nonclosure of mesenteric defects during laparoscopic Roux-en-Y gastric bypass. Obes Surg. 2009;19(5):549–52.
11. Ortega J, Cassinello N, Sanchez-Antunez D, et al. Anatomical basis for the low incidence of internal hernia after a laparoscopic Roux-en-Y gastric bypass without mesenteric closure. Obes Surg. 2013;23(8):1273–80.
12. Facchiano E, Lucchese M, Iannelli A. Anatomical basis for the low incidence of internal hernia after a laparoscopic Roux-en-Y gastric bypass without mesenteric closure. Obes Surg. 2013;23(12):2110–1.

Emergencies in Bariatric Surgery: Highlights for the General Surgeon

26

Carlo Bergamini, Giovanni Alemanno, Enrico Facchiano, and Marcello Lucchese

26.1 Introduction

Bariatric surgery is safely performed in specialized centers: complications are <1 % in almost all published experiences, with <0.35 % in some specialized centers, similar to cholecystectomy [1]. These complications are treated by the original bariatric center, where the required skills and knowledge are available. However, acute complications might require emergency treatment in a local district hospital [2–4].

The physiological effects of bariatric surgery, the knowledge about its anatomic reconstruction, and even the management of the health consequences of morbid obesity are not traditionally included in general surgery training programs. However general surgeons, regardless of their specific interest in obesity surgery, should develop a basic anatomical, clinical, and surgical understanding of these procedures because they may be called to face acute complications of bariatric surgery during their activity.

C. Bergamini (✉) • G. Alemanno
General, Emergency and Mini-Invasive Surgery Unit, Largo Brambilla, 3, Florence 50132, Italy
e-mail: drcarlobergamini@gmail.com; g.alemannomd@gmail.com

E. Facchiano • M. Lucchese
Department of Surgery, Bariatric and Metabolic Surgery Unit, Azienda Sanitaria Firenze, Santa Maria Nuova Hospital, Piazza Santa Maria Nuova, 1, Florence 50122, Italy
e-mail: enricofacchiano@yahoo.it; mlucch@iol.it

At present, scientific societies are far to have reached strict evidence-based recommendations on these topics. However, in this chapter, we tried to outline an up-to-date guide about specific acute complications that may occur early or late after laparoscopic bariatric surgery, which may happen to be diagnosed and managed by the general surgeon, even without specific bariatric experience.

26.2 General Clinical Management

When an emergency occurs, the evaluation of the bariatric patient follows a typical stepwise approach. Assessment and treatment of patient's ABC (airway, breathing, circulation) should precede any specific consideration; no change to cardiac arrest resuscitation treatment algorithms for obese patients is justified [5, 6]. After resuscitation, a complete evaluation should consider bariatric surgery-related complications. History is essential to find out details about the procedure; that being said, at the beginning of the evaluation, a consultation with a bariatric surgeon (possibly the surgeon who performed the procedure) should be obtained.

The presence of vital sign instability must take into account the possibility of pulmonary embolism and sepsis. Pulmonary embolism is the leading cause of death among bariatric surgery

M. Lucchese, N. Scopinaro (eds.), *Minimally Invasive Bariatric and Metabolic Surgery: Principles and Technical Aspects*, DOI 10.1007/978-3-319-15356-8_26,

patients; its incidence is low with appropriate prophylaxis, but it deserves maximal consideration in this group of patients. Most venous thrombo-embolism events may occur after the initial hospital discharge [7, 8].

Sepsis and peritonitis can represent the final stage of a suture or anastomotic leak; an intra-abdominal infection from a leaking anastomosis is the most common cause of mortality within the first 12 weeks after surgery [9]. Fever, hypotension, tachycardia, tachypnea, decreased urine output, and hypoxia (with tachycardia being the most sensitive sign [10]), should alert the physician for the research of a bariatric surgery-related causes of sepsis. The knowledge of the type of surgery in the patient history will guide among the septic procedure-specific complications.

Evaluation of gastrointestinal (GI) bleeding, abdominal pain, nausea, and vomiting should take into account the specific procedure complications, examined in later paragraphs. Prompt fluid resuscitation should be started with non-glucose-containing intravenous solutions administration. These patients require particular attention because they often show atypical features (physical constitution may interfere with the assessment of signs and symptoms). Peculiarities in their management are often appropriate: (a) supine position should be avoided due to possible respiratory problems caused by excess skin and adipose tissue; (b) if endotracheal intubation is necessary, anesthesiologists should be aware of the potential intubation difficulties [11, 12]; (c) nasogastric or orogastric intubation should consider the changed anatomy of the upper GI tract and has to be achieved very carefully, possibly avoiding blind placement; (d) drugs that can induce gastric mucosa damage (NSAIDs, ASA, steroids) should be avoided; and (e) a possible thiamine deficiency, due to malnutrition or altered food habits, must be considered. If fluid replacement is indicated, start infusing non-glucose-containing solutions (normal saline or Ringer's lactate), and administer thiamine before infusing glucose to avoid an acute onset of Wernicke's syndrome [13, 14].

26.3 Procedure-Specific Acute Complications

26.3.1 Adjustable Gastric Banding

Laparoscopic adjustable gastric banding (LAGB) is still performed worldwide and represents the bariatric procedure with the lower reported incidence of short- and mid-term adverse events [15]; however, long-term data show a higher incidence of postoperative acute complications leading to band repositioning or removal and eventually conversion to other procedures. The major complications are pouch dilation (acute or chronic) often referred to as "slippage," erosion, and permanent or recurrent outlet obstruction [16–18].

26.3.1.1 Slippage

Slippage is the most common LAGB complication and the leading cause of reoperation. It can develop early or late during the postoperative course. Its reported incidence of 1–20 %, in the published series, dropped (even to 0.9 %) after the surgical technique, and the prosthesis evolved during the years [19, 20]. It consists in the dilatation of the gastric pouch, above the band, in three different modalities: anterior, posterior, or symmetrical. Chronic pouch dilation presents with a gradual onset of symptoms as food intolerance, dysphagia, decrease in satiety, and sense of restriction. Its diagnosis and treatment is usually managed by the bariatric surgeon. An acute slippage is characterized by persistent abdominal pain, vomiting, and eventually obstructive symptoms. The incidence of acute slippage dropped to about 2–10 % after the positioning technique of the band through the pars flaccida has been generally adopted (24 % with the initial peri-gastric technique) [21]. The radiological diagnosis is based on the modified orientation of the band on plain abdominal X-ray, associated with an enlarged gastric pouch at the upper GI series. Band position, connection tube location, and continuity with the access port should be always checked both on plain and contrast X-ray. Nausea, vomiting, and reduction of oral intake can be so severe to result in severe dehydration with changes in the cardiovascular status and vital signs. Emergency treatment consists in complete band deflation through the subcutaneous port system, nasogastric tube positioning in the pouch (possibly under radiographic control), and intravenous administration of fluids, antiemetics, and proton pump inhibitors [22]. This should determine a significant improvement of the condition and allow time to refer the patient to the bariatric center. Good results can be achieved with conservative treatment, especially in the symmetrical dilation, but if symptoms persist for more than 3–5 days, surgical treatment is needed to prevent gastric pouch ischemia. Gastric necrosis after late slippage is, in fact, a rare but life-threatening reported complication [23, 24]; persistence or worsening of the initial symptoms, tachycardia, raised lactate levels, and acidosis should orientate the diagnosis.

The general surgeon without prior bariatric surgery experience, when encountering acute slippage, after a short course of conservative treatment as described earlier, must remove the band in order to treat the emergency when gastric outlet stenosis is evident. Laparoscopic approach in case of acute slippage is effective in over 95 % of the cases and is the standard choice, provided that no gastric necrosis is found [18]. During surgery, the band is exposed, following the connecting tube, and cut to remove the obstruction of the gastric outlet. The surgeon should be aware of the possible fixation of the band with two to four gastro-gastric sutures. In case of gastric necrosis, appropriate resection should be performed after the band removal.

26.3.1.2 Complicated Intra-gastric Band Migration

Intra-gastric band migration (incidence 0.8–4 %) is usually diagnosed at the radiological or endoscopic follow-up and usually is not a surgical emergency [25, 26]. Intra-operative gastric wall trauma and tight band placement may account for early erosion; high band pressure, band overinflation, and dietary noncompliance can cause late band erosion. Band removal is mandatory because of the risk of complications as hemorrhage or perforation but is part of a standard approach in a bariatric center, which includes serial upper GI endoscopies. Most cases do not require emergency surgery. Chronic melena, with chronic anemia, in the absence of abdominal symptoms and with a stop of weight loss or even weight regain, is a sign of latent band erosion and possible intragastric migration.

26.3.2 Laparoscopic Sleeve Gastrectomy

Laparoscopic sleeve gastrectomy (LSG) is today recognized as a stand-alone procedure that originates from the two-stage approach of the biliopancreatic diversion with duodenal switch (BPD–DS). It is one of the most popular procedures and consists in a calibrated, longitudinal/vertical gastrectomy, performed alongside the small curvature, using linear staplers, with complete removal of the gastric fundus and body and part of the antrum. Early staple line complications are rare but most feared; bleeding and/or leaks are usually managed by the bariatric center in the immediate postoperative days. Depending on the local regional circumstances, more and more bariatric procedures, including sleeve gastrectomy, are performed nowadays on a very short hospitalization, with early discharge as standard of care. Therefore, the general surgeon can be confronted even with early complications like bleeding or acute leaks.

26.3.2.1 Leaks

Suture line leakage rate after LSG ranges between 0.7 and 7 %, depending on the series and the patient characteristics, with a risk ranging between 1.5 and 2.4 % in recent systematic reviews and meta-analysis [27–29]. Revisional surgery after initial bariatric procedure (conversion of gastric banding or vertical gastroplasty to LSG or gastric bypass) can increase the fistula rate up to 20 %. The critical areas for leakage are the top of the suture line, near the gastroesophageal junction (89 %), and the transition point between sequential cartridges. Postoperative leaks may be classified into acute, late, very late, and chronic [28, 30, 31]. The general surgeon, in an emergency setting, is rarely involved in evaluating and taking care of either an acute or a chronic leak, generally treated by the bariatric center. They might face, however, an obese patient with a "late" or "very late" leak, developed after an initial uneventful postoperative course, as almost 80 % of the postoperative fistulas appear after discharge from the bariatric center.

Symptoms and signs suggestive of a localized or generalized peritonitis (pain, fever, tachycardia, tachypnea, often left pleural effusion, and pain in the left shoulder) in a patient who recently had bariatric surgery are likely due to a late fistula. Abdominal plain X-rays and contrast X-ray studies may assist in the diagnosis, but in all suspected cases, a CT scan with oral Gastrografin is essential. Misdiagnosis will worsen the patient's future evolution.

The CT scan usually shows three possible pictures:

1. High staple line fistula (esophago-gastric junction) along with a left sub-diaphragmatic collection
2. "Bubbles" in the peri-gastric fat near the staple line and a peri-gastric fluid collection without evidence of contrast medium leak

26.3.2.2 Multiple Leaks and Diffuse Fluid Collection

In the latter case, an emergency laparoscopy/laparotomy (according to the local skill) may be indicated to carry out a lavage of the upper abdominal cavity and drainage as a first emergency surgical step. Conservative treatment including bowel rest, fluid resuscitation, antibiotics, aspiration of esophageal and gastric secretions, nutritional support, analgesia, endoscopic stent, and transfer to the bariatric unit is appropriate, but experienced intensive care, endoscopy, and radiology units may be required. Surgical emergency treatment should be considered in a hemodynamically unstable patient with severe, persistent symptoms and an acute fistula or a late fistula with diffuse fluid collection. Laparoscopic approach is the best option if experience is available and can accomplish extensive peritoneal washout, identification of the fistula site (check first the esophago-gastric junction), and multiple drainage. No attempt of correction of the staple line defect is usually indicated. Three main objectives are pursued: sepsis control, prevention of abdominal recontamination, and nutritional (parenteral and enteral) support [32–34].

All other cases of late staple line fistula, if stable, should be referred to the bariatric center where the best management strategy can be adopted. Their treatment is based on percutaneous drainage plus parenteral/enteral nutrition and antibiotics. An endoscopic prosthesis can be positioned in selected cases and/or endoscopic fibrin glue applied [35].

26.3.3 Laparoscopic Gastric Bypass

Gastric bypass (GBP) represents the gold standard of the surgical treatment of morbid obesity and includes the creation of an upper small gastric pouch of 25–30 ml using linear staplers, with a Roux-en-Y gastro-jejunostomy reconstruction

26.3.3.1 Anastomotic Leak

Anastomotic leak after GBP is a life-threatening complication (incidence 0–6.1 %) [36]. It presents the same problems of the superior polar sleeve gastrectomy leak discussed earlier: timing (early or late), clinical presentation (from subclinical to sepsis), diagnosis (Gastrografin swallows, CT scan, and blood counts), and treatment (conservative, including fluid resuscitation, antibiotics, analgesia, endoscopic stent, and transfer to the bariatric unit when possible). Surgical emergency treatment should be considered in a hemodynamically unstable patient with severe, persistent symptoms: intense washout of the abdominal cavity and multiple drain placement should be considered. Laparoscopic approach is the best option if the surgeon is experienced. Final surgical treatment should be referred to the bariatric center.

26.3.4 Laparoscopic Biliopancreatic Diversion and Duodenal Switch

Biliopancreatic diversion along with its variations is the bariatric/metabolic procedure with the higher reported estimated weight loss. Patients require particular attention, especially in the emergency room setting, for the changes in their gastrointestinal (GI) anatomy and physiology following surgery. Early or late complications of BPD or DS are rare and often require the experience of a bariatric surgery team for their prompt resolution. Specific late complications, even if not surgical, might be observed in an emergency setting: protein malnutrition (often not properly treated in a nonspecialized center), severe anemia, and Wernicke's encephalopathy [37–39]. Stabilization of the patient is usually possible in order to transfer the patient to a specialized bariatric center. Particular attention should be addressed to appendicitis or cholelithiasis after BPD or DS. Initial BPD included cholecystectomy, appendectomy, and hepatic biopsy, but after the introduction of laparoscopy and technical evolution to DS, these procedures are no longer routinely performed.

26.4 Non-procedure-Specific Acute Complications

26.4.1 Bleeding

Bleeding can be a consequence of the staple line or other sources. Trocar site bleeding, splenic injury, or liver lacerations from retractor injury are rare but possible hemorrhage sources. Usually these complications appear in the first 48 h after surgery, when the patient is still under bariatric specialist surveillance, but routine early discharge policies can bring an early postoperative bleeding to the attention of a general surgeon or an emergency physician. Although the clinical picture of bleeding often leaves no room for doubts (anemia, hypotension, tachycardia, hematemesis, and melena), the site of bleeding and the corresponding control can be a challenge.

Early bleeding from a staple or suture line can be extra-or intra-luminal. Most early upper gastrointestinal, intra-luminal hemorrhage will manifest with hematemesis and melena, and their treatment does not differ from any other upper GI bleeding in a non-bariatric patient. In all cases, management includes serial blood counts, good intravenous access, fluids administration, stop of anticoagulants, monitoring of vital signs, and upper GI endoscopy. If the endoscopist is familiar with the anatomic changes related to the bariatric procedure, endoscopy may reveal the bleeding point from the inner side of the staple line and control it by adrenaline injection, electro-coagulation, or endoclips if good visualization is obtained. The endoscopic examination for perforation at the bleeding site should not be omitted. Late bleeding in a gastric bypass can present relevant peculiarities. A significant amount of later hemorrhage in a gastric bypass is related to a marginal ulcer. Severe hemorrhage or perforation can be faced by a general surgeon as reported [40]. Endoscopic management is essential, and only its failure can indicate an angiography (selected cases) or surgical exploration.

The jejuno-jejunal anastomosis of a gastric bypass or the ileo-ileal anastomosis in a biliopancreatic diversion can also be responsible for bleeding. Spiral angio-CT scan or selective angiography can assess bleeding at these sites. Bleeding in a GBP can originate also from erosion or ulcerations of the gastric remnant or even from duodenal or jejunal ulceration [41]. Refractory bleeding from the gastric remnant or other sites with no access for endoscopy can entail surgical revision.

Upper gastrointestinal bleeding can occur anytime after LAGB positioning due to erosions or ulcers. Peptic ulcer, Mallory–Weiss tear, erosive gastritis, and esophagitis can also be sources of bleeding in patients with LAGB. Acute upper GI bleeding, occurring in late follow-up, could be the result of an active ulcer, and careful endoscopy should recognize and even treat it.

The initial treatment of upper GI bleeding after LAGB, as of any other gastrointestinal bleeding, is conservative (adequate resuscitation, close monitoring, assessment of the severity of bleeding, blood transfusions, and emergency endoscopy when necessary). When surgery becomes necessary, the patient should be referred to the bariatric center, when the clinical situation permits it. Extraluminal bleeding could be shown by the drain when present and still functional; otherwise, an acute drop of hematocrit, with hypotension and tachycardia, would indicate unstable hemodynamic condition that may require reoperation for lavage, identification of the source, and hemostasis. At surgery, the bleeding source (staple line, retrogastric vessels, short gastric vessels, omentum dissection line, splenic or liver injury, trocar site, etc.) will often no longer be active; intense abdominal washout, multiple drainage, and supportive intensive care will suffice. Laparoscopic approach is recommended, but only where experience is available.

26.5 Small Bowel Obstruction (SBO) After Bariatric Procedures

Evaluation and treatment of SBO is one of the most common tasks that a general surgeon or an emergency physician has to face. About 16 % of surgical admissions and more than 300,000 operations annually in the USA are related to SBO [42]. The standard management algorithm, commonly practiced for SBO, includes an initial trial of nonoperative treatment using nasogastric decompression, bowel rest, fluid resuscitation, and close monitoring. A substantial number of cases are treated only with such conservative measures in the absence of signs suggesting impending or ongoing bowel ischemia. In patients with a history of bariatric surgery, the outcome of commonly adopted protocols could be affected by several factors related to the new anatomy and physiology of the gastrointestinal tract. Physicians who are not adequately familiar with these alterations may be misled in their evaluation. The nasogastric decompression may be ineffective on a substantial portion of the gastrointestinal tract (gastric remnant, biliopancreatic limb) and prolonged nonoperative management may be futile and dangerous. If a Roux reconstruction is present, a portion of the bowel is excluded from the alimentary flow; the evaluating physician must consider that obstipation may then be absent even in a complete obstruction and that the risk of a closed-loop bowel obstruction is higher than in non-bariatric patients. Finally, it may be difficult to identify small incisional hernias (trocar site hernias) in an obese patient, and the incidence of internal hernia is higher.

The most common cause of SBO in the bariatric population is an abdominal wall or internal hernia [43]. Port site hernia could be determined by the ≥10-mm trocar abdominal fascial defects left unclosed at the end of the laparoscopic bariatric procedures. A trocar site hernia is an uncommon complication of laparoscopic surgery; however, it is necessary to take into consideration this possibility in the bariatric patient: a recent review showed that higher BMI is a significant risk factor for its development even if its incidence after bariatric surgery does not seem to be higher [44]. The identification of small incisional hernia can be exceedingly difficult in obese patients. Emergency treatment for partial or complete bowel obstruction allows rapid reduction of the herniated content. A laparoscopic approach is recommended if adequate experience is available; bowel resection might be necessary in case of perforation or bowel ischemia. The closure of the abdominal wall defect completes the operation. Internal hernia is widely recognized as the most frequent cause of SBO (>50 %) in bariatric patients [45]. SBO after GBP or BPD is determined mainly by internal hernia. There are three classic locations where SBO can occur after GBP: Petersen's space (between Roux limb's mesentery and transverse mesocolon), at the transverse mesocolon defect (for retrocolic bypasses), and at the jejuno-jejunostomy. Obstruction can involve the alimentary limb, the biliopancreatic limb, or the common channel, with incidence between 0.4 and 7.5 % [46–48]. Symptoms can suggest the site of obstruction: heartburn and vomiting are associated with the common channel or alimentary limb's obstruction; bilious vomiting originates from the common channel obstruction; distension of the gastric remnant or biliopancreatic limb suggests common channel and biliopancreatic limb obstruction.

Diagnosis is based on clinical presentation, plain abdominal X-ray, and upper gastrointestinal studies. CT scan is a standard diagnostic tool and can demonstrate the dilatation of the Roux limb, of the gastric remnant, or of the biliopancreatic limb, depending on localization. Even sophisticated imaging (multislice CT spiral scan), however, will fail to disclose internal hernia in up to two of three cases. This has led to an increasing acceptance for immediate laparoscopic/laparotomic exploration in bariatric patients with subtle symptoms of SBO. Symptom persistence, acidosis, lactate rise, or signs of an acute abdomen should prompt exploration. Laparoscopy is the best choice (if previous bariatric surgery was also laparoscopic) where expertise is available. Small bowel assessment and handling are not easy, regardless of the access. As in any laparoscopic exploration for SBO, a retrograde examination of the bowel starting from the ileo-cecal valve is easier and less risky [49–52].

In case of positive identification of an internal hernia, a gentle reduction should be done, followed by the closure of the mesenteric defect. Patients with history of bariatric procedures, who also had other abdominal surgery (cholecystectomy, incisional hernia repair, gynecological operation, etc.), should always be checked for potential mesenteric defects in other areas. Symptoms can also evolve chronically, with intermittent and recurrent abdominal pain associated with nausea and vomiting but without a clear obstructive picture. This can be misinterpreted as food intolerance, marginal ulcer, or gastroesophageal reflux disease (GERD). Quite often, the intermittent pinching of a loop of bowel in an internal hernia defect can induce chronic, intermittent abdominal pain; the mechanism underlying the symptom may remain unknown, not discovered even by the most sophisticated imaging techniques, unless a very high degree of suspicion is maintained. Any patient with previous GBP or BPD who presents with chronic, intermittent abdominal pain or recurrent signs of a SBO should be suspected of having an internal hernia, and a referral to a bariatric center for a laparoscopic exploration may be warranted. Early diagnosis and intervention are imperative in order to reduce morbidity and mortality associated with intestinal necrosis.

Acute SBO can be life-threatening in the post-bariatric patients who have undergone a Roux-en-Y reconstruction. In fact, an obstruction point along the biliary limb or at the small bowel anastomosis will result in a closed-loop obstruction that can be rapidly fatal if not recognized and decompressed. An invasive procedure (emergency surgery or percutaneous CT-guided gastrostomy) is the only option to achieve decompression because nasogastric suctioning is precluded by the anatomical changes. A closed-loop obstruction can also result from an obstruction distal to the jejuno-jejunostomy if an effective decompression is not obtained through the alimentary channel.

The closed-loop obstruction of the biliopancreatic channel has been defined as "bypass obstruction" by Mason. He maintained that a universally recognized denomination of this dangerous nosologic entity could facilitate recognition, study, prevention, and early treatment. In gastric bypass, the syndrome may include "gastric remnant dilatation," with potential gastric necrosis, or gastric obstruction with perforation. When presenting as an acute, rapidly evolving complication, a complete bypass obstruction has one of the shortest "time to treat" (TTT) [53]. This is due to the large volume of digestive fluids accumulated in the upper digestive tract, with possible evolution to gastric wall necrosis and/or perforation. Hypovolemic shock (evidenced by tachycardia) is thus complicated by peritonitis and sepsis due to perforation. A chronic presentation is also described, with symptoms including abdominal pain, nausea, hiccup, vomiting, and tachycardia. Elevated hepatic functional markers and pancreatic enzymes can be related to the increased duodenal pressure. CT scan may show the dilatation of the gastric remnant. The evaluation of the stomach remnant after GBP is attainable also by virtual gastro-duodenoscopy [53]. Revision of the jejunostomy may be needed. In the emergency setting, when an interventional radiologist is not available, it is imperative to decompress the stomach, and subsequently, through the gastric access, it is possible to obtain X-ray contrast studies or endoscopy.

26.6 Biliary Tract Lithiasis After Bariatric Surgery

After bariatric surgery, the risk of gallstone formation increases if weight loss rate exceeds 1.5 kg/week or when there has been excess weight loss of more than 24 % [54]. Most gallstones form in the first 6 months after surgery, with a symptomatic onset after a mean period of 10.2 months. A recent meta-analysis confirmed the effectiveness of ursodeoxycholic acid prophylaxis. Symptomatic gallstones, including acute cholecystitis in a patient with a history of bariatric surgery, should not constitute a problem for the general surgeon. The presence of choledocholithiasis can be difficult to diagnose and treat after gastric or intestinal bypass due to the anatomical changes and the lack of endoscopic access using endoscopic retrograde cholangio-pancreatography (ERCP). Diagnosis can be based on ultrasound, computed tomography, or magnetic resonance cholangio-pancreatography. Before cholecystectomy for symptomatic gallstones, a careful evaluation of the common bile duct (CBD) with noninvasive imaging techniques should be obtained, and a larger use of intraoperative cholangiogram is warranted. Once common bile duct obstruction is diagnosed, the endoscopic/surgical treatment depends on the surgeon's experience and the patient's status. The problem of approaching bypassed structures is not new, and different access techniques have been described. The options include laparoscopic or open CBD exploration, percutaneous transhepatic instrumentation of the biliary tree, transgastric ERCP, transenteric endoscopic cholangio-pancreatography, and ERCP using specialized endoscopes [55, 56].

The success rate reported using a retrograde approach is 65 % in standard RYGBP but nearly impossible in a long-limb RYGBP or BPD. In a GBP, it is possible to reach the biliary tree by advancing the endoscope through the gastric remnant, but the inability to distend it with air makes an imaging-guided access challenging. The use of double-balloon enteroscopy to perform an endoscopic-assisted placement of a trocar into the remnant stomach was recently reported. An open gastrostomy is the easiest approach to access the residual stomach. Some studies describe a minimally invasive technique to access the bypassed stomach after RYGBP: a laparoscopic gastrostomy is obtained after induction of carbon dioxide pneumo-peritoneum, and a 15-mm trocar is placed into the stomach to allow the insertion of the endoscope. When the endoscopic procedure is completed, the gastrostomy is closed with a running suture or a linear stapler. The procedure can be performed at the same time of the laparoscopic cholecystectomy. Possibility to reach the papilla after BPD through a surgical jejunostomy has been reported [57–59].

References

1. Kremen AJ, Linner JH, Nelson CH. An experimental evaluation of the nutritional importance of proximal and distal small intestine. Ann Surg. 1954;140(3):439–48.
2. Boru C, Silecchia G. Bariatric emergencies: what the general surgeon should know. Chir (Bucur). 2010; 105(4):455–64.
3. Kirshtein B, Lantsberg L, Mizrahi S, Avinoach E. Bariatric emergencies for non-bariatric surgeons: complications of laparoscopic gastric banding. Obes Surg. 2010;20(11):1468–78.
4. Monkhouse SJ, Morgan JD, Norton SA. Complications of bariatric surgery: presentation and emergency management—a review. Ann R Coll Surg Engl. 2009; 91(4):280–6.
5. Morrison LJ, Deakin CD, Morley PT, Callaway CW, Kerber RE, Kronick SL, Lavonas EJ, Link MS, Neumar RW, Otto CW, Parr M, Shuster M, Sunde K, Peberdy MA, Tang W, Hoek TL, Böttiger BW, Drajer S, Lim SH, Nolan JP; Advanced Life Support Chapter Collaborators. Part 8: Advanced life support: 2010 International Consensus on Cardiopulmonary Resuscitation and Emergency Cardiovascular Care Science With Treatment Recommendations. Circulation. 2010; Oct 19;122 (16 Suppl 2):S345–421. doi:10.1161/CIRCULATIONAHA.110.971051.
6. Böttiger BW, Drajer S, Lim SH, Nolan JP, Advanced Life Support Chapter Collaborators. Part 8: advanced life support: 2010 International Consensus on Cardiopulmonary

Resuscitation and Emergency Cardiovascular Care Science with Treatment Recommendations. Circulation. 2010;122(16 Suppl 2):S345–421.
7. Sapala JA, Wood MH, SchuhKneckt MP, Sapal MA. Fatal pulmonary embolism after bariatric operations for morbid obesity: a 24 year retrospective analysis. Obes Surg. 2003;13:819–25.
8. Becattini C, Agnelli G, Manina G, Noya G, Rondelli F. Venous thromboembolism after laparoscopic bariatric surgery for morbid obesity: clinical burden and prevention. Surg Obes Relat Dis. 2012;8(1):108–15.
9. Smith MD, Patterson E, Wahed AS, Belle SH, Berk PD, Courcoulas AP, Dakin GF, Flum DR, Machado L, Mitchell JE, Pender J, Pomp A, Pories W, Ramanathan R, Schrope B, Staten M, Ude A, Wolfe BM. Thirty-day mortality after bariatric surgery: independently adjudicated causes of death in the longitudinal assessment of bariatric surgery. Obes Surg. 2011;21(11):1687–92.
10. Gagnière J, Slim K. Don't let obese patients be discharged with tachycardia after sleeve gastrectomy. Obes Surg. 2012;22(9):1519–20.
11. Loder WA. Airway management in the obese patient. Crit Care Clin. 2010;26(4):641–6.
12. Kristensen MS. Airway management and morbid obesity. Eur J Anaesthesiol. 2010;27(11):923–7.
13. Kazemi A, Frazier T, Cave M. Micronutrient-related neurologic complications following bariatric surgery. Curr Gastroenterol Rep. 2010;12(4):288–95.
14. Galvin R, Bråthen G, Ivashynka A, Hillbom M, Tanasescu R, Leone MA, EFNS. EFNS guidelines for diagnosis, therapy and prevention of Wernicke encephalopathy. Eur J Neurol. 2010;17(12):1408–18.
15. Manzanares W, Hardy G. Thiamine supplementation in the critically ill. Curr Opin Clin Nutr Metab Care. 2011;14(6):610–7.
16. Becker DA, Balcer LJ, Galetta SL. The neurological complications of nutritional deficiency following bariatric surgery. J Obes. 2012;2012:608534. doi:10.1155/2012/608534.
17. O'Brien PE. Bariatric surgery: mechanisms, indications and outcomes. J Gastroenterol Hepatol. 2010; 25(8):1358–65.
18. Silecchia G, Bacci V, Bacci S, Casella G, Rizzello M, Fioriti M, Basso N. Reoperation after laparoscopic adjustable gastric banding: analysis of a cohort of 500 patients with long-term follow-up. Surg Obes Relat Dis. 2008;4(3):430–6.
19. Spivak H, Abdelmelek MF, Beltran OR, Ng AW, Kitahama S. Long-term outcomes of laparoscopic adjustable gastric banding and laparoscopic Roux-en-Y gastric bypass in the United States. Surg Endosc. 2012;26(7):1909–19.
20. Himpens J, Cadière GB, Bazi M, Vouche M, Cadière B, Dapri G. Long-term outcomes of laparoscopic adjustable gastric banding. Arch Surg. 2011;146(7):802–7.
21. Bueter M, Maroske J, Thalheimer A, Gasser M, Stingl T, Heimbucher J, Meyer D, Fuchs K-H, Fein M. Short- and long-term results of laparoscopic gastric banding for morbid obesity. Langenbecks Arch Surg. 2008;393(2):199–205.
22. Angrisani L, Furbetta F, Doldi S, Basso N, Lucchese M, Giacomelli F, Zappa M, Cosmo L, Veneziani A, Turicchia G, et al. Lap Band® adjustable gastric banding system. Surg Endosc. 2003;17(3):409–12.
23. Iannelli A, Facchiano E, Sejor E, Baqué P, Piche T, Gugenheim J. Gastric necrosis: a rare complication of gastric banding. Obes Surg. 2005;15(8):1211–4.
24. Landen S, Majerus B, Delugeau V. Complications of gastric banding presenting to the ED. Am J Emerg Med. 2005;23(3):368–70.
25. Campbell NA, Brown WA, Smith AI, Skinner S, Nottle P. Small bowel obstruction creates a closed loop in patients with a laparoscopic adjustable gastric band. Obes Surg. 2008;18(10):1346–9.
26. Egberts K, Brown WA, O'Brien PE. Systematic review of erosion after laparoscopic adjustable gastric banding. Obes Surg. 2011;21(8):1272–9.
27. Aurora AR, Khaitan L, Saber AA. Sleeve gastrectomy and the risk of leak: a systematic analysis of 4,888 patients. Surg Endosc. 2012;26(6):1509–15.
28. Tan JT, Kariyawasam S, Wijeratne T, Chandraratna HS. Diagnosis and management of gastric leaks after laparoscopic sleeve gastrectomy for morbid obesity. Obes Surg. 2010;20(4):403–9.
29. Parkish M, Issa R, McCrillis A, Saunders JK, Ude-Wecome A, Gagner M. Strategies that may decrease leak after laparoscopic sleeve gastrectomy: a systematic review and meta-analysis of 9991 cases. Ann Surg. 2013;257(2):231–7.
30. Csendes A, Burgos AM, Braghetto I. Classification and management of leaks after gastric bypass for patients with morbid obesity: a prospective study of 60 patients. Obes Surg. 2012;22(6):855–62.
31. Bruce J, Krukowski ZH, Al-Khairy G, Russell EM, Park KG. Systematic review of the definition and measurement of anastomotic leak after gastrointestinal surgery. Br J Surg. 2001;88:1157–68.
32. Ballesta C, Berindoague R, Cabrera M, Palau M, Gonzales M. Management of anastomo tic leaks after laparoscopic Roux-en-Y gastric bypass. Obes Surg. 2008;18(6):623–30.
33. Yurcisin BM, DeMaria EJ. Management of leak in the bariatric gastric bypass patient: reoperate, drain and feed distally. J Gastrointest Surg. 2009;13(9):1564–6.
34. Morales MP, Miedema BW, Scott JS, De la Torre RA. Management of postsurgical leaks in the bariatric patient. Gastrointest Endosc Clin N Am. 2011;21(2): 295–304.
35. Eubanks S, Edwards CA, Fearing NM, Ramaswamy A, De la Torre RA, Thaler KJ, Miedema BW, Scott JS. Use of endoscopic stents to treat anastomotic complications after bariatric surgery. J Am Coll Surg. 2008;206(5):935–8.
36. Bendewald FP, Choi JN, Blythe LS, Selzer DJ, Ditslear JH, Mattar SG. Comparison of hand-sewn, linear-stapled, and circular-stapled gastrojejunostomy in laparoscopic Roux-en-Y gastric bypass. Obes Surg. 2011;21(11):1671–5.
37. Scopinaro N, Marinari G, Camerini G, Papadia F, 2004 ABS Consensus Conference. Biliopancreatic

diversion for obesity: state of the art. Surg Obes Relat Dis. 2005;1:317–28.
38. Cossu ML, Meloni GB, Alagna S, Tilocca PL, Pilo L, Profili S, Noya G. Emergency surgical conditions after biliopancreatic diversion. Obes Surg. 2007;17(5):637–41.
39. Silecchia G, Rizzello M, Casella G, Fioriti M, Soricelli E, Basso N. Two-stage laparoscopic biliopancreatic diversion with duodenal switch as treatment of high-risk super-obese patients: analysis of complications. Surg Endosc. 2009;23(5):1032–7.
40. Sacks BC, Mattar SG, Qureshi FG, Eid GM, Collins JL, Barinas-Mitchell EJ, Schauer PR, Ramanathan RC. Incidence of marginal ulcers and the use of absorbable anastomotic sutures in laparoscopic Roux-en-Y gastric bypass. Surg Obes Relat Dis. 2011;2(1):11–6.
41. Ruutiainen AT, Levine MS, Williams NN. Giant jejunal ulcers after Roux-en-Y gastric bypass. Abdom Imaging. 2008;33(5):575–8.
42. Maung AA, Johnson DC, Piper GL, Barbosa RR, Rowell SE, Bokhari F, Collins JN, Gordon JR, Ra JH, Kerwin AJ. Evaluation and management of small-bowel obstruction: an Eastern Association for the Surgery of Trauma practice management guideline. J Trauma Acute Care Surg. 2012;73(5 Suppl 4):S362–9.
43. Martin MJ, Beekley AC, Sebesta JA. Bowel obstruction in bariatric and nonbariatric patients: major differences in management strategies and outcome. Surg Obes Relat Dis. 2011;7(3):263–9.
44. Owens M, Barry M, Janjua AZ, Winter DC. A systematic review of laparoscopic port site hernias in gastrointestinal surgery. Surgeon. 2011;9(4):218–24.
45. Husain S, Ahmed AR, Johnson J, Boss T, O'Malley W. Small-bowel obstruction after laparoscopic Roux-en-Y gastricbypass: etiology, diagnosis, and management. Arch Surg. 2007;142(10):988–93.
46. Higa KD, Ho T, Boone KB. Internal hernias after laparoscopic Roux-en-Y gastric bypass: incidence, treatment and prevention. Obes Surg. 2003;13:350–4.
47. Tucker ON, Escalante-Tattersfield T, Szomstein S, Rosenthal RJ. The ABC system: a simplified classification system for small bowel obstruction after laparoscopic Roux-en-Y gastric bypass. Obes Surg. 2007; 17:1549–54.
48. Silecchia G, Boru CE, Mouiel J, Rossi M, Anselmino M, Morino M, Toppino M, Gaspari A, Gentileschi P, Tacchino R, Basso N. The use of fibrin sealant to prevent major complications following laparoscopic gastric bypass: results of a multicenter, randomized trial. Surg Endosc. 2008;22(11):2492–7.
49. Iannuccilli JD, Grand D, Murphy BL, Evangelista P, Roye GD, Mayo-Smith W. Sensitivity and specificity of eight CT signs in the preoperative diagnosis of internal mesenteric hernia following Roux-en-Y gastric bypass surgery. Clin Radiol. 2009;64(4):373–80.
50. Reddy SA, Yang C, McGinnis LA, Seggerman RE, Garza E, Ford 3rd KL. Diagnosis of transmesocolic internal hernia as a complication of retrocolic gastric bypass: CT imaging criteria. AJR Am J Roentgenol. 2007;189(1):52–5.
51. Onopchenko A. Radiological diagnosis of internal hernia after Roux-en-Y gastric bypass. Obes Surg. 2005;15(5):606–11.
52. Shwetambara P, Soto E, Merola S. Diagnosis and management of internal hernias after laparoscopic gastric bypass. Obes Surg. 2007;17:1498–502.
53. Mason EE, Renquist KE, Huang YH, Jamal M, Samuel I. Causes of 30-day bariatric surgery mortality: with emphasis on bypass obstruction. Obes Surg. 2007;17:9–14.
54. Li VK, Pulido N, Fajnwaks P, Szomstein S, Rosenthal R, Martinez-Duartez P. Predictors of gallstone formation after bariatric surgery: a multivariate analysis of risk factors comparing gastric bypass, gastric banding, and sleeve gastrectomy. Surg Endosc. 2009;23(7):1640–4.
55. Ahmed AR, Husain S, Saad N, Patel NC, Waldman DL, O'Malley W. Accessing the common bile duct after Roux-en-Y gastric bypass. Surg Obes Relat Dis. 2007;3(6):640–3.
56. Levitzky BE, Wassef WY. Endoscopic management in the bariatric surgical patient. Curr Opin Gastroenterol. 2010;26(6):632–9.
57. Ceppa FA, Gagné DJ, Papasavas PK, Caushaj PF. Laparoscopic transgastric endoscopy after Roux-en-Y gastric bypass. Surg Obes Relat Dis. 2006;3(1): 21–4.
58. Dapri G, Himpens J, Buset M, Vasilikostas G, Ntounda R, Cadière GB. Video. Laparoscopic transgastric access to the common bile duct after Roux-en-Y gastric bypass. Surg Endosc. 2009;23(7):1646–8.
59. Mergener K, Kozarek RA, Traverso W. Intraoperative ERCP: case reports. Gastrointest Endosc. 2003;58: 461–3.

Part IV

Outcomes

27 Nutritional Outcomes

Giovanni Camerini

27.1 Introduction

The employment of surgery to treat morbid obesity is increasing all over the world due to the growing prevalence of obesity, the usual failure of conservative treatment in providing an important and a long-lasting weight loss, and the development of minimally invasive surgery.

Current bariatric operations are classified as simply gastric restrictive procedures, including adjustable silicone gastric banding (ASGB), vertical banded gastroplasty (VBG), and sleeve gastrectomy (SG), malabsorptive procedures, including biliopancreatic diversion with duodenal switch (BPD-DS) or without duodenal switch (standard-BPD) and restrictive–malabsorptive procedures, including Roux-en-Y gastric bypass (RYGBP). The number of "malabsorptive" operations is increasing each year, because of better and more durable results in weight loss and resolution of comorbidities.

After ASGB, according to the laparoscopic Cadière technique [1], and after VBG, according to the MacLean technique [2], the stomach is divided into two parts, creating a proximal small pouch (approximately 30 mL in size), with a small outlet (10–12 mm in diameter). Sleeve gastrectomy is, on the other hand, a longitudinal gastric resection leaving a pouch of about 100 mL, that takes the shape of a sleeve.

Purely restrictive procedures, by decreasing the gastric capacity, induce an early and prolonged satiety, thereby reducing the daily volume of food intake. After these operations, which leave the normal absorptive physiology of the small bowel intact, selective nutritional deficiencies are unusual. However, some factors may cause nutritional deficiencies also even after restrictive surgery such as developed intolerance to certain types of food (red meat, milk, fiber), poor eating behaviors, a too rapid and significant weight loss or the occurrence of surgical complications.

Standard-BPD consists of a distal gastrectomy with a long Roux-en-Y reconstruction, with the enteroenterostomy placed 50 cm proximal to the ileocecal valve and the gastroenteric anastomosis created 250 cm proximal to the ileocecal valve [3]. The BPD-DS is a modification of the BPD where a sleeve gastrectomy is fashioned, the pylorus is left intact, and the proximal duodenum is anastomosed to the ileum 250 cm proximal to the ileocecal valve [4]. After BPD, the bypass of the duodenum and of the entire jejunum results in a selective and permanent limitation of intestinal absorption for fat and starches, and thus energy. Both procedures, decreasing significantly the absorptive surface area, are associated with serious risks of deficiencies, unless followed with appropriate supplementation.

G. Camerini
Department of Surgery, University of Genoa, School of Medicine, Genoa, Italy
e-mail: camerini@unige.it

M. Lucchese, N. Scopinaro (eds.), *Minimally Invasive Bariatric and Metabolic Surgery: Principles and Technical Aspects*, DOI 10.1007/978-3-319-15356-8_27,

In RYGBP, a small proximal gastric pouch (approximately 15–30 mL in size) with a 75–150 cm Roux-en-Y reconstruction is anastomosed 30–50 cm distally to the ligament of Treitz, combining two mechanisms promoting weight loss, restriction, and malabsorption [5]. The bypass of the distal stomach, duodenum, and proximal jejunum causes a greater reduction of absorption of nutrients, a greater weight loss and a greater risk of nutrient deficiency, the longer the Roux limb is.

All bariatric operations entail a profound change in digestive physiology, either restricting ingestion or reducing absorption. After any bariatric operation, a negative energy balance occurs, the body distribution of carbohydrates, proteins, and lipid is altered and hormonal and enzymatic functions are modified. Indeed, in order to reach a reduction of energy intake and a consequent weight loss, the creation of another disease is required, namely "controlled starvation." Therefore, nutritional and metabolic complications can appear, for both supplemented and non-supplemented operated patients, in the short and in the long term, the deficits most frequently observed regarding iron, vitamin B12, calcium, vitamin D, and proteins. The importance of nutritional complications may result from several factors besides the type of operation performed, such as subclinical deficiencies preexisting surgery, the compliance with recommended modification of the eating behaviors, and nutrient supplementation on the development of postoperative complications.

27.2 Deficiencies Preexisting to Surgery

Obese subjects, though having an excess of stores of energy, are paradoxically quite often not well nourished. If adequately screened, obese patients already reveal subclinical nutritional deficiencies before surgery between 40 and 80 %. The reported prevalence for vitamin D deficiency is between 50 and 80 %, for folate 20–30 %, for selenium 10–20 %, and for iron 25–40 %. Several studies confirm these findings [6–9]. This state of "high calorie malnutrition" is caused by poor food quality and eating behaviors and by the chronic dieting cycles of obese people. Therefore, independently of the bariatric procedure planned, a complete nutritional assessment including serum levels of vitamins and minerals is suggested, in order to correct deficiencies before surgery. Indeed such deficiencies are more difficult to correct in the postoperative period, may be theoretically worsened by malabsorptive procedures and, furthermore, may interfere with the healing process after surgery.

27.3 Modifications of Eating Behavior

Following bariatric surgery, depending on the procedure involved, different modifications in eating behavior are required, in order to obtain good weight results and to minimize postoperative problems.

After purely restrictive procedures, patients must take small meals, reducing the food volume, chew very well, separate fluids and foods, eat slowly, stop eating when they feel full. The non-adherence to these recommendations results in regurgitation, vomiting, and food blockages.

After RYGBP and SG, which combine a reduction of gastric volume with hormonal changes, the avoidance of simple sugars and drinking no beverages during meals avoid regurgitation and dumping syndrome.

After malabsorptive operations, protein-rich food should be preferred and the consumption of highly refined sugars should be avoided, in order to improve weight loss and to prevent dumping syndrome. High-fat foods and skimmed milk should also be avoided to prevent excessive steatorrhea, diarrhea, and meteorism.

It is recommended that all operated patients receive an accurate dietary education. The non-compliance of such postoperative alimentary rules is the primary reason of failure of reaching a good weight loss and of occurrence of nutritional and metabolic problems following bariatric surgery.

27.4 Supplementation

It is unanimously thought that after bariatric surgery a lifelong multivitamin supplementation is required. The typical supplementation model contains at least 1,200–2,000 mg/day of calcium citrate D, 400–800 UI/day of vitamin D, 50–100 mg/day of elemental iron, 300–350 μg/day of folic acid, and 100–350 μg/day of vitamin B12. Such regimen supplementations are planned for lifelong daily supplementation and not to treat deficiencies.

The fact is that daily supplementation with commercially available multivitamin preparations is often insufficient to prevent nutritional deficiencies, so that additional iron, vitamin B12, calcium plus vitamin D supplements are indispensable after malabsorptive procedures.

Gasteyger confirmed that standard multivitamin supplementation is not adequate after RYGBP: almost 60 % of patients 6 months after surgery and 100 % after 24 months needed one or more nutritional supplements in his study [10].

The American Society for Metabolic and Bariatric Surgery (ASMBS) recommends a supplementation for all nutrients consisting of a dosage double compared with the normal amount, beginning as soon as possible after the operation. However, controlled trials are still lacking supporting the adequacy of this model of supplementation [11].

27.5 Nutritional Surveillance

Since evidence-based data remain scarce, the dietary strategies, the frequency of postoperative visits and laboratory tests, as well as the dose of mineral and vitamin supplementation of operated patients, are at the moment still empirical. The only three things that are certain in the follow-up of operated patients are that it must be stratified according to the specific surgical technique, performed by a trained multidisciplinary staff (bariatric surgeon, obesity specialist, and the dietician) and maintained throughout life.

Frequent clinical visits are necessary after restrictive procedures, in order to achieve and maintain a good weight loss.

After malabsorptive operations, the clinical follow-up is lighter than after purely restrictive procedures, as upper gastrointestinal (GI) symptoms are infrequent and weight loss is, as a rule, good. Nevertheless, the clinical and laboratory surveillance should be anyway frequent, in this case in order to prevent, detect, and correct nutritional complications.

This is why European guidelines recommend after both categories of bariatric operations the similar following protocol: checkup after 1 month, a minimal follow-up every 3 months for the first year, every 6 months for the second year and annually thereafter [12]. Similarly, in respect of laboratory tests, according to Pournaras, it should be worthwhile monitoring calcium, vitamin B12, ferritin, folate, and iron indices with blood tests at 3, 6, 12, 24 months postoperatively, and yearly thereafter for all patients submitted to bariatric operations [13].

27.6 Postoperative Complications

Vomiting and diarrhea are the most frequent gastrointestinal symptoms following bariatric surgery. They, in turns, may generate an insufficient oral intake or an excess of intestinal losses, both potential causes of malnutrition, respectively, after restrictive and malabsorptive operations.

Vomiting occurs in one third of operated patients, typically during the first 6 months after surgery and is the most common complaint after bariatric surgery [14]. During this period, the causes of vomiting are usually related to the inability to modify the eating behaviors, and include insufficient chewing, drinking during meals, too large meals, and food intolerance. If vomiting persists for more than 6 months after surgery, an outlet mechanical problem should be suspected, such as a stenosis, a displacement, or slippage in case of ASGB or a stenosis of the gastroenterostomy or a marginal ulceration in case of BPD or RYGBP.

Gastroesophageal reflux disease, symptomatic gallstones and medications are additional causes of late vomiting.

Table 27.1 Micronutrients recommended dietary allowances, micronutrients supplementation for prevention, and treatment of postsurgical nutritional deficiencies

Micronutrients	R. D. A.	Supplementation	Treatment
Vitamin B1	1–1.3 mg	100 mg	1,500 mg 250 mg i.v.
Folic acid	400 μg	800–1,000 μg 1 mg/day (pregnant women)	1–5 mg
Vitamin B12	2.4 μg	350 μg/day p.o. 1,000 μg/m i.m.	1,000–2,000 μg 1,000 μg/w i.m.
Vitamin C	75–90 mg	75–90 mg	
Vitamin A	900 μg (3,000 UI)	10,000 UI/day	25,000 UI/day
Vitamin D	5 μg (200 UI)	400–800 UI/day	50,000 UI/week
Vitamin E	15 mg	150 UI/day	800–1,200 UI/day
Vitamin K	150 μg	150 μg	5–20 mg a day
Calcium	800 mg/day	1,200–2,000 mg/day	1.2 g
Iron	8–18 mg	60–120 mg	180 mg
Selenium	55 μg	55 μg	
Zinc	8–11 mg	8–11 mg	220 mg

After BPD and RYGBP, diarrhea related to dumping syndrome, lactose intolerance, bacterial overgrowth or any intestinal infection provokes an excess of intestinal energy and nitrogen loses, and can impair the nutritional status in any patient submitted to malabsorptive operations.

We should always bear in mind that after any bariatric surgery, the insurgence of any complication, as well as the occurrence of any disease, can easily result in a catabolic state and in a metabolic impairment in an otherwise well-nourished patient.

Regarding this aspect, Faintuch analyzed the circumstances associated with the occurrence of severe malnutrition in 11 of 236 (4.7 %) patients submitted to RYGBP on average 18 months after surgery, and observed that exogenous precipitating factors were present in 64 % of them [15] (Tables 27.1 and 27.2).

27.7 Specific Deficiencies

27.7.1 Macronutrient Deficiencies

The purpose of obesity surgery is the reduction of energy intake. After surgery, the modification of the energy balance occurs as a consequence of a major reduction in intake, or absorption, of the three energy-rich macronutrients: proteins, starches, and fats. This can result in a deficiency most frequently of proteins and seldom of essential fatty acids.

27.7.1.1 Protein Depletion and Protein–Energy Malnutrition

After BPD, the reduction of protein digestion, resulting from the reduction of the time of contact between digestive enzymes and the bolus (due to asynchronia and the delayed meeting between the alimentary bolus and the biliopancreatic secretions, the reduction of enzyme secretion, the faster intestinal transit time, and limited contact with the brush border of enterocytes) and the reduction of intestinal absorption area, causes a decrease in protein absorption of around 30 %. Furthermore, Scopinaro demonstrated in BPD subjects an endogenous nitrogen loss of about 5 g/day, which greatly exceeds what is considered to be the maximum normal in intact GI tract individuals. Both events play a significant role in the pathogenesis of protein malnutrition (PM) after BPD [16].

Protein malnutrition represents a dangerous potential complication of malabsorptive operations. Scopinaro describes two types of protein malnutrition: the sporadic and the recurrent one.

Table 27.2 Clinical presentation of nutritional problems after bariatric surgery

Deficiency	Causal factors	Complication	Diagnosis
Vitamin B1	Recurrent vomiting, glucose intravenous infusion	Beriberi, dry beriberi, Wernicke's encephalopathy	Low serum thiamine level, reduced erythrocyte transketolase activity
Folic acid	Low intake	Fatigue, dyspnea, fetal neural-tube defects	Serum folate <3 ng/mL, megaloblastic anemia
Vitamin B12	Reduced intake of meat or milk products, decreased of intrinsic factor, bypass of duodenum, rapid transit time in the ileum	Macrocytic anemia, neuropathy, paresthesias, sensory abnormalities, spastic paraparesis, visual loss	B12 <200 pg/mL, elevated methylmalonic acid homocysteine concentrations
Vitamin A	Low intake, malabsorption	Night blindness, conjunctival xerosis, keratitis, corneal scarring, dry skin, pruritus	Vitamin A <1.6 μmol/L
Vitamin D	Low intake, malabsorption	Osteomalacia, osteoporosis	Low serum 25-hydroxyvitamin D
Vitamin E	Low intake, malabsorption	Hemolytic anemia, pigmented retinopathy, areflexia, ataxia	Vitamin E <7 μmol/L
Vitamin K	Low intake, malabsorption	Bleeding disorder	Vitamin K <0.3 nmol/L
Calcium	Bypass of duodenum and proximal jejunum, vitamin D deficiency, bacterial overgrowth	Osteomalacia, osteoporosis myalgias, bone pain, increased risk of fracture	Low serum calcium augmentation of alkaline phosphatase and parathyroid hormone
Iron	Low meat intake, bypass of antrum, duodenum and proximal jejunum, gastrointestinal blood loss	Fatigue, dyspnea, pale conjunctiva, koilonychia	Microcytic anemia, low serum iron, high TIBC, low serum ferritin
Selenium	Low intake	Cardiomyopathy, arrhythmia, osteoarthritis, hair loss, impaired immunity, low thyroid function	Selenium <0.7 umol/L
Zinc	Reduced intake, chronic diarrhea	Alopecia epithelial eruption, glossitis, nail dystrophy, and immune deficiencies	

The *sporadic protein malnutrition* can occur in the early postoperative period, because of too drastic protein intake reduction or the preference for carbohydrate intake, and at any time after the operation, because of prolonged diarrhea or reduced food intake for any reason. Of much greater importance is the *recurrent form of protein malnutrition*. A number of different factors, alone or in combination, can lead to this condition. *Patient-dependent factors* are insufficient protein intake, insufficient protein absorption per unit of intestinal surface, and excessive loss of endogenous nitrogen. *Operation-dependent factors* are too small stomach (causing too rapid emptying and too rapid intestinal transit with permanently reduced absorption) and too short alimentary limb (causing insufficient protein absorption). One or more of these factors can be responsible for the complication. The concept is that specific operation as it is, in that specific subject as he/she is, is incompatible with good protein nutritional status. After two or more episodes of protein malnutrition, the decision for surgical revision is made, consisting of elongation of the common limb. Because, protein absorption depends on the length of the small bowel from the GEA to the ICV, the elongation must not be done along the alimentary limb, but along the biliopancreatic one. The standard which in our hands guarantees the solution of all protein nutritional problems is to add 150 cm, for a final total length of 400 cm. This obviously entails the restabilization of body weight at an average level which corresponds to about 25 % regain of the original excess weight [3].

The incidence of PM in the initial series of Scopinaro is included between 7 and 21 % [17].

On the contrary, another study by Trotte on 180 patients submitted to standard-BPD demonstrated a protein deficiency, requiring parenteral nutrition and the elongation of the common limb, only in two patients [18].

Marinari in 2004 reviewed the experience of our group, in the last 858 patients with "ad hoc stomach ad hoc alimentary limb" BPD, 5 years after the operation, and found mild hypoalbuminemia in 11 % and severe in 2.4 % of BPD patients. Reoperations were performed in 6 % of the total patient population, mainly for late recurrent protein malnutrition [19].

Nanni found that the main specific complication after "ad hoc stomach ad hoc alimentary limb" BPD was PM, which was observed in 3.4 % of operated patients [20].

According to Marceau, the BPD-DS procedure, due to the conservation of antrum and pylorus, would be expected to reduce diarrhea and risk of PM, when compared with standard-BPD. On the contrary, the author observed a high incidence of protein deficiency 79 months after BPD (11 % of the patients revealed albumin levels <3.5 g/dL, and 2.4 % <3.2 g/dL), needing revisional surgery in 6 % of them [21].

Dolan also found that 18 % of patients were hypoalbuminemic at a median follow-up of 28 months with no significant differences between BPD and BPD-DS with a common channel length of 50 cm [22].

Rabkin, in a study on 589 consecutive patients, showed that after BPD-DS, protein metabolism markers were normal within the first 3 postoperative years, but with a common channel of 100 cm [23].

Marceau had similar results, with the length of the common channel of 100 cm instead of 50 cm, in a subsequent study on 465 patients who underwent BPD-DS at 4 years [4].

In condition of normal GI anatomy, half of protein absorption occurs in the duodenum, the majority of protein uptake occurring within the mid-jejunum. It is therefore obvious that protein deficiency may occur after RYGBP as well.

This complication, indeed quite rare after standard RYGBP (with 75–150 cm Roux limb lengths), is observed more frequently after longer Roux limbs, with a reported incidence of 7–12 % [24].

In the randomized series of Brolin, no protein deficit was showed at a minimum of 2 years after standard RYGBP, while 13 % of the patients submitted to a distal RYGBP had PM [25].

Kalfarentzos confirmed this difference with a 5.9 % protein deficiency rate 20 months after distal RYGBP, but no deficiency after the standard RYGBP [26].

After standard and distal RYGBP, 1.4 and 3 % of patients, respectively, showed an albumin level <3 g/dL in the study of Skroubis [27].

Clinical manifestations of PEM are hypoalbuminemia, asthenia, anemia, loss of muscle mass, anomalies of the skin mucosa and nails (hair loss, striated nails, dermatitis), and edema. Protein depletion is very easy to recognize by following albumin (albumin <3.5 g/dL).

An intake of 1.0–1.5 g/kg ideal body weight (60–80 g/day total protein) in the early postoperative period is recommended after any bariatric operation. Due to the loss of endogenous nitrogen greater than normal, alimentary protein requirements in BPD patients have to be increased by 30 %, that is approximately 90 g/day. During the postoperative visits, the assessment of protein intake has to be performed, and protein supplementation should be given when protein intake remains inferior to 60 g/day.

Mild-to-moderate cases of PM are usually corrected by more frequent dietetic counseling and increased protein intake [27].

In case of severe PM, a prompt rehospitalization and the initiation of parenteral nutrition is mandatory. Three weeks of total parenteral nutrition (TPN) are usually sufficient to correct the acute problem, whether PM occurs after the BPD or RYGBP.

27.7.1.2 Essential Fatty Acids

In condition of normal GI anatomy, while bile salts are absorbed only in the terminal ileum, fat and fat-soluble vitamins absorption occur all along the small intestine, the majority of lipids uptake occurring in the proximal two thirds of the jejunum.

Following BPD and distal RYGBP, the meeting between the food and biliopancreatic secretions and the absorption occurs in the common channel, resulting in a reduction of lipid absorption of around 70 %. Based on this, Scopinaro showed, after standard-BPD, a maximum threshold of 40 g/day of the dietary fat absorption.

If it is true that the shorter the length of the common channel (generally varying between 50 and 100 cm), the greater the fat malabsorption, the consequent weight loss and maintenance are, it is equally true that longer common channels are better tolerated, being associated with less steatorrhea and diarrhea.

Fat-soluble vitamins and essential fatty acid deficiencies are common following malabsorptive procedures. Linoleic and α-linoleic acids are fundamental components for the prostaglandin and leukotriene synthesis. Therefore, deficit of essential fatty acids can induce anemia, thrombocytopenia, alopecia, and dermatitis, even if this topic has not been studied in depth.

Fat malabsorption, clinically expressed by steatorrhea, never present after ASGB and SG, frequently present after RYGBP, is always present after BPD, being the principal mechanism by which BPD promotes weight loss. Therefore, special attention to the quality of alimentary fat should be given after any malabsorptive operation.

27.7.2 Micronutrient Deficiencies

27.7.2.1 Iron

Ingested iron is solubilized, ionized, and reduced from the alimentary ferric form to its ferrous form by acid gastric juices, and subsequently actively transported into the cell. Iron absorption may occur throughout the small bowel, but it is best absorbed in the duodenum and in upper jejunum.

There are several mechanisms that cause iron malabsorption after RYGBP and BPD, including a relatively achlorhydric gastric pouch, with limited exposure of food to acid, and the exclusion of duodenum and proximal jejunum (where iron is maximally absorbed) from digestive continuity. After gastric restrictive procedures, a reduction of red meat intake, the major source of heme, and of iron-rich foods can be an important factor in such deficiency.

SG, entailing the removal of most of the stomach, so reducing the production of hydrochloric acid, is followed by iron deficiency [28]. Indeed, hemoglobin and hematocrit were less than normal in, respectively, 28.6 and 25 % of the 82 patients submitted to SG at 5 years, in a study by Saif et al. [29]. A Dutch study confirmed a decrease in iron levels in 43 % of patients 1 year after SG [30]. On the contrary, a report from Saudi Arabia showed no occurrence of iron deficiency 1 year after sleeve gastrectomy [31].

Although there is no solid data regarding iron deficiency after purely restrictive operations, this complication occurs surely after RYGBP and BPD.

The American Society of Bariatric Surgery surgeons showed the incidence of iron deficiency of 14–16 % after RYBG and 21–26 % after BPD [32].

Brolin demonstrated an iron deficiency in 49–52 %, and anemia in 35–74 % in a series of 298 superobese patients, 3 years after RYGBP, depending on the Roux limb length [25].

Skroubis found an iron deficiency after RYGBP increasing from 26 % preoperatively, to 39 % at 4 years, and then decreasing to 25 % at 5 years [27].

BPD also reduces the iron absorption, and many studies showed a higher prevalence of iron deficiency when compared with other bariatric operations, particularly in young women [23].

In the aforementioned study by Skroubis, iron deficiency rates increased from 32.6 % preoperatively to 44.4 % at 4 years and 100 % at 5 years, following BPD [27].

Marceau after BPD-DS showed abnormal ferritin levels (<20 μg/L) in 4 % of the 92 patients preoperatively, and in 25–40 % at 5 years [21].

Dolan reported an iron deficiency in 22.9 % of his patients at mean follow-up of 28 months. This complication was similar in patients submitted to BPD with or without a duodenal switch, in spite of the respect of antrum, pylorus, and a cuff of duodenum entailed with the latter operation [22].

Skroubis demonstrates no differences in the incidence of iron deficiency, in a study comparing patients submitted to RYGBP or BPD at a 5-year follow-up [27].

Brolin demonstrated a significant decline in the iron status in 63 % of 140 subjects followed for 2 years after RYGBP in spite of a correct standard supplementation. This suggests that additional prophylactic iron supplements should be provided for women to prevent iron deficiency, in addition to the standard supplementation [33].

The laboratory diagnosis for iron deficiency includes anemia with a low MCV, low serum iron, high TIBC, and low serum ferritin level.

Subjective manifestations are fatigue, reduced exercise tolerance and dyspnea. On examination, the patient has pale conjunctiva, koilonychia (spoon nails), hair loss, and possibly atrophic glossitis.

Though malabsorption is the obvious reason to explain any iron deficiency after bariatric surgery, an additional mechanism for iron deficiency after RYGBP and BPD is the gastrointestinal blood loss. Typical sites of bleeding are a marginal ulcer (on the anastomosis between the jejunum or ileum and the gastric pouch), an iron-losing enteropathy of bypassed loop, an overgrowth of intestinal bacteria phenomenon in the small bowel excluded, or hemorrhoids. But any pathology of the GI tract (such as a gastrointestinal cancer) should be excluded in refractory cases.

Oral treatment usually consists of 325 mg of ferrous sulfate or 200 mg of ferrous fumarate (providing about 65 mg of iron), one to two tablets a day as prophylaxis, and three to four tablets a day to correct iron deficiency. The bypass of the antrum and duodenum makes the iron absorption very difficult in deficient patients. Preparations containing elemental iron complexed with a polysaccharide are well absorbed and can be assumed in single daily doses of 100–200 mg. The dosage may be increased if iron parameters do not improve within a few months of starting therapy. The addition of vitamin C enhances the absorption.

Sometimes, parenteral iron infusion with iron dextran, ferric gluconate, or ferric sucrose is needed either in patients who have poor response to oral iron therapy or in case of intolerance or noncompliance. Intramuscular iron is not tolerable in the long run. On the contrary, intravenous iron dextran can be well tolerated by patients, also as an outpatient procedure, and can be used regularly.

After bariatric surgery, iron deficiency can occur early after surgery or after some time. Patients submitted to RYGBP and BPD require postoperative screening for iron status, including blood count with MCV, serum iron, ferritin, and TIBC. After the first year, these values should be checked yearly or biyearly throughout life.

27.7.2.2 Vitamin B1

Thiamin absorption is maximal in the small bowel, thanks to a mechanism of active transport, mediated by a specific sodium and energy-dependent carrier, and a mechanism of passive diffusion. The vitamin B1 deficiency has a low prevalence: only 29 cases were identified in a study on 168,010 bariatric operations, (0–0.002 %) [34], but it is a major complication of all bariatric operations.

As vitamin B1 is contained in all aliments, the deficit occurs as a consequence of the association of frequent episodes of vomiting and a reduced intake. It is not evident if the decreased absorption plays a role in the development of the deficiency. Symptomatic thiamine deficiency has been observed both after restrictive and malabsorptive procedures. The small amount of liver thiamine stored (which last approximately 30 days) contributes to this deficiency weeks or months after surgery.

Since vitamin B1 is involved in carbohydrate metabolism, administration of intravenous glucose or dextrose in patients complicated or dehydrated from vomiting, who have low vitamin B1 reserves, has been reported to be a precipitating factor for Wernicke's encephalopathy (bariatric beriberi).

A few cases of the deficiency have been reported after ASGB [35].

Low levels of thiamine were demonstrated in 0–11 % of patients 1 year after SG and in 31 % of patients after 5 years [36].

In a series of 141 patients submitted to RYGBP, the prevalence of thiamine deficiency was 18 % after 1 year and 11 % after 2 years [37].

A study on 1,663 patients submitted to BPD demonstrated an incidence of 0.18 % of Wernicke's encephalopathy 3–5 months after the operation [38].

The laboratory diagnosis for deficiency includes a low serum thiamine level and a reduced erythrocyte transketolase activity.

Wernicke's encephalopathy classically presents with a clinical triad: ocular manifestations, (such as nystagmus and ocular palsies), ataxia, and mental disturbances such as confusion. More often, an isolated peripheral neuropathy is described (dry beriberi) with symptoms of pain, burning, or tingling in the distribution of the affected sensory nerves, or peripheral extremity weakness in case of motor impairment.

In case of suspected deficiency, prompt recognition and immediate treatment with 50–100 mg of parenteral thiamine every 8 h can resolve ocular symptoms within a few days, but neurologic sequelae need months to completely regress, and are often not totally reversible.

In patients with protracted vomiting, aggressive supplementation with thiamine for 1 month after surgery avoids the deficiency.

Compliance to a multivitamin supplement is usually sufficient to prevent thiamine deficiency in most of the cases.

The presence of a bacterial overgrowth in the bypassed bowel must be considered when patients do not respond to an adequate oral therapy, due to an increased consumption. In these cases, the diagnosis can be confirmed by elevation of serum folate level or by the increase in hydrogen or methane in breath after an oral load of glucose.

27.7.2.3 Vitamin B9 (Folate)

Folate deficiency, defined as serum folate levels <3 ng/mL, is the most common nutrient deficiency after gastric restrictive procedures, usually caused by a decrease in the intake of vegetables in the immediate postoperative period. After RYGBP and BPD, the deficiency is produced by a reduction of acid and pepsinogen secretion (responsible for the vitamin bioavailability) and the lack of contact of food with the duodenum and the proximal third of the jejunum, primary sites of its absorption.

Gasteyger found a significant decrease in serum folate in 44 % of 36 women submitted to ASGB 2 years after surgery [39].

Folate deficiency has an incidence of 9–35 % after bypass surgeries [40].

Halverson demonstrated that 1 year after gastric bypass, 63 % of patients have folate deficiency [41].

Another study by Brolin showed folate deficiency in 22 % of patients 2 years after the operation [33].

On the contrary, the risk of folate deficiency is negligible in the long term, because an important bacterial synthesis of the vitamin occurs in the small intestine, progressively colonized after most bariatric operations.

Clinical manifestations of folate deficiency are megaloblastic anemia or a normocytic anemia, characterized by increased red cell distribution width. On the contrary, high serum folate levels are a specific marker for intestinal bacterial overgrowth.

Unlike iron and vitamin B12, routine multivitamin preparation (400 μg/day) is sufficient to maintain a good folate status.

The correction of folate deficit consists of oral folic acid 1–5 mg daily, even if the deficiency is as a rule corrected with multivitamin supplements alone.

A folate supplement of 1 mg/day is particularly important in pregnant women, in order to avoid risks of fetal neural-tube defects in case of deficiency.

27.7.2.4 Vitamin B12

Vitamin B12 deficiency is a common consequence both of restrictive procedures and malabsorptive ones, and involves multifactorial origin.

RYGBP and BPD, but also SG, excluding the majority of parietal cell mass and chief cells, primarily located in the fundus and body of the stomach, cause a significant vitamin B12 bioavailability reduction and a decreased production of intrinsic factor, a glycoprotein produced by parietal cells, required for absorption of the vitamin in the terminal ileum.

Further potential mechanisms for the vitamin malabsorption after RYGBP and BPD are the bypass of duodenum and the rapid transit time in the ileum. The risk of B12 deficiency is also increased after purely restrictive surgery, if patients reduce their intake of meat or milk products.

In a group of 100 patients planned for bariatric surgery, the incidence of vitamin B12 deficiency has been demonstrated in 5 % of subjects [42].

SG should have a more important effect on B12 status, compared with other restrictive procedures, due to resection of the fundus and the body of the stomach. Indeed, deficiencies in vitamin B12 have been showed at 1 and 3 years following SG [28], but not in the study by Saif [29].

Abnormal serum B12 levels (<180 pg/mL) were observed in 154 of 429 patients (36 %) at an average of 22 months after gastric bypass surgery in a study [43].

Another study confirmed that 33 % of patients have vitamin B12 deficiency (<250 pg/mL) 1 year after gastric bypass [41].

Brolin also showed vitamin B12 deficiency in 37 % of patients 2 years after gastric bypass [33].

Comparing 45 and 25 patients submitted, respectively, to BPD-DS and RYGBP at 2 years, Breton showed that vitamin B12 deficiency was more common in patients with gastric bypass [44].

The prevalence of vitamin B12 deficiency after bariatric surgery ranges from 4 to 62 % [45], whereas clinical symptoms are less common. This variability from study to study can be explained both by the different length of follow-up of studies, conditioning the time necessary to deplete the considerable body storage of vitamin, and by the differences in regime and adherence to supplementation.

Vitamin B12 is synthesized by bacteria and it is present in all forms of animal tissues, but not in fruits and vegetables. The recommended dietary intake is about 5 μg per day. The normal human body storage of the vitamin is about 2,000 μg, so the deficiency occurs years after surgery.

Clinical manifestations of vitamin B12 deficiency are the pernicious (megaloblastic) anemia and development of disorders of both CNS and PNS. These can include paresthesias, sensory abnormalities, spastic paraparesis, visual loss, cognitive, and neuropsychiatric manifestation.

Levels of vitamin B12 <200 pg/mL can indicate the presence of deficiency. Measurement of serum methylmalonic acid and homocysteine concentrations, the preferred marker of B12 status, can for certain confirm the deficiency.

The optimal dosage has not yet been demonstrated, but 350–1,000 μg a day generally corrects low levels of vitamin B12 in 95 % of patients. After RYGBP, oral supplementation with crystalline vitamin B12 corrects deficiency in most cases, as ileal absorption of crystalline B12 remains normal. Probably in BPD patients, nasal or sublingual preparations of vitamin B12, widely promoted nowadays, are better absorbed than oral forms to normalize vitamin levels [46]. Parenteral treatment with cyanocobalamin 1,000 μg every month, or 3,000 μg every 6 months, is necessary if oral supplementation is not adequate to sustain a sufficient blood level of the vitamin.

Evaluation of vitamin B12 deficiency is indispensable in all patients submitted to RYGBP, BPD, and SG every year. Indeed, since symptoms are frequently absent, ongoing B12 deficiency in the long term causes considerable risks of irreversible neurological damage.

27.7.2.5 Vitamin D and Calcium

It has been reported that calcium and vitamin D deficiency occurs in 25–75 % of obese patients even prior to surgery. A negative correlation between BMI and vitamin D levels was demonstrated by Buffington [47].

Another study on 213 patients candidate for surgical treatment of obesity showed that hyperparathyroidism was present in 25 % of subjects, and that 21 % of patients had abnormally low levels of 25-hydroxyvitamin D, PTH being positively correlated with BMI [48].

The possible explanations are a storage and sequestration of vitamin D in adipose tissue, a reduction of physical activity, an insufficient exposure to solar ultraviolet radiations with a decreased skin production, and a lowered hepatic hydroxylation of the vitamin in obese population.

Following bariatric surgery, the rapid weight loss liberates vitamin D from adipose tissue, with a temporary increase in vitamin D hematic concentrations. Recent studies confirm that plasma concentrations of vitamin D_2 increase at 1 month after surgery and have a decreasing trend over the following months [49].

Calcium is absorbed with a specific mechanism of active transport, mediated by a specific carrier, in the duodenum and proximal jejunum, and with a mechanism of passive diffusion in the remaining small bowel and colon. Vitamin D is absorbed in the jejunum and ileum. After RYGBP and BPD, calcium and vitamin D malabsorption results from the loss of acid action, and from the exclusion of duodenum and proximal jejunum (the primary sites for calcium absorption), from digestive continuity. Vitamin D deficiency is an additional cause of calcium malabsorption. Bacterial overgrowth in the bypassed small intestine can further interfere with vitamin D absorption.

Patients submitted to restrictive bariatric surgery can be afflicted by bone mass abnormalities as well as due to a restriction of calcium intake, even if conclusive data are lacking in respect of the association of ASGB or SG and of altered calcium and vitamin D homoeostasis [50].

On the other hand, it is well known that patients with a rapid weight loss from any cause are prone to bone mass loss, even in the presence of normal vitamin D and parathyroid hormone levels.

Literature shows a prevalence of the deficiency ranging from 7 to 60 % after RYGBP [37, 49], longer bypass limb lengths being followed by lower vitamin D levels [51]. Johnson confirmed a linear reduction of vitamin D concentration and a linear increase in PTH increasing the Roux limb length in RYGBP [52].

Calcium and vitamin D deficiency appears even more severe after BPD. Metabolic bone disease was present in 30 patients (73 %) in one study by Compston et al. [53].

Levels of vitamin D lower than normal are reported in 57 and 63 %, respectively, 1 and 4 years after BPD, with a corresponding increase in PTH levels in 69 % of patients at 4 years [54]. Another study on 82 subjects submitted to BPD showed that 25 % were hypocalcemic, 50 % had low vitamin D and 63 % had elevated PTH, at median follow-up of 32 months [55].

The duodenal switch does not improve the vitamin D status compared with standard-BPD [22], while reducing the degree of fat malabsorption by lengthening the common channel produces a lower incidence of vitamin D deficiency and hypocalcemia [6, 56].

Marceau showed only modest changes of the bone mineral density analysis 4 and 10 years after BPD, provided that there is appropriate supplementation and close surveillance to avoid for specific long-term disturbances [57].

The alterations in bone metabolism following bariatric surgery are associated in the long term with loss of bone mass and osteomalacia with complaints of myalgias, difficulty walking, bone pain, back pain, or aching of the limbs, and an increased risk of fracture [58]. Larger scale investigations are needed to associate with certainty the deficit of vitamin D to peripheral vascular disease, rheumatoid arthritis, diabetes, and cancer [59].

As calcium decreases in the blood, parathyroid hormone levels increase, with releasing of calcium from bone and consequently osteoporosis. Hence serum calcium measurement is not a reliable marker in the follow-up of postoperative calcium metabolism. Operated patients maintain normal serum calcium levels while bone loss and osteoporosis are in progress. Therefore, calcium, phosphorus, alkaline phosphatase, parathyroid hormone, and 25-hydroxyvitamin D should be monitored every 6 months in patients submitted to RYGBP or BPD.

It is not known if calcium 1.2–1.5 g/day and vitamin D 800 UI/day, contained in standard supplementation, are adequate to prevent deficiencies in the long run. What is certainly proven is that these amounts did not always normalize markers of bone resorption and secondary hyperparathyroidism [56]. Anyway, the dosage may be increased if calcium parameters do not improve within a few months.

Since calcium from carbonate is not available in the absence of gastric acidity, calcium citrate is more easily absorbed after bariatric surgery and it is the preferred preparation for replacement.

In case of important serum deficiency, the global dose for treatment is at least 600,000 IU of vitamin D2 (ergocalciferol), usually 50,000 IU taken orally once per week for 6–8 weeks.

A great prudence should be used in performing bariatric surgery in patients previously submitted to thyroid or parathyroid operations, because intractable symptomatic hypocalcemia was described years after BPD [60, 61].

27.7.2.6 Selenium

Selenium is a nutritional essential trace element, a fundamental component of glutathione peroxidase (GTP), an enzyme active against oxygen-derived free radicals. Severe selenium deficiency can induce cardiomyopathy, arrhythmia, muscle wasting, osteoarthritis, hair loss, loss of skin and hair pigmentation, impaired immunity, low thyroid function, and progressive encephalopathy. The evidence linking selenium deficiency and an increased incidence of cancer is conflicting.

Due to the reduction in food intake, and the fact that most selenium is absorbed in condition of normal GI anatomy in the duodenum, patients submitted to BPD and RYGBP can be prone to disturbances of selenium and GTP homeostasis.

Few clinical studies concerning selenium deficiency after bariatric surgery have been published.

Abnormal levels of selenium status were reported preoperatively in 30 %, and 1 year after RYGBP in 36 % of patients in one study [42] .

In another study by Freeth, a significant reduction of serum selenium level was demonstrated 3 months after GB and RYGBP, while the level trended back toward baseline values at 12 months, without any supplementation [62].

Dolan found that 14.5 % of patients were deficient in selenium (<0.7 umol/L), at a median follow-up of 28 months with no significant differences between BPD and BPD-DS with a common channel length of 50 cm and no clinical consequences [22].

There are insufficient data to justify both routine screening for selenium deficiency and selenium supplementation at higher levels than the current recommended dietary allowances (RDA) (55 mcg/day) in patients submitted to bariatric surgery.

27.7.2.7 Zinc

Zinc has a role in reducing the oxidative processes, protecting protein sulfhydryls, reducing the hydroxyradical formation, or inducing in the liver, gut, and kidney the synthesis of the metallothioneins, a group of amino acids that have been shown to scavenge free radicals and bind some oxidants. Therefore, zinc deprivation results in an increased sensitivity to oxidative stress.

Zinc absorption occurs throughout the length of the small intestine, the majority of zinc uptake occurring in the jejunum and depending on lipids absorption.

Low zinc concentrations have been described after gastric restrictive procedures by reason of a reduced intake.

Since zinc absorption depends on fat absorption, low zinc concentrations are observed in patients submitted to RYGBP and BPD.

Vanderhoof showed no differences in either hair or serum zinc levels between 14 patients submitted to BPD 12–56 months earlier and 11 obese patients [63].

Madan found abnormal levels of zinc in 36 % of 33 patients 1 year after RYGBP [42].

After BPD with or without the duodenal switch, zinc deficiency was demonstrated in 10.8 % of patients, despite the fact that more than 80 % took correct supplementation [22]. Slater showed a zinc deficiency in half of 170 patients 4 years after BPD-DS [54].

Despite these findings, clinical consequences of zinc deficiency, such as alopecia epithelial eruption, glossitis, nail dystrophy, and immune deficiencies are seldom reported.

Indeed the transient hair loss, very often occurring a few months after bariatric surgery, has a controversial pathogenesis (including the “stress of weight loss,” or iron or protein sparing), and is not always is imputable to zinc deficiency [64].

One study reported resolution of alopecia after supplementation with zinc sulfate in patients submitted to VBG [65].

In case of deficiency, the treatment consists of oral zinc sulfate (220 mg/day).

27.7.2.8 Other Fat-Soluble Vitamins

Vitamin A

Vitamin A complex is a family of essential fat-soluble compounds, formed by carotenoids, retinols, and β-carotenes, required for cell proliferation and differentiation, growth, reproduction, and vision. The normal human liver generally stores a quantity, sufficient for 1 year of vitamin A requirement.

Common manifestations of vitamin A deficiency are night blindness, conjunctival xerosis, keratitis, corneal scarring, possibly leading to blindness, dry skin, dry hair, and pruritus. Other uncommon symptoms are decreased visual acuity and reduced resistance to infections.

Ledoux showed a prevalence of vitamin A deficiency of 25.5 % in the ASGB group compared with 52.5 % in the RYGBP group ($P<0.01$) in one study [66].

Brolin reported a deficiency in 10 % of patients, 4 years after distal RYGBP, in spite of vitamin A correct supplementation [33].

Several studies showed vitamin A deficiency manifestations after BPD [67–69].

Dolan demonstrated low levels of vitamin A (<1.6 μmol/L) in 61 % of patients submitted to BPD with or without duodenal switch at a mean 28 months follow-up, despite an 80 % compliance rate with multivitamin supplementation [22].

An incidence of vitamin A deficiency of 69 % 4 years after BPD-DS, with a progressive increase in the incidence and severity of hypovitaminemia was reported in another study [54].

Marceau showed a deficiency of vitamin A in 12 % of 233 patients 8 years after standard-BPD, and in 5 % of 457 patients 4 years after BPD-DS despite a prophylactic supplementation [4].

A daily supplementation of 10,000 IU of vitamin A is recommended.

In case of deficiency oral replacement with vitamin A, 10,000 UI/day normalizes the visual acuity within few months.

Vitamin E

Vitamin E is a collective name for all tocol and tocotrienol molecules, which have the activity of α-tocopherol. This vitamin has antioxidant properties, preventing the propagation of free radical damage within the cell membranes. Vitamin E deficiency should be considered, particularly following malabsorptive operations, in patients with hemolytic anemia, pigmented retinopathy, hypo or areflexia, ataxia, and skeletal myopathy.

Ledoux found a prevalence of vitamin E deficiency of 11.8 % in the ASGB group compared with 22.5 % in the RYGBP group ($P<0.05$) [66].

Dolan demonstrated low levels of vitamin E (<7 μmol/L), only in 5 % of patients, the majority taking supplements, at an average of 28 months after BPD [22].

Another study showed an incidence of 4 % of vitamin E deficiency not increasing at 1 and 4 years after BPD-DS in patients taking vitamin supplements [54].

Vitamin E deficiency is not common, and has not been shown to be clinically significant in patients following supplementation protocol [70].

If demonstrated, the treatment of vitamin E deficiency consists of oral vitamin E 800–1,200 IU a day.

Vitamin K

Vitamin K includes a cluster of compounds, all containing 2-methyl-1,4-naphthoquinone nucleus, involved in the formation of the seven vitamin K-dependent coagulation proteins (prothrombin, factors VII, IX, and X, protein C, Z, and S), all fundamentals for blood clotting. The vitamin has a widespread distribution, in plants and animal tissues, and the intestinal flora of the normal gut contributes to most of the daily requirements. The total body pool of vitamin K is surprisingly small and the turnover rapid. Its deficiency can entail abnormalities of coagulation and increased bleeding tendency.

Dolan compared the BPD with and without the duodenal switch and showed that half of his patients were deficient in vitamin K, with no significant differences between the two operations [22].

An incidence of vitamin K deficiency (<0.3 nmol/L) in 68 % of patients, with a progressive increase in the incidence and severity with time after BPD, was found in another study [54].

Table 27.3 Recommended follow-up of the operated patient

	1 month	3 months	6 months	12 months	24 months	Annually
Chemistry panel	All operations	All operations	All operations	All operations	All operations	All operations
Blood count	All operations	All operations	All operations	All operations	All operations	All operations
Vitamin B1	All operations (persistent vomiting)	All operations (persistent vomiting)	RYGBP, BPD	RYGBP, BPD	RYGBP, BPD	RYGBP, BPD
Vitamin B12	–	–	RYGBP, BPD	All operations	All operations	All operations
Folic acid	All operations	–	RYGBP, BPD	RYGBP, BPD	–	–
Vitamin A	–	–	RYGBP, BPD	RYGBP, BPD	RYGBP, BPD	RYGBP, BPD
Vitamin D	–	RYGBP, BPD	RYGBP, BPD	RYGBP, BPD	All operations	All operations
Vitamin E	–	–	–	Optional	Optional	Optional
Vitamin K	–	–	–	Optional	Optional	Optional
Iron	–	RYGBP, BPD	RYGBP, BPD	RYGBP, BPD	All operations	All operations
Selenium	–	–	–	RYGBP, BPD	Optional	Optional
Zinc	–	–	–	RYGBP, BPD	RYGBP, BPD	RYGBP, BPD
Parathyroid hormone	–	–	–	RYGBP, BPD	RYGBP, BPD	RYGBP, BPD
Bone density	–	–	–	RYGBP, BPD	RYGBP, BPD	RYGBP, BPD

In spite of this, clinical manifestations of vitamin K deficiency have seldom reported after bariatric surgery. Nevertheless, it is strongly suggested to regularly monitor serum fat-soluble vitamins before and after BPD.

A daily supplementation of 300 μg of vitamin K is recommended.

In case of vitamin K deficiency, the therapy consists of oral vitamin K 5–20 mg/day [13] (Table 27.3).

Conclusion

Modern bariatric surgery has a major role in the control of weight and of obesity-related comorbidities; it can be safely performed in selected patients, and decreases mortality rates in surgically treated obese patients. However, the majority of studies suggest a long-term pattern of nutritional and metabolic complications following bariatric surgery. The type of operation suggests which metabolic problem and deficiencies are to be expected, with malabsorptive procedures being most often implicated. The incidence of nutritional deficiencies is related to the amount of weight loss, presence of clinical symptoms suggesting complications and adherence to the suggested supplementation. Great attention should be paid to patients reaching extreme weight loss and to patients with frequent vomiting or poor food intake, even after SG or ASGB. Any deficiency can be prevented by a correct monitoring of operated patients and by an adequate nutritional supplementation strategy. Significant nutritional complications are uncommon and are, as a rule, easily corrected, on condition that a prompt diagnosis and an adequate therapy are performed by a multidisciplinary team. Even if experts have recently developed and compiled practical recommendations and a few clinical guidelines, the long-term nutritional outcome data are presently poor, and consensus is still lacking on many critical issues. Further randomized prospective trials are needed to develop more appropriate guidelines for follow-up and supplementation of operated patients.

References

1. Favretti F, Cadiere GB, Segato G, et al. Laparoscopic placement of adjustable silicone gastric banding: early experience. Obes Surg. 1995;5:71–3.
2. MacLean L, Rhode BM, Forse RA. A gastroplasty that avoids stapling in continuity. Surgery. 1993;113:380–8.
3. Scopinaro N, Adami GF, Marinari GM, et al. Biliopancreatic diversion. World J Surg. 1998;22: 936–46.

4. Marceau P, Hould FS, Simard S, Lebel S, Bourque RA, Potvin M, Biron S. Biliopancreatic diversion with duodenal switch. World J Surg. 1998;22(9):947–54.
5. Griffen Jr WO, Young VL, Stevenson CC. A prospective comparison of gastric and jejunoileal bypass procedures for morbid obesity. Ann Surg. 1977;186(4):500–9.
6. Hamoui N, Kim K, Anthone G, et al. The significance of elevated levels of parathyroid hormone in patients with morbid obesity before and after bariatric surgery. Arch Surg. 2003;138(8):891–7.
7. Sanchez Hernandez J, Ybarra J, Gich I, et al. Effects of bariatric surgery on vitamin D status and secondary hyperparathyroidism: a prospective study. Obes Surg. 2005;15(10):1389–95.
8. Compston JE, Vedi S, Ledger JE, et al. Vitamin D status and bone histomorphometry in gross obesity. Am J Clin Nutr. 1981;34(11):2359–63.
9. Bell NH, Epstein S, Greene A, et al. Evidence for alteration of the vitamin D endocrine system in obese subjects. J Clin Invest. 1985;76(1):370–3.
10. Gasteyger C, Suter M, Gaillard RC, Giusti V. Nutritional deficiencies after Roux-en-Y gastric bypass for morbid obesity often cannot be prevented by standard multivitamin supplementation. Am J Clin Nutr. 2008;87:1128–33.
11. Allied Health Sciences Section Ad Hoc Nutrition Committee, Aills L, Blankenship J, et al. ASMBS Allied Health Nutritional Guidelines for the surgical weight loss patient. Surg Obes Relat Dis. 2008;4:S73–108.
12. Fried M, Hainer V, Basdevant A, Buchwald H, Deitel M, Finer N, et al. Interdisciplinary European guidelines on surgery of severe obesity. Int J Obes (Lond). 2007;31:569–77.
13. Pournaras DJ, le Roux CW. After bariatric surgery, what vitamins should be measured and what supplements should be given? Clin Endocrinol (Oxf). 2009;71(3):322–5.
14. Ukleja A, Stone RL. Medical and gastroenterologic management of the postbariatric surgery patient. J Clin Gastroenterol. 2004;38(4):312–21.
15. Faintuch J, Matsuda M, Cruz ME, et al. Severe protein–calorie malnutrition after bariatric procedures. Obes Surg. 2004;14(2):175–81.
16. Scopinaro N, Marinari GM, Camerini G, et al. Energy and nitrogen absorption after biliopancreatic diversion. Obes Surg. 2000;10:436–41.
17. Scopinaro N, Gianetta E, Adami GF, et al. Biliopancreatic diversion for obesity at eighteen years. Surgery. 1996;119:261–8.
18. Totte E, Hendrickx L, van Hee R. Biliopancreatic diversion for treatment of morbid obesity: experience in 180 consecutive cases. Obes Surg. 1999;9:161–5.
19. Marinari GM, Murelli F, Camerini G, et al. A 15-year evaluation of biliopancreatic diversion according to the Bariatric Analysis Reporting Outcome System (BAROS). Obes Surg. 2004;14:325–8.
20. Nanni G, Balduzzi GF, Capoluongo R, et al. Biliopancreatic diversion: clinical experience. Obes Surg. 1997;7:26–9.
21. Marceau S, Biron S, Lagace M, et al. Biliopancreatic diversion, with distal gastrectomy, 250 cm and 50 cm limbs: long-term results. Obes Surg. 1995;5:302–7.
22. Dolan K, Hatzifotis M, Newbury L, et al. A clinical and nutritional comparison of biliopancreatic diversion with and without duodenal switch. Ann Surg. 2004;240:51–6.
23. Rabkin RA, Rabkin JM, Metcalf B, et al. Nutritional markers following duodenal switch for morbid obesity. Obes Surg. 2004;14:84–90.
24. Byrne TK. Complications of surgery for obesity. Surg Clin North Am. 2001;81:1181–93.
25. Brolin RE, LaMarca LB, Kenler HA, et al. Malabsorptive gastric bypass in patients with superobesity. J Gastrointest Surg. 2002;6:195–203.
26. Kalfarentzos F, Dimakopoulos A, Kehagias I, et al. Vertical banded gastroplasty versus standard or distal Roux-en-Y gastric bypass based on specific selection criteria in the morbidly obese: preliminary results. Obes Surg. 1999;9:433–42.
27. Skroubis G, Sakellaropoulos G, Pouggouras K, et al. Comparison of nutritional deficiencies after Roux-en-Y gastric bypass and after biliopancreatic diversion with Roux-en-Y gastric bypass. Obes Surg. 2002;12:551–8.
28. Himpens J, Dapri G, Cadière GB. A prospective randomized study between laparoscopic gastric banding and laparoscopic isolated sleeve gastrectomy: results after 1 and 3 years. Obes Surg. 2006;16:1450–6.
29. Saif T, Strain GW, Dakin G, Gagner M, Costa R, Pomp A. Evaluation of nutrient status after laparoscopic sleeve gastrectomy 1, 3, and 5 years after surgery. Surg Obes Relat Dis. 2012;8(5):542.
30. Gehrer S, Kern B, Peters T, Christoffer-Courtin C, Petersli R. Fewer nutrient deficiencies after laparoscopic sleeve gastrectomy (LSG) than after laparoscopic Roux-en-Y gastric bypass (LRYGB). Obes Surg. 2010;20:447–53.
31. Hakeam HA, O'Regan PJ, Salem AM, Bamchriz FY, Eldali AM. Impact of laparoscopic sleeve gastrectomy on iron indices: 1 year follow up. Obes Surg. 2009;19:1491–6.
32. Brolin RE, Leung M. Survey of vitamin and mineral supplementation after gastric bypass and biliopancreatic diversion for morbid obesity. Obes Surg. 1999;9:150–4.
33. Brolin RE, Gorman RC, Milgrim LM, Kenler HA. Multivitamin prophylaxis in prevention of postgastric bypass vitamin and mineral deficiencies. Int J Obes. 1991;15:661–7.
34. Chang CG, Adams-Huet B, Provost DA. Acute postgastric reduction surgery (APGARS) neuropathy. Obes Surg. 2004;14:182–9.
35. Chaves L, Faintuch J, Kahwage S, et al. A cluster of polyneuropathy and Wernicke–Korsakoff syndrome in a bariatric unit. Obes Surg. 2002;12:328–34. [43] Sola E, Morillas C, Garzon S, et al. Rapid onset of Wernicke's encephalopathy following gastric restrictive surgery. Obes Surg. 2003;13:661–2.
36. Aarts EO, Janssen IMC, Berends FJ. The gastric sleeve: losing weight as fast as micronutrients? Obes Surg. 2011;21:207–11.

37. Clements RH, Katasani VG, Palepu R, Leeth RR, Leath TD, et al. Incidence of vitamin deficiency after laparoscopic Roux-en-Y gastric bypass in a university hospital setting. Am Surg. 2006;72:1196–202.
38. Primavera A, Brusa G, Novello P, et al. Wernicke–Korsakoff encephalopathy following biliopancreatic diversion. Obes Surg. 1993;3:175–7.
39. Gasteyger C, Suter M, Calmes JM, Gaillard RC, Giusti V. Changes in body composition, metabolic profile, and nutritional status 24 months after gastric banding. Obes Surg. 2006;16:243–50.
40. Brolin RE. Gastric bypass. Surg Clin North Am. 2001;81:1077–95.
41. Halverson JD. Micronutrient deficiencies after gastric bypass for morbid obesity. Am Surg. 1986;52:594–8.
42. Madan AK, Orth WS, Tichansky DS, et al. Vitamin and trace mineral levels after laparoscopic gastric bypass. Obes Surg. 2006;16:603–6.
43. Marcuard SP, Sinar DR, Swanson MS, et al. Absence of luminal intrinsic factor after gastric bypass surgery for morbid obesity. Dig Dis Sci. 1989;34:1238–42.
44. Ocon Breton J, Perez Naranjo S, Gimeno Laborda S, Benito Ruesca P, Garcia Hernandez R. Effectiveness and complications of bariatric surgery in the treatment of morbid obesity. Nutr Hosp. 2005;20:409–14.
45. Ziegler SO, Sirveaux MA, Brunauda L, Reibel N, Quilliot D. Medical follow up after bariatric surgery: nutritional and drug issues general recommendations for the prevention and treatment of nutritional deficiencies. Diabetes Metab. 2009;35:544–57.
46. Aasheim ET, Johnson LK, Hofso D, Bohmer T, Hjelmesaeth J. Vitamin status after gastric bypass and lifestyle intervention: a comparative prospective study. Surg Obes Relat Dis. 2012;8:169–75. [50] Rhode BM, Arseneau P, Cooper BA, Katz M, Gilfix BM, MacLean LD. Vitamin B-12 deficiency after gastric surgery for obesity. Am J Clin Nutr. 1996;63:103–9.
47. Buffington CK, Walker B, Cowan GS, et al. Vitamin D deficiency in the morbidly obese. Obes Surg. 1993;3:421–4.
48. Hamoui N, Anthone G, Crookes PF. Calcium metabolism in the morbidly obese. Obes Surg. 2004;14:9–12.
49. Lin E, Armstrong-Moore D, Liang Z, Sweeney JF, Torres WE, et al. Contribution of adipose tissue to plasma 25-hydroxyvitamin D concentrations during weight loss following gastric bypass surgery. Obesity. 2011;19:588–94.
50. Mechanick JI, Kushner RF, Sugerman HJ, Gonzalez-Campoy JM, Collazo-Clavell ML, Spitz AF, et al. American Association of Clinical Endocrinologists, The Obesity Society, and American Society for Metabolic & Bariatric Surgery medical guidelines for clinical practice for the perioperative nutritional, metabolic, and nonsurgical support of the bariatric surgery patient. Obesity. 2009;17:1–70.
51. Jin J, Stellato TA, Hallowell PT, Schuster M, Graf K, Wilhelm S. Utilization of preoperative patient factors to predict postoperative vitamin D deficiency for patients undergoing gastric bypass. J Gastrointest Surg. 2009;13:1052–7.
52. Johnson JM, Maher JW, Demaria EJ, et al. The long-term effects of gastric bypass on vitamin D metabolism. Ann Surg. 2006;243(5):701–4.
53. Compston JE, Vedi S, Gianetta E, Watson G, Civalleri D, Scopinaro N. Bone histomorphometry and vitamin D status after biliopancreatic bypass for obesity. Gastroenterology. 1984;87:350–6.
54. Slater GH, Ren CJ, Siegel N, et al. Serum fat-soluble vitamin deficiency and abnormal calcium metabolism after malabsorptive bariatric surgery. J Gastrointest Surg. 2004;8:48–55.
55. Newbury L, Dolan K, Hatzifotis M, et al. Calcium and vitamin D depletion and elevated parathyroid hormone following biliopancreatic diversion. Obes Surg. 2003;13:893–5.
56. Larrad Jimenez A, Sanchez Cabezudo C, de Quadros Borrajo PP, et al. Course of metabolic syndrome following the biliopancreatic diversion of Larrad. Obes Surg. 2004;14:1176–81.
57. Marceau Marceau P, Biron S, Lebel S, et al. Does bone change after biliopancreatic diversion? J Gastrointest Surg. 2002;6:690–8.
58. Viegas M, Vasconcelos RS, Neves AP, Diniz ET, Bandeira F. Bariatric surgery and bone metabolism: a systematic review. Arq Bras Endocrinol Metabol. 2010;54:158–63.
59. Holick MF. The vitamin D epidemic and its health consequences. J Nutr. 2005;135:2739S–48.
60. Manco M, Nanni G, Tondolo V, et al. Hypocalcemia complicating near-total thyroidectomy in patients with coexisting lipid malabsorption due to biliopancreatic diversion. Obes Surg. 2004;14:1429–34.
61. Rojas-Marcos PM, Rubio MA, Kreskshi WI, et al. Severe hypocalcemia following total thyroidectomy after biliopancreatic diversion. Obes Surg. 2005;15:431–4.
62. Freeth A, Prajuabpansri P, et al. Assessment of selenium in Roux-en-Y gastric bypass and gastric banding surgery. Obes Surg. 2012;22(11):1660–5.
63. Vanderhoof JA, Scopinaro N, Tuma DJ, Gianetta E, Civalleri D, Antonson DL. Hair and plasma zinc levels following exclusion of biliopancreatic secretions from functioning gastrointestinal tract in humans. Dig Dis Sci. 1983;28:300–5.
64. Fujioka K. Follow up of nutritional and metabolic problems after bariatric surgery. Diabetes Care. 2005; 28:481–4.

65. Neve HJ, Bhatti WA, Soulsby C, Kincey J, Taylor TV. Reversal of hair loss following vertical gastroplasty when treated with zinc sulfate. Obes Surg. 1996;6: 63–5.
66. Ledoux S, Msika S, Moussa F, et al. Comparison of nutritional consequences of conventional therapy of obesity, adjustable gastric banding, and gastric bypass. Obes Surg. 2006;16:1041–9.
67. Spits Y, De Laey JJ, Leroy BP. Rapid recovery of night blindness due to obesity surgery after vitamin A repletion therapy. Br J Ophthalmol. 2004;88:583–5.
68. Hatizifotis M, Dolan K, Newbury L, Fielding G. Symptomatic vitamin A deficiency following biliopancreatic diversion. Obes Surg. 2003;13:655–7.
69. Quaranta L, Nascimbeni G, Semeraro F, Quaranta CA. Severe corneo conjunctival xerosis after biliopancreatic bypass for obesity (Scopinaro's operation). Am J Ophthalmol. 1994;118:817–8.
70. Vazquez C, Morejon E, Munoz C, et al. Nutritional effect of bariatric surgery with Scopinaro operation. Analysis of 40 cases. Nutr Hosp. 2003;18: 189–93.

Long-Term Follow-Up After Bariatric Surgery

28

Konstantinos Spaniolas and Walter J. Pories

28.1 The Birth of Metabolic Surgery

Bariatric surgery was initially devised as the surgical means for weight loss in patients whose weight was deemed extremely abnormal. Since that time, the obesity epidemic has lead to continuously increasing the numbers of severely obese people, with more than a third of the western population being obese. Since the birth of bariatric surgery in the middle of the previous century, more bariatric procedures are being performed over time. Even though weight loss was the primary focus of this field early on, alterations in metabolism were commonly seen, and attributed to malabsorption associated with intestinal bypasses [1, 2]. Over time, the metabolic and hormonal effects associated with bariatric procedures have led to the transformation of the field and the birth of metabolic surgery.

28.2 Weight Loss

The weight-loss effects of bariatric surgery have been well established. The Swedish Obese Subjects (SOS) study prospectively followed 2,010 patients undergoing bariatric surgery, and compared them with 2,037 matched controls who underwent medical management of obesity [3]. Even though the majority of patients underwent a bariatric procedure that has been subsequently found to be suboptimal and abandoned, long-term follow-up results are available up to 20 years after intervention. With a median follow-up of 15 years and a baseline BMI of 42, the mean weight loss was 18 % of baseline. The weight-loss curves for all procedures demonstrate a common pattern: dramatic loss during the first year, followed by minimal gradual weight regain for the subsequent few years until plateau.

In order to address the low percentage of Roux-en-Y gastric bypass (RYGB) in the SOS study and complement its results, the Longitudinal Assessment of Bariatric Surgery (LABS) study was designed as a prospective nonrandomized study at six clinical centers in the United States. This is one of the few high-volume cohorts on bariatric patients undergoing currently accepted weight-loss procedures. Reports from the 3-year follow-up of 1,738 patients who underwent RYGB and 610 adjustable gastric banding (AGB), demonstrate median weight loss at 31.5 and 15.9 % of baseline for the two groups, respectively [4].

K. Spaniolas • W.J. Pories (✉)
Department of Surgery, Brody School of Medicine, East Carolina University, 600 Moye Boulevard, Greenville, NC 27858, USA
e-mail: SpaniolasK@ecu.edu; PoriesW@ecu.edu

M. Lucchese, N. Scopinaro (eds.), *Minimally Invasive Bariatric and Metabolic Surgery: Principles and Technical Aspects*, DOI 10.1007/978-3-319-15356-8_28,

Table 28.1 Long-term weight loss with bariatric surgery

Study	Procedure/ sample size	Design	BMI	Follow up (years)	Weight loss
SOS [3]	AGB: 376 VBG: 1,369 RYGB: 265	Prospective, matched, nonrandomized	42.4	14.7	18 % of baseline weight
LABS [4]	RYGB: 1,738 AGB: 610	Prospective, nonrandomized	46	3	RYGB: 31.5 % of baseline AGB: 15.9 % of baseline
Buchwald meta-analysis [5]	RYGB: 7,074 AGB: 3,873 VBG: 1,568 DS: 4,035	Meta-analysis	46.9	Variable	61.2 % EBWL (AGB 47.5 %, RYGB 61.6 %, VBG 68.2 %, DS 70.1 %)
Utah Obesity Study [6]	RYGB: 418	Retrospective	45.9	6	27.7 % of baseline weight
East Carolina University [7]	RYGB: 608	Retrospective	49.7	7.6 years: 317 at 5 years 158 at 10 years 10 at 14 years	32.5 % of baseline weight at 5-years 32.3 % at 10-years

AGB adjustable gastric banding, *VBG* vertical band gastroplasty, *RYGB* Roux-en-Y gastric bypass, *DS* duodenal switch, *BMI* body mass index, *EBWL* excess body weight loss

Table 28.1 lists long-term weight-loss results with multiple bariatric procedures, based on multiple studies with different research methodologies.

28.3 Diabetes

Diabetes remission as a concept became a focus of interest as a result of outcomes with bariatric surgery. Since this is a chronic condition, and long-term data are lacking, "cure" as a term is seldom used. Normalization of blood glucose and HgA1c in the absence of antiglycemic medications defines remission. This has been historically a rare occurrence with medical therapy, but bariatric surgery has led to the International Diabetes Federation suggesting surgical therapy as a valid option for the treatment of diabetes.

A recent meta-analysis of 19 different studies revealed that bariatric surgery overall is associated with a 0.33 risk reduction for the presence of type 2 diabetes postoperatively [8]. As multiple single-institution studies have previously shown (Table 28.2), this meta-analysis again underlines a significant difference in risk reduction between RYGB/biliopancreatic diversion (BPD) and AGB (0.26 vs 0.44, $p<0.0001$). A few recent randomized controlled trials have assessed the effect of bariatric surgery on diabetes control and have provided high quality data in this topic. The first one evaluated 150 obese (BMI > 27) patients with poorly controlled diabetes [9]. Patients were randomized to intense medical therapy, consisting of lifestyle counseling, weight management programs, incretin analogs, and frequent visits with an endocrinologist, vs bariatric surgery, and the purpose of the study was to achieve diabetes control. Diabetes control (12 % vs 42 % vs 37 %) and remission (0 vs 42 % vs 27 %) at 12-months after surgery were significantly more common in the bariatric surgery groups than medical treatment. A similar study from Italy on 60 severely obese patients with poorly controlled diabetes, randomized patients to intense medical therapy vs RYGB vs BPD [10]. Diabetic remission at 48 months after surgery was significantly higher after RYGB (75 %) and BPD (95 %) compared to medical treatment (nil). The intensity of medical therapy is illustrated on the fact that it led to an 8 % decrease in BMI and discontinuation of antihypertensive medications in 70 % of the group.

The effect of bariatric surgery on diabetes is not only about remission, but also about preventing its development in the severely obese. In the SOS study, the adjusted odds ratio for new-onset diabetes was 0.25 in the surgery group compared to the medically treated group [18]. The prevalence at 10 years after surgery was 5–10 %. In

Table 28.2 The effect of bariatric surgery on diabetes remission and improvement during follow-up

Study	Procedure/ sample size	Design	BMI	Follow-up (years)	Diabetes
LABS [4]	RYGB: 1,738 (320 diabetics) AGB: 610 (98 diabetics)	Prospective, nonrandomized	46	3	RYGB: 67 % partial remission AGB: 28.6 % partial remission
SOS [11]	AGB: 376 VBG: 1,369 RYGB: 265 (323 diabetics)	Prospective, matched, nonrandomized	42.4	2 10	72 % 36 %
Buchwald meta-analysis [5]	RYGB: 7,074 AGB: 3,873 VBG: 1,568 DS: 4,035 (2,331 diabetics)	Meta-analysis	46.9	Variable	76.8 % remission (AGB 47.9 %, RYGB 83.7 %, VBG 71.6 %, DS 98.9 %) 85.4 % improvement
Utah Obesity Study [6]	RYGB: 418 (93 diabetics)	Retrospective	45.9	6	62 % remission
East Carolina University [7]	RYGB: 608 (165 diabetics, 165 IFG)	Retrospective	49.7	Variable (–14)	82.9 % remission 99 % normalization of IFG
Virginia Commonwealth University [12]	RYGB: 1,025 (154 diabetics)	Retrospective	51	Variable (91 % 2)	83 % resolution
Fresno, CA [13]	RYGB: 242 (45 diabetics)	Retrospective	NR	Variable (51 at 10)	83 % resolution or improvement at 2 years 67 % at 10 years
University of Pittsburgh [14]	RYGB: 191 (177 diabetics, 14 IFG)	Retrospective	50.1	20 months	83 % remission 17 % improvement
San Diego, CA [15]	RYGB: 500 (85 diabetics)	Retrospective	NR	Variable	97 % resolution
University of Oslo [16]	RYGB: 184 (49 diabetics)	Retrospective	46	5	67 % remission 20 % improvement
Cleveland Clinic [9]	RYGB: 50 SG: 41 (all diabetic)	Randomized controlled	36	1	42 % remission for RYGB 27 % remission for SG (no statistical difference between the groups)
Università Cattolica del Sacro Cuore [10]	RYGB: 19 BPD: 19 (all diabetic)	Randomized controlled	45	2	75 % remission for RYGB 95 % remission for BPD
Monash University Medical School [17]	AGB: 30 (all diabetic)	Randomized controlled	37	2	73 % remission with AGB vs 13 % for medical therapy

AGB adjustable gastric banding, *VBG* vertical band gastroplasty, *RYGB* Roux-en-Y gastric bypass, *DS* duodenal switch, *BMI* body mass index, *IFG* impaired fasting glucose, *NR* nonreported

comparison, the Framingham Study addressed the question of the effect of medical weight loss on diabetes prevention [19]. Overweight patients (total 618) who lost at least 1 lb/year were compared to patients with weight regain and ones with weight stable in this time period. Adjusting for years of follow-up, diabetes at the weight-stable patients occurred in 8.1 per 1,000 person-years; sustained weight loss led to a 37 % lower risk of diabetes development (relative risk 0.63). Similarly, the Diabetes Prevention Program study randomized over 3,000 overweight and obese (mean BMI of 34) patients with pre-diabetes to intense lifestyle changes vs metformin vs placebo [20]. The incidence of diabetes in this high-risk group at 10 years was 40 %. Lifestyle modification (including low-caloric low-fat diet, moderate physical activity, and one-to-one educational sessions) was associated with a significant decrease in the prevalence of diabetes (OR 0.42), but less to what is achieved with bariatric surgery.

28.4 Hypertension

The effect of bariatric surgery on hypertension is variable, but all studies universally demonstrate improvement after surgery. In a comparison analysis of 418 patients undergoing RYGB, hypertension remission was reported in 53 % of the 169 hypertensive patients at 2 years after bariatric surgery, and 42 % at 6 years [6]. Using meta-analytic methods on almost 7,000 bariatric patients, hypertension resolved postoperatively in 65.6 % and improved in 81.8 % [5]. There was a significant difference between the stapling procedures (RYGB and DS) and AGB, with almost a twofold difference in the rate of hypertension remission after intervention. A more recent analysis reported similar findings with 0.52 risk reduction for hypertension after bariatric surgery [8]. Similarly, another meta-analysis with a total of 243 randomized bariatric patients and almost 17,000 observed nonrandomized patients found hypertension improvement or resolution in 75 and 74 %, respectively [21].

Prospective long-term data on remission of hypertension show a less pronounced impact compared to diabetes. In the 3-year follow-up of the LABS study, 38.2 and 17.4 % of the patients who underwent RYGB and AGB, respectively, had remission of hypertension [4]. The SOS study showed that at 2 years after bariatric surgery (mostly VBG), hypertension resolution occurred in 34 % of the patients, while this number dropped to 19 % at 10 years. Given the established relationship between advancing age and the prevalence of hypertension, this drop in hypertension resolution at 10 years after intervention should not be viewed as failure of bariatric surgery to control this comorbidity, but rather as an evolution of the nature process of aging.

28.5 Dyslipidemia

Abnormalities in lipids, lipoproteins, and triglycerides are common. They are a substantial contributor to the metabolic syndrome and represent a major risk factor for cardiovascular disease in diabetic and nondiabetic patients. Metabolic surgery allows for improvement in the lipid profiles in the majority of patients. In a large meta-analysis from 2004, improvements in hypertriglyceridemia, hypercholesterolemia, and hyperlipidemia occurred in 92.8 % (912 of 983), 86.6 % (1,777 of 2,051), and 83 % (846 of 1,019), respectively [5]. These numbers for RYGB and DS exceeded 90 % for all measures. A more recent meta-analysis evaluating overall cardiovascular risk reduction after surgery, reported a hyperlipidemia risk reduction of 0.39 for patients undergoing bariatric surgery; RYGB and BPD were associated with a risk reduction of 0.26 [8]. A second recent review of 25 bariatric studies reporting on lipid outcomes found resolution or improvement of dyslipidemia in 76 % of patients participating in a bariatric surgery randomized control trial and 68 % of patients included in observational studies [21].

Long-term assessment of lipid profiles after RYGB demonstrates sustained improvement in dyslipidemia with surgery [6]. Normalization for HDL, LDL, and triglycerides 6 years after RYGB was seen in 67, 53, and 71 % of patients, respectively. Again, there were minimal differences in these rates from year 2 to year 6 after RYGB. Recent data from the LABS study shows that at 3 years from RYGB, the majority of patients normalize their LDL (59.7 %), HDL (85.6 %), and triglycerides (85.8 %). Improvements to a lesser degree were also seen after AGB (22.7, 67.3, and 62.1 %, respectively) [4]. Long-term data are also available from the SOS study [11]. Normalization of LDL, HDL, and triglycerides 10 years after bariatric surgery were found in 21, 73, and 46 % of patients, respectively. Interestingly, there were no significant differences in the rates of resolution for HDL and LDL abnormalities between year 2 and year 10 after surgical intervention, suggesting that the benefit with bariatric surgery is seen early and is long lasting.

28.6 Obstructive Sleep Apnea

There is a strong association between obesity and the development of obstructive sleep apnea. The crowded posterior oropharynx in the severely obese leads to obstructive sleep apnea in up to 70 % of this patient population. This leads to fatigue and poor quality of life (QOL). There seems to be a profound improvement in symptomatology with bariatric surgery, which appears to be mediated directly by weight loss. A meta-analysis from 2,004 included 1,921 patients with obstructive sleep apnea who underwent bariatric surgery [5]. Resolution and improvement of symptoms were reported in over 80 % of this subgroup of patients. In a similar meta-analysis with a total of 44 patients who participated in a randomized trial and 9,845 patients included in an observational study, sleep apnea improvement or resolution was reported in 96 and 90 %, respectively [21].

28.7 Cardiovascular Risk

With long-lasting improvements in dyslipidemia, diabetes, and hypertension, the cardiovascular risk of severely obese individuals is also expected to be reduced after bariatric surgery. A single-institution study of 184 patients with a 5-year follow-up after RYGB, reported on 112 patients who met criteria for the metabolic syndrome pre-operatively [16]. At the end of the follow-up period, 67 % of these patients were relieved of the metabolic syndrome. In this same cohort, the Framingham risk score significantly decreased with RYGB, representing an absolute risk reduction of 1 % and a relative risk reduction of 18.3 %. Furthermore, the SOS study, with a median follow-up of 14.7 years, has demonstrated that bariatric surgery is associated with a significantly lower incidence of cardiovascular events and cardiovascular-specific deaths [3].

28.8 Cancer Risk and Overall Survival

Large epidemiologic studies have illustrated that obesity is associated with higher mortality. The first study to suggest a survival benefit with bariatric surgery retrospectively compared 154 patients who underwent RYGB with 78 patients who were evaluated for bariatric surgery but were denied for surgery by their insurance company [22]. With a mean follow-up of 9 years in the surgical group and 6.2 years in the controls, all-cause mortality was 9 % vs 28 %. In a large comparison of almost 10,000 patients who underwent bariatric surgery with a cohort of nonsurgically treated severely obese patients [23] with a mean follow-up of 7.1 years, there was a 40 % decrease in overall adjusted mortality in bariatric surgery patients. Cause-specific mortality for diabetes and cardiac disease decreased by 92 and 56 %, respectively. Interestingly, cancer-specific mortality decreased by 60 %. The SOS study verified the survival benefit with bariatric surgery in a large prospective cohort [24]. With a mean follow-up of 10.9 years for over 4,000 obese patients (split between surgery and medical management of obesity), the adjusted for age, gender, and comorbidities hazard ratio was 0.71 for bariatric surgery. The most common causes of death were cardiac events and cancer. Both of these studies surprisingly illustrated a benefit in terms of cancer for bariatric surgery patients.

In a follow-up analysis of the SOS study, a significant reduction in cancer incidence was seen with bariatric surgery [25]. The overall cancer incidence in the surgery group decreased with an odds ratio of 0.67. With subgroup analysis, this effect was significant for female patients, and was independent of weight loss. Similarly, using data from the Utah Cancer Registry, cancer incidence was assessed with a mean follow-up of 12.5 years in a bariatric surgery cohort [26]. Cancer incidence and cancer-specific mortality were significantly decreased in the bariatric surgery group (hazard ratio 0.75 and 0.54, respectively). Another observational study compared 1,035 bariatric surgery patients with a control group matched for age and gender [27]. Cancer-related office and hospital visits were significantly lower in the bariatric surgery group (relative risk 0.22) over a 5-year follow-up. Even though multiple theories exist to explain this effect, there have been no definitive studies to date to support the mechanism behind it.

28.9 Quality of Life

Severely obese individuals have severe impairments in QOL, and any modality to treat obesity warrants evaluation in this regard. Multiple studies have shown improvement in QOL after bariatric surgery. Fifty one patients after RYGB completed a bariatric-specific QOL questionnaire, which incorporates self-esteem and activity of daily living, among objective changes in medical conditions, and only seven (14 %) were deemed as failures [13]. In a recent study from Norway, 177 patients 5 years after RYGB completed QOL questionnaires [16]. Significant improvements were seen in all categories of a generic questionnaire after RYGB. Using an obesity-specific questionnaire, there were significant benefits at 5 years, with marked improvements in the psychosocial functioning of these patients. Preoperatively, 74 % of patients had severe psychosocial impairment, compared to 12 % of patients 5 years after bariatric surgery.

Furthermore, physical capacity is improved even as early as 3 months after bariatric surgery. In a study of 67 patients with a mean preoperative BMI of 51, significant improvements were seen in objective measurements of walking, transfer capacity, and functional independence in activities of daily living [28].

The SOS study demonstrated, using a series of generic, obesity, and comorbidity-specific questionnaires, that improvements in QOL were associated with the grade of weight loss [29]. Peak improvements in patients after bariatric surgery were seen during the first postoperative year, followed by small gradual decline the subsequent 5 years, and stability thereafter for the remaining 10-year follow-up period. Compared with the medically managed group, bariatric surgery at 10 years was associated with a significant improvement in QOL, health perception, social interaction, psychosocial functioning, and depression.

28.10 Malnutrition and Vitamin Deficiencies

The detrimental nutritional effects of the jejunoileal bypass in the 1960s and 1970s led to many patients developing liver or kidney failure, with subsequent mortality or need for transplantation or reversal. Bariatric surgeons have since learned the risk of malnutrition, the dangers of extensive malabsorptive procedures and the necessity for nutrition assessment and supplementation in all patients. The RYGB, which is the most common bariatric procedure performed at present, is not without malnutrition risks.

Most of the malnourished patients have no clinical symptoms but many bariatric patients report symptomatology suggestive of nutrient deficiencies. A study including 49 RYGB patients, reported clinical symptoms of malnutrition in 59 %; hair loss and/or dry skin in 39 %, paresthesias in 12 %, and myalgias in 16 % [30]. These symptoms were seen despite the lack of measured deficiencies in iron, ferritin, calcium, vitamin B1, vitamin B6, folate, vitamin B12, vitamin C, A, or E, suggesting the involvement of protein or mineral metabolism.

Protein deficiencies have been mostly reported with long distal bypasses. In RYGB, protein deficits are infrequent and are in part attributed to poor intake [31]. In a study of 236 banded-RYGB patients, severe malnutrition with hypoproteinemia was identified in 11 (4.7 %) [32]. Most of these patients experienced strictures requiring re-interventions or persistent emesis without abnormal endoscopic findings. It is noteworthy that cause-specific mortality was 2/11 (18 %). Reporting on 174 patients after bariatric surgery (79 RYGB and 95 BPD) patients, Skroubis et al. found only three patients with hypoalbuminemia over 3 years for an incidence of 1.72 % [33]. In a large study of 824 patients who underwent BPD with 15-year follow-up, the reoperation rate – mostly for protein malnutrition – was 6.3 % [34]. The authors found that the reoperation rate was affected by the length of the alimentary limb.

Vitamin deficiencies – especially vitamin B12 – are commonly found after RYGB. It is difficult to know if this is related to inherent properties of the operations or poor compliance with prescribed supplementation after surgery. In a retrospective study of 136 patients after laparoscopic RYGB who had nutrition testing done, 66 % were found to have a nutritional deficiency [13]. Vitamin B12 deficiency was identified in 71 %, anemia in 39 %, abnormal vitamin B6 in

15 % and hypocalcemia in 14 % of the assessed patients. These abnormalities were evenly distributed throughout the 10-year postoperative follow-up, and more frequent in the superobese individuals. Another study of 170 patients with a 3-year follow-up after RYGB, found an increase in folic acid, vitamin B12, and iron at the end of follow-up, with 72.4 % of patients maintaining vitamin supplementation at 3 years [35]. Anemia was found in 6.5 % of patients preoperatively and 33.5 % of patients at 3 years; low folic acid level was found in 6.5 % of patients before surgery and only 0.6 % of patients at the end of follow-up. In a retrospective single-institution study of 75 RYGB patients with at-least 5 years follow-up, long-term vitamin deficiencies were common; 32.1 % had hypomagnesemia, 50.8 % anemia, 30 % low iron, 40.5 % low zinc, 61.8 % vitamin B12 deficiency and 60.5 % abnormal vitamin D3 levels [36]. It is noteworthy that only one third of the patients took their prescribed multivitamins daily. Hypoalbuminemia was only seen in 5.3 % of this patient population. Interestingly, the biochemical workup 2 years after bariatric surgery correlated with final excess weight loss. Fat-soluble vitamin (A, D, E, K) deficiencies are uncommon after RYGB, but can be frequency seen in BPD patients [37].

Mineral deficiencies are also not infrequent after bariatric surgery. In a cohort of 141 bariatric surgery patients (52 RYGB, 89 BPD), subclinical low copper levels were found in 50.6 % of the BPD patients and 3.8 % of the RYGB patients [38]. All but one of the BPD patients had at least one measurement of low zinc, and at different timepoints, the prevalence of hypozincemia ranged between 44.9 and 74.2 %. In the RYGB group, for the first 3 years after surgery, the prevalence of hypozincemia decreased compared to preoperative, but this increased over the following 2 years, reaching 21.2 % at 5 years after surgery. No symptoms developed due to low zinc values. Another retrospective study on 136 patients after RYGB found 9.6 % prevalence of copper deficiency [39]. Of those patients, hematologic abnormalities were seen in 61 %, fatigue in 38 % and neurologic symptoms in 38 %. When 16 patients were followed prospectively after RYGB, three developed zinc deficiency at 2 years for an incidence of 18.8 %.

Although routine vitamin supplementation is essential in the postoperative long-term care of the bariatric patient, this practice does not eliminate the risk of vitamin deficiencies. In a retrospective study with a 2-year follow-up of 137 RYGB patients undergoing routine supplementation with a standardized vitamin and mineral preparation, 59 % of patients at 6-months, 86 % at 12-months and 98 % at 24-months were receiving at least one additional supplement [40]. Vitamin B12 was the most frequent additional supplement (80 % at 2 years), followed by iron (60 %), calcium/vitamin D (60 %) and folic acid (45 %).

Conclusion

Metabolic surgery has progressed beyond a set of operations to induce weight loss. The four current operations also produce full and durable remission of the metabolic syndrome (severe obesity, hypertension, type 2 diabetes, and hyperlipidemia) in addition to a broad array of related co-morbidities such as sleep apnea, polycystic ovary disease, pseudotumor cerebri as well as those that are due to excessive weight such as arthritis of weight-bearing joints. Now that the operations can be done with the same low mortality and morbidity rates as routine cholecystectomy, metabolic surgery offers an effective, indeed the most effective, therapy for the most costly diseases of the developed world. The most important contribution of metabolic surgery, however, is that it provides new, safe, and ethical approaches to study obesity, diabetes, and the other expressions of the metabolic syndrome, research that eventually and hopefully, will provide approaches including prevention and medications to make surgery obsolete.

References

1. Shibata HR, MacKenzie JR, Long RC. Metabolic effects of controlled jejunocolic bypass. Arch Surg. 1967;95(3):413–28.
2. Scott Jr HW, Dean R, Shull HJ, Abram HS, Webb W, Younger RK, Brill AB. Considerations in use of jejunoileal bypass in patients with morbid obesity. Ann Surg. 1973;177(6):723–35.
3. Sjöström L, Peltonen M, Jacobson P, Sjöström CD, Karason K, Wedel H, Ahlin S, Anveden Å, Bengtsson C, Bergmark G, Bouchard C, Carlsson B, Dahlgren

S, Karlsson J, Lindroos AK, Lönroth H, Narbro K, Näslund I, Olbers T, Svensson PA, Carlsson LM. Bariatric surgery and long-term cardiovascular events. JAMA. 2012;307(1):56–65.
4. Courcoulas AP, Christian NJ, Belle SH, Berk PD, Flum DR, Garcia L, Horlick M, Kalarchian MA, King WC, Mitchell JE, Patterson EJ, Pender JR, Pomp A, Pories WJ, Thirlby RC, Yanovski SZ, Wolfe BM, Longitudinal Assessment of Bariatric Surgery (LABS) Consortium. Weight change and health outcomes at 3 years after bariatric surgery among individuals with severe obesity. JAMA. 2013;310(22):2416–25.
5. Buchwald H, Avidor Y, Braunwald E, Jensen MD, Pories W, Fahrbach K, Schoelles K. Bariatric surgery: a systematic review and meta-analysis. JAMA. 2004;292(14):1724–37.
6. Adams TD, Davidson LE, Litwin SE, Kolotkin RL, LaMonte MJ, Pendleton RC, Strong MB, Vinik R, Wanner NA, Hopkins PN, Gress RE, Walker JM, Cloward TV, Nuttall RT, Hammoud A, Greenwood JL, Crosby RD, McKinlay R, Simper SC, Smith SC, Hunt SC. Health benefits of gastric bypass surgery after 6 years. JAMA. 2012;308(11):1122–31.
7. Pories WJ, Swanson MS, MacDonald KG, Long SB, Morris PG, Brown BM, Barakat HA, de Ramon RA, Israel G, Dolezal JM, et al. Who would have thought it? An operation proves to be the most effective therapy for adult-onset diabetes mellitus. Ann Surg. 1995;222(3):339–50.
8. Ricci C, Gaeta M, Rausa E, Macchitella Y, Bonavina L. Early impact of bariatric surgery on type II diabetes, hypertension, and hyperlipidemia: a systematic review, meta-analysis, and meta-regression on 6,587 patients. Obes Surg. 2013;10.
9. Schauer PR, Kashyap SR, Wolski K, Brethauer SA, Kirwan JP, Pothier CE, Thomas S, Abood B, Nissen SE, Bhatt DL. Bariatric surgery versus intensive medical therapy in obese patients with diabetes. N Engl J Med. 2012;366(17):1567–76.
10. Mingrone G, Panunzi S, De Gaetano A, Guidone C, Iaconelli A, Leccesi L, Nanni G, Pomp A, Castagneto M, Ghirlanda G, Rubino F. Bariatric surgery versus conventional medical therapy for type 2 diabetes. N Engl J Med. 2012;366(17):1577–85.
11. Sjöström L, Lindroos AK, Peltonen M, Torgerson J, Bouchard C, Carlsson B, Dahlgren S, Larsson B, Narbro K, Sjöström CD, Sullivan M, Wedel H, Swedish Obese Subjects Study Scientific Group. Lifestyle, diabetes, and cardiovascular risk factors 10 years after bariatric surgery. N Engl J Med. 2004;351(26):2683–93.
12. Sugerman HJ, Wolfe LG, Sica DA, Clore JN. Diabetes and hypertension in severe obesity and effects of gastric bypass-induced weight loss. Ann Surg. 2003;237(6):751–6.
13. Higa K, Ho T, Tercero F, Yunus T, Boone KB. Laparoscopic Roux-en-Y gastric bypass: 10-year follow up. Surg Obes Relat Dis. 2011;7(4):516–25.
14. Schauer PR, Burguera B, Ikramuddin S, Cottam D, Gourash W, Hamad G, Eid GM, Mattar S, Ramanathan R, Barinas-Mitchel E, Rao RH, Kuller L, Kelley D. Effect of laparoscopic Roux-en-Y gastric bypass on type 2 diabetes mellitus. Ann Surg. 2003;238(4):467–84.
15. Wittgrove AC, Clark GW. Laparoscopic gastric bypass, Roux-en-Y- 500 patients: technique and results, with 3–60 month follow-up. Obes Surg. 2000;10(3):233–9.
16. Aftab H, Risstad H, Søvik TT, Tomm Bernklev PD, Hewitt S, Kristinsson JA, Mala T. Five-year outcome after gastric bypass for morbid obesity in a Norwegian cohort. Surg Obes Relat Dis. 2014;10:71–8.
17. Dixon JB, O'Brien PE, Playfair J, Chapman L, Schachter LM, Skinner S, Proietto J, Bailey M, Anderson M. Adjustable gastric banding and conventional therapy for type 2 diabetes: a randomized controlled trial. JAMA. 2008;299(3):316–23.
18. Sjöström L. Review of the key results from the Swedish Obese Subjects (SOS) trial – a prospective controlled intervention study of bariatric surgery. J Intern Med. 2013;273(3):219–34.
19. Moore LL, Visioni AJ, Wilson PW, D'Agostino RB, Finkle WD, Ellison RC. Can sustained weight loss in overweight individuals reduce the risk of diabetes mellitus? Epidemiology. 2000;11(3):269–73.
20. Diabetes Prevention Program Research Group, Knowler WC, Fowler SE, Hamman RF, Christophi CA, Hoffman HJ, Brenneman AT, Brown-Friday JO, Goldberg R, Venditti E, Nathan DM. 10-year follow up of diabetes incidence and weight loss in the Diabetes Prevention Program Outcomes Study. Lancet. 2009;374(9702):1677–86.
21. Chang SH, Stoll CR, Song J, Varela JE, Eagon CJ, Colditz GA. The effectiveness and risks of bariatric surgery: an updated systematic review and meta-analysis, 2003–2012. JAMA Surg. 2014;149:275–87.
22. MacDonald Jr KG, Long SD, Swanson MS, Brown BM, Morris P, Dohm GL, Pories WJ. The gastric bypass operation reduces the progression and mortality of noninsulin-dependent diabetes mellitus. J Gastrointest Surg. 1997;1(3):213–20.
23. Adams TD, Gress RE, Smith SC, Halverson RC, Simper SC, Rosamond WD, Lamonte MJ, Stroup AM, Hunt SC. Long-term mortality after gastric bypass surgery. N Engl J Med. 2007;357(8):753–61.
24. Sjöström L, Narbro K, Sjöström CD, Karason K, Larsson B, Wedel H, Lystig T, Sullivan M, Bouchard C, Carlsson B, Bengtsson C, Dahlgren S, Gummesson A, Jacobson P, Karlsson J, Lindroos AK, Lönroth H, Näslund I, Olbers T, Stenlöf K, Torgerson J, Agren G, Carlsson LM, Swedish Obese Subjects Study. Effects of bariatric surgery on mortality in Swedish obese subjects. N Engl J Med. 2007;357(8):741–52.
25. Sjöström L, Gummesson A, Sjöström CD, Narbro K, Peltonen M, Wedel H, Bengtsson C, Bouchard C, Carlsson B, Dahlgren S, Jacobson P, Karason K, Karlsson J, Larsson B, Lindroos AK, Lönroth H, Näslund I, Olbers T, Stenlöf K, Torgerson J, Carlsson LM, Swedish Obese Subjects Study. Effects of bariatric surgery on cancer incidence in obese patients

in Sweden (Swedish Obese Subjects Study): a prospective, controlled intervention trial. Lancet Oncol. 2009;10(7):653–62.
26. Adams TD, Stroup AM, Gress RE, Adams KF, Calle EE, Smith SC, Halverson RC, Simper SC, Hopkins PN, Hunt SC. Cancer incidence and mortality after gastric bypass surgery. Obesity (Silver Spring). 2009;17(4):796–802.
27. Christou NV, Lieberman M, Sampalis F, Sampalis JS. Bariatric surgery reduces cancer risk in morbidly obese patients. Surg Obes Relat Dis. 2008;4(6):691–5.
28. Vargas CB, Picolli F, Dani C, Padoin AV, Mottin CC. Functioning of obese individuals in pre- and postoperative periods of bariatric surgery. Obes Surg. 2013;23(10):1590–5.
29. Karlsson J, Taft C, Rydén A, Sjöström L, Sullivan M. Ten-year trends in health-related quality of life after surgical and conventional treatment for severe obesity: the SOS intervention study. Int J Obes (Lond). 2007;31(8):1248–61.
30. Coupaye M, Puchaux K, Bogard C, Msika S, Jouet P, Clerici C, Larger E, Ledoux S. Nutritional consequences of adjustable gastric banding and gastric bypass: a 1-year prospective study. Obes Surg. 2009;19(1):56–65.
31. Moize V, Geliebter A, Gluck ME, Yahav E, Lorence M, Colarusso T, Drake V, Flancbaum L. Obese patients have inadequate protein intake related to protein intolerance up to 1 year following Roux-en-Y gastric bypass. Obes Surg. 2003;13(1):23–8.
32. Faintuch J, Matsuda M, Cruz ME, Silva MM, Teivelis MP, Garrido Jr AB, Gama-Rodrigues JJ. Severe protein–calorie malnutrition after bariatric procedures. Obes Surg. 2004;14(2):175–81.
33. Skroubis G, Sakellaropoulos G, Pouggouras K, Mead N, Nikiforidis G, Kalfarentzos F. Comparison of nutritional deficiencies after Roux-en-Y gastric bypass and after biliopancreatic diversion with Roux-en-Y gastric bypass. Obes Surg. 2002;12(4):551–8.
34. Marinari GM, Murelli F, Camerini G, Papadia F, Carlini F, Stabilini C, Adami GF, Scopinaro N. A 15-year evaluation of biliopancreatic diversion according to the Bariatric Analysis Reporting Outcome System (BAROS). Obes Surg. 2004;14(3):325–8.
35. Blume CA, Boni CC, Casagrande DS, Rizzolli J, Padoin AV, Mottin CC. Nutritional profile of patients before and after Roux-en-Y gastric bypass: 3-year follow up. Obes Surg. 2012;22(11):1676–85.
36. Dalcanale L, Oliveira CP, Faintuch J, Nogueira MA, Rondó P, Lima VM, Mendonça S, Pajecki D, Mancini M, Carrilho FJ. Long-term nutritional outcome after gastric bypass. Obes Surg. 2010;20(2):181–7.
37. Slater GH, Ren CJ, Siegel N, Williams T, Barr D, Wolfe B, Dolan K, Fielding GA. Serum fat-soluble vitamin deficiency and abnormal calcium metabolism after malabsorptive bariatric surgery. J Gastrointest Surg. 2004;8(1):48–55.
38. Balsa JA, Botella-Carretero JI, Gómez-Martín JM, Peromingo R, Arrieta F, Santiuste C, Zamarrón I, Vázquez C. Copper and zinc serum levels after derivative bariatric surgery: differences between Roux-en-Y Gastric bypass and biliopancreatic diversion. Obes Surg. 2011;21(6):744–50.
39. Gletsu-Miller N, Broderius M, Frediani JK, Zhao VM, Griffith DP, Davis Jr SS, Sweeney JF, Lin E, Prohaska JR, Ziegler TR. Incidence and prevalence of copper deficiency following Roux-en-y gastric bypass surgery. Int J Obes (Lond). 2012;36(3):328–35.
40. Gasteyger C, Suter M, Gaillard RC, Giusti V. Nutritional deficiencies after Roux-en-Y gastric bypass for morbid obesity often cannot be prevented by standard multivitamin supplementation. Am J Clin Nutr. 2008;87(5):1128–33.

MIX
Papier aus verantwortungsvollen Quellen
Paper from responsible sources
FSC® C105338

If you have any concerns about our products,
you can contact us on
ProductSafety@springernature.com

In case Publisher is established outside the EU,
the EU authorized representative is:
Springer Nature Customer Service Center GmbH
Europaplatz 3, 69115 Heidelberg, Germany

Printed by Libri Plureos GmbH
in Hamburg, Germany